Assisting in Long-Term Care

FOURTH EDITION

Assisting in
Long-Term Care

FOURTH EDITION

Barbara R. Hegner, MS, RN (deceased)
Former Professor Emeritus
Nursing and Life Science
Long Beach City College (CA)

Contributing author:
Joan F. Needham, MSEd, RNC
Consultant and Educator for
Long-Term Care and Gerontology

DELMAR
THOMSON LEARNING ™

Australia   Canada   Mexico   Singapore   Spain   United Kingdom   United States

Assisting in Long-Term Care, 4th Edition
by Barbara R. Hegner, Esther Caldwell, Joan F. Needham

Acquisitions Editor:
Sherry Gomoll

Technology Project Manager:
Laurie Davis

Health Care Publishing Director:
William Brottmiller

Executive Editor:
Cathy L. Esperti

Developmental Editor:
Marjorie A. Bruce

Project Editor:
Mary Ellen Cox

Editorial Assistant:
Jennifer Conklin

Production Coordinator:
Nina Lontrato

Art/Design Coordinator:
Jay Purcell

Executive Marketing Manager:
Dawn F. Gerrain

For permission to use material from this text or product, contact us by
Tel   (800) 730-2214
Fax (800) 730-2215
www.thomsonrights.com

Library of Congress Cataloging-in-Publication Data

Hegner, Barbara R.
    Assisting in long-term care / Barbara R. Hegner, contributing author, Joan R. Needham.— 4th ed.
        p. ; cm.
    Includes bibliographical references and index
    ISBN 0-7668-3479-4 (alk. paper)
    1. Long-term care of the sick.   2. Nurses' Aides.   3. Nursing home care.
        [DNLM: 1. Long-term Care—method.   2. Nurses' Aides.   3. Nursing Care—method.   4. Nursing Homes. WY 152 H464a 2002] I. Caldwell, Ester.   II. Needham, Joan Fritsch.   III. Title.
    RT120.L64 H44   2002
    362.1′6—dc21   2001042441

NOTICE TO THE READER

Dedication

This text is dedicated to the memory of Barbara R. Hegner. Barbara was a visionary who saw the need for formalized instructional materials to help educate and develop skilled nursing assistants. She was committed to this unique and important group of health care professionals and her compassion, honesty, and integrity will be greatly missed.

Table of Contents

About the Authors   xix

Preface   xxi

Acknowledgments   xxiii

About This Book   xxiv

Section 1 The Long-Term Care Setting   1

LESSON 1   **The Long Term Care Facility**   3
    Community Health Care Facilities   4
    Types of Long-Term Care Facilities   8
    Functional Areas in a Long-Term Care Facility   10
    Standards and Regulations   14
    OBRA Legislation   14
    Financing in Long-Term Care   15
    The Survey   16

LESSON 2   **The Caregivers**   21
    The Interdisciplinary Team Members   22
    Administrative Organization   28
    Educational Services   29

LESSON 3   **The Nursing Assistant in Long-Term Care**   33
    Professionalism   34
    Personal Characteristics   34
    Attitude   35
    Personal Hygiene   36
    Uniforms   36
    Duties and Responsibilities: The Job Description   37
    Staff Relations   39
    Assignments   40
    Specific Duties   40
    Organization of Time   41
    Violence in the Workplace   42
    Self-Care   43
    Sexual Harassment   44
    Continue to Grow   44

Section 2 Communication Skills   49

LESSON 4   **Communication and Interpersonal Skills**   51
    The Communication Process   52
    Communicating with Staff Members   53
    Oral Communications   53

Written Communications 55
Communicating with Residents 56
Guidelines for Communicating with Residents 58
Communicating Through the Use of Touch 60
Communicating with Residents Who Have Special Needs 61
Communicating with the Potentially Violent Resident 64

LESSON 5   **The Language of Health Care** 67
The Language of Health Care 68
Word Parts 68
Expanding Your Vocabulary 69
Common Word Parts 69
Common Abbreviations 72
Understanding the Body 76
Anatomic Terms 76
Organization of the Body 78
Cells 78
Tissues 79
Organs 79
Systems 79
Membranes 79
Cavities 81

LESSON 6   **Observation, Documentation, and Reporting** 85
Observation 86
Reporting 91
Documentation 92
The Interdisciplinary Health Care Team Process 94

Section 3   **Protecting Residents' Rights and Safety** 99

LESSON 7   **Residents' Rights** 101
Purpose of the Residents' Rights Document 102
Residents' Rights 103
Legal Aspects of Health Care 117
Ethics and the Health Care Provider 118

LESSON 8   **Safety** 123
Safety in Health Care Facilities 124
Employee Safety 124
Guidelines for Using Ergonomic Techniques to Reduce the Risk of Having an Incident 125
Hazards in the Work Environment 127
Resident Safety 130
Guidelines for the Use of Restraints 132
Wheelchair Safety 135
Fire Safety 135

LESSON 9   **Emergencies**   139
General Measures to Follow for Emergencies   140
    Guidelines for Responding to an Emergency   140
Cardiac Arrest   141
Foreign Body Airway Obstruction (Choking)   142
The Recovery Position   143
Early Defibrillation   143
PROCEDURE   1 Assisting the Conscious Person with Obstructed
    Airway—Heimlich Maneuver   143
PROCEDURE   2 Obstructed Airway, Unconscious Person   145
PROCEDURE   3 One-Rescuer CPR, Adult   147
PROCEDURE   4 Positioning the Resident in the Recovery Position   148
Hemorrhage   148
Resident Falls   148
Seizures   148
PROCEDURE   5 Hemorrhage   149
PROCEDURE   6 Care of Falling Resident   150
Burns   151
Orthopedic Injuries   152
Accidental Poisoning   152
Fainting   152

LESSON 10   **Infection**   155
Infectious Disease   156
Microbes   156
The Chain of Infection   157
Body Flora   158
Natural Body Defenses Against Disease   158
Immunity   159
Inmmunizations   160
Serious Infections in Health Care Facilities   160
Bacterial Infections   160
Viral Infections   162
Other Important Infections   165
Why the Elderly in Long-Term Care Are at Risk for Infections   165
General Measures to Prevent Infections   166
Outbreak of Infectious Disease in a Long-Term Care Facility   167

LESSON 11   **Infection Control**   169
Medical Asepsis   170
Handwashing   172
PROCEDURE   7 Handwashing   172
Protecting Yourself   174
Standard Precautions   174
    Guidelines for Standard Precautions   175
    Guidelines for Environmental Procedures   176
Transmission-Based Precautions   178
PROCEDURE   8 Putting on a Mask and Gloves   183

PROCEDURE 9 Removing Contaminated Gloves   183
PROCEDURE 10 Putting on a Gown   184
PROCEDURE 11 Removing Contaminated Gloves, Mask,
              and Gown   185
PROCEDURE 12 Caring for Linens in Isolation Unit   188
PROCEDURE 13 Measuring Vital Signs in Isolation Unit   188
PROCEDURE 14 Serving a Meal Tray in Isolation Unit   189
PROCEDURE 15 Specimen Collection from Resident
              in Isolation Unit   190
PROCEDURE 16 Transferring Nondisposable Equipment Outside
              of Isolation Unit   192
PROCEDURE 17 Transporting Resident to and from
              Isolation Unit   192
Disinfection and Sterilization   193
Sterile Procedures   194
PROCEDURE 18 Opening a Sterile Package   194

Section 4   **Characteristics of the Long-Term Care Resident**   197

LESSON 12   The Long-Term Care Resident   199
About Aging   200
The Process of Normal Aging   200
Changes Caused by Aging   200
Illness and Disability   203
Stereotypes and Myths   205
The Younger Resident in the Long-Term Care Facility   208
       Guidelines for Caring for Younger Residents   209
Comfort, Rest, and Sleep   209

LESSON 13   The Psychosocial Aspects of Aging   213
Basic Human Needs   214
Cultural Influences   216
Spirituality   216
Religion   217
Sexuality and Intimacy   217
Major Challenges to Adjustments   219
Using Defense (Coping) Mechanisms   220
Meeting Residents' Psychosocial Needs   221
Stress Reactions   222
Reactive Behaviors   222

LESSON 14   Alternative Health Practices   227
Scientific (Western) Approach to Health Care   228
Alternative and Adjunctive Therapies   228
Importance for the Nursing Assistant   232

Section 5 **Meeting the Residents' Basic Needs** **235**

LESSON 15 **Care of the Residents' Environment** 237
Resident Environment 238
Personal Space 238
Resident Unit 239
Extended Resident Environment 240
  Guidelines for Ensuring a Safe and Comfortable Environment 242
Critical Procedure Actions 242
Bedmaking 245
  Guidelines for Handling Linens and Making the Bed 245
PROCEDURE 19 Unoccupied Bed: Changing Linens 246
PROCEDURE 20 Occupied Bed: Changing Linens 250

LESSON 16 **Caring for the Residents' Personal Hygiene** 255
Epidermis 256
Dermis 256
Skin Functions 257
Skin Changes Caused by Aging 257
Skin Lesions 257
  Guidelines for Preventing Skin Breakdown 261
Backrub 264
Bathing Residents 264
PROCEDURE 21 Backrub 265
PROCEDURE 22 Bed Bath Using Basin and Water 267
PROCEDURE 23 Bed Bath Using a Rinse-Free Cleanser and Moisturizer 270
PROCEDURE 24 Tub Bath or Shower 271
PROCEDURE 25 Partial Bath 272
PROCEDURE 26 Female Perineal Care 274
PROCEDURE 27 Male Perineal Care 275
Daily Hair Care 276
Facial Hair 277
PROCEDURE 28 Daily Hair Care 278
PROCEDURE 29 Shaving Male Resident 279
Hand and Fingernail Care 279
PROCEDURE 30 Hand and Fingernail Care 280
Foot and Toenail Care 280
PROCEDURE 31 Foot and Toenail Care 281
Oral Hygiene 281
PROCEDURE 32 Assisting Resident to Brush Teeth 283
PROCEDURE 33 Cleaning and Flossing Resident's Teeth 284
PROCEDURE 34 Caring for Dentures 285
PROCEDURE 35 Assisting with Oral Hygiene for the Unconscious Resident 286
Dressing Resident 286
PROCEDURE 36 Dressing and Undressing Resident 287

LESSON 17   Meeting the Residents' Nutritional Needs   291
The Digestive System   292
The Digestive Process   293
Aging Changes   295
Nutrients   295
Electrolyte Balance   296
Food Groups   297
Nutritional Status   299
Dehydration   300
Intake and Output (I&O)   301
PROCEDURE 37 Measuring and Recording Fluid Intake   302
Diets   303
Nursing Assistant Responsibilities   305
PROCEDURE 38 Assisting the Resident Who Can Feed Self   307
PROCEDURE 39 Feeding the Dependent Resident   309
Nourishments and Supplements   310
Alternate Methods of Feeding   311
Disorders of the Digestive System   312

LESSON 18   Meeting the Residents' Elimination Needs   319
Introduction   321
The Continent Resident   321
Equipment to Assist Elimination   321
PROCEDURE 40 Giving and Receiving the Bedpan   323
PROCEDURE 41 Giving and Receiving the Urinal   325
PROCEDURE 42 Assisting with Use of the Bedside Commode   326
PROCEDURE 43 Assisting Resident to Use the Bathroom   326
Elimination from the Lower Digestive Tract   327
The Resident with Constipation   328
Bowel Aids   328
PROCEDURE 44 Giving an Oil-Retention Enema or Commercially
              Prepared Enema   330
PROCEDURE 45 Giving a Soapsuds Enema   331
Rectal Tube and Flatus Bag   337
PROCEDURE 46 Inserting a Rectal Tube and Flatus Bag   338
Ostomies   338
PROCEDURE 47 Giving Routine Stoma Care (Colostomy)   340
Fecal Incontinence   342
Collecting a Stool Specimen   343
PROCEDURE 48 Collecting a Stool Specimen   343
Urinary System   344
Changes in the Urinary System Caused by Aging   346
Urine Elimination   347
Urinary Retention and Incontinence   347
Internal Urinary Catheter Drainage   347
PROCEDURE 49 Giving Indwelling Catheter Care   349
PROCEDURE 50 Emptying a Urinary Drainage Unit
              and Disconnecting the Catheter   352

Intake and Output (I&O)   352
PROCEDURE 51 Measuring and Recording Fluid Output   353
Leg Bag Drainage   356
PROCEDURE 52 Connecting Catheter to Leg Bag and Emptying the Leg Bag   357
PROCEDURE 53 Collecting a Routine or Clean-Catch Urine Specimen   360
External Urinary Drainage (Male)   361
PROCEDURE 54 Applying a Condom for Urinary Drainage   362
Common Conditions   363

Section 6   Special Nursing Assistant Activities   359

LESSON 19   Measuring and Recording Residents' Data   361
Measuring Vital Signs   362
Temperature   363
PROCEDURE 55 Measuring an Oral Temperature (Glass Thermometer)   365
PROCEDURE 56 Measuring a Rectal Temperature (Glass Thermometer)   367
PROCEDURE 57 Measuring an Axillary Temperature (Glass Thermometer)   368
PROCEDURE 58 Measuring an Oral Temperature (Electronic Thermometer)   369
PROCEDURE 59 Measuring a Rectal Temperature (Electronic Thermometer)   369
PROCEDURE 60 Measuring an Axillary Temperature (Electronic Thermometer)   370
PROCEDURE 61 Measuring a Tympanic Temperature   371
Pulse and Respiration   372
PROCEDURE 62 Counting the Radial Pulse Rate   373
PROCEDURE 63 Counting the Apical-Radial Pulse   374
PROCEDURE 64 Counting Respirations   375
Blood Pressure   376
Guidelines for Preparing to Measure Blood Pressure   378
PROCEDURE 65 Taking Blood Pressure   379
Weighing and Measuring the Resident   380
PROCEDURE 66 Weighing and Measuring the Resident Using an Upright Scale   383
PROCEDURE 67 Measuring Weight with an Electronic Wheelchair Scale   384
PROCEDURE 68 Weighing the Resident in a Chair Scale   385
PROCEDURE 69 Measuring and Weighing the Resident in Bed   385
Recording Vital Signs   386

LESSON 20   Admission, Transfer, and Discharge   389
Admitting the Resident   390
PROCEDURE 70 Admitting the Resident   393

Transferring the Resident   395
Discharging the Resident   398
PROCEDURE 71 Transferring the Resident   398
PROCEDURE 72 Discharging the Resident   399

LESSON 21   **Warm and Cold Applications**   405
Safety   406
Commercial Preparations   406
Use of Warm Applications   407
PROCEDURE 73 Applying an Aquamatic K-Pad®   408
Use of Cold Applications   409
PROCEDURE 74 Applying a Disposable Cold Pack   409
PROCEDURE 75 Applying an Ice Bag   410
PROCEDURE 76 Assisting with the Application of a Hypothermia
              Blanket   411

Section 7   Introduction to Restorative Care   415

LESSON 22   **Restorative/Rehabilitative Care of the Resident**   417
Restorative Care and the Interdisciplinary Health Team   419
Purposes of Restorative/Rehabilitative Care   420
Preventing Complications from Inactivity   421
Activities of Daily Living   423
Setting Up Restorative Programs   424
The Restorative/Rehabilitative Environment   426
        Guidelines for Nursing Assistant Responsibilities
        in General Restorative Program   430
Progressive Mobilization   431
Range of Motion   431
        Guidelines for Passive Range of Motion Exercises   432
PROCEDURE 77 Passive Range of Motion Exercises   434
Self Range of Motion Exercises   441
Active Range of Motion Exercises   441
Positioning the Resident   442
        Guidelines for Positioning   442
Turning the Dependent Resident with a Turning Sheet   446
PROCEDURE 78 Moving the Resident in Bed   446
PROCEDURE 79 Turning the Resident to the Side   448
PROCEDURE 80 Logrolling the Resident onto the Side   449
Positioning the Dependent Resident   450
PROCEDURE 81 Supine Position   451
PROCEDURE 82 Semisupine or Tilt Position   452
PROCEDURE 83 Lateral (Side-Lying) Position   452
PROCEDURE 84 Lateral Position on the Affected Side   453
PROCEDURE 85 Semiprone Position   454
PROCEDURE 86 Fowler's Position   454
PROCEDURE 87 Chair Positioning   456

PROCEDURE 88 Repositioning a Resident in a Wheelchair — 457

PROCEDURE 89 Wheelchair Activities to Relieve Pressure — 458

Independent Bed Movement — 459

PROCEDURE 90 Assisting with Independent Bed Movement — 459

Continuing with Progressive Mobilization — 460

Bowel and Bladder Programs — 460

Guidelines for Bowel and Bladder Programs — 461

LESSON 23 **Restoring Residents' Mobility** — 467

Transfers — 468

Guidelines for Transfers — 469

PROCEDURE 91 Using a Transfer Belt (Gait Belt) — 469

PROCEDURE 92 Bringing the Resident to a Sitting Position at the Edge of the Bed — 471

PROCEDURE 93 Assisted Standing Transfer — 472

PROCEDURE 94 Transferring the Resident from Chair to Bed — 473

PROCEDURE 95 Assisted Standing Transfer/Two Assistants — 474

PROCEDURE 96 Wheelchair to Toilet and Toilet to Wheelchair Transfers — 475

PROCEDURE 97 Transferring to Tub Chair or Shower Chair — 476

PROCEDURE 98 Transferring a Nonstanding Resident from Wheelchair to Bed — 477

Using Mechanical Lifts — 478

PROCEDURE 99 Transferring Resident with a Mechanical Lift — 478

Sliding Board Transfer — 480

Guidelines for Sliding Board Transfers — 481

PROCEDURE 100 Sliding Board Transfer — 481

Ambulation — 481

Guidelines for Ambulation — 485

PROCEDURE 101 Ambulating a Resident — 486

PROCEDURE 102 Assisting Resident to Ambulate with Cane or Walker — 486

Using a Wheelchair — 487

Special Maneuvers with Wheelchairs — 488

Positioning the Dependent Resident in the Wheelchair — 491

Wheelchair Activity — 493

Section 8 **Residents with Specific Disorders** — 497

LESSON 24 **Caring for Residents with Cardiovascular System Disorders** — 499

Introduction — 500

The Heart — 501

Blood Vessels — 503

Lymph — 503

The Blood — 503

Disorders of the Blood — 504

Disorders of the Blood Vessels and Circulation — 506

**Guidelines for Caring for Residents
with Peripheral Vascular Disease** 508
Heart Disease 510
PROCEDURE 103 Applying Elasticized Stockings 512

LESSON 25   **Caring for Residents with Respiratory System Disorders** 517
Introduction 518
The Respiratory Organs 518
Voice Production 519
Changes in the Respiratory System Caused by Aging 519
Introduction to Pathology 519
PROCEDURE 104 Collecting a Sputum Specimen 521
Chronic Obstructive Pulmonary Disease 522
Treatment and Care of Residents with COPD 523
PROCEDURE 105 Refilling the Humidifier Bottle 525

LESSON 26   **Caring for Residents with Endocrine System Disorders** 529
Introduction 530
Endocrine Glands 530
Aging Changes 532
Glucose Metabolism 532
Diabetes Mellitus 533

LESSON 27   **Caring for Residents with Reproductive System Disorders** 539
Introduction 540
The Male Reproductive System 540
The Female Reproductive System 541
Menstrual Cycle 543
Menopause 544
Changes in the Reproductive System as a Result of Aging 544
Related Conditions 544
Sexually Transmitted Diseases 545

LESSON 28   **Caring for Residents with Musculoskeletal System Disorders** 551
The Musculoskeletal System 552
Changes in the Musculoskeletal System Caused by Aging 553
Conditions Affecting the Musculoskeletal System 555

LESSON 29   **Caring for Residents with Nervous System Disorders** 565
Components of the Nervous System 567
Central Nervous System 568
Autonomic Nervous System 570
Sense Organs 570
Changes in the Nervous System Caused by Aging 572
Causes of Severe Vision Impairment 572
PROCEDURE 106 Care of Eyeglasses 572
Guidelines for Assisting Visually Impaired Residents 573
Hearing Loss 574

PROCEDURE 107 Applying and Removing In-the-Ear
or Behind-the-Ear Hearing Aids 575
Nervous System Disorders 576
Guidelines for Caring for Residents with Parkinson's
Disease 577
Guidelines for Caring for Residents Who Have Had
a Stroke 579
Guidelines for Caring for Residents with Multiple
Sclerosis 580
Guidelines for Caring for Residents
with Huntington's Disease 581
Guidelines for Caring for Residents Who Have
Amyotrophic Lateral Sclerosis 582
Guidelines for Caring for Residents Who Have
Myasthenia Gravis 583

Section 9   Residents with Special Needs **587**

LESSON 30   **Alzheimer's Disease and Related Disorders
(Caring for the Cognitively Impaired Resident)** 589
Definition of Alzheimer's Disease 590
Stages and Symptoms of Alzheimer's Disease 591
Caring for Residents with Dementia 593
Guidelines for Caring for Residents with Alzheimer's
Disease 595
Guidelines for Activities of Daily Living 597
Special Problems 599
Special Management Techniques 601

LESSON 31   **Caring for Residents with Developmental Disabilities** 605
Characteristics of a Developmental Disability 606
Mental Retardation 607
Other Forms of Developmental Disabilities 609
Caring for Residents with Developmental Disabilities 611

LESSON 32   **Caring for the Dying Resident** 615
Introduction 616
Hospice Care 616
The Dying Process 617
Signs of Approaching Death 622
Postmortem Care 622
PROCEDURE 108 Giving Postmortem Care 623

LESSON 33   **Caring for the Person in Subacute Care** 627
Description of Subacute Care 628
Special Procedures Provided in the Subacute Care Unit 629
Care of the Surgical Patient 629

Pulse Oximetry   629
Intravenous Therapy   630
Pain Management Procedures   631
   **Guidelines for Caring for Residents with Intravenous
Lines**   632
PROCEDURE 109 Changing a Gown on a Resident
      with a Peripheral Intravenous Line in Place   632
Caring for Residents with Tracheostomies   634
Caring for the Resident Receiving Dialysis Treatments   634
Oncology Treatments   635

Section 10 Employment   639

LESSON 34   Seeking Employment   641
Congratulations Are in Order   641
Step I—Self-Appraisal   642
Step II—Possibility Search   642
Step III—The Résumé   643
Step IV—References   644
Step V—Taking the Step   644
Step VI—The Interview (Putting Your Best Foot Forward)   644
Keeping the Job   646
Growing   646
Resigning   647

Glossary   651
Index   671

About the Authors

Barbara R. Hegner

Barbara Robinson Hegner, RN, MSN, was a graduate of a three-year diploma nursing program where direct and total care was the focus. She earned a BSN at Boston College and an MS in nursing from Boston University, with a minor in biologic sciences. She was Professor Emeritus of Nursing and Life Sciences at Long Beach City College, Long Beach (CA).

Throughout her professional career, she had a deep interest in both hospital-based and long-term care nursing.

Ms. Hegner believed that to ensure the rights and well-being of residents in long-term care requires the care of competent, caring nursing assistants under the supervision of professional nurses. The nursing assistants who provide this care should be thoroughly trained and consistently encouraged, evaluated, and given the opportunity for continued learning. Providing the tools to prepare these health care providers in the most effective and efficient way is the goal of *Assisting in Long-Term Care*, fourth edition. Other texts by Barbara R. Hegner, also from Delmar Publishers are: *Geriatrics, A Study of Maturity*, fifth edition, and *Nursing Assistant, A Nursing Process Approach*, eighth edition.

Joan F. Needham

Joan Fritsch Needham, MSEd, RNC, is a contributing author to the fourth edition of *Assisting in Long-Term Care*. She also graduated from a three-year diploma nursing program. She received her BS from the College of Saint Francis and her MS from Northern Illinois University. She is certified by the American Nurses Association in Gerontological Nursing. Ms. Needham was Director of Education at a long-term care facility where she was responsible for staff development, curriculum development and instruction for basic and advanced nursing assistant training, and development and instruction in continuing education courses for licensed nurses. In addition, she is a consultant on nursing assistant education and nursing continuing education.

She contributed to *Nursing Assistant, A Nursing Process Approach*, sixth, seventh, and eighth editions and is the author of *Gerontological Nursing—A Restorative Approach* (Delmar) and *Plans of Care for Specialty Practice, Gerontological Nursing* (Delmar).

Preface

INTRODUCTION

Long-term care facilities provide services to an ever-changing population that includes:

- The elderly
- People who have had an acute illness and still require nursing care during recuperation and restoration before returning home
- People of various ages who need assistance and supervision because of developmental disabilities or mental incapacity
- Those who have experienced severe trauma and have been transferred from an acute care facility for continued care and rehabilitation
- People with chronic illnesses that interfere with their ability to live independently

These residents need well-trained and highly motivated people to provide care. Nursing assistants provide the majority of direct personal care and are in a unique position to enhance the quality of life for residents.

The goal of *Assisting in Long-Term Care* is to serve as a critical resource in the education and training of nursing assistants as essential care providers. The text stresses core concepts and provides clearly written explanations of principles. Examples, illustrations, guidelines, and procedures serve to reinforce the principles and help learners gain a firm understanding of topics and develop competence in essential skills. The text also helps learners appreciate their value to the interdisciplinary health care team that is the basis of care in the long-term care facility.

ELEMENTS OF THE TEXT

The text is designed to enhance the learning process. Among the elements provided are the table of contents with the procedures identified for OBRA content or a video component, Clinical Focus in each unit, objectives, vocabulary lists with phonetic pronunciations, highlighted vocabulary terms in the text content, guidelines, procedures, photos and line drawings, cultural awareness notes, On the Job boxes, lesson synthesis, and lesson reviews. Refer to the section

"About This Book" following the acknowledgments for an explanation of each of these features and how they contribute to enhanced learning.

CHANGES FOR THE FOURTH EDITION

The goal of the fourth edition of *Assisting in Long-Term Care* is to address the changes that occur continually in nursing assistant practice in long-term care. The major changes for this edition include:

- In all lessons, added "On the Job" boxes to contrast the ideal concepts of the classroom with the realities of practice in the workplace.
- Lesson 1—added OBRA legislation, the National Nurse Aide Assessment Program, financing of care in long-term care (Medicare and Medicaid), and facility surveys with responsibilites of nursing assistants during survey
- Lesson 2—new content on professionalism with guidelines for nursing assistant conduct and violence in the workplace with recommendations for dealing with situations involving residents, families of residents, staff, and visitors
- Lesson 4—new content on communicating with potentially violent residents with guidelines for the nursing assistant
- Lesson 6—new table on signs/symptoms of illness by body system with reportable nursing assistant observations
- Lesson 7—expanded ethics content with guidelines for ethical behavior by nursing assistants
- Lesson 9—new content on the cardiac chain of survival, revised obstructed airway and CPR procedures to reflect 2000 American Heart Association guidelines, and using the automatic external defibrillator (AED)
- Lesson 10—updated content on drug resistant microorganisms; added content on external parasites (lice and scabies)
- Lesson 11—new content on facility exposure control training programs mandated by OSHA

(exposure to infectious pathogens) with lists of infections/diseases requiring specific types of transmission-based isolation precautions

- Lesson 12—added content on the general characteristics of aging/normal process of aging, expanded content on working with younger residents in long-term care, and new content on assisting residents to meet physical needs of comfort, rest, and sleep
- NEW Lesson 14 provides basic introduction to alternative health care practices (compared to traditional scientific [Western] approach to health care) to help nursing assistants recognize the importance of these practices to residents who use them
- Lesson 16—new content on waterless bathing using rinse-free cleanser and moisturizer products
- Lesson 17—new content on the Food Guide Pyramid for people 70 years and older, signs/ symptoms of malnourishment/dehydration with recommendations for nursing assistant actions, and introduction to "Nutrition Care Alerts" developed for long-term care facilities
- Lesson 19—revised measuring blood pressure procedure based on latest American Heart Association guidelines
- Lesson 22—new content on use of goniometer to test residents for contractures/functional (motion) capacity and four stages of contracture development
- Lesson 30—new content on purpose/organization of specialized Alzheimer's disease units in long-term care facilities
- Lesson 32—new content on philosophy/ services of hospice care for terminally ill residents and their families and expanded content on coping with grief and assisting others to cope
- Lesson 34—new content on health care registries that provide health care workers, including nursing assistants, to facilities for long term or part-time employment; added

typical questions asked during the employment interview that nursing assistants should be prepared to answer

SUPPLEMENTS

The supplements package consists of an Instructor's Manual, Student Workbook, Instructor's Resource Kit, and Computerized Test Bank. Also available is the third edition of Delmar's Nursing Assistant Video Series.

- The Instructor's Manual consists of teaching strategies, teaching and learning resources, supplementary learning aids, answers to end of lesson reviews, answers to workbook exercises, procedure evaluation forms, and transparency masters.
- The Student Workbook consists of information on the learning process, tips on studying effectively, student activities, exercises, student performance record form, procedure evaluation forms, and medical terminology flash cards.
- The Instructor's Resource Kit contains teaching methods and strategies, resource materials (including internet addresses), lesson plans, clinical situations, classroom activities, procedure guidelines, curriculum guides, and quizzes and final examination with answer keys.
- The Computerized Test Bank with additional questions organized by lesson. Question types include multiple choice, true and false, completion, brief answer, and matching. Instructors have the capability of generating a multitude of combinations of questions for testing purposes.

Join us on the web: www.DelmarAlliedHealth.com for the latest information on health care assisting and related topics.

Acknowledgments

The revision was aided by a dedicated group of instructors who reviewed content at different stages of the revision process. For their valuable suggestions and corrections, we thank:

Barbara Acello, MS, RN
Innovations in Health Care, Denton, TX

Alison P. Bell, RNC, BSN
Eastern Maine Technical College, Bangor, ME

Casey J. Blumenthal, MHSA, RN
Whitefish, MT

Ellen Reed Riley, RNC, MA
Southwestern Oregon Community College, Coos Bay, OR

Ann E. Sims, RN
Albuquerque Technical Vocational Institute, Albuquerque, NM

Margaret Toth, RNC, CRRN
HCR-Manor Care, Inc., Newton Falls, OH

About this **Book**

Inside Cover Content

The listings of beginning and ending procedure actions give the essential steps to be performed before beginning any direct resident care procedure. These steps assure the rights of the resident and the safety of the resident and you, the nursing assistant. The ending procedure actions are performed at the end of each procedure to ensure that the resident is comfortable and safe, the resident's environment is clean, all equipment used is cleaned or discarded according to facility policy, and the proper documentation is completed.

Table of **Contents**

The table of contents lists, for each lesson, the lesson title, major topic headings, general guidelines for specific areas of care or topics of importance to the nursing assistant, and resident care procedures.

Lesson Opening Page

The **Clinical Focus** presents a common resident care situation and asks you to think about ways to address the situation as the lesson content is studied.

The **Objectives** help you know what is expected of you as you read the text. Your success in achieving each objective is measured by your completion of the unit end reviews.

The **Vocabulary** list alerts you to new terms presented in the lesson. When each term is first presented in the text, it is highlighted in boldface and color. (The color of the term in the vocabulary list matches the color of the term in the text.) Each term is defined at this point. Read the definition and note the context of the term until you feel comfortable using the term.

The vocabulary list also contains the **phonetic pronunciation** for each new term. This is a system in which common sounds are used consistently to indicate the pronunciation. The part of the word that receives the primary emphasis is shown in **boldface** and **CAPITAL LETTERS**. The part or parts that receive the secondary emphasis is in boldface lower case letters.

Building Cultural Awareness

These brief examples are designed to help you become aware of the differences between people from different groups. They help you recognize that people react differently to health and sickness and that their reactions are determined largely by the culture of which they are a part. The text suggests that if you observe, listen and learn and accept people as they are, you will provide a high level of caring service.

Procedures

The text contains 109 clinical procedures that provide step-by-step directions for a specific aspect of care. Each procedure reminds you to perform the beginning procedure actions. A list of equipment and supplies needed for the procedure follows. Any notes or cautions about performing the precaution are given. The steps take you carefully through the procedure, emphasizing at all times the need to work safely and to protect the resident's dignity. At the end, you are reminded of the procedure completion actions (refer to the inside back cover to refresh your memory of these actions).

Three icons may be used with the procedures:

 OBRA to indicate an essential procedure required for certification

 gloves to indicate the need to observe Standard Precautions and wear personal protective equipment

 video to indicate that there is a companion video segment for the procedure in *Delmar's Nursing Assistant Video Series, 3rd edition*

Guidelines

The table of contents identifies the guidelines included in each lesson. These guidelines highlight important points that you need to remember for specific situations or types of care. They are presented in an easy to use format that you can refer to repeatedly until you know the actions you must take when confronted with the situation.

Lesson Synthesis: Putting it all Together

At the end of each lesson, you are asked to return to the situation presented in the **Clinical Situation** at the beginning of the lesson. Based upon what you have learned from the lesson, you are to answer a series of questions related to the resident or nursing assistant discussed. This exercise helps you to integrate what you have learned and apply it to a common clinical situation.

Review

A variety of review questions tests your understanding of the lesson content. For additional activities and exercises to reinforce your learning, refer to the Student Workbook. Your instructor has the answers to the Lesson Reviews and the Workbook Activities (exercises) in the accompanying Instructor's Guide. Your instructor may give you additional questions and tests from the Instructor's Resource Kit or the Computerized Test Bank accompanying this text.

SECTION 1

The Long-Term Care Setting

LESSONS

1 **The Long-Term Care Facility**

2 **The Caregivers**

3 **The Nursing Assistant in Long-Term Care**

The Long-Term Care Facility

Clinical Focus

Think about the different types of agencies and facilities available to provide care and services to people with health needs. Consider how the services are paid for and regulated and how people may move from one agency or facility as their health needs change.

*R*udolph McCarver. Mr. McCarver is recovering from a stroke. He is 79 years old and is eligible for Medicare. Although he no longer needs the services of an acute care hospital, he will still require weeks of rehabilitation in long-term care before he can return to his home. His facility is expecting surveyors to visit within the next month.

OBJECTIVES

After studying this lesson, you should be able to:

- Define and spell vocabulary words and terms.
- Name community facilities that offer health care services.
- Explain the differences in services offered by health care facilities.
- List names applied to types of long-term care facilities.
- Describe the functional areas and equipment related to a long-term care facility.
- Describe state and federal licensing standards and regulations.
- State the importance of OBRA regulations to nursing assistant certification.
- Identify the role Medicare plays in helping to finance the care of long-term care residents.
- Explain the importance of records related to regulation and reimbursements.
- Describe the survey process, stating the assistants' responsibilities and the consequences of an unsatisfactory survey.

3

VOCABULARY

assignment   *(ah-**SIGHN**-ment)*

certification   *(**sir**-tih-fih-**KAY**-shun)*

client   *(**KLIGH**-ent)*

communal   *(kum-**MYOU**-nul)*

compliance   *(kom-**PLY**-ans)*

confidential   *(kon-fih-**DEN**-shul)*

day room   *(day room)*

decline   *(dih-**KLINE**)*

deficiencies   *(dee-**FISH**-en-seez)*

delegation   *(deh-leh-**GAY**-shun)*

emesis basin   *(**EM**-eh-sis **BAY**-sin)*

geriatric   *(jer-ee-**AT**-rick)*

Kardex   *(**KAR**-dex)*

licensure   *(**LIE**-sen-shur)*

long-term care facility   *(lawng turm kair fah-**SILL**-ih-tee)*

Medicaid   *(**MEH**-dih-kaid)*

Medicare   *(**MEH**-dih-kare)*

nurses' station   *(nur-ses **STAY**-shun)*

OBRA   *(**OH**-brah)*

patient   *(**PAY**-shent)*

policy book   *(**POL**-ah-see book)*

procedure book   *(proh-**SEE**-jur book)*

rehabilitation   *(ree-hah-**BILL**-ih-**tay**-shun)*

resident   *(**REZ**-ih-dent)*

resident unit   *(**REZ**-ih-dent **YOU**-nit)*

restoration   *(reh-stor-**AY**-shun)*

skilled nursing facility   *(skilled **NUR**-sing fah-**SILL**-ih-tee)*

subacute care   *(**sub**-ah-**KYOOT** kair)*

survey   *(**SIR**-vay)*

surveyor   *(sir-**VAY**-er)*

terminal   *(**TER**-mih-nul)*

Nursing assistants make valuable contributions in providing health care. Nursing assistants are trained to care for people who are ill or need help in caring for themselves. The care given is always under the guidance and supervision of licensed health care providers such as nurses or physicians.

COMMUNITY HEALTH CARE FACILITIES

The health needs of the nation are met in various community settings (Figure 1-1). Although trained nursing assistants may work in any type of agency or facility, they find their greatest opportunity for employment in agencies or facilities that provide:

- Assisted living facilities
- Health and personal care for people in their homes
- Hospice care for the terminally ill
- Care for the developmentally disabled
- Health services in acute care hospitals
- Extended (long-term) care
- Subacute care services

Each care setting provides basic care in addition to special services to meet individual needs. Figure 1-2 compares some of the characteristics of three care settings where nursing assistants are employed.

Home health care, assisted living facilities, hospices, and homes for the developmentally disabled offer similar services:

- They are conducted in a homelike setting.
- They stress supportive psychosocial services.
- They provide for physical needs.
- They assist clients to maintain and achieve the maximum level of personal control and functioning.

Home Health Care

Home health services provide for the health and daily living activity needs of people who are ill or have disabilities when family members cannot provide the necessary care in the home.

The care needed is assessed and planned by the nurse along with other health care specialists.

On the Job

Although many health care services are available, people are not always able to access the services necessary to meet their health needs. This is a critical problem in health care delivery.

FIGURE 1-1 Different types of health care facilities are needed to meet the nation's health needs.

- Acute care hospitals
- Facilities for the mentally ill
- Physicians' offices
- Clinics of various kinds
- Hospices for the terminally ill
- Facilities for the developmentally disabled
- Facilities for long-term care

- Rehabilitation facilities
- Assisted living facilities
- Community nursing centers
- Subacute care facilities
- Residential care facilities for the elderly
- Adult day care facilities
- Group homes
- Adult foster care

FIGURE 1-2 Comparison of the health care provided in different health care settings

Facility	Care Recipient	Length of Stay	Characteristics/Service	Nursing Assistant Participation
Acute care	Patient	Few days to weeks	Cure-oriented; frequent physician visits; high-level skilled nursing; high-technology equipment; multiple support services; multiple support departments; multiple personnel; may be specialized according to patient needs; care of acutely ill persons; limited term.	Employed by the hospital; may or may not require certificate; gives basic care under direct supervision; assists professionals in more complex care; carries out special techniques under supervision and for which they have been specially educated; contributes to nursing care plan or clinical pathway through observing and reporting.
Long-term care	Resident	Weeks, months, years	Subacute care; restoration, maintenance-oriented; assistance with activities of daily living; rehabilitative techniques; less sophisticated equipment; stress on social and psychological needs; fewer physician visits; professional nursing supervision; long-term care of chronically ill, infirmed, and developmentally disabled; pediatric and in some cases psychiatric services.	Requires certification; encourages self-care when possible; provides complete personal care for those who are unable to help themselves; participates in rehabilitative efforts; contributes to nursing care plan through observing and reporting.

(continues)

FIGURE 1-2 *(continued)*

Facility	Care Recipient	Length of Stay	Characteristics/ Service	Nursing Assistant Participation
Home health care	Client	Intermittent, may have periodic hospital stays	Some procedures may be assigned and monitored by the RN. Other procedures may be **delegated** (assigned to another care provider) and supervised periodically.	Employed by the agency; time spent with a client may range from 1 hour to a full 8-hour shift; may visit several clients in one day for 1–3 hours each; must interact with family members to provide required services to client; offers emotional support to family; carries out basic care under indirect supervision; promotes self-care and rehabilitation; contributes to the nursing care plan by observing, reporting, and documenting; keeps records related to reimbursements.

The nursing assistant, who works for the home health care agency, carries out the care in the person's home. The person who receives the care is called a **client**. The home care nursing assistant is supervised by professionals but usually works alone with clients. The client is assisted in performing activities of daily living (ADL) and needed personal and basic nursing care is given. The nursing assistant reports directly to the supervising nurse and is involved in the planning, implementation, and documentation of care.

Hospice Care

Hospice care is provided in a special area of a hospital, in a nursing home, in the client's own home, or in a special hospice facility (Figure 1-3). The nursing assistant helps meet the physical and psychosocial needs of the person who has a limited life span, usually less than 6 months. Lesson 32 gives a fuller description of hospice and hospice care.

Care for the Developmentally Disabled

Services for the developmentally disabled are designed to assist in the care and training of persons whose mental and physical limitations affect self-care (Figure 1-4).

Many developmentally disabled clients live in a long-term care facility. Some clients live at home but spend time daily in the facility for care and training, such as in ADL. The nursing assistant who works with this group of clients also needs basic nursing and interpersonal skills.

FIGURE 1-3 Hospice care assists people with a limited life span.

FIGURE 1-4 People with developmental disabilities have a limited ability to care for themselves.

Acute Care Hospitals

People receiving care in an acute care hospital are called **patients**. These people are usually seriously ill or injured, or they have some special health need. They require a high level of skilled professional care. Nursing assistants provide basic care and are supervised as they perform special technical skills that they have been taught. Patients stay in hospitals for a limited time and may then be transferred to long-term care facilities or home as their conditions change.

Because the patients in an acute care facility need closer attention and more care, the nursing assistant is assigned to care for a specific number of people at a time and is always under the direct supervision of a professional health provider. The nursing assistant working in an acute care facility needs basic nursing skills and interpersonal relationship skills and may

be trained by the facility in special technical skills.

Physicians' Offices/Clinics

People visit physicians' offices for acute short-term care and referrals. Nursing assistants may assist the professional staff by receiving patients and performing basic procedures such as measuring temperature, pulse, respiration, and blood pressure. Nursing assistants may be asked to measure and weigh patients and record and report the information. Selected nursing assistants are trained to do other special procedures under the direct supervision of the physician or nurse.

Facilities for the Mentally Ill

Patients are admitted to facilities for mental illness to receive care and therapy. Some patients may stay for a short time, whereas others are admitted for long periods of time. The trend today is to move patients out of institutions as soon as possible and into community-based outpatient programs. Nursing assistants employed by the facility perform basic care skills and make a major contribution to the nursing care plan through careful observation and reporting of the patients' behavior and response to care.

Rehabilitation Clinics

Patients visit rehabilitation clinics as outpatients. The focus is on evaluating, maintaining, and restoring the patients' mobility and independence in carrying out ADLs. Generally, the patients make many visits over a period of weeks to months. Nursing assistants work with nurses and therapists in positioning patients, caring for equipment, and providing emotional support and encouragement. For example, a person who is recovering from a fractured leg received in an automobile accident may live at home but receive rehabilitation therapy as an outpatient.

Community Nursing Centers

These outpatient centers offer short-term care and staff see clients on a regular basis. Nurses in the centers provide health teaching and monitor chronic conditions such as diabetes and high blood pressure (hypertension). They also offer weight control counseling. The centers may provide reproductive health services, breast and cervical cancer screening, immunizations, well baby clinics, and AIDS testing and counseling. Nursing assistants provide basic skills such as measuring and weighing clients and taking vital signs. They may also help with examinations and care for equipment and records.

Long-Term Care Facilities

The person cared for in a **long-term care facility** is called a **resident**. The facility becomes this person's home for an extended period. This period may be for weeks or months as the resident is restored to health. In some cases the facility may become the resident's permanent home.

People are discharged from an acute care facility because they no longer need the specialized care provided there. However, they may still require skilled care and not be ready to return home. Often they are admitted to the **subacute care** unit in a long-term care facility. Here, they receive short-term nursing care until they are ready to go home.

The different types of long-term care facilities employ many nursing assistants who play a vital role in the success of the care given. Nursing assistants who work in long-term care must be certified. This text is designed to help students become successful certified nursing assistants.

TYPES OF LONG-TERM CARE FACILITIES

Several different names are applied to long-term care (LTC) facilities. Some of the names you will hear include:

- Nursing home
- Nursing facility (NF)
- Intermediate care facility (ICF)
- Skilled nursing facility
- Rehabilitation care center
- Assisted living facility
- Alzheimer's care center

People who need long-term care are those who:

- Need to regain the ability to care for themselves (restoration or rehabilitation)
- Cannot, because of illness or disability, care for themselves, and have no one else to provide such care
- Are elderly and frail and need continuous nursing care (**geriatric** care)

FIGURE 1-5 Health care facility functions
All long-term care facilities provide:
• Physical care
• Emotional care
• Help with activities of daily living (ADLs)
• Restorative care
• Safety and security
• Opportunities for social interaction
• Spiritual/religious activities
• Access to voting

All long-term care facilities provide housing, protection, and assistance as needed to meet individual needs (Figure 1-5). Some also provide skilled nursing care. Placement in a specific long-term care facility is determined by the level of care and type of services needed (Figure 1-6). Much of the service is supported by governmental funds such as Medicare and Medicaid.

The Skilled Nursing Facility

The **skilled nursing facility** (SNF) offers professional nursing care to chronically ill or disabled persons and those who are recovering but do not require the high-cost services of an acute hospital setting. Many of these people are elderly; some are in the **terminal** (last) stage of life. They have many needs and require the services of many skilled professionals. Highly trained team members provide this specialized care. Physicians, professional nurses, and pharmacy services are readily available. Other support personnel and specialists are available as required.

Skilled nursing facilities are able to provide many of the services offered in the acute hospital setting. The care is aimed at maintenance and **restoration (rehabilitation)** (Figure 1-7). Maintenance is aimed at preventing further loss and limitations.

Restoration or rehabilitation is the process of assisting residents to do as much as they can, as well as they can, for as long as they can for themselves. Residents of any age who are admitted primarily for rehabilitation usually stay about 3 months before they are discharged. The cost of

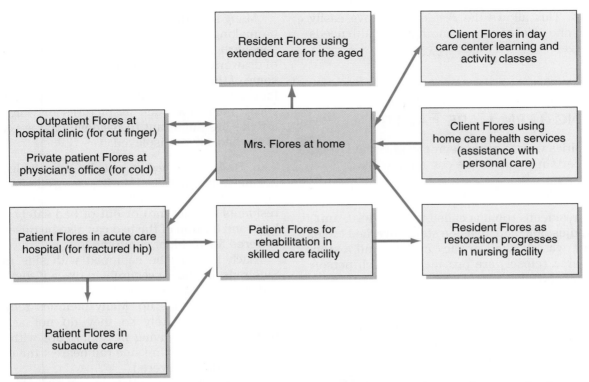

FIGURE 1-6   People move from one health care service to another as their needs change.

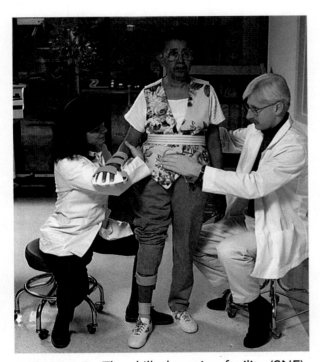

FIGURE 1-7   The skilled nursing facility (SNF) provides technical nursing care and emphasizes rehabilitation.

care in such an SNF is higher than for some other types of extended care because more services are available. As soon as appropriate, residents are transferred, usually to a less expensive care setting such as a nursing facility or to their homes.

The Nursing Facility

In the nursing facility (NF), the restorative effort is continued, but at a less intensive level, requiring fewer specialists. Supervision and care are still provided, however, on a 24-hour basis. When a person in an NF has made as much progress toward self-care as possible, that person is again transferred. It might be to his or her own home or, if further help is necessary, to a still less intensive care facility such as an assisted living facility.

Assisted Living Facility

Residents in this type of facility can provide most of their own care. Services include meals, assistance with medications, and housekeeping. These facilities are often associated with skilled care facilities, subacute units, or acute care hospitals. This allows the resident to move easily from one level of care to another as health needs change.

FUNCTIONAL AREAS IN A LONG-TERM CARE FACILITY

Facilities vary to some degree in physical layout, but certain elements are common to all.

The Resident Room

The resident's room is called the **resident unit**. An adjustable bed, bedside stand, overbed table, chair, wastebasket, privacy curtain, and a storage area (closet) are provided for each person (Figure 1-8).

Resident rooms may be designed for occupancy by a single individual, but usually accommodate two persons. In some instances several residents share a single room.

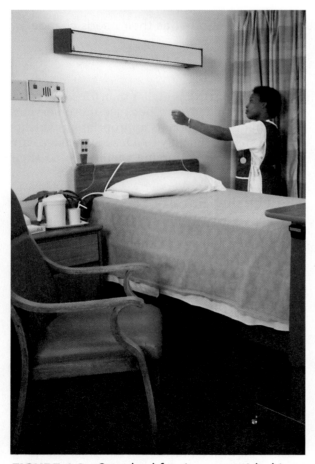

FIGURE 1-8 Standard furniture provided in a resident unit

Many facilities encourage residents who will be making the facility their home to bring personal articles as space permits. A familiar chest of drawers, a lamp, or bedside table may replace some of the facility's equipment to add a sense of familiarity and security for the resident. Personal mementos such as pictures or religious articles are important to residents and are kept at the bedside or displayed.

The Bed. The bed is usually adjustable for height. It can be raised during care (eliminating bending for the caregiver) and lowered so that residents can get into or out of bed safely. The head and bottom of the bed can also be raised or lowered for resident comfort.

Each bed can be equipped with side rails. Side rails should be securely in place if they are ordered for a specific resident. Not all residents need the side rails up. Many facilities remove side rails completely so they do not act as restraints. When giving personal care with the bed elevated, only the side rail nearest the caregiver should be lowered.

Some beds are electric; others are adjusted by hand with a crank. The assistant should be thoroughly familiar with the bed controls before attempting to operate them.

Personal Equipment. The bedside stand in each unit is equipped with articles for the resident's personal care and use. Many of the articles are purchased by the resident or the resident's family. These articles should not be shared with other residents.

The equipment included in each unit is kept in two areas of the bedside stand. These items should be clearly marked with the resident's name. The top shelf and two drawers (Figure 1-9) are "clean areas" and hold the following:

- Resident's personal toilet articles
- Wash basin
- Kidney-shaped emesis (vomit) basin
- Soap/dish

The **emesis basin** is usually used when performing personal care procedures such as brushing the teeth.

The drawer holds personal toilet articles such as:

- Toothbrush
- Toothpaste
- Denture cup
- Comb and hairbrush
- Lotion
- Makeup

FIGURE 1-9   The top two areas of a bedside stand (either drawers or shelves) contain clean equipment.

The toothbrush and toothpaste should be kept in plastic, away from the comb and hairbrush.

The bottom drawer is a "dirty area" and holds the:

• Bedpan or bedpan and urinal
• Toilet tissue

In some facilities these are stored in the bathroom.

Call Lights.   Each unit has a signaling device, such as a call light (Figure 1-10). Call lights may be attached to the wall or may be part of a more complex panel attached to the side rail. The panel may also control a radio, television, or telephone. Call lights are also located in the bathroom and shower area. The shower and bathroom lights blink differently, indicating the need for immediate attention. When a resident needs help and uses the call signal, a light at the nurses' station comes on, showing the room number of the resident who called (Figure 1-11).

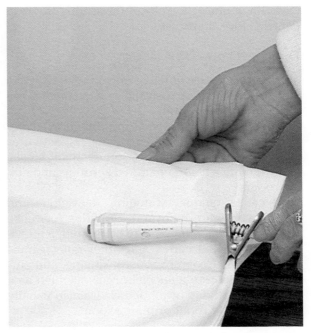

FIGURE 1-10   Each resident unit has a way for the resident to signal for assistance.

The call light should always be within reach of the resident.

An overbed table, which is adjustable in height, may be placed over the bed, providing a place to serve meals or hold equipment during

FIGURE 1-11   When the resident pushes the button of his or her signaling device, a light shows at the communications center at the nurses' station and over the door of the resident's room to indicate which resident is calling for assistance.

care. Each unit has a closet for storing the resident's personal articles.

Dining Room/Day Room

Residents who are able are encouraged to eat in a **communal** (group) setting, so each facility has a common dining room.

Dining rooms can sometimes function as **day rooms** where residents can meet for activities and socialization at times other than meals. Many facilities have separate day rooms and dining rooms.

Because talking, watching television, and playing cards are enjoyable activities for those whose physical abilities may be limited, a television set, playing cards, and other quiet games are available. Group exercises, singing, and parties that celebrate a special occasion, such as a resident's birthday or a holiday, are also usually held in the day room or dining room.

Nurses' Station

Every facility has an area where records of care are kept. This area is called the **nurses' station**. Part of the nurses' station is set aside for the control and dispensing of medications; unauthorized persons are not permitted in this area. Authorized persons include the physician, the pharmacist, the registered nurse, and the licensed vocational/practical nurse (LVN or LPN). This part of the nurses' station is kept locked when unattended.

Medications are delivered to residents by the medication nurse using a medicine cart. Residents are not permitted near an unattended medication cart because a confused resident might be hurt by accidentally sampling medications. Medication carts must always be locked when unattended.

Reports of residents' needs and care are usually given within the nurses' station. This is **confidential** (private, personal) information and should not be discussed within hearing of the residents or guests. This information should never be discussed outside the facility. Nursing assistants use this area to report and record their observations and the care given. Directions and **assignments** (list of duties) are received at the nurses' station.

Records. Important records are found in the nurses' station. They are the:

1. Procedure book
2. Policy book
3. Resident's chart
4. Kardex or resident profile

FIGURE 1-12 The policy book outlines the rules of the facility.

5. Assignment sheet
6. Care plans
7. Fire and safety manual
8. Logs for ongoing records
9. Disaster plan
10. Material Safety Data Sheets
11. Infection control manual

The **procedure book** explains how care is to be given. The **policy book** (Figure 1-12) outlines the rules for the facility and explains what will be done for the residents. The resident's chart contains a record of the care given and the progress reported, as well as information about the resident. The resident profile or **Kardex** contains information about the specific daily care to be given to a particular resident. The information on the Kardex reflects a plan called the interdisciplinary care plan that has been developed for each resident. The assignment sheet lists the specific assignments and duties for the staff for the shift. The fire and safety manual outlines procedures to follow if a fire or accident occurs in the facility.

Computers

Computers are used in health care facilities to:

- Maintain records such as care plans, nursing assessments, physicians' orders, and required reports to state and federal agencies
- Inventory supplies
- Record medications and treatments
- Schedule appointments
- Set work schedules

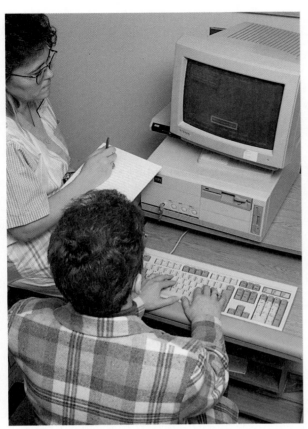

FIGURE 1-13 Computers provide immediate access to resident information.

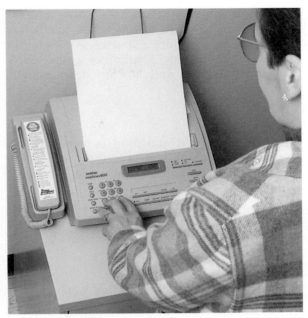

FIGURE 1-14 Fax machines make it possible to transmit information rapidly from one place to another.

If your facility uses computers to process information, you may be asked to use one. You will be trained to use the computer and then be supervised until you can operate it properly.

Computers have a central processing unit, a drive, a display screen, and a keyboard. The keyboard is like the keyboard of a typewriter. The information typed appears on the screen. Information can be stored in the drive of the computer or on disks. A disk has a menu that lists the files of information on the disk. Once information is entered and named, the file name can be selected on the menu and opened. The information can then be reviewed and revised as needed.

Computers provide ready access to essential information that can be used to make medical and nursing decisions (Figure 1-13).

Fax Machines

Fax machines (Figure 1-14), allow you to send information from printed sheets over telephone lines to other locations. These locations may be within the same building, the same city, across the United States, or in another country. The sending and receiving of information by fax machines can be accomplished in a few minutes. To operate the fax machine, you dial a telephone number that prepares a machine at the other end to receive and print the message.

Areas for Specific Rehabilitation

To make it easier to work with residents, facilities have special areas devoted to the rehabilitation process.

- In the physical therapy department, physical therapists and physical therapy aides focus on exercises to strengthen the residents' larger muscles. Residents are also taught to use prostheses (artificial limbs), canes, walkers, or crutches to increase their mobility and independence.
- In the occupational therapy department, occupational therapists and occupational therapy aides focus on improving the flexibility of the smaller muscles of the residents' hands and arms and focus on specific tasks. This is especially helpful when a resident has arthritis and for rehabilitation after a stroke.
- In the speech therapy department, residents are evaluated for speech and swallowing problems. Speech therapists assist residents to improve their written and oral communication abilities.

• In the respiratory therapy department, residents are helped to make the most efficient use of their breathing capacity. For example, they may be taught respiratory exercises to clear the airway and how to do pursed-lip breathing.

Kitchen

Meals are prepared and food is stored in the kitchen. Meals are then delivered to residents in the day room, dining room or, when necessary, in their rooms.

Both regular and special diets are prepared for residents in this area and then delivered in special carts.

Laundry

Some facilities have laundries that wash and dry residents' personal clothes. Basic linens needed in resident care may be commercially laundered and delivered to the facility and soiled laundry and clothing may be picked up for cleaning. Some facilities may handle all laundry needs on the premises.

STANDARDS AND REGULATIONS

All facilities must adhere to standards that are set by official public agencies. These standards govern the:

• Qualifications of the caregivers
• Care that is given
• Safety of the facility
• Sanitary conditions

OBRA LEGISLATION

In 1987, the first **OBRA** (Omnibus Budget Reconciliation Act) was passed. This legislation was designed to improve the quality of care, health, life, and safety of residents living in long-term care facilities. It also established training and evaluation standards for nursing assistants working in such facilities. A new OBRA is passed each year. This legislation requires all nursing assistants to complete an evaluation program and be entered into a state registry before they can work in long-term care.

OBRA also requires the:

• Promotion of resident independence
• Elimination of restraints
• Promotion of improved quality of life, care, health, and safety for all residents

OBRA legislation focuses on all aspects of the resident's social, mental, physical, and spiritual life. Facilities and nursing assistants must follow the OBRA rules and regulations to be in **compliance** (accord) with the law.

Nursing Assistant Certification Under the Omnibus Budget Reconciliation Act

Nursing assistants must be certified by the state before they can work in long-term care. State regulations for the training and certification of nursing assistants are guided by the OBRA. Since October 1, 1990, all persons working as nursing assistants must complete a competency evaluation program or approved course.

The National Nurse Aide Assessment Program

The National Nurse Aide Assessment Program (NNAAP) is an examination made up of two parts: a written (or oral) examination and a skills examination. These examinations test the aide's ability to safely perform entry-level job skills and demonstrate the related knowledge and ability to support such care. Both parts of the examination must be passed for the aide to be certified and to become listed in the nurse aide registry.

Areas of testing include:

• Physical care skills, including activities of daily living, basic nursing skills, and restorative services
• Psychosocial care skills, including meeting emotional, mental health, and spiritual needs
• Role of the nurse aide, including communication, residents' rights, ethical behavior, and being a member of the health care team

Nursing assistants who are not certified have three opportunities to meet the requirements for certification. In some states a new training and competency evaluation program must be completed by nursing assistants who previously finished such a program but have not performed nursing-related services for pay for a continuous 24-month period. Certified nursing assistants must complete at least 12 hours of continuing education per year. In some states, the continuing education requirement is 24 hours per year.

The OBRA regulations are important because they:

• Give nursing assistants recognition through certification and listing on the state registry
• Help define the scope of nursing assistant practice

- Ensure better uniformity of care by nursing assistants
- Promote educational standards for nursing assistants

Be sure you are familiar with any specific state regulations or legislation that relate to your job as a nursing assistant.

FINANCING IN LONG-TERM CARE

Long-term care is paid for in several ways, such as through:

- Private sources—residents pay the costs out of their own funds
- Prepaid insurance—residents pay premiums to insurance companies that, in turn, pay providers for care
- A Preferred Provider Organization (PPO)—members are given a list of providers from which to choose a primary care provider
- Health maintenance organizations (HMO)
- Charitable organizations and community agencies
- Medicare
- Medicaid

Most long-term care is paid for through Medicare and Medicaid programs. Not all facilities accept Medicare payment, but those that do must follow Medicare rules and regulations to receive reimbursement.

Medicaid

Medicaid (Title XIX) is a state and federally funded program designed to provide health care for eligible low-income individuals. Federal money is issued to the states, which then determine how to distribute the money to health care facilities. Facilities must be approved (certified) to participate in the program. Not all facilities choose to participate.

Medicare

The **Medicare** program is federally funded and is under the administration of the Health Care Financing Administration (HCFA). Facilities must be approved to participate in the program. Medicare is divided into two parts: A and B.

Part A.   To be eligible for Part A, the resident must:

- Be a complex case
- Need professional care and assessment daily
- Require a physician's order for skilled therapy

- Be over 65 years of age or disabled for more than 2 years, except for those who are in renal failure or on dialysis
- Reside in a skilled care facility

Part A pays for certain services in hospital long-term care and home health settings for a fee. These services include room, board, all care, supplies, and rehabilitative services. Safety is a major consideration.

Most long-term care services are not considered skilled care according to Medicare criteria.

Part B.   Medicare beneficiaries may pay an additional premium monthly which makes them eligible for additional services, such as some diagnostic tests, splints, braces, prosthetics, therapy evaluation, limited rehabilitation services, and other outpatient care.

Medicare Reporting Regulations.   To be in compliance and receive reimbursement, specific reports must be submitted to show that the facility is assisting the resident to function at the highest possible level.

The government developed a Resident Assessment Instrument (RAI) to help with the assessment and reporting process. The nursing care plan guides the resident's care using the data from the RAI.

Resident Assessment Instrument.   The RAI has been in use since the early 1990s. New regulations require that information gathered for the RAI be sent electronically to the state. The state then transmits the data to the federal government. Medicare and Medicaid payments are made to the facility based on the residents' conditions and needs as identified on the RAI. (See Figure 1-15.)

The information is also used to track resident **declines** within the facility. Too many declines can trigger an unannounced survey.

The RAI consists of three parts:

- The Minimum Data Set (MDS2.0)
- Triggers
- Resident Assessment Protocols (RAPs) (18 in all)

The RAI is used to:

- Set payment to the facility
- Identify resident problems, needs, and risks
- Develop a care plan that maintains or improves the resident's condition
- Coordinate facility staff to better meet resident needs

Minimum Data Set (MDS2.0).   This form focuses on the resident's ability to perform activities of daily living and the degree of assistance

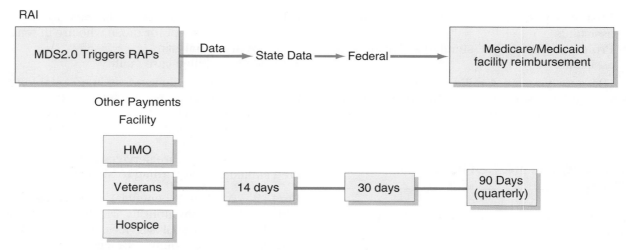

FIGURE 1-15 Reimbursement for resident care services in long-term care

required. The MDS2.0 also evaluates several other areas of the resident's function, such as bowel and bladder habits, sleep habits, and sensory abilities.

Triggers. Completion of the MDS2.0 may reveal a condition that requires review. These are called *triggers.* Triggers alert the staff to problems that warrant further investigation, including possible care plan intervention. For example, the resident may have an actual condition, such as loss of weight, with the potential for complications or an infection that could cause his or her health to worsen. It might be that the resident is a candidate for a restorative program. Triggers lead to resident assessment protocols (RAPs).

Resident Assessment Protocols. Resident Assessment Protocols (RAP) link the MDS2.0 with care plan goals. They are lists of problem-oriented information and guidelines. The staff uses them to identify problems and in care planning and treatment decisions.

Reporting Times. To be in compliance and receive reimbursement, reports (MDS2.0, trig-gers, RAP) must be completed and submitted on time (Figure 1-16). OBRA requires that an RAI be completed within 14 days of admission of a new resident. An additional 7 days are allowed for the staff to develop a care plan. Specific reporting periods are required for compliance. Care plans may change if the MDS2.0 assessment changes.

THE SURVEY

All health care facilities must be licensed to provide care. The license is awarded by the agency that regulates care. In most states this is the Department of Public Health.

Facilities that receive Medicare funds participate in a **certification** process. One **survey** is usually done for both **licensure** and certification. All health care facilities undergo surveys on a regular basis.

A team of health care professionals (**survey-ors**) is responsible for conducting the survey. The team determines if the facility is following all state and federal regulations and that the

FIGURE 1-16	Required reporting periods			
Report	**RAI**	**MDS2.0**	**Short Version MDS2.0**	**New MDS2.0***
Due	Within 14 days of resident admission	Days 5–14 30–60 90	Quarterly	Annually and when significant changes in resident's condition occur

*A new MDS2.0 is necessary if resident shows decline or improvement in two or more ADLs

facility is in compliance (doing what it is supposed to do). Surveyors may make their visits unannounced.

Purpose

The purpose of the survey is to:

- Review the quality of life for the residents
- Review the quality of care given to residents
- Review cleanliness and sanitation of the environment
- Review food preparation, quality, and service
- Evaluate facility safety
- Determine areas of deficient care
- Review policies and procedures

Survey Process

Surveyors make judgments about a facility by:

- Gathering information prior to the visit
- Identifying
  —areas of concern
  —special features of the facility, such as Alzheimer's units
  —residents and families to interview
  —contacting the facility ombudsman to learn about reported complaints
- During the survey,
  —making observations
  —asking questions of staff members
  —interviewing residents and their families
  —reviewing residents' medical records and care plans
  —reviewing facility manuals and records
  —touring the facility (signs are placed around the facility indicating that a survey is taking place)

Nursing Assistant Responsibilities During a Survey

During a survey there is always a higher level of tension and anxiety among caregivers. You give your best level of care if you always use good work habits and:

- Be calm and confident
- Know the residents you care for

- Know and follow the care plan for each resident in your care
- Cooperate with the surveyors
- Keep all work areas clean and tidy
- Perform each procedure as outlined in the facility procedure manual
- Know the policies that affect you in your facility
- Know how to operate all equipment properly
- Respect the residents' rights
- Report for duty where and when assigned and carry out your normally assigned tasks
- Attend inservice education programs and cooperate in presurvey audits conducted by the quality assurance committee of the facility
- Answer surveyor questions honestly
- If the surveyor asks you a question you cannot answer, you might say "I do not know the answer, but I will find out for you." Be sure you know where to find the requested information. Do not give excuses such as:
- "I don't usually work on this floor."
- "No one ever told me that."
- "I'm new here."

Do not try to outsmart a surveyor. Answer only the questions they ask you.

Survey Completion

The findings of the survey are important and are discussed with the facility administration during an exit conference. If **deficiencies** are found, the facility is usually given 10 days to prepare a plan to correct them. Up to 60 days are allowed for the facility to correct the deficiencies.

Serious deficiencies can result in:

- Fines of up to $10,000 per day until all deficiencies are corrected
- A stop on payment for Medicare and Medicaid
- Loss of certification
- Loss of approval to educate CNAs for two years
- Loss of licensure to operate as a long-term care facility and loss of your job

Nursing assistants are important to the success of the survey!

LESSON SYNTHESIS: Putting It All Together

You have just completed this lesson. Now go back and review the Clinical Focus at the beginning of the lesson. Try to see how the Clinical Focus relates to the concepts presented in the lesson. Then answer the following questions.

1. Why would Mr. McCarver not remain in the acute care facility until he had entirely recovered?

2. What services would be provided for Mr. McCarver in the long-term care facility?

3. How does the organization of the long-term care facility and the equipment provided for each resident contribute to the comfort, safety, and well-being of the resident?

4. How does Medicare relate to the financing of Mr. McCarver's health care? What is the importance of the records that must be kept?

REVIEW

A. Match each term with the proper definition.

a. geriatric care
b. long-term care facility
c. resident
d. restoration
e. terminal

1. _____ rehabilitation

2. _____ last or final

3. _____ care concerned with the medical problems and nursing care of the elderly

4. _____ person cared for in long-term care

5. _____ skilled care facility

B. List five community health agencies that provide health care.

6. _____

7. _____

8. _____

9. _____

10. _____

C. Select the one best answer for each of the following.

11. Mr. Jackson has cancer and is not expected to live more than 3 months. He probably would be cared for in
    (A) an acute care hospital
    (B) a hospice program
    (C) a long-term care facility
    (D) an outpatient clinic

12. A person being cared for in a long-term care facility is usually called the
    (A) patient
    (B) resident
    (C) client
    (D) recipient

13. The care in a skilled care facility is aimed at
    (A) acute short-term care
    (B) terminal care
    (C) restoration
    (D) providing a homelike atmosphere

14. Which articles are kept in the "dirty" area of the bedside table?
    (A) denture cup
    (B) comb
    (C) toothbrush and toothpaste
    (D) bedpan, urinal

15. The resident's room is called the
    (A) resident's space
    (B) resident's bedroom
    (C) resident's area
    (D) resident's unit

16. The nurses' station is the area where
    (A) personal care is given
    (B) food is stored
    (C) residents' records and charts are kept
    (D) residents' clothes are laundered

17. All of the following contain confidential resident records except
    (A) resident's chart
    (B) Kardex
    (C) care plans
    (D) policy book

18. OBRA regulations
    (A) give nursing assistants recognition through certification and listing in the state registry
    (B) require nursing assistants to report on duty on time
    (C) require nursing assistants to have some home health experience before working in an acute care facility
    (D) allow people with no previous education to work as nursing assistants

19. The expense of long-term care is mostly paid by
    (A) private funds
    (B) health maintenance organizations
    (C) Preferred Provider Organizations
    (D) Medicare and Medicaid

20. Surveyors observe to see that standards are being met for everything except
    (A) safety
    (B) infection control
    (C) residents' rights
    (D) employee pay scales

21. The Resident Assessment Instrument (RAI) requires facilities to transmit information gathered from the
    (A) Minimum Data Set (MDS2.0)
    (B) triggers
    (C) Resident Assessment Protocols (RAPs)
    (D) A, B, and C

22. During a survey, how should the nursing assistant answer questions asked by the surveyor?
    (A) I'm new here
    (B) No one ever told me that
    (C) Answer questions honestly
    (D) I don't usually work here

D. **Indicate where each of the following areas is found by selecting from the list (items a.–d.). (More than one answer may apply.)**

a. nurses' station   c. resident unit
b. dining room   d. day room

23. _____ bedside stand

24. _____ medication storage

25. _____ meal service area

26. _____ emesis basin

27. _____ bed

28. _____ group activities area

29. _____ television

30. _____ reports

31. _____ resident's health record

32. _____ Kardex

E. **Clinical Experience**

Amelia Walters, 85, has lived in the same community all of her life. She has lived alone since her husband died 3 years ago. Her only living relative, a daughter, lives some distance away. The daughter has little contact with her mother.

Mrs. Walters had frequent upper respiratory infections and received care from her neighborhood physician.

During wet weather, Mrs. Walters fell and broke her right ankle and both wrists. Mrs. Walters is unable to perform personal care. She requires full-time care. Healing is slow and her generally frail health makes it impossible for her to live independently. Despite care, her condition declines.

Tests ordered by her physician reveal advanced cancer of the colon, a terminal condition. Mrs. Walters insists that she wants to go home and remain there as long as possible. Answer the following questions relating to Mrs. Walters. Select your answers from the list provided.

a. hospice care
b. acute care hospital
c. skilled nursing facility
d. physician's office
e. home care

33. _____ Mrs. Walters received care here for her upper respiratory infections.

34. _____ Care was given here when Mrs. Walters fell, breaking an ankle and both wrists.

35. _____ Mrs. Walters received restorative care here as her ankle and wrists healed.

36. _____ What help may make it possible for Mrs. Walters to go home once more?

37. _____ What kind of care is available to Mrs. Walters during the final stage of her life?

LESSON 2

The Caregivers

Clinical Focus
Think about how staff members contribute their special knowledge and expertise to the resident's well-being as you study this lesson and meet:

*M*s. Esther Patterson, who is 74 years old, and complains every time her shoes are put on her feet and she is assisted to walk. You are asked to help the podiatrist who is visiting her. Consider how this care will help Ms. Patterson become more active.

OBJECTIVES
After studying this lesson, you should be able to:

- Define and spell vocabulary words and terms.
- Name three or more members of the interdisciplinary team.
- Describe the purpose of the interdisciplinary team.
- List the members of the nursing staff.
- State the purpose of the organizational chart.

VOCABULARY

activities of daily living (ADL) *(ack-TIV-ih-tees of DAY-lee LIV-ing)*
adaptive device *(ah-DAP-tiv dih-VICE)*
administrator *(ad-MIN-iss-tray-tor)*
ambulation *(am-byou-LAY-shun)*
assessment *(ah-SESS-ment)*
assistive device *(ah-SIS-tiv dih-VICE)*
audiologist *(awe-dee-OL-oh-jist)*
care plan conference *(kair plan KON-fer-ens)*

consultant *(kon-SUL-tant)*
dental hygienist *(DEN-tal high-JEE-nist)*
dentist *(DEN-tist)*
diagnosis *(die-ag-NOH-sis)*
dietitian *(die-eh-TISH-un)*
environmental services *(en-vire-un-MEN-tal SIR-vuh-sez)*
interdisciplinary health care team *(in-ter-DISS-sih-plin-air-ee health kair team)*

VOCABULARY

licensed practical nurse *(LICE-enst PRACK-tih-kul nurs)*

mobility *(moh-BILL-ih-tee)*

nursing assistant *(NUR-sing ah-SIS-tant)*

occupational therapist *(ock-you-PAY-shun-al THER-ah-pist)*

ophthalmologist *(off-thal-MOL-oh-jist)*

optometrist *(op-TOM-eh-trist)*

orthotic device *(or-THAW-tick dih-VICE)*

physical therapist *(FIZ-ih-kul THER-ah-pist)*

podiatrist *(poh-DYE-ah-trist)*

registered nurse *(REJ-is-terd nurs)*

rehabilitation aide *(ree-hah-BILL-ah-tay-shun ayd)*

social worker *(SO-shul WERE-ker)*

speech-language pathologist *(speech LAN-gwehj pah-THOL-oh-jist)*

support services *(sup-PORT SIR-vuh-sez)*

therapeutic diet *(ther-ah-PEW-tick DIE-et)*

therapeutic recreational specialist *(ther-ah-PEW-tick reck-ree-AY-shun-al SPEH-shul-ist)*

total care *(TOH-tal kair)*

THE INTERDISCIPLINARY TEAM MEMBERS

Many workers help care for the resident. These caregivers represent many professions or "disciplines," and each has a specific function. As a group they are called the **interdisciplinary health care team** (Figure 2-1). Each member of the interdisciplinary health care team helps plan the care of the residents. This process is completed at the resident's **care plan conference.** You will learn more about this in Lesson 6. The team members who attend the care plan conference include the:

- Resident
- Resident's family (if resident gives permission)
- Members of the nursing staff
- Members of the rehabilitation staff
- Social worker
- Activities director
- Dietitian or dietary supervisor

By using the interdisciplinary team approach, the residents receive **total care**. This considers the emotional, spiritual, physical, and social needs of each person. The resident and the resident's family are also considered members of the team. Most of the direct care is given by the nursing staff. Figure 2-2 defines the jobs of peo-

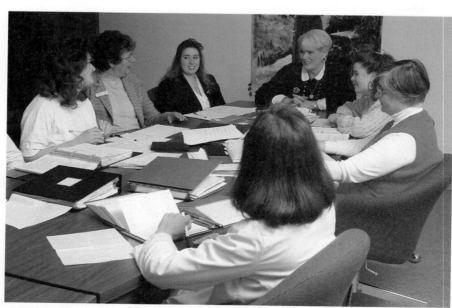

FIGURE 2-1 The interdisciplinary health care team is responsible for the care of the resident.

FIGURE 2-2   Who's who on the interdisciplinary health care team

Each of these disciplines requires a specified course of study (usually a minimum of a college degree and clinical training). Most require either licensing by a state agency or certification from a professional association. Requirements for some disciplines may vary from state to state.

Activities director:	Requirements vary. Plans and implements activities for residents to meet the goals on the care plan.
Administrator:	Licensed and meets state requirements to provide general administration and supervision of a long-term care facility.
Audiologist:	Certified in audiology and qualified to test hearing and prescribe hearing aids.
Chaplain:	Provides services to meet the spiritual needs of residents.
Dental hygienist:	Licensed by the state and provides dental services under the supervision of a dentist.
Dentist:	Licensed by the state to provide services for the prevention and treatment of diseases and disorders of the teeth and oral cavity.
Dietitian:	Licensed by the state and responsible for the provision of all nutritional assessments and food services for residents.
Licensed practical nurse (LPN or LVN):	Licensed by the state and provides direct resident care under the supervision of a registered nurse. Sometimes called licensed vocational nurse.
Medical record practitioner:	Certified or licensed to review and audit all medical records.
Nursing assistant:	Has completed at least 75 hours of a state-approved course and is certified to provide direct resident care under the supervision of a licensed or registered nurse.
Occupational therapist:	Licensed to provide rehabilitative services to evaluate and treat persons with physical injury or illness, psychosocial problems, or developmental disabilities. Occupational therapy assistants and aides have completed specified courses of study and work under the supervision of an occupational therapist.
Optometrist:	Licensed by the state to examine eyes and prescribe glasses.
Orthotist:	Licensed by the state and designs and fits braces and splints for the extremities.
Pharmacist:	Licensed by the state and fills prescriptions for medications as ordered by the physician. Resource to nurses and physicians for updates on new medications and for maintaining safe drug therapy for residents.
Physical therapist:	Licensed by the state to provide rehabilitative services to evaluate and treat persons with neuromuscular and musculoskeletal problems due to disease, injury, or developmental disability. Physical therapy assistants and aides have completed specified courses of study and work under the supervision of a physical therapist. *(continues)*

FIGURE 2-2 *(continued)*	
Physician:	Licensed by the state to diagnose and treat disease and to prescribe medications. The many specialty areas within medicine require additional education.
Podiatrist:	Licensed by the state to treat diseases and disorders of the feet.
Prosthetist:	Licensed by the state to design and fit artificial limbs for persons who have had amputations.
Registered nurse (RN):	Licensed by the state to make assessments, plan, implement, and evaluate nursing care. Supervises other nursing staff and may coordinate the interdisciplinary health care team. The many specialty areas within nursing require additional education.
Rehabilitation aide, Restorative nursing assistant (RNA):	A certified nursing assistant with additional training to perform procedures under the direction of the licensed physical therapist and licensed occupational therapist.
Resident:	The most important member of the interdisciplinary team and has input into the planning and implementation of care. The family may participate with the resident or in place of the resident if the resident is unable to do so.
Respiratory therapist:	Licensed by the state to evaluate and treat diseases and problems associated with breathing and the respiratory tract.
Social worker:	Licensed by the state to assess and provide services for the nonmedical, psychosocial needs of residents.
Speech-language pathologist:	Licensed by the state to evaluate and provide services for residents with problems in hearing, language, speech production, and swallowing.
Therapeutic recreational specialist:	Certified to evaluate and provide recreational services to treat mental and physical disorders.
Unit secretary:	Certified nursing assistant with additional training, responsible for clerical duties of nursing staff; may also be a person with no previous health care experience who is trained as a unit secretary for a specific period of time.

In addition to these members of the interdisciplinary health care team, many other employees in the long-term care facility provide services that benefit the quality of life for residents.

- Environmental services staff maintain a clean, comfortable, and homelike environment. These services may include housekeeping, laundry, and building and grounds maintenance.
- The business office handles the personal funds of residents as well as the financial affairs of the facility.
- Assistants in all departments provide services to residents as part of the interdisciplinary team.
- Volunteers may provide direct services to residents and may raise funds to provide equipment for resident care.

ple who are commonly part of the interdisciplinary health care team.

The Nursing Staff

The nursing staff in a long-term care facility includes **registered nurses** (RNs), **licensed practical nurses** (LPNs), and **nursing assistants**. (In some states LPNs are called licensed vocational nurses or LVNs.)

The *director of nursing* must be a registered nurse. This person has had, besides nursing school, some additional training in administration. The director of nurses is the head of the nursing staff and is responsible for all nurses, nursing assistants, and residents in the facility. If the facility is very large, there may also be an assistant director of nursing and supervisors, as well as other nurses in charge of education, infection control programs, and quality assurance. These programs ensure that all residents receive appropriate care.

An *assistant director of nursing* works with the director. *Supervisors* are in charge of the entire building during a specific shift. *Charge nurses* are responsible for a nursing unit. There may be one or several nursing units within a facility. *Staff nurses* are in charge of a specific number of residents. They pass medications, perform treatments, and supervise the residents' direct care (Figure 2-3). There may be a *rehabilitation nurse* who coordinates activities between the therapists and the nurses and restorative care. The nursing assistants are responsible for carrying out most of the personal resident care (Figure 2-4).

The use of advance practice nurses is becoming more common. An *advance practice nurse* has completed additional educational programs leading to a master's degree or doctoral degree. The course of study qualifies them to work as nurse practitioners or clinical nurse specialists.

The *unit secretary* is responsible for the clerical tasks of the nursing staff. These duties include answering the telephone, writing out daily reports, filing, entering reports into the medical records, making out assignment sheets, and ordering supplies.

Social Services

The social services department provides for many of the nonmedical needs of the residents (Figure 2-5). The department works closely with the nursing staff. In many facilities they are

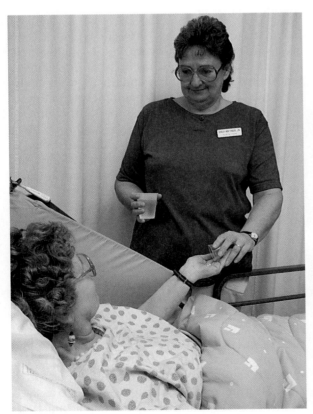

FIGURE 2-3 Staff nurses pass medications and perform treatments.

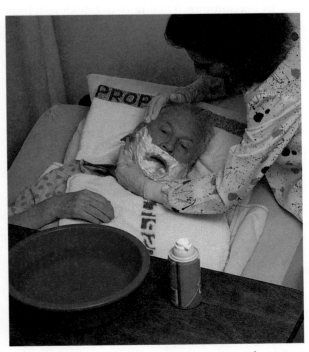

FIGURE 2-4 Nursing assistants provide most of the resident's personal care.

FIGURE 2-5   The social services department is responsible for the admission of new residents.

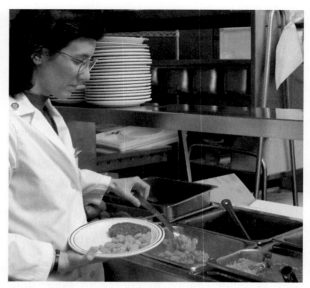

FIGURE 2-6   The dietitian supervises the nutritional services of the facility.

responsible for the admission of new residents. **Social workers** plan the discharge for residents going home. This may involve coordination of community services for the resident, such as making arrangements for homemaking services or for the services of a home health agency. The social workers may arrange for appointments with dentists, podiatrists, audiologists, or mental health consultants. They may organize religious services and other programs with local religious groups or leaders. Social workers care for residents with behavior problems, depression, and psychosocial needs.

The Physician

Each resident has a physician who makes the medical **diagnosis** and writes medical orders for the resident. In addition to writing new orders, the physician evaluates the health and well-being of the residents. The physician may also participate in care plan conferences.

The Dietitian

A **dietitian** plans and supervises the preparation of resident meals and therapeutic diets (Figure 2-6). The dietitian performs a nutritional **assessment** for each resident. Monitoring residents' weights is another duty of the dietitian. Special meals and supplements are provided for residents requiring **therapeutic diets** (special diets designed to meet a resident's specific

needs). Therapeutic diets are ordered by the physician. (Lesson 17 has more details on therapeutic diets.)

Special Therapists

In large facilities many different types of therapists are in the facility every day. In smaller facilities, the therapists may be **consultants**. Consultants come to the facility regularly to evaluate the residents' conditions and recommend treatment.

The **physical therapist** works to improve the **mobility** (ability to move) of the resident (Figure 2-7). After an initial evaluation, a plan is developed to restore and maintain optimum body functioning. This may include teaching the resident how to use an **assistive device**. Canes and walkers are examples of assistive devices. Many times the nursing assistant helps to carry out the program prescribed by the therapist. For example, range of motion exercises are part of daily care. These are ordered by the physician but they are done by the nursing assistant or in the rehabilitation department.

The **occupational therapist** helps residents learn new ways of doing basic self-care (**activities of daily living** or **ADL**). For example, the therapist may teach the resident to dress or eat with the use of **adaptive devices**. An adaptive device is a piece of equipment designed to assist a resident to carry out ADL. The occupational therapist may evaluate and fit an **orthotic device** (splint) for a resident's hand. Orthotic devices are

FIGURE 2-7   The physical therapist works to improve the resident's mobility.

FIGURE 2-8   The occupational therapist applies an orthotic device to support the resident's weak right hand and wrist.

appliances used to protect and support a body part. Such a device can hold a paralyzed hand in position to prevent contractures (permanent deformities) from forming (Figure 2-8).

There may be other members of the rehabilitation team. Physical therapy assistants and occupational therapy assistants must complete 2 years of an approved educational program. They work under the direct supervision of the therapists. Restorative nursing assistants work under the direction of the registered nurse. Some states allow occupational and physical **rehabilitation aides** to perform some of the less complex, routine procedures. They also work under the direction and supervision of the therapists. The rehabilitation aides are nursing assistants who have taken additional courses to prepare them for this job.

The occupational therapist or **therapeutic recreational specialist** may direct recreational, educational, spiritual, artistic, or social activities for the resident. Activities aides also work with the resident in doing the activities.

The **speech-language pathologist** (speech therapist) works with residents who have speech and language problems. The speech-language pathologist may help a resident regain the ability to talk. If a resident is unable to do this, the resident will be taught other means of communication. Speech-language pathologists also work with residents who have trouble swallowing. They do swallowing evaluations and suggest techniques for feeding residents.

Consultants

Some of the services provided by the facility are not needed on a daily basis. Not all residents need all of the services. Consultants are hired to perform these services.

The **audiologist** tests and evaluates hearing. For residents with impaired hearing, the audiologist may prescribe a hearing aid.

Dentists or **dental hygienists** examine and clean teeth. They also evaluate the resident's dental health. Maintaining good nutrition is diffi-

Clinical Focus

The podiatrist is visiting Ms. Patterson. Think about the role of the podiatrist and what you can do to help Ms. Patterson feel more comfortable during the examination. What can you do to assist the podiatrist?

cult when teeth are in poor condition. The dentist will recommend dentures or denture repair when needed. Choking is always a concern with improperly fitting dentures.

The **podiatrist** is another special caregiver who visits periodically. Many older persons have foot and toenail problems that make **ambulation** (walking) difficult. The podiatrist examines and may treat foot problems, such as bunions, hammer toes, calluses, and corns. This increases the resident's comfort and mobility because these conditions are very painful.

An **ophthalmologist** examines the resident's eyes and prescribes glasses. The ophthalmologist may also perform surgery to correct or improve vision problems. The **optometrist** is licensed by the state to examine eyes and prescribe glasses.

Support Services

Many other workers provide **support services**. These workers:

- Maintain the building and grounds
- Perform housekeeping duties

BUILDING CULTURAL AWARENESS

The health care facility is staffed with persons from many different ethnic groups. It is important that you examine your ideas about persons who may have different values and traditions from yours. The team effort requires that all persons work together harmoniously.

- Do the laundry
- Work in the kitchen
- Handle administrative duties
- Manage the financial affairs of the facility

Buildings and grounds, housekeeping, and laundry departments are sometimes called **environmental services**.

ADMINISTRATIVE ORGANIZATION—

Each facility has an organizational chart that shows the line of authority or command (Figure 2-9). Each department is represented on the chart. All employees are recognized within these departments. The organizational chart is also used as a guide for communication so all employees know to whom they should report.

The **administrator** of the long-term care facility provides leadership for all departments and employees.

The facility is managed and directed by a Board of Directors that delegates authority for day-to-day operation to the administrator and department heads.

Your immediate supervisor is the instructor, charge nurse, or staff nurse designated for this role. The supervising nurse will give you your assignment and you will report your observations and the completion of the assigned tasks to this person.

Any questions about your assignment should be directed to your supervising nurse for clarification. *Never attempt to carry out an assignment for which you have not been trained or an assignment you do not fully understand.* Inform the supervisor and ask for help. Never feel embarrassed. It is better to ask for help than to injure a resident.

On the Job

Remember that there are many variations in long-term care facilities. Smaller facilities have fewer staff members and may not employ all the types of workers described in this lesson.

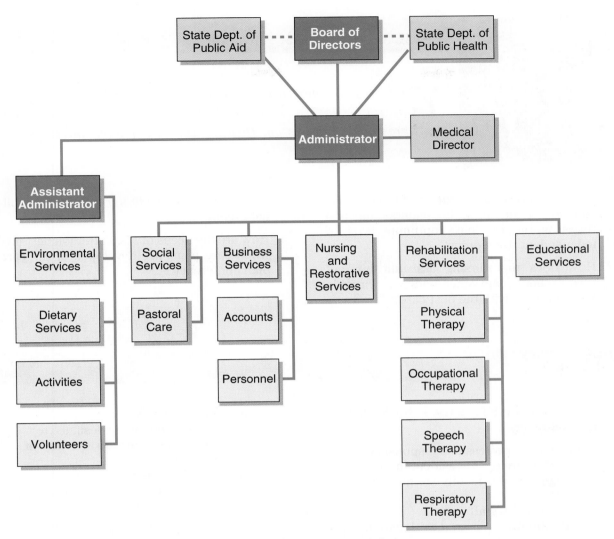

FIGURE 2-9 Organizational chart

EDUCATIONAL SERVICES

The term *educational services* includes all forms of educational programs within the health care facility. Resident education, community education, and staff education may all be responsibilities of this department. Employers must provide their staff members with continuing education programs.

All staff members are expected to participate in continuing education programs. This is called *staff development*. Some of the programs will be attended by all members of the interdisciplinary team. Other programs may be presented specifically for nursing assistants. OBRA requires that all nursing assistants participate in a minimum of 12 hours of continuing education each year. Some states may require more than 12 hours. At these programs, you will learn about:

- New facility policies
- New procedures involving resident care
- Use of new equipment
- Caring for residents with unusual diagnoses or problems
- Issues in health care
- Topics related to residents' rights, safety, and infection control

The more you learn, the better you can care for the residents and the more you will enjoy your work.

LESSON SYNTHESIS: Putting It All Together

You have just completed this lesson. Now go back and review the Clinical Focus. Try to see how the Clinical Focus relates to the concepts presented in the lesson. Then answer the following questions.

1. What role does each member of the interdisciplinary team play in maintaining and restoring the resident's optimum level of independent functioning?

2. How does the nursing assistant interact with other team members to provide Ms. Patterson with the best care?

3. How do consultants fit into the interdisciplinary team?

4. How are the needs of Ms. Patterson best met when care plans are developed at the care plan conference?

REVIEW

A. Select the one best answer for each of the following.

1. The many professions responsible for the care of the resident in the long-term care facility are members of the
   (A) medical staff
   (B) interdisciplinary health care team
   (C) employee council
   (D) residents' council

2. Employees who attend the resident's care plan conference include
   (A) the resident
   (B) activities director
   (C) members of the nursing staff
   (D) A, B, and C

3. The person who is responsible for helping residents learn new ways of doing the activities of daily living is the
   (A) occupational therapist
   (B) physician
   (C) pharmacist
   (D) physical therapist

4. An adaptive device is a
   (A) piece of equipment designed to assist a resident with activities of daily living
   (B) cane or walker
   (C) hearing aid
   (D) set of dentures

5. A splint is a device that
   (A) helps the resident walk
   (B) prevents deformities in an extremity
   (C) helps the resident breathe
   (D) restrains the resident

6. The social worker may be responsible for
   (A) admission and discharge of residents
   (B) giving medications
   (C) giving physical therapy
   (D) supervising nursing assistants

7. Most of the direct care of residents is given by the
   (A) director of nursing
   (B) nursing assistants
   (C) administrator
   (D) dietitian

8. The purpose of the organizational chart is to
   (A) indicate the lines of authority
   (B) provide a guide for communication
   (C) indicate the chain of command
   (D) A, B, and C

9. The housekeeping, laundry, and maintenance departments may be referred to as
   (A) rehabilitation services
   (B) food services
   (C) environmental services
   (D) nursing services

10. The Omnibus Budget Reconciliation Act (OBRA) requires that all nursing assistants participate in
    (A) a minimum of 12 hours of in-service education each year
    (B) annual college courses
    (C) providing social services
    (D) food preparation

11. Nursing assistants report to:
    (A) the resident's physician
    (B) the housekeeping supervisor
    (C) the administrator
    (D) a registered nurse or a licensed practical nurse

B. Match the team members (items a.–j.) with their responsibilities.

a. physician
b. dietitian
c. physical therapist
d. respiratory therapist
e. administrator
f. audiologist
g. dentist
h. podiatrist
i. ophthalmologist
j. housekeeper

12. _____ cares for residents with mobility problems

13. _____ provides leadership to staff

14. _____ performs housekeeping duties

15. _____ examines and cleans teeth

16. _____ provides eye examinations and prescriptions

17. _____ defines the medical diagnosis and writes orders

18. _____ treats diseases associated with breathing

19. _____ cares for foot problems

20. _____ plans and supervises preparation of meals

21. _____ tests and evaluates residents' hearing

LESSON 3

The Nursing Assistant in Long-Term Care

Clinical Focus

Think about the characteristics that are needed to be a successful nursing assistant as you study this lesson and meet:

*R*ay Rodriquez, who is 20 years old. He did not finish high school because he needed to earn money to help at home. Ever since he was a little boy he has known responsibility and the need to be prompt and dependable. While growing up, he helped his mother care for an elderly grandmother and younger brothers and sisters. He learned to be patient as he helped his grandmother eat. Ray comes from a very close and loving family and is putting his skills to positive use.

OBJECTIVES

After studying this lesson, you should be able to:

- Define and spell vocabulary words and terms.
- List five personal characteristics needed to be a successful nursing assistant in long-term care.
- Describe how to dress properly for work.
- Define the job description.
- List 10 duties that the nursing assistant performs.
- Explain how interpersonal relations influence the effectiveness of resident care.
- List five ways to use time efficiently.
- Identify signs of increasing resident stress
- State ways to deal with violent situations
- State the responsibilities the nursing assistant has for personal and clinical growth.

VOCABULARY

accuracy (*ACK-your-ah-see*)

assignment (*ah-SIGHN-ment*)

attitude (*AT-ih-tood*)

burnout (*BURN-out*)

dependability (*dee-pen-dah-BILL-ih-tee*)

empathy (*EM-pah-thee*)

harmony (*HAR-mun-ee*)

job description (*job dih-SKRIP-shun*)

maturity (*mah-CHUR-rih-tee*)

procedure (*proh-SEE-jur*)

professionalism (*proh-FEH-shun-ul-izm*)

sensitivity (*sen-sih-TIV-ih-tee*)

violence (*VY-oh-lenz*)

PROFESSIONALISM

Nursing assistants are expected to function in a professional manner at all times. Professionalism does not come from having a stethoscope around your neck or one or more degrees following your name, although many professional people carry this equipment and have these credentials.

Professionalism is demonstrated by:

- The security with which you carry out your tasks
- Keeping up to date and current with the latest information in your field by reading, taking classes, and attending in-service programs
- The careful way you perform the skills you have been taught
- Paying attention to the safety and comfort of the resident and remembering to protect the resident's dignity
- The gentle way you relate to the resident during care
- Protecting the resident's privacy and offering the resident choices whenever possible
- Keeping all information confidential
- Completing your assignments fully, correctly, and in a timely manner

PERSONAL CHARACTERISTICS

Nursing assistants working in long-term care are very special people. They feel pride in themselves when they fulfill their role with enthusiasm and dedication. They will be successful if they:

- Possess maturity and sensitivity
- Are dependable and accurate
- Can be satisfied with small gains
- Bring a positive attitude to their job
- Carry out an **assignment** (work to be completed during the shift). Each task is to be performed as it has been taught and in a safe manner

Not everyone can be a successful, satisfied long-term care nursing assistant. Nursing assistants care for many people who cannot care for themselves. Some of these residents may be confused; others need a great deal of patience and assistance in carrying out even the most intimate parts of their own personal hygiene.

Sensitivity and Maturity

Because residents have so many needs, the nursing assistant must have the **sensitivity** to recognize the needs that are expressed and those that are not expressed. The need for dry, clean linen is obvious if the bed is wet. The need for a close human relationship may be less obvious. It is just as important to be aware of and to meet residents' emotional needs as their physical needs (Figure 3-1).

The sensitive, mature care provider quickly recognizes both the physical and emotional needs of residents and willingly reaches out. **Maturity** means that you can control your emotions. Angry responses have no place in the facility. You must relate to residents and coworkers with courtesy, kindness, and respect. The mature individual can accept and learn from constructive evaluation and criticism. Maturity and sensitivity are also required to make the observations (assessments) that are part of a nursing assistant's job. Maturity is not a matter of age; it is one of attitude.

In the acute care hospital, patients who have been very ill or who have had extensive surgery can make rapid, dramatic gains as their health improves. They look forward to returning home. In the past, the resident in a long-term care facility made small strides—for example, relearning to hold a spoon or walking a corridor with the help of a cane. The facility became their home, and often the staff became their only family and friends. The enthusiasm and patience that the nursing assistant brought to work spread like sunshine throughout the unit. A smile or the

FIGURE 3-1 The nursing assistant must be sensitive to the resident's needs.

FIGURE 3-2 Reporting for duty on time demonstrates responsibility and dependability.

therapeutic use of touch in the recognition of a resident's successful efforts brightened the day for those being cared for. However, this scenario changed in long-term care facilities in the 1990s as patients left acute care hospitals earlier and sicker, and required levels of care not available to them at home. These patients were and are being admitted to skilled care facilities for rehabilitation or stabilization of their conditions until they are ready to return home. Once home, they may need continued care but at a reduced level until they are able to take care of themselves.

Insurance companies and HMOs promote this extension of acute care services. It is also more economical for private-pay patients who do not have Medicare or private insurance.

Dependability and Accuracy

Dependability and **accuracy** are also essential qualities of the nursing assistant. You demonstrate these qualities when you:

- Arrive for duty on time (Figure 3-2)
- Come prepared to do your job
- Carry out your assignment correctly
- Keep a positive attitude

Empathy

The ability to put yourself in another person's position is called **empathy**. Being able to see a

situation from another person's viewpoint helps you become more sensitive to that person.

Just for a moment, pretend you are one of the residents. What qualities do you want in the nursing assistants who care for you? Imagine what it must be like to:

- Have to sit for hours in a geri-chair
- Have thoughts you cannot express in words
- Need to go to the toilet and have to wait for help
- Need help to take a bath
- Not be able to feed yourself
- Have a tube in your bladder to drain urine
- Be separated from family and friends
- Be demeaned by wearing a protective brief for incontinence

As you do this, you will begin to understand the situation of the residents, and your empathy for those in your care will grow.

ATTITUDE

The most important characteristic that you bring to your job is your **attitude** (Figure 3-3). The other characteristics described here are an outer reflection of your inner feelings, of your attitude about yourself and others.

Residents have the right to be cared for in a calm, unhurried atmosphere. Your attitude and behavior are critical in providing such an environment.

Attitudes are contagious. To promote a high quality of care and therapeutic relationships

FIGURE 3-3 Therapeutic relationships with residents in long-term care result when caregiving skills are combined with a positive, caring attitude. Factors affecting the outcome include trust, respect, competent and compassionate care, and promotion of normalcy.

with residents, caregiving skills must be combined with a positive, caring attitude. The factors that facilitate these goals include trust, respect, competent and compassionate care, and promotion of normalcy.

Your attitude is reflected in the way you relate to your coworkers as well. Each time you willingly help another worker, you show your shared concern for each other and for the welfare of the residents.

PERSONAL HYGIENE

The work of a long-term care nursing assistant is physically demanding. Because you will be in close contact with the residents, your personal hygiene and grooming must be the very best (Figure 3-4). Good grooming starts with a daily bath or shower and the use of a deodorant to control body odor. Careful attention to the cleanliness of teeth and nails is also important; teeth should be cleaned at least twice each day and fingernails kept trimmed and smooth. (Long nails are unsafe for two reasons: (1) they can injure a resident, and (2) they promote the growth of potentially harmful germs.) Hair should be neatly arranged and controlled. Hair should not fall over the face or shoulders. It should be pulled up or back neatly. Beards and mustaches should be neatly trimmed. Makeup should be moderate.

Strongly scented aftershave lotions and perfumes can bother many people and cause allergic reactions in others. Do not use them while you are on duty.

FIGURE 3-4 Good grooming starts with a daily bath or shower and the use of a deodorant. It also includes teeth that are brushed and clean hair arranged in a neat style.

UNIFORMS

The uniform of nursing assistants in long-term care facilities is often a matter of preference. If your facility has a dress code and specifies how nursing assistants should dress, you must follow that code (Figure 3-5).

The uniform includes shoes and stockings or socks. Shoes are usually white and should be cleaned daily, and white shoelaces should be laundered frequently. Because nursing assistants spend many hours on their feet, good, comfortable, well-fitting shoes are required.

Wear your uniform only while on duty. When you arrive home, remove your uniform, fold it inside out so that the dirtiest part is on the inside, and put it in the laundry. When doing the laundry, use bleach if possible to kill the bacteria that may be present on the uniform.

Wear a fresh, clean uniform each day that you report to work. Make sure that the uniform is

FIGURE 3-5   Well-groomed nursing assistants wear a fresh, clean uniform each day.

presentable, with no broken zippers, missing buttons, hanging hems, or tears.

Do not smoke while in uniform. Clothing and breath absorb the odor of tobacco, which is offensive to many people. If you do smoke, storing clean uniforms in plastic garment bags at home will help reduce the exposure to smoke.

Accessories

Bracelets, rings, earrings, and necklaces are not to be worn (although most facilities do permit the wearing of a wedding ring and small stud earrings). Jewelry tends to harbor germs, may scratch or injure a resident, and can easily be lost.

A watch with a second hand and an identification badge are part of your official uniform. You will need the watch to do certain procedures. The identification badge lets other staff members know who you are and helps residents remember your name. It should always be worn when you are in uniform.

You should keep a pen and a small notepad in your uniform pocket to jot down your observations of the residents and their responses to care.

Pride in Appearance

Always remember that your appearance declares your professionalism and your pride in yourself and your work. Remember that you are a repre-

sentative of your facility to residents and visitors. You are ready to work if you:

- Demonstrate personal cleanliness
- Use an antiperspirant or deodorant
- Wear an appropriate, clean uniform
- Wear clean shoes and stockings or socks, including clean shoelaces
- Arrange your hair so that it is neat and controlled
- Neatly trim your beard and mustache (if you are a man)
- Trim fingernails smoothly; do not use colored polish
- Do not use strong perfumes or aftershave lotion
- Wear a watch with a second hand
- Carry a pen and notepad in your uniform pocket
- Properly pin identification badge on your uniform
- Do not smoke while in uniform

DUTIES AND RESPONSIBILITIES: THE JOB DESCRIPTION

The duties and responsibilities of nursing assistants in long-term care are stated in the policy book as a **job description**. During the preemployment interview, you should review the

On the Job

You may find that procedures are carried out in the facility in ways that differ greatly from those you learned in the classroom. You must adapt and learn the procedures according to facility guidelines. Remember, you are responsible for performing all procedures correctly.

job description to be sure you can perform the work required before you accept employment. As you learned in Lesson 1, each facility has:

- A policy book that describes what will be done
- A procedure book that describes how each task should be performed
- Job description that states who will do specific tasks

Find each of these books in your unit and become familiar with them. Both books are usually found in the nurses' station.

Basic **procedures** may be varied in some ways to meet individual needs. You must know any differences in basic procedures preferred by your facility. Differences in procedure may be explained during the orientation period after you are hired. You can also check the procedure book for exact details of how procedures are to be performed.

Be willing to learn new techniques and different ways to perform tasks, taking instruction from your charge nurse or staff development coordinator. If you are asked to perform a procedure that you have not learned but is within the scope of practice for nursing assistants, ask for a demonstration. You will be supervised until both you and your supervisor are confident in your ability to do the procedure correctly and safely.

The job description is the basis for specific assignments (Figure 3-6).

FIGURE 3-6 Typical nursing assistant tasks. Specific tasks will vary depending on state regulations and facility policy.

Some of the tasks performed by nursing assistants include activities that:

1. Protect the rights of residents
   a. Treat resident with respect.
   b. Protect resident's privacy and maintain confidentiality.
   c. Keep call bells within resident's reach and answer promptly.
   d. Give resident choices whenever possible.
   e. Assist in recreational and spiritual activities of resident's choice.

2. Help the unit function smoothly
   a. Report for duty on time and ready to work.
   b. Cooperate with other team members.
   c. Communicate effectively with residents, their families, and other members of the interdisciplinary health care team.
   d. Follow facility policies.
   e. Know and carry out assignments.

3. Protect the safety of residents
   a. Keep units clean and clutter-free.
   b. Know how to operate equipment properly.
   c. Use standard precautions for routine care.
   d. Follow the principles of medical asepsis, including transmission-based isolation precautions when appropriate.
   e. Make beds properly.
   f. Report potential hazards as soon as noted.
   g. Use bed side rails and restraints properly.
   h. Know and practice the fire safety plan of the facility.
   i. Know and practice the disaster plan of the facility.

(continues)

FIGURE 3-6 *(continued)*

    j. Know and practice emergency procedures for obstructed airway (Heimlich maneuver) and cardiopulmonary resuscitation.
    k. Follow oxygen precautions carefully.

4. Help residents by observing and collecting data
    a. Measure and record vital signs (temperature, pulse, respirations, and blood pressure).
    b. Measure weight and height.
    c. Measure intake and output.
    d. Collect specimens.
    e. Document and report observations of resident's condition.

5. Help residents meet personal hygiene needs
    a. Bathe residents.
    b. Give oral hygiene.
    c. Provide denture care.
    d. Provide nail and hair care.
    e. Assist residents to dress and undress.
    f. Shave residents.
    g. Apply support hose.

6. Help residents meet nutritional needs
    a. Check food trays.
    b. Serve food trays.
    c. Assist residents who can help themselves.
    d. Feed dependent residents.
    e. Provide fresh water, nourishments, and supplements.

7. Help residents meet elimination needs
    a. Assist with bedpans, urinals, and commodes.
    b. Empty urine collection bags.
    c. Give enemas.
    d. Assist with colostomy care.

8. Help residents with restoration and mobility
    a. Turn and position residents in bed, wheelchair, or geri-chair to prevent complications of immobility.
    b. Assist in transfer activities.
    c. Carry out range of motion exercises.
    d. Help with ambulation.
    e. Assist with restorative activities.
    f. Encourage independence.

9. Help in carrying out special procedures (as defined by the facility)
    a. Admitting, transfer, and discharge.
    b. Warm and cold applications.
    c. Catheter care.
    d. Ostomy care.

Staff Relations

All members of the interdisciplinary health care team are expected to be friendly and to cooperate with each other. This kind of relationship promotes a sense of **harmony**, which is important to create a calm atmosphere. Older residents are adversely affected by any discord among staff members. While you are in the facility, you must be supportive of and pleasant to everyone.

If a staff member or resident complains to you about another nursing assistant, tactfully refuse to comment. Never criticize your coworkers to the residents. Suggest that the matter be referred to the charge nurse.

Listen to residents and offer to help with legitimate problems according to facility policy. Always remember that the effectiveness of care is affected by interpersonal relationships. Good relationships improve care; poor ones can harm the quality of care.

ASSIGNMENTS

The charge nurse makes out assignments based on the needs of residents and availability of staff. At times your care load will be lighter than usual and at times much heavier. Remember that the staff works as a team. Develop a positive attitude and be ready to help when someone needs it.

Your assignment must be carried out with the resident's personal wishes in mind. Talk with the resident about the care plan so that the resident is involved in making decisions about how and when the plan can best be carried out.

Although you will be responsible for the care of specific residents, do not ignore a resident who needs help but is not part of your assignment. Never allow any resident to be uncomfortable or in danger. For example, a resident who needs assistance to walk becomes impatient waiting in the day room for her assistant to help her return to her room. She stands up and starts unsteadily down the hall. You see potential danger and without hesitation assist her to her room even though she is not part of your specific assignment (Figure 3-7).

Unfinished Assignments

Be sure to report any difficulty you have in performing a procedure or finishing an assignment. Tell the charge nurse of any tasks that are not completed at the time indicated. This can be very important. For example, you are assigned to have a resident dressed and ready to leave for a physician's appointment before 10:00 AM. You have been very busy with a new admission and will not be able to do this task on time. Tell the charge nurse right away so the resident can receive the necessary care. Always tell the nurse if you believe that you might not be able to complete any part of your assignment. Plan ahead so

FIGURE 3-7 A nursing assistant saw that a resident needed help and moved quickly to assist.

that someone else may be assigned to take care of it and will have time to do the task.

SPECIFIC DUTIES

The duties of a nursing assistant can be divided into four groups of activities:

1. Assisting in the activities of daily living (ADL)
2. Carrying out special procedures
3. Performing support services
4. Documenting (keeping records)

Activities of Daily Living

Much of the nursing assistant's duties are centered on helping residents carry out the ADL that meet their physical, emotional, spiritual, and social needs. The major physical needs of the resident include:

- Cleanliness
- Proper exercise and positioning
- Proper nourishment (Figure 3-8)
- Elimination of wastes

Remember that each time residents participate in their own care or are able to contribute to making decisions, the residents feel they have some control over their own lives, which fosters independence.

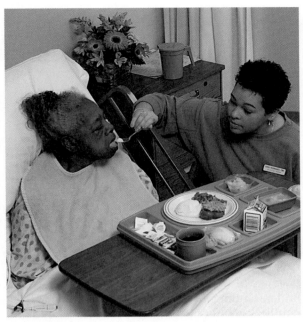

FIGURE 3-8 Feeding dependent residents is a required nursing assistant task that provides an essential ADL.

FIGURE 3-9 Placing and removing food trays is a nursing assistant function.

Special Procedures

Special procedures are required to care for residents with special needs. Special procedures include:

- Catheter care
- Ostomy care
- Measuring urine
- Giving enemas
- Collecting specimens

Support Services

The third group of tasks does not necessarily involve resident contact. These tasks support the nursing care and include:

- Supplying drinking water
- Placing and removing meal trays (Figure 3-9)

On the Job

As a nursing assistant, you will be performing intimate procedures for residents. It is important that you accept these tasks and be able to perform them in an objective manner.

- Making beds
- Caring for equipment
- Carrying messages

Each activity makes the nursing care better and more effective. For example, elderly persons often do not drink enough fluids, and part of your assignment is to encourage them to drink more liquids. Offer them liquids each time you enter the room.

Documentation

The fourth group of nursing assistant tasks involves documentation of observations. These tasks are described in Lesson 6.

ORGANIZATION OF TIME

Nursing assistants have many tasks to carry out during their on-duty time. The better organized you are, the more easily you will complete your tasks. You can become more organized by:

- Reporting for duty on time
- Listening to report
- Planning your work
- Working while on duty
- Trying to improve your performance
- Being observant at all times

Report for Duty at the Correct Time

Your job is your first responsibility. People are depending on you. If you are ill, you must call the facility as soon as you know that you will be unable to work, so that someone can cover your responsibilities. If you have personal responsibilities that might affect your availability, you should discuss these with your employer when you are hired. Be sure that you and your employer agree as to how these responsibilities are to relate to your on-duty time.

Know who you should call if you cannot report for duty. Keep the telephone number and name beside your home telephone and in your wallet.

Listen to the Report/Review Your Assignment

Note any changes in the care plans and any special orders that are to be followed. Make special note of orders that must be carried out at a specific time. Do not assume that because a resident has been at the facility for a long time, orders remain the same.

Plan Your Work and Improve Your Efficiency

Take a few moments to rearrange your plans if something unexpected develops during your shift. Refer to your plan frequently so that you can reorganize if necessary. *Remember that you are employed and paid to work for a whole shift.* Do not waste time chatting with coworkers. Be on time returning from breaks and lunch and do not leave early without permission. At the end of your shift, review your assignment. Think of ways you might have used your time and energy more efficiently. Learn to organize activities and tasks in order of importance.

Violence in the Workplace

Part of your responsibility is to maintain a calm, peaceful environment in the facility. However, from time to time, conflict and **violence** may occur in the facility between residents, residents and staff, residents and family members or other visitors, staff, and staff and visitors.

Staff members should be constantly aware of any rising tension, such as increased volume or pitch of voices before actual violence occurs (Figure 3-10).

Avoidance of violence is always preferable to dealing with violence once it erupts.

FIGURE 3-10 Signs of rising stress
Verbal outbursts
Pacing
Swearing
Increased complaining
Increased body movements
Changes in facial expressions

Disagreements Between Staff

Conflicts can arise between staff members because of work load, specific assignments, misunderstandings, or for personal reasons. These conflicts should be handled out of the sound and sight of residents or visitors.

- Seek the help of the supervisor and speak in private.
- Be factual.
- Be open to the other person's point of view, listening carefully.
- Try to solve the problem cooperatively, with each party contributing to the solution.
- Plan to meet again if the solution is ineffective.
- Put the agreed-upon solution into action.
- Thank the supervisor for meeting with you.

In some facilities there may be a grievance committee to help with severe conflicts.

An Isolated Incident

There may be a single incident in which a resident, feeling frustrated by some event, becomes upset and behaves in an angry way. Try to assess the situation in light of the resident's usual behavior. For example, a resident returns from a tiring therapy session and is feeling despondent about his progress. At this time, his lunch tray is delivered. In a sudden violent response he throws the tray on the floor. You know this is not typical of this resident. Recognize the situation as a temporary emotional response to frustration and stress. Sit with the resident to offer emotional support and provide the resident with an opportunity to express his feelings.

The Violent Resident

If a resident becomes agitated or violent, signal for help. Some health care facilities have security personnel who can be called for assistance.

FIGURE 3-11 Controlling violence in the workplace

- Stay calm

- Always know the location of signal alarms or other security devices

- Make sure you have a clear pathway to an exit

- Know and follow the facility policy for response to violence or disasters

- Report potential problems promptly

- Complete a report, following agency policy

- Participate in classes to learn how to manage residents with uncontrolled behavior

Move other residents out of the area to safety. Maintain a safe distance between yourself and the disturbed resident. Make sure that you have a safe exit route. Use a calm voice and simple words when speaking to the resident. Do not argue with or contradict the resident. Leave the room and make a report as soon as possible. Refer to Figure 3-11.

Visitors Who Become Violent

Visitors who become violent can be asked to leave the facility. The assistance of security personnel may be necessary. Do not take sides in any dispute between residents and their visitors. However, you must be firm and courteous in your insistence that the environment of the facility remain calm.

SELF-CARE

Caregivers may get so involved in caring for others that they do not pay enough attention to their own well-being. You must take care of your own mental and physical health if you are to have the energy and enthusiasm to work successfully. When people are tired or stressed, they may find it hard to be cooperative, patient, and pleasant. Mistakes are more likely to be made. For your own sake and that of the residents in your care, you need to be at your best.

You will spend much of your time on your feet—walking corridors, pushing wheelchairs, handling equipment, and moving, supporting, and lifting residents—and carrying out detailed procedures. In addition you will be offering emotional support in a variety of situations. All of these activities require physical and emotional energy. To stay fit you will need:

- Sufficient rest
- Good nutrition
- Balanced recreation

There are some additional actions that you can take to promote your own well-being:

- Have regular physical examinations, including immunizations.
- Limit alcohol intake; do not drink alcohol while on duty or before reporting for duty.
- Limit or stop smoking.
- Always use proper body mechanics.
- Wear a support belt.
- Get help and use mechanical lifts when residents are heavy.
- Practice safe sex.

Career Health

Nursing assistants also need to care for their careers. A nursing assistant who feels insecure in skills and knowledge cannot perform at a high level. You can increase your confidence when you:

- Follow procedures as they are taught
- Do only those activities that are within your job description
- Attend staff development programs
- Seek other opportunities to increase your nursing care knowledge and skills

Emotional Health

You give so much of yourself to those in your care that you face the risk of burnout.

Burnout is mental and emotional—and sometimes physical—fatigue. People who work with the sick or infirm often experience burnout because of the emotional and physical demands of providing care. You can reduce the stress that leads to burnout by balancing your work with rest and recreation.

You can also learn stress-reducing techniques. Food and cigarettes are used by some people to reduce stress, but these can cause other serious health problems. To reduce stress try the following:

- Exercise at least three to five times a week, doing something you enjoy.
- Sit for a few moments with your feet up.

- Shut your eyes and take deep breaths.
- With your eyes shut, picture a special place you like, and be there in your mind.
- Take a warm relaxing bath.
- Listen to some quiet music.
- Carry out a specific relaxation exercise.
- Make yourself a cup of herbal tea and sip it slowly.
- Find a hobby that you really enjoy.
- Take a few minutes to talk with a friend (Figure 3-12).
- Meditate on your higher power or value belief system.

SEXUAL HARASSMENT

People cannot perform at their best when they are subjected to insensitive remarks or inappropriate behavior by coworkers or supervisors. The anxiety these situations produce is increased by the fear of losing their jobs if they take action against the person responsible.

Sexual harassment may be expressed by actions, words, or implied threats. These behaviors create an environment that is hostile and nonproductive. Examples of sexual harassment include:

- The administrator makes sexual advances when you deliver reports to the office.
- A coworker rubs your neck as you document your completed tasks in the nurses' station.
- A coworker repeatedly tells off-color jokes in your presence even though you have asked him not to do so.

- A coworker makes remarks related to the size of your breasts, buttocks, or genitalia.
- Sexually explicit cartoons are posted on the staff bulletin board.
- A coworker reads and shows pornographic magazines during lunch.
- A supervisor tells you that your performance evaluation will be better if you are more "friendly."
- A charge nurse tells you that your assignments will be reduced if you agree to a date.

It is important to understand that you have the right to work in an environment that is free of sexual harassment. However, handling these situations requires sensitivity and tact. First, be sure that the situation is truly sexual harassment. Then:

- Tell the offender that you are displeased with the action.
- Document the incident so the details stay fresh in your mind.
- Report the situation to your supervisor.
- If the offender is your supervisor, follow the chain of command upward.

CONTINUE TO GROW

Your training program prepares you to perform as a beginning level nursing assistant. You have a responsibility to continue your education and personal growth (Figure 3-13). If you

FIGURE 3-12 A quiet moment relaxing with a friend is a good way to reduce stress.

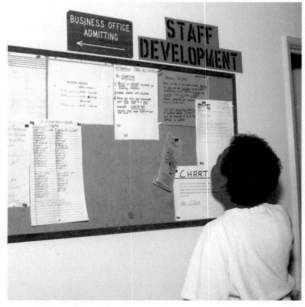

FIGURE 3-13 Once employed, take advantage of staff development programs to advance your education.

are willing to do so, you may learn much from team leaders, charge nurses, and other nursing assistants.

The procedure and policy books kept at the nursing station are ready references when you have questions about a new procedure or how to handle a new situation. Become familiar with each of these sources and with the medical dictionary on your unit. Use the dictionary to look up and learn the correct spelling of medical words. Learn at least two new words each week and practice using them. Remember, always ask for help when in doubt. Always be ready to learn.

Many facilities have professional magazines for staff use. Take advantage of this opportunity to increase your knowledge.

Care planning conferences can be an excellent way to expand your knowledge. Listen carefully. Remember, learning is a lifelong challenge.

LESSON SYNTHESIS: Putting It All Together

*Y*ou have just completed this lesson. Now go back and review the Clinical Focus. Try to see how the Clinical Focus relates to the concepts presented in the lesson. Then answer the following questions.

1. How do Ray's attitude and maturity affect the level of care the residents receive?

2. How does the pride Ray has in himself show in his own appearance and work?

3. What important contributions do nursing assistants make to the well-being of residents through the activities they perform?

4. What responsibility does a nursing assistant have to maintain personal mental and physical health?

REVIEW

A. Match each term (items a.–e.) with the proper definition.

a. accuracy   d. empathy
b. attitude   e. harmony
c. burnout

1. _____ friendly, cooperative atmosphere

2. _____ ability to put yourself in another person's position

3. _____ total emotional and mental fatigue

4. _____ outer reflection of inner feelings

5. _____ performing correctly

B. Select the one best answer for each of the following.

6. Recognizing needs that are expressed and those that are not expressed shows that the nursing assistant is
   (A) dependable
   (B) mature
   (C) sensitive
   (D) accurate

7. Maturity is related to
   (A) age
   (B) attitude
   (C) accuracy
   (D) energy

8. The nursing assistant should bathe
   (A) daily
   (B) once a week
   (C) twice each week
   (D) every other day

9. Which of the following is a proper part of your uniform?
   (A) earrings
   (B) bracelets
   (C) identification badge
   (D) necklace

10. The nursing assistant is ready for work when
    (A) fingernails are polished bright red
    (B) strong aftershave lotion is applied
    (C) wearing a watch with a second hand
    (D) wearing bracelets

11. The activities and responsibilities of nursing assistants are
    (A) stated in the procedure manual
    (B) called a job description
    (C) located in the nurses' manual
    (D) the same all over the country

12. Nursing assistant assignments are based on
    (A) the needs of the assistant
    (B) the needs of the residents
    (C) the wishes of visitors
    (D) the wishes of social workers

13. The nursing assistant's uniform is
    (A) worn on shopping trips
    (B) worn for 3 days without washing it
    (C) folded so the dirtiest side is on the outside when it is put into the laundry
    (D) worn only on duty

14. The nursing assistant notices that a resident who is not assigned to him is walking unsteadily down the hall. He should
    (A) ignore the situation
    (B) assist the resident as needed
    (C) notify the supervisor
    (D) inform the assigned nursing assistant of the situation

15. The nursing assistant has not had the time to carry out the exercises that had been ordered for a resident. It is now time to go off duty. She should
    (A) tell another assistant to do the exercises

(B) go off duty because it is not really important that the exercises be done
(C) tell the supervisor right away
(D) plan to do double the amount of exercises the next day

16. Mrs. Angdon is very upset. Her voice is rising and she is swearing (something she never does under ordinary circumstances). She is also making threats. Roseanne, the nursing assistant, should
    (A) speak loudly
    (B) hold Mrs. Angdon in her chair
    (C) make sure there is a clear exit for herself
    (D) ask her roommate to help

17. Peter and Doug are angry with one another because Doug feels Peter's assignment is lighter than his. This situation is best handled by
    (A) discussing it with a resident
    (B) discussing it in the hall
    (C) discussing it in the dining room
    (D) discussing it with the supervisor in private

C. **For each of the following duties, indicate if it is a duty of the nursing assistant by answering yes (Y) or no (N).**

18. Y   N   giving bed baths

19. Y   N   measuring temperatures

20. Y   N   serving trays

21. Y   N   starting intravenous fluids

22. Y   N   making beds

23. Y   N   applying sterile dressings

24. Y   N   calling physicians for orders

25. Y   N   weighing residents

26. Y   N   carrying messages

D. **Clinical Experiences**

Read each case history and answer the questions.

27. Mary was assigned to make the bed of a resident who was able to get out of bed. The supervisor was not satisfied with the way the bed was made and told Mary she would have to remake the

bed. Mary was very angry. After the supervisor left, she complained to the resident.
a. Did Mary show maturity in her reaction?
b. How should Mary have reacted?

28. Mrs. Randolph is a very slow eater. She had a stroke and lost the use of her left side. She is naturally left-handed. Star, the nursing assistant, can feed Mrs. Randolph faster than she can feed herself, but Star lets Mrs. Randolph feed herself.
a. Do you think Star has a special reason for letting Mrs. Randolph feed herself?
b. What do you think her purpose is?

29. John did not complete his assignment on time and his supervisor told him he must plan more carefully. John said nothing but slammed the door on the way out of the office.
a. Do you think John responded in a mature way?
b. How can you tell?
c. Is maturity a matter of age or attitude?

30. Even though they can feed themselves slowly, Carrie feeds her residents to save time.
a. Is her method of feeding best?
b. Is it more or less satisfying to the resident to be fed?
c. What benefit is there in allowing residents to feed themselves?

31. Eric always comes to work on time, has a pleasant attitude, and finishes his assignment correctly.
a. What important characteristic does Eric show by arriving on time?
b. What characteristic does he show by being sure his assignments are done correctly?

32. Lois is very patient with the residents in her care because she says she would find it so hard to need help to go to the bathroom or to have to sit all day.
a. By her actions Lois is showing what important characteristic?

SECTION 2

Communication Skills

LESSONS

4 **Communication and Interpersonal Skills**

5 **The Language of Health Care**

6 **Observation, Documentation, and Reporting**

LESSON 4

Communication and Interpersonal Skills

Clinical Focus

Think about how successful messages are sent and received and how people communicate with one another as you study this lesson and meet:

*D*oris Greene, age 83, who broke her hip and had no one to care for her at home. She has been a resident in long-term care for 4 years. She has no immediate family and her only sister lives 3,000 miles away. The staff and residents have become her family and friends.

OBJECTIVES
After studying this lesson, you should be able to:

- Define and spell vocabulary words and terms.
- Identify barriers to effective communications with residents.
- State two ways in which people communicate.
- Describe situations when nursing assistants must communicate with other staff members.
- List general guidelines for communicating with residents.
- Describe ways in which a nursing assistant can improve communications with residents who have impaired hearing, impaired vision, aphasia, or disorientation.

VOCABULARY

aphasia *(ah-FAY-zee-ah)*
articulation *(are-tick-you-LAY-shun)*
body language *(BAH-dee LAN-gwihj)*
Braille *(brayl)*

care plan *(kair plan)*
communication *(kom-myou-nih-KAY-shun)*
disorientation *(dis-oh-ree-en-TAY-shun)*
medical chart *(MED-ih-kul chart)*

VOCABULARY

memo   *(**MEM**-oh)*

nonverbal communication   *(**NON**-ver-bal
    kom-**myou**-nih-**KAY**-shun)*

shift report   *(shift ree-**PORT**)*

symbol   *(**SIM**-bull)*

verbal communication   *(**VER**-bal kom-
    myou-nih-**KAY**-shun)*

THE COMMUNICATION PROCESS

Communication involves the exchange of information (Figure 4-1). For successful **communication**, you must have a:

*   Sender
*   Message
*   Receiver

As a nursing assistant, you can assist in this process by using effective methods of communication with residents and coworkers. Some of the residents you care for will have barriers to effective communication. These may be caused by difficulties in hearing, seeing, or understanding what is being communicated. You can improve the quality of life for residents by communicating

On the Job

As a health care worker, you may be communicating with persons who are not able to talk or hear, with persons who speak a different language, or with persons who are disoriented. Communication is the foundation for successful health care.

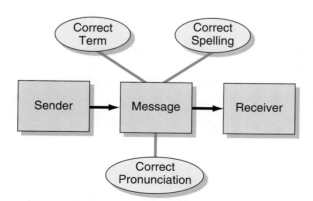

FIGURE 4-1   The message can be interpreted correctly only if the words are chosen carefully and pronounced and spelled correctly.

appropriately with each one (Figure 4-2). When residents speak a different language, you may need an interpreter to communicate effectively.

The two ways to communicate are:

*   Verbally—using spoken language
*   Nonverbally—using **body language** and **symbols**

Verbal Communication

Verbal communication includes more than the words you speak. How you say the words also sends a message to the listener. When communicating verbally with others, be aware of:

*   The tone of your voice
*   Loudness (volume) of your voice
*   Articulation
*   Words or phrases with double meanings or cultural meanings
*   Swearing or the use of slang

The tone of voice you use and its volume can convey a message of happiness, anger, sadness, or caring. Keep the volume of your voice at a

FIGURE 4-2   The nursing assistant is listening to the resident.

moderate level. A harsh, loud voice is disturbing to others.

Articulation is the clarity with which you pronounce words. If you do not articulate (speak clearly), others will not be able to understand you.

You will be caring for residents from many cultures and ethnic groups. Remember that certain words in your culture may have an entirely different meaning to someone else. Swearing is never permissible in a health care facility and slang is not to be used.

Nonverbal Communication

Your **nonverbal communication** or body language can sometimes say more than words. Be aware of the message that is being sent through your:

- Body posture/position
- Body movements
- Facial expressions
- Activity level
- Overall appearance

Your body movements send messages that can give the receiver either a negative or positive reaction about you. Your appearance gives others their first impression about you. This impression is usually lasting; it is important that it be positive. As you work in the facility, be aware that your body language is sending messages to those around you (Figure 4-3). Remember that residents may be looking at you when you are not aware of their attention.

FIGURE 4-3 The social worker's body language shows caring and interest in the resident's message.

COMMUNICATING WITH STAFF MEMBERS

In Lesson 2 you learned that the organizational chart is a guide for communication. The organizational chart tells you the lines of authority. All facilities have an organizational chart that illustrates how each department relates to other departments. Some larger departments, such as nursing, have their own chart that indicates the line of authority within the nursing department (Figure 4-4). You will need to develop methods of communication with other staff members in nursing and with members of other departments.

ORAL COMMUNICATIONS

When you first come on duty, you will listen to **shift report**. The nurse who worked the previous shift will report to staff coming on duty. This report will include:

- Changes in residents' conditions
- Information about new residents
- Names of residents who were discharged or died
- Any incidents that occurred to residents
- Physicians' new orders
- Special events for the residents that will occur during your shift

Listen carefully to the report because it will help you plan your assignment (Figure 4-5). Your assignment includes:

- The residents you will care for during your shift
- The procedures you will need to do for these residents

Your supervising nurse will then give you additional information about your assignment based on the shift report. This information may include orders to complete procedures for specific residents:

- Take temperature, pulse, and respirations on designated residents
- Obtain weights on designated residents
- Allow a resident to remain in bed because of a change in condition
- Make observations on a resident who has had a change of condition

Many skilled nursing facilities are eliminating the shift report. If your facility does not use shift reports, you must go to the team

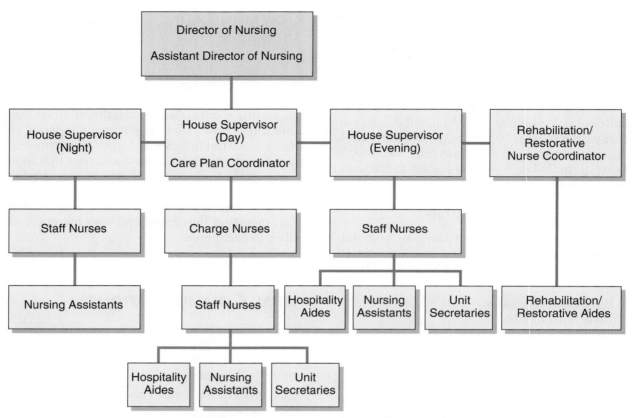

FIGURE 4-4 Nursing organizational chart

leader for assignments. At this time, you may ask about any unusual occurrences or admissions that took place while you were away from the facility.

During your shift you will give oral reports to the nurse about procedures you have completed and observations you have made. At the end of the shift you will summarize your assignment to

CNA ASSIGNMENT SHEET									DATE	4-18-XX
Rm.	Resident	Bath	Pos. Sched.	PROM	V.S.	WT.	B+B	ADL Prog.	Transfer	Safety
101ᴬ	J. Damski	X	X	X			X	X	2+TB	X
101ᴮ	G. Jones		X	X	X	X			Mech Lift	
102ᴬ	C. Hernandez	X				X			Indep.	
102ᴮ	R. Lattini	X	X	X			X		2+ TB	X
103	N. Goldberg	X			X	X	X		SBA	
104ᴬ	M. Welch		X	X					Mech Lift	
104ᴮ	L. Ordoni		X	X			X	X	1+TB	X
105	B. Brinzoski	X			X		X		Indep.	
106ᴬ	A. Feinstein	X				X		X	1+TB	
106ᴮ	D. Farmell		X	X	X		X	X	2+TB	
107	T. Green	X	X	X		X	X		2+TB	
108ᴬ	H. Johnson	X	X	X	X			X	2+TB	
108ᴮ	B. Miller		X	X		X			1+TB	X

FIGURE 4-5 The assignment sheet gives directions for the tasks to be completed.

the nurse so that the information can be included in the shift report for the employees coming on duty when you leave. When leaving the nursing unit for any reason during your shift, always report to the nurse.

At the end of the shift, be sure that you have fully documented the care you provided to residents. Sign each entry. Remember that if the care is not charted, it is considered not done.

Answering the Telephone

Many telephone calls come into a long-term care facility. Families call to ask about the condition of a loved one. Physicians call to leave new medical orders. The laboratory may call to give results of diagnostic tests. Remember that nursing assistants are not allowed to take physician's orders or results of diagnostic tests or to give information to families. You must call the nurse to do this. If you answer the telephone:

- Smile as you answer the telephone; it will give your voice a pleasant, professional sound to the person listening.
- Identify the nursing unit: "third floor, north," for example.
- Identify yourself and your position: "Mary Smith, nursing assistant, how may I help you?"
- Ask the caller's name and ask the caller to wait while you locate the person called.

- If the person is unavailable, take a message (Figure 4-6) and write down the following information:
  - Date and time of call
  - Caller's name and telephone number
  - Message left by caller
  - Whether the person is to return the call or whether the caller will telephone again later
  - Your signature

Some facilities have more complex telephone systems. You will be taught how to transfer calls or to voice page. Most facilities do not allow employees to make or receive personal telephone calls while they are on duty.

WRITTEN COMMUNICATIONS

Many situations rely on written communications. The ability to accurately write or read the communication is essential to the care of the resident.

Memos

A **memo** (Figure 4-7) is a brief communication that informs or reminds employees of:

- Changes in policies or procedures
- Upcoming meetings or staff development classes
- Admission of new residents
- Promotions of staff members

Be sure you know where memos are posted so that you will be aware of the facility activities.

FIGURE 4-6 Telephone messages must be accurate and clear.

FIGURE 4-7 Memos are brief but contain important information.

Manuals

All facilities have several manuals that provide information about policies and procedures (Figure 4-8). These may include:

- Employee personnel handbook—describes all the personnel policies and benefits
- Disaster manual—gives directions for actions to take for fire or other disasters
- Procedure manual—gives directions for all procedures performed for residents
- Quality assurance manual—describes all quality control policies and procedures
- Nursing policy manual—describes rules and regulations pertaining to care of residents
- Dietary manual—explains therapeutic diets

You are not expected to memorize all the information contained in the manuals, but you should know where they are kept on the nursing unit and be able to look up information when it is needed.

The Resident Care Plan

Each resident has a **care plan** that has been developed by the interdisciplinary health care team (Figure 4-9). The care plan:

- Lists the resident's medical diagnoses
- Identifies the resident's problems

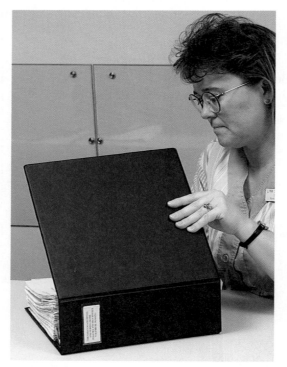

FIGURE 4-8 The procedure manual gives information on all nursing procedures performed in the facility.

- Gives directions for resolving the resident's problems
- Lists the expected outcomes for resolving the problems
- Is updated regularly

Your assignment is based on the resident's care plan. You will learn more about the care plan in Lesson 6.

The Resident's Medical Chart

Each resident has a **medical chart** or record (Figure 4-10, page 58). The medical chart contains:

- The physician's medical orders for that resident—medications, treatments, diagnostic tests
- The medical history of the resident—summary of all past illnesses and surgeries
- Results of physical examinations
- Results of all diagnostic tests—blood tests and x-rays
- Progress notes from the physician and from all disciplines involved in the resident's care—brief, periodic descriptions of the resident's condition and response to treatment
- Assessments from all disciplines—identifies the resident's problems
- Nursing notes—information that describes the resident's condition, nursing care given, and the resident's response to the care

The information entered into the chart is called *documentation*. The chart is a legal document. It may be used to:

- Determine payments by insurance companies
- Determine settlement of lawsuits

This means that all entries must be made in blue or black ink and signed. The entries are considered permanent.

COMMUNICATING WITH RESIDENTS

The ability to communicate with a resident is a skill that will develop with experience. It is not always the words you choose that are important, but the way in which they are said. Your tone of voice, facial expression, and even the way you touch a resident, all communicate a sense of honest caring, or lack of caring, to the resident. Looking directly at the resident as you speak and addressing the person respectfully by name are also indications of caring.

Listening actively is a special skill requiring more than just being physically present. When

MARYSVILLE CARE CENTER	CARE PLAN	02/06/2002
		FORM # 280L

PROBLEM	SHORT TERM GOAL	APPROACH

(1) Potential for impaired skin integrity
  a) Related to altered circulation in legs
  b) Related to flexion contracture of neck
 	
  ONSET TARGET RESOLVE
  02/06/2002 05/07/2002 / /
	(1) Will remain ulcer free (legs) through 05/07/2002
	
	  BEGIN TARGET RESOLVE
	  02/06/2002 05/07/2002 / /
	
	(2) Skin intact lower neck through 05/07/2002
	
	  BEGIN TARGET RESOLVE
	  02/06/2002 05/07/2002 / /
		(1) R.N. check legs q a.m.
		  DISC: NSG
		
		(2) Elevate legs when up in w/c.
		  DISC: NA
		
		(3) Wash and dry area b.i.d.
		  DISC: NA
		
		(4) Apply 4 x 4 to separate skin surfaces.
		  DISC: NSG NA
		
		(5) Use Mycalog cream for increased redness prn.
		  DISC: NSG

(2) Alteration in comfort
  a) Related to impaired circulation
  b) Related to joint pain
 	
  ONSET TARGET RESOLVE
  02/06/2002 05/07/2002 / /
	(1) 2 nocs/week without leg cramps by 05/07/2002
	
	  BEGIN TARGET RESOLVE
	  02/06/2002 05/07/2002 / /
	
	(2) States relief of pain with heat packs through 05/07/2002.
	
	  BEGIN TARGET RESOLVE
	  02/06/2002 05/07/2002 / /
		(1) Administer Procardia as ordered and assess effectiveness.
		  DISC: NSG
		
		(1) Heat packs to neck, shoulder, knees 5x/wk.
		  DISC: RA

PHYSICIAN / ALT. PHYSICIAN	PHONE NO.	ALLERGIES / NOTES				
WASHINGTON, JAMES M.D. KEELEY, JANICE M.D.	(555) 555-8888	PENICILLIN, ASPIRIN				
RESIDENT	STATION / ROOM / BED	ADMISSION NUMBER / DATE	SEX	DATE OF BIRTH	CARE PLAN DATE	PAGE #
JAMES, FIONA	NORTH-122-B	33652 10/18/1995	F	(73) 02/28/1923	02/06/2002	1

FIGURE 4-9 The care plan gives information for the resident's care.

you listen actively, all of your attention is focused on the speaker. You maintain eye contact and do not interrupt while the other person is speaking. You ask questions that encourage the speaker to continue and respond to specific questions being asked. To communicate effectively:
- Face the resident.
- Speak slowly.
- Maintain eye contact.

FIGURE 4-10 The medical chart is a tool for communication.

BUILDING CULTURAL AWARENESS

You should be aware that not all cultures view direct eye contact as meaning interest, attention, and courtesy. Some Asian and Native American cultures view sustained, direct eye contact as rude. People from these cultures normally would not look at a speaker directly for any length of time, nor would they stare at a person they were addressing. To do so is considered a sign of disrespect in their cultures. Do not make assumptions about the behavior of the residents in your care. If they are not of your culture, find out as much as you can about their culture. Refer to the resident assessment and care plan for information that is resident-specific. This may be done if people from specific cultures are residents in the facility.

- Listen carefully.
- Be patient and take your time.
- Use touch appropriately.
- Be aware of your body language.
- Do not sit or stand too close to the resident.
- Avoid finishing their sentences for them.

*G*uidelines for
Communicating with Residents

Remember these guidelines when you are communicating with residents.

Sending a Message

First, be aware of the message you are sending to the resident:

1. Use nonthreatening words or gestures.
   - Be calm. Avoid rapid, jerky movements.
   - Speak clearly and courteously.
   - Use a pleasant tone of voice.
   - Use the name of the resident's choice. Some residents may wish to be called

   by Mr., Mrs., or Miss with the last name. Others will ask you to use their first names. Avoid using names like "dear" or "honey."

2. Use appropriate body language.
   - This includes your general appearance. Think about the first impression that you make. Do your uniform and grooming show pride in yourself and your work?
   - Your posture and movements will tell the residents whether or not you are enthusiastic about your work.

(continues)

Guidelines *(continued)*

3. Show interest and concern when the resident is talking.
   - Use eye contact that is natural.
   - Try to communicate at eye level. Many residents use wheelchairs, so you may need to squat down or sit to do this.
   - Remain at a comfortable distance from the resident. For most people, this is about 2 feet away. If a resident is disoriented, this may be too close (Figure 4-11).

FIGURE 4-11 Remain a comfortable distance from the resident.

4. Be considerate when you are working with residents.
   - Do not talk as if the resident is not present. Include the resident in the conversation.
   - Do not discuss personal activities with other staff members in the presence of the residents.
   - Do not interrupt when the resident is speaking.
   - Ask for clarification if you do not understand the resident.

5. Give the resident only factual information, not your personal feelings, opinions, or beliefs. Your responsibility as a nursing assistant is to listen in a nonjudgmental manner. Remember:
   - Do not give orders or advice to residents.
   - Do not use threats or warnings to get residents to do what you want them to do.
   - Do not criticize or make fun of residents' beliefs or ideas.

6. Information concerning the resident's condition, medications, and treatments should be given only by the nurse.

Receiving a Message

Be sensitive to the message you are receiving from the resident.

1. Be alert to the resident's needs to communicate with you. Allow time for the resident to talk and respond.
2. Observe the resident's body language. This is especially important if a resident is unable to communicate verbally.
   - Does the resident's posture indicate the presence of pain?
   - Do the resident's gestures and movements indicate that the resident may be anxious or frightened? (Figure 4-12)

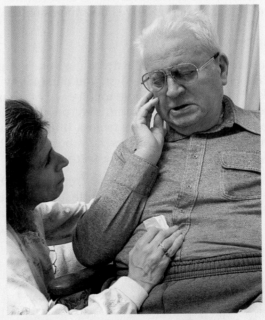

FIGURE 4-12 This resident's body language indicates fear and anxiety.

3. Consider whether the resident can see and hear you. A resident may have difficulty paying attention if there are many distractions in the environment. This

(continues)

---

*G*uidelines *(continued)*

includes other people, televisions, and radios.

4. Report problems to the nurse if you are concerned about the resident's statements. Do not argue or try to talk a resident out of a belief.

5. Ask for clarification if you are unsure of what the resident is saying.
6. Reflect the feelings and thoughts of the resident by rewording the resident's statements into questions.

COMMUNICATING THROUGH THE USE OF TOUCH

All human beings have a need to touch and be touched by others. Infants go through a "bonding" process when they are held close to another human being. This human contact is essential to the growth and development of infants and children. The need for touching is never outgrown. However, as people age, there are fewer opportunities for touching. Many older people no longer have a spouse. As one gets older, the circle of friends and relatives becomes smaller.

Appropriate Touch

Nursing assistants can learn to use touch appropriately with residents. First, you must know the residents. The way people touch each other may mean different things to different people. This is because everyone comes from a different background. Cultural meanings may be attached to touching. Be aware of these factors:

1. You will touch residents frequently while you are giving care. Be gentle and patient.
2. Touching others is not just physical contact. We touch others with our eye contact, facial expressions, and body language.

Clinical Focus

Think about Doris Greene and how you might use the sense of touch to communicate with her.

3. Some residents may have been physically abused in the past. They may associate all forms of physical contact with abuse. It may be difficult for them to accept nonthreatening forms of touch.
4. Some individuals view touching only as a preliminary to sexual intercourse. You will need to avoid touching these individuals in a way that can be misinterpreted.
5. Touching can be patronizing. An example of this is patting a resident on the head.
6. Holding a resident's hand can demonstrate a sense of caring (Figure 4-13).
7. For some residents, a hug may be suitable (Figure 4-14).
8. Disoriented residents may be startled if you touch them unexpectedly. They may react aggressively. Be sure they are aware of your approach.

FIGURE 4-13 Holding a resident's hand can show a sense of caring.

FIGURE 4-14 Some residents may appreciate a hug.

9. Touching residents appropriately can increase their self-esteem. It gives the message that you accept and care about them.

COMMUNICATING WITH RESIDENTS WHO HAVE SPECIAL NEEDS

Some residents may have difficulty communicating with you. This may be caused by:

- Hearing impairment
- Vision impairment
- Aphasia
- Disorientation

Always check the care plan before attempting to communicate with a resident who has special communication needs. Specific approaches may be established for all staff members to use with the resident. Lack of consistency in the use of these approaches is confusing and frustrating to the resident.

Communicating with Residents Who Have Hearing Impairment

Many older adults lose some of their hearing. Some of them may wear hearing aids. Even those who do may still have problems understanding others when they speak.

1. Get the resident's attention first.
   - Make sure the resident sees you.
   - Touch the resident lightly to indicate you wish to speak.
2. If the resident uses a hearing aid, be sure the resident is wearing it and that the hearing aid is on.
3. If the resident has a "good" ear, stand or sit on that side when you are talking.
4. Do not chew gum, eat, or cover your mouth while you are talking.
5. The light should be behind the resident, so your face can be clearly seen.
6. Face the resident; many persons with hearing impairments can read lips or interpret your facial expressions.
7. Reduce outside distractions. Turn off the television and move the resident to a quieter place.
8. Speak quietly and calmly.
9. Keep your voice pitch low.
10. Speak slowly, distinctly, and naturally.
11. Start conversation with a key word or phrase to identify the topic for the resident.
12. Form words carefully, use familiar words, and keep sentences short.
13. Rephrase words as needed.
14. Shouting, exaggerating words, or speaking very slowly only make it harder for the resident to understand you.
15. Use facial expressions, gestures, and body language to help express your meanings.
16. Some residents with hearing impairment use sign language. Signing depends on hand and finger movements and facial expressions. It is a skill that requires learning and practice. There are different forms of sign language just as there are different spoken languages. Recognizing some basic signs may be helpful (Figure 4-15).
17. Residents who have been hearing impaired for several years may have speech that is difficult to understand.
18. Some persons with hearing impairment are embarrassed to tell you when they do not understand you. Watch the resident's facial expressions. You may be able to tell whether or not your message was understood.
19. People who cannot hear may appear confused when they are not.

Communicating with Visually Impaired Residents

As people age, vision changes usually occur. These can generally be corrected with glasses. However, some older people have eye diseases that may seriously impair their vision. Even though they are not completely blind, they may be unable to see clearly.

Having a visual impairment does not necessarily mean the resident will have problems with communication. However, some actions you can take will make the resident feel more at ease.

1. When approaching a resident who has a visual impairment, address the person by name and then touch him or her lightly on the hand or arm to avoid startling.
2. After you speak to the resident, identify yourself and explain why you are there. "Hello, Mr. Smith. My name is Mary Jones and I would like to check your blood pressure."
3. Be specific when giving directions: "I am putting your mail on the right side of your bedside stand."
4. When giving directions for locating an area in the building, tell the resident how many doors to pass and when the resident should turn right or left.
5. When you leave the resident, make sure you announce your departure, "I am leaving your room now. May I get you anything else?"

A. HURT, PAIN, ACHE, SORE   B. NO

(REPEAT MOVEMENT)

C. HELLO, HI!   D. GOOD MORNING

FIGURE 4-15 Signing: A. Palms facing chest, index fingers extended toward, but not touching, one another. Thrust them toward one another several times: *hurt, pain, ache, sore*. B. Extend index and middle fingers, bringing them down to meet the thumb in two quick movements: *no*. C. Start with the index finger of the right hand at the right temple, palm forward and fingers pointing up. Bring the hand outward to the right: *hello, hi*. D. Start with the fingertips of the right open hand toward face. Touch lips and bring hand down, bending elbow. Touch inner elbow with left open hand as the right hand is brought upward: *good morning*.

6. Offer to read mail to residents who have visual impairments (Figure 4-16).
7. Help the resident use a telephone by counting the numbers on the dial or otherwise guiding the resident verbally to make calls.
8. Tactfully inform a person who has visual impairment if clothing is soiled, unmatched, or in need of repair.
9. Encourage the resident to listen to the radio or television to keep up with news and current events.
10. Make sure the resident is aware of talking book machines. Inform social services or activities departments if the resident wishes to use these.
11. Describe the environment and objects around the resident. This helps avoid disorientation.
12. Describe the food served to the resident. Use an example of a clock. "Your meat is at 12:00, the peas are at 3:00, and the potato is at 9:00."

Using Braille. Some residents with impaired vision may know how to read **Braille**. This is a system in which each letter of the alphabet and numbers 0 through 9 are translated into a unique pattern of raised dots. Rather than reading the printed letters with their eyes, those who know Braille "read" with their fingers as they touch the

FIGURE 4-16 Offer to read mail to residents who have visual impairments.

raised dots and spell out words. Many books and other printed materials are produced in Braille. In addition, most elevator controls are marked in Braille. Braille telephones are also available. Room numbers in facilities may also be marked in Braille and residents with visual impairments may have their names marked in Braille outside their rooms.

Communicating with Residents Who Have Aphasia

Aphasia is a condition that results from damage to the area of the brain that controls speech. This can happen after a stroke or a severe brain injury. Some chronic diseases can also cause aphasia, and this impairment can take many forms. Some residents with aphasia:

- Have trouble expressing themselves.
- Express themselves better than they can understand others.
- May have lost control of the muscles needed for speech.
- May not be able to understand what is said.
- May have intact muscle control, but lack the memory of how to say the word.
- May understand what is said but not have the ability to communicate accurately.
- Be confused; other residents with aphasia are not confused but may not be able to speak clearly and correctly.

Be patient with anyone who has a communication impairment.

Aphasia can be frustrating to the resident and the caregivers. To communicate more effectively with residents who have aphasia, follow these suggestions:

1. Face the resident and make eye contact before speaking.
2. Say the resident's name and include a social greeting ("Good morning, Mrs. Jones.") before asking questions or giving instructions.
3. Speak slowly and clearly. Use short, complete sentences.
4. Pause between sentences to allow the resident time to understand and interpret what you said.
5. Check the resident's comprehension before you proceed. Ask a question based on information you just gave the resident.
6. Use nonverbal cues to reinforce spoken communication. Gestures, facial expressions, or pictures are helpful.
7. Ask questions that require only short responses or answers that can be made nonverbally.

8. Repeat what the resident just said to help her keep focused on the conversation.
9. Find out if the speech therapist has devised methods of nonverbal communication, such as communication boards or picture books.
10. Do not avoid talking to persons with aphasia. Do not shout to try and make them understand.
11. If you sense frustration, let the resident know that you are aware of the frustration. Suggest that you talk about something else for a while and then try again.

Communicating with Residents Who Are Disoriented

Some residents in long-term care facilities are disoriented. **Disorientation** means the resident is not aware of time and place. This may be permanent, as a result of a mental impairment such as Alzheimer's disease. Sometimes disorientation is temporary. This is common in new residents until they get used to their new surroundings. Residents who have an acute illness such as an infection may also be temporarily disoriented. You can improve communication with disoriented residents when you:

1. Begin a conversation by identifying yourself and calling the resident by name. Do not ask the resident if he remembers you or knows who you are. This puts the resident "on the spot" and may embarrass him.
2. Talk to the resident at eye level and maintain eye contact.
3. Maintain a pleasant facial expression while you are talking and listening.
4. Place a hand on the resident's arm or hand unless this causes agitation.
5. Make sure the resident can hear you.
6. Use a lower tone of voice.
7. Provide a calm and quiet environment.
8. Use short, common words and short, simple sentences.
9. Give the resident time to respond.
10. Ask only one simple question at a time. If you must repeat it, say it exactly the same way.
11. Ask the resident to do only one task at a time.
12. Residents with dementia will eventually be unable to understand any verbal communication.

   - Use pictures; point, touch, or hand things to the resident.
   - Demonstrate the action when you want the resident to complete a task. For example, put the washcloth in your hand and make face-washing movements. Then

instruct the resident to do the same. If this does not work, use a hand-over-hand technique.

13. Understand the word substitutes used by the resident. If these are consistent, find out what they mean. Use them yourself to see if the resident understands you better.
14. Avoid abstract, common expressions that may be misunderstood. For example, "You can hop into bed now," may mean just that to the resident. The resident may really try to "hop" into bed.
15. Repeat the resident's last words to help stay on track during conversation.
16. Do not try to force the resident to understand. Avoid lengthy explanations and excessive verbal communication. This tends to agitate people who are disoriented.
17. Use nonverbal praise freely and always respect the resident's feelings.

COMMUNICATING WITH THE POTENTIALLY VIOLENT RESIDENT

You may be assigned to work with residents who have the potential for aggressive behavior. Residents may have this tendency because they:

- Become frustrated at their inability to complete certain tasks.
- Have a condition in which the brain cells that modify behavior are damaged by dementia or a stroke.
- Have a mental disorder.
- Are affected by a form of chemical abuse.

Check with your supervisor to find out if the medical record indicates what causes the behavior. Sometimes certain events can trigger aggressive behavior. For example, a person with dementia may become frustrated when he is not able to button his shirt. A person who has had a stroke may become frustrated when her caregivers cannot understand what she is saying. An individual with a mental disorder may believe that others are planning to harm him, so he strikes out in self-defense.

To avoid aggressive behavior:

1. Prevent situations that you know may trigger this behavior.
2. Do not expect or ask more from the resident than he or she is capable of.
3. Always use a calm approach and avoid surprising or startling the resident.
4. If you cannot understand what the resident is saying to you, ask your supervisor for assistance.
5. Maintain a calm, quiet environment.
6. Learn to identify the signs that a resident may become violent. For example, constant pacing, excessive talking, and defensive behavior may all be indications of escalating behavior. Report these signs to your supervisor.

The way in which you communicate with residents can make a difference in their lives. Be caring, considerate, and sensitive to their feelings and needs.

LESSON SYNTHESIS: Putting It All Together

You have just completed this lesson. Now go back and review the Clinical Focus. Try to see how the Clinical Focus relates to the concepts presented in the lesson. Then answer the following questions.

1. How can Doris Greene meet her physical, emotional, and social needs if communications with the staff are ineffective?

2. How can the nursing assistant improve the flow of communication or make it more difficult?

3. What special situations may make communications especially difficult with this resident?

4. What can the nursing assistant do to improve communications in the situations listed for question 3?

5. Why is it especially important for communications to be open with Doris Greene?

REVIEW

A. Select the one best answer for each of the following.

1. Successful communication requires all but which of the following?
   (A) sender
   (B) message
   (C) receiver
   (D) telephone

2. Verbal communication includes
   (A) talking and listening
   (B) facial expressions
   (C) writing reports
   (D) using a fax machine

3. Verbal communication is influenced by all but which of the following?
   (A) tone of voice
   (B) choice of words used
   (C) handwriting
   (D) articulation

4. Examples of nonverbal communication include
   (A) gestures and body language
   (B) answering the telephone
   (C) listening to shift report
   (D) conversing with residents

5. A nursing assistant may give or take which information over the telephone?
   (A) report of a resident's condition
   (B) physician's orders
   (C) results of laboratory tests
   (D) name of person leaving the message

6. The shift report is given by the
   (A) administrator
   (B) physician
   (C) nurse who worked the previous shift
   (D) director of nursing

7. The purpose of the shift report is to
   (A) give information about all the residents on the nursing unit
   (B) discuss the social activities of the staff
   (C) tell the nursing assistants when they are scheduled for days off
   (D) rest before starting work

8. You must report to the nurse when you
   (A) take a break or go to lunch
   (B) have completed each assigned task
   (C) wash your hands
   (D) have any contact with a resident

9. One purpose of a memo is to inform staff of
   (A) meetings or educational programs
   (B) residents' conditions
   (C) physicians' new orders for specific residents
   (D) weather conditions

10. Examples of manuals that are found on nursing units include
    (A) salary manual
    (B) disaster manual
    (C) employee evaluation manual
    (D) physician's procedure manual

11. The resident's care plan provides information for
    (A) the nursing assistant assignments
    (B) employee benefits
    (C) procedure for fire drills
    (D) dietary procedures

12. The resident's medical record or chart is
    (A) used only by the physician
    (B) used by all members of the interdisciplinary health care team
    (C) a temporary record
    (D) a report of the nursing assistant's competencies

13. Which of the following is an example of verbal communication?
    (A) The resident is crying.
    (B) The resident is sleeping.
    (C) The resident states, "I am having chest pain."
    (D) The resident is writing a letter to her daughter.

14. If a resident is disoriented, it means the resident is
    (A) mentally ill
    (B) unaware of the environment and the time
    (C) unable to communicate with you
    (D) unable to hear

15. Aphasia means the resident
    (A) has an infection of the respiratory tract
    (B) is hearing-impaired
    (C) is disoriented
    (D) is unable to speak or to understand the spoken language of others

16. When working with residents who have hearing impairments, you should
    (A) speak in a calm, quiet manner
    (B) talk louder
    (C) avoid speaking if possible
    (D) speak very slowly

17. When working with residents with aphasia, it is best to
    (A) use only hand gestures to communicate
    (B) speak louder
    (C) avoid communication if at all possible
    (D) face the resident and make eye contact before speaking

18. Residents who are visually impaired should
    (A) stay in their rooms to avoid getting lost in the facility
    (B) have identification on their clothing so everyone realizes they are visually impaired
    (C) learn to use sign language
    (D) be given directions for locating various areas in the building

19. When working with residents who are disoriented, you should
    (A) ask the resident if she remembers you or knows who you are
    (B) try to make the resident understand you
    (C) avoid distractions of noise and activity when communicating with them
    (D) get as close as possible to the resident when talking or giving care

20. Touching the resident can be a successful method of communication if you
    (A) are gentle and caring
    (B) use stern gestures and facial expressions
    (C) restrain a resident's hand
    (D) avoid eye contact

B. Fill in the blanks by selecting the correct word or phrase from the list provided.

aphasia   medical chart
body language   memo
Braille   nonverbal communication
care plan   shift report
disorientation   verbal communication

21. Persons who cannot express themselves verbally or understand verbal communications have _____.

22. Loss of recognition of time, place, location, or person is called _____.

23. The exchange of information given by the nurse going off duty to those coming on duty is called the _____.

24. The _____ is a legal document.

25. A brief, written message that provides information is a _____.

26. _____ is an example of nonverbal communication.

27. The record that contains a description of the resident's problems, the goals for resolving the problems, and the approaches used is the _____.

28. Sign language is an example of _____.

29. Talking orally is _____.

30. _____ is used by persons who are visually impaired.

LESSON 5

The Language of Health Care

Clinical Focus

Think about how your knowledge of the language of health care and the human body can improve your understanding of the conditions of the residents in your care as you study this lesson and meet:

Georgina England, 74 years old, who has just been admitted to your facility because she can no longer care for herself. Her Hx reveals long-term arthritis, cardialgia, and recurrent cystitis. Her current admission Dx is ASHD, arthritis, and UTI. Part of her care plan includes: ass't c̄ ADL, Amb & Ass't c̄ cath care, I & O, VS q4h.

OBJECTIVES

After studying this lesson, you should be able to:

- Define and spell vocabulary words and terms.
- Use combining forms to develop new words.
- Recognize the meanings of common suffixes and prefixes.
- Write terms and abbreviations commonly used in health care communications and documentation.
- Locate body parts and organs, using the proper anatomic terms.
- Explain the organization of the body into cells, tissues, organs, and systems.
- List body systems and their functions.

VOCABULARY

abbreviation   *(ah-**BREE**-vee-**ay**-shun)*

abdominal   *(ab-**DOM**-ih-nal)*

anatomic position   *(**an**-ah-**TOM**-ick poh-**ZISH**-un)*

anatomy   *(ah-**NAT**-oh-mee)*

anterior   *(an-**TEER**-ee-or)*

cardiac muscle   *(**KAR**-dee-ack **MUS**-ell)*

cavity   *(**KAV**-ih-tee)*

VOCABULARY

cell *(sell)*

combining form *(kom-**BUY**-ning form)*

connective tissue *(kuh-**NECK**-tiv **TISH**-you)*

connective tissue cell *(kuh-**NECK**-tiv **TISH**-you sell)*

cutaneous membrane *(kyou-**TAY**-nee-us **MEM**-brain)*

distal *(**DIS**-tal)*

dorsal *(**DOR**-sal)*

epithelial cell *(ep-ih-**THEE**-lee-al sell)*

epithelial tissue *(ep-ih-**THEE**-lee-al **TISH**-you)*

gerontology *(jer-on-**TOL**-oh-jee)*

inferior *(in-**FEER**-ee-or)*

kidney *(**KID**-nee)*

lateral *(**LAT**-er-al)*

medial *(**MEE**-dee-al)*

medical terminology *(**MED**-ih-kul ter-mih-**NOL**-oh-jee)*

membrane *(**MEM**-brain)*

meninges *(meh-**NIN**-jeez)*

mucous membrane *(**MYOU**-kus **MEM**-brain)*

mucus *(**MYOU**-kus)*

muscle cell *(**MUS**-ell sell)*

muscle tissue *(**MUS**-ell **TISH**-you)*

nerve cell *(nurv sell)*

nervous tissue *(**NUR**-vus **TISH**-you)*

organ *(**OR**-gan)*

pancreas *(**PAN**-kree-as)*

pathology *(pah-**THOL**-oh-jee)*

pericardium *(**pair**-ih-**KAR**-dee-um)*

peritoneum *(**pair**-ih-toh-**NEE**-um)*

physiology *(**fiz**-ee-**OL**-oh-jee)*

pleura *(**PLOOR**-ah)*

posterior *(pos-**TEER**-ee-or)*

prefix *(**PREE**-fix)*

proximal *(**PROX**-ih-mal)*

quadrant *(**KWAHD**-rant)*

serous membrane *(**SEE**-rus **MEM**-brain)*

skeletal muscle *(**SKEL**-eh-tal **MUS**-ell)*

skin *(skin)*

smooth muscle *(smooth **MUS**-ell)*

suffix *(**SUF**-fix)*

superior *(soo-**PEE**-ree-or)*

synovial membrane *(sih-**NOH**-vee-al **MEM**-brain)*

system *(**SIS**-tum)*

tissue *(**TISH**-you)*

umbilicus *(um-**BILL**-ih-kus)*

ventral *(**VEN**-tral)*

word root *(werd root)*

THE LANGUAGE OF HEALTH CARE

The study of **medical terminology** can aid you in understanding the names of specific diseases or conditions that residents may experience. You have learned that people communicate information to one another in different ways. It is important that the sender and receiver understand the same message.

Two ways to help keep the message clear in written and oral communications are:

- Choosing the correct word or term to express the message
- Spelling or pronouncing the word properly

Health care has its own language and sometimes a single letter can change the entire meaning.

For example:

- *Ilium* is part of the pelvic bone.
- *Ileum* is part of the intestinal tract.

- *Perineum* is an area of the body between the vagina and anus.
- *Peritoneum* is a membrane that lines one of the body cavities.

You can see how important it is to use the correct scientific terms and to spell them accurately.

WORD PARTS

The language of health care is formed by building on common word parts (Figure 5-1).

On the Job

Poor communications can result in injury to a resident and liability for you.

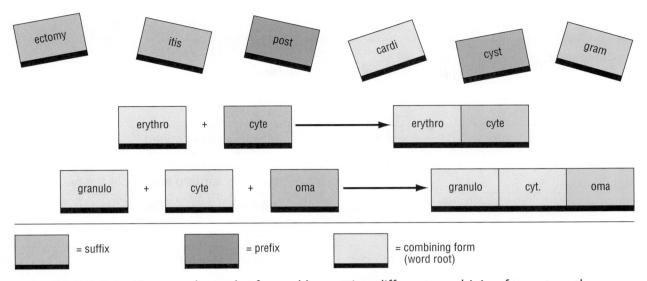

FIGURE 5-1   New words can be formed by putting different combining forms together.

These parts include:

- **Word root**—the body or main part of the word; it usually refers to the part of the body or condition being treated.
- **Combining form**—combination of root word and another form. Sometimes a vowel is added at the end of the root to make it easier to connect another word part.
- **Prefix**—word part found at the beginning of a word to change or add to its meaning.
- **Suffix**—word part found at the end of a word to change or add to its meaning.
- **Abbreviation**—shortened form of word(s) (often just letters).

For example, the word form *cyte* means cell. It is a common combining form because the human body is made up of many different kinds of cells. *Cyte* is seen in different positions in many words and the letter *C* may refer to cell in abbreviations.

Look at the following examples carefully:

- *Cyt*ology—(prefix) study of the cell
- Erythro*cyte*—(suffix) red blood cell
- Granulo*cyt*oma—(root word) a tumor made up of cells called granulocytes
- WB*C*—(abbreviation) white blood cell

EXPANDING YOUR VOCABULARY—

During your career you will continue to add to your understanding and ability to use scientific terms. Here are some ways to help yourself.

- Use the facility medical dictionary to check new words.
- Look up new words; note spelling, meaning, and pronunciation.
- Get a medical dictionary and keep it available at home.
- Keep a notebook of new words, writing down:
  - Definitions
  - Spelling
  - Pronunciation
- Practice writing new words until you spell them correctly without checking your notebook or the dictionary.
- Try to use each new term correctly three times in the next month. If you succeed, you can claim it as your own. You might do this in your conversation, in your documentation, or by explaining the word to a coworker.
- Be willing to accept your teacher's or supervisor's suggestions as to proper pronunciation and usage. Remember, this is a learning process and everyone needs a guide.

COMMON WORD PARTS—

Combining Forms

The basic combining forms listed in Table 5-1 will serve as a foundation for your learning. Your teacher may make selections from this list. Study each set carefully and do the exercises in the text and workbook and you will have started on a path of lifelong learning.

TABLE 5-1 Combining Forms

Combining Form	Meaning	Example	Meaning
abdomin (o)	abdomen	abdominal	portion of body between the thorax and the pelvis
arthr (o)	joint	arthritis	inflammation of a joint
bronch (i)(o)	bronchus	bronchiectasis	abnormal enlargement of passageways that carry air into and out of the lungs
cardi (o)	heart	cardialgia	pain in the region of the heart
cephal (o)	head	cephalic	pertaining to the head
cerebr (o)	brain	cerebro-vascular accident	another name for a stroke
chol (e)	bile	cholecystitis	inflammation of the gallbladder
col (o)	colon, large intestine	colectomy	excision of the colon
crani (o)	skull	craniotomy	opening of the skull
cyst (o)	bladder, cyst	cystitis	inflammation of the bladder
cyt (o)	cell	cytology	study of cells
dent (i) (o)	tooth	dentist	person licensed to practice dentistry
dermat (o)	skin	dermatitis	inflammation of the skin
enter (o)	small intestine	enteritis	inflammation of the intestines
gastr (o)	stomach	gastritis	inflammation of the lining of the stomach
glyc (o)	sugar	glycemia	sugar in the blood
hem (o), hemat (o)	blood	hematuria	discharge of blood in urine
hepat (o)	liver	hepatitis	inflammation of the liver
hydr (o)	water	dehydration	not having adequate water
hyster (o)	uterus	hysterectomy	surgical removal of the uterus
laryng (o)	larynx	laryngectomy	partial or total removal of the larynx by surgery
mast (o)	breast	mastitis	inflammation of the breast
men (o)	menstruation	menstrual	pertaining to menstruation
my (o)	muscle	myalgia	muscular pain

(continues)

TABLE 5-1   Combining Forms *(continued)*

Combining Form	Meaning	Example	Meaning
nephr (o)	kidney	nephrolithiasis	presence of renal calculi
neur (o)	nerve	neuropathy	any disease of the nervous system
oste (o)	bone	periosteum	specialized connective tissue covering all bones of the body
ot (o)	ear	otitis media	inflammation of the middle ear
pharyng (o)	throat, pharynx	pharyngitis	inflammation of the pharynx
pneum (o)	lung, air, gas	pneumonectomy	resection of lung tissue
proct (o)	rectum	proctoscopy	rectal exam with a proctoscope
psych (o)	mind	psychology	study of human behavior
pulm (o)	lung	pulmonary	pertaining to the lungs
py (o)	pus	pyogenic	producing pus
rect (o)	rectum	rectocele	hernial protrusion of part of the rectum into the vagina
thorac (o)	chest	thoracotomy	opening of the chest
thromb (o)	clot	thrombosis	formation of blood clots inside a blood vessel
trache (i) (o)	trachea	tracheotomy	incision of the trachea
ur (o)	urine	urinalysis	analysis of the urine
urin (o)	urinary tract	urinopathy	disease in any part of the urinary system

TABLE 5-2   Common Prefixes

Prefix	Meaning	Example	Meaning
a-	without	asepsis	without infection
ante-	before	antemortem	before death
anti-	against, counteracting	antidote	substance that counteracts the effects of a poison
brady-	slow	bradycardia	slow heart rate
dys-	pain or difficulty	dysuria	painful urination
hyper-	above, excessive	hypertension	high blood pressure

(continues)

TABLE 5-2	Common Prefixes *(continued)*		
Prefix	**Meaning**	**Example**	**Meaning**
hypo-	low, deficient	hypotension	low blood pressure
poly-	many	polyuria	excessive urine
post-	after	postoperative	after surgery
pre-	before	premenstrual	before the menses
tachy-	fast	tachycardia	pulse rate above normal

TABLE 5-3	Common Suffixes		
Suffix	**Meaning**	**Example**	**Meaning**
-ectomy	excision of	mastectomy	excision of a breast
-emia	blood	anemia	lacking sufficient quality or quantity of blood
-gram	record	electro-cardiogram	record produced by electrocardiography
-itis	inflammation of	bronchitis	inflammation of the bronchi
-logy	study of	hematology	study of blood
-oma	tumor	fibroma	a tumor containing fibrous tissue
-otomy	incision	tracheotomy	incision of the trachea
-plegia	paralysis	hemiplegia	paralysis of one side of the body
-pnea	breathing, respiration	apnea	temporary cessation of breathing
-scope	examination instrument	otoscope	instrument for inspecting the ear
-scopy	examination using a scope	proctoscopy	rectal exam with a proctoscope

COMMON ABBREVIATIONS

Lists of abbreviations and their meanings are given in Table 5-4. They have been grouped according to most common usage for easier learning.

Specific abbreviations may have different meanings in different parts of the country and in different facilities. For example, drg in one facility may mean *drainage*, yet in another facility it is used to mean *dressing*. Both facilities may use IDDM to mean *insulin-dependent diabetes mellitus*. Lists of facility-approved terms and abbreviations are usually found in the policy or procedure manual.

TABLE 5-4   Common Abbreviations

Body Parts

abd abdomen	**GU** genitourinary
AU auditory	**lt (L)** left
AX axillary	**os** mouth
bld blood	**sh** shoulder
GI gastrointestinal	**vag** vagina, vaginal

Diagnoses

AIDS acquired immune deficiency syndrome

AKA above-knee amputation

ASHD arteriosclerotic heart disease

BKA below-knee amputation

CA cancer

CAD coronary artery disease

CHD coronary heart disease

CHF congestive heart failure

COPD chronic obstructive pulmonary disease

CVA cerebrovascular accident; stroke

DJD degenerative joint disease

FUO fever of unknown origin

Fx fracture

HBV hepatitis B virus (infection)

HIV human immune deficiency virus (infection)

IDDM insulin-dependent diabetes mellitus

KS Kaposi's sarcoma

MI myocardial infarction; refers to the death of heart tissues due to loss of blood supply (heart attack)

(continues)

Diagnoses *(continued)*

MRSA methicillin-resistant *Staphylococcus aureus*

MS multiple sclerosis

NIDDM non–insulin-dependent diabetes mellitus

NSU nonspecific urethritis

PID pelvic inflammatory disease

PVD peripheral vascular disease

RF renal failure

SDAT senile dementia of Alzheimer's type

STD sexually transmitted disease

TIA transient ischemic attack

URI upper respiratory infection

UTI urinary tract infection

Patient Orders and Charting

ā before

ADL activities of daily living

ad lib. as desired

adm admission

ADT admission, discharge, transfer

amb ambulate, ambulatory

ASAP as soon as possible

as tol as tolerated

B.M., bm bowel movement

BP blood pressure

B.R. bed rest, bathroom

BRP bathroom privileges

BSC bedside commode

c̄ with

(continues)

TABLE 5-4 Common Abbreviations *(continued)*

Patient Orders and Charting *(continued)*	Patient Orders and Charting *(continued)*
cath catheterize/catheter	**neg** negative
CBB complete bed bath	**NGT** nasogastric tube
CBR complete bed rest	**NPO** nothing by mouth
ck check	**N & V** nausea and vomiting
cl liq clear liquid	**NVD** nausea, vomiting, diarrhea
c/o complains of	**O** oral
CP care plan	**O₂** oxygen
DAT diet as tolerated	**OOB** out of bed
DC, D/C discontinue	**p̄** after
disch discharge	**per** by
DNR do not resuscitate	**p.o. (per os)** by mouth
DR doctor	**PPE** personal protective equipment
drg dressing, drainage	**p.r.n.** whenever necessary
DSD dry, sterile dressing	**pt** patient; pint (500 mL)
Dx diagnosis	**Px** prognosis (prog)
E enema	**q.s.** sufficient quantity
GT gastrostomy tube	**qt** quiet
HOB head of bed	**R** rectal
HOH hard of hearing	**rehab** rehabilitation
ht height	**resp** respiration
Hx history	**rt (R)** right, routine
I & O intake and output	**Rx** treatment
irrig irrigation	**s̄** without
isol isolation	**sm** small
IV intravenous	**spec** specimen
lg large	**SSE** soap suds enema
liq liquid	**stat** at once, immediately
MDS minimum data set	**Sx** symptoms
N/C no complaints *(continues)*	**TIAN** toilet in advance of need *(continues)*

TABLE 5-4 Common Abbreviations *(continued)*

Patient Orders and Charting *(continued)*

TPN total parenteral nutrition

TPR temperature, pulse, respiration

TWE tap water enema

Tx traction

TY tympanic

ung. ointment (oint)

VS vital signs

w/c wheelchair

wt weight

Tests

AFB acid-fast bacillus

CBC complete blood count

FBS fasting blood sugar

GTT, gtt glucose tolerance test

S & A sugar and acetone

UA urinalysis

Places or Departments

CS central supply

Lab laboratory

MRD medical record department

OT occupational therapy

PT physical therapy

Time Abbreviations

a.c. before meals

AM morning   *(continues)*

Time Abbreviations *(continued)*

b.i.d. twice a day

h hour

h.s. hour of sleep (bedtime)

noc, noct night

p.c. after meals

PM evening or afternoon

qd every day

qh every hour

q2h every 2 hours

q.i.d. four times a day

qm (qAM) every morning

qn every night

qod every other day

t.i.d. three times a day

WA while awake

Roman Numerals

I 1		**VI** 6	
II 2		**VII** 7	
III 3		**VIII** 8	
IV 4		**IX** 9	
V 5		**X** 10	

Measurements and Volume

cc cubic centimeter

mL milliliter

L liter

(continues)

TABLE 5-4 Common Abbreviations *(continued)*		
Weight/Height		**Temperature**
kg kilogram		**F** Fahrenheit
lb pounds		**C** Celsius
in inches		**°** degree

UNDERSTANDING THE BODY

The reasons for the type of care given to residents are based on an understanding of how the body is made, how it functions normally, and the changes caused by age and disease.

These reasons, or principles, are derived from four sciences:

- **Anatomy:** the study of structure
- **Physiology:** the study of function
- **Gerontology:** the study of aging
- **Pathology:** the study of disease

ANATOMIC TERMS

Special terms are used to describe the location and relationship of body parts and organs. Knowing these terms will help you to study and learn more easily. You will also be able to communicate more accurately as you report and record your observations.

The Anatomic Position

Health care providers must use the same frame of reference when describing the resident's body, the position of the resident, and actions to be taken. For example, everyone who works with the resident must understand and describe precisely where the back of the resident's left wrist is and which is the resident's right hand.

It is helpful to view the resident as if he or she were standing in the **anatomic position.** This means the resident:

- Is standing
- Is facing the observer
- Has hands at the sides
- Has palms forward (Figure 5-2)

This means that the heels will always be toward the back, even if the resident is resting on the abdomen or lying on the side. The

FIGURE 5-2 In the anatomic position, the person is standing, facing forward, with palms forward.

breasts will always be described as facing front even if she is sitting in a wheelchair or walking away from you. Notice also that the resident's left hand will be on the same side as your right hand. It is the same as looking at a mirror image.

Descriptive Terms

Imaginary lines drawn through the body (Figure 5-3) can provide us with other reference terms.

- A line drawn down the center of the body from head to foot divides the body into equal right and left sides. This line is called the *midline* or *midsagittal line.* Note that the body has the same parts on either side. For example, there is an arm, a leg, an eye, and half of a nose on each side of the line.
- Parts close to this line are **medial** to the line.

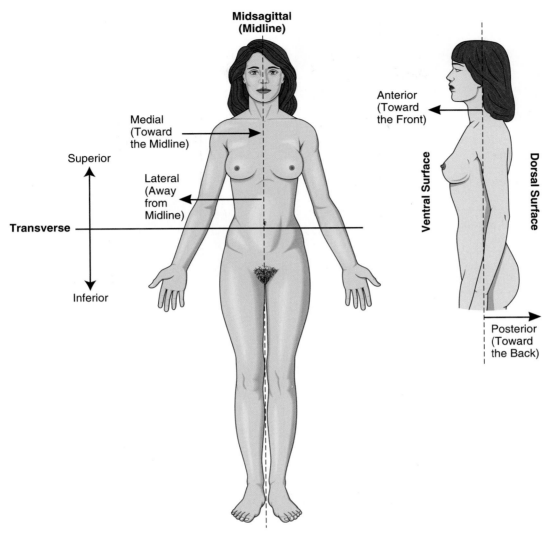

FIGURE 5-3 Imaginary lines can be used to section the body to make it easier to locate parts.

- Parts farther away from the line are **lateral** to the line.
- For example, in the anatomic position, the thumbs are more lateral to the line and the little fingers are more medial to the line.

Another line drawn parallel to the floor divides the body into upper and lower parts. This line can be drawn at any level on the body as long as it is parallel to the floor. This is the *transverse line.*

- Parts located above this line are **superior** to the line.
- Parts located below this line are **inferior** to the line.
- For example, if the line is drawn between the knees and ankles, the knees are superior to the ankles and the ankles are inferior to the knees.

A third line can be drawn to divide the body into front and back.

- Parts in front of this line are **anterior** or **ventral** to the line.
- Parts in back of this line are **posterior** or **dorsal** to the line.

Points of Attachment

The arms and legs are called the *extremities* of the body. The arms are attached to the body at the shoulders. The legs are attached to the body at the hips. Two terms are used to describe the relationship between the parts of the extremities and their points of attachment to the body.

- **Proximal**—means closest to the point of attachment

FIGURE 5-4 Summary of terms relating to the anatomic position and the location of parts

- **Anterior** or **ventral** refers to the front.

- **Posterior** or **dorsal** refers to the back.

- **Lateral** refers to the side (away from the midline).

- **Medial** refers to the center of the body (midline).

- **Proximal** means closest to the point of attachment.

- **Distal** refers to the point farthest away from the point of attachment.

- **Midsagittal** refers to an imaginary line that divides the body into equal right and left sides.

- **Transverse** refers to an imaginary line that divides the body into upper and lower areas.

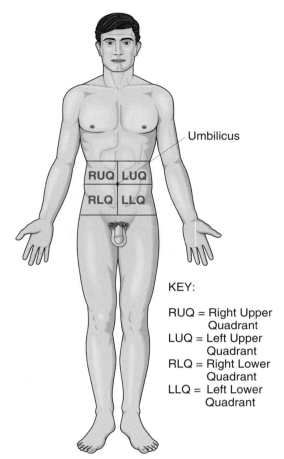

Umbilicus

KEY:

RUQ = Right Upper Quadrant
LUQ = Left Upper Quadrant
RLQ = Right Lower Quadrant
LLQ = Left Lower Quadrant

FIGURE 5-5 The abdominal quadrants

- **Distal**—means farthest away from the point of attachment

Because the upper arm is closest to the shoulder, where it is attached, this part is described as proximal when compared to the fingers, which are farthest away. The fingers are distal or farthest away from the point of attachment of the upper extremity. Figure 5-4 presents a summary of terms.

Abdominal Quadrants

If a resident places his or her hand on the anterior **abdominal** wall, complaining of pain, you must be able to describe the area in proper terms. For reference, the anterior wall of the abdomen is divided into four parts or **quadrants** (Figure 5-5). The center of the area is the **umbilicus**. The abdomen can also be described as having regions (Figure 5-6).

ORGANIZATION OF THE BODY

All parts of the body are interdependent. The basic unit of the body is the **cell**. Groups of similar cells are organized into **tissues**. Differ-

ent tissues form **organs**. The organs are organized into **systems** that perform the body functions.

CELLS

Each cell performs the same basic functions that the total body performs, but on a smaller scale. These functions are breathing (respiration), reproduction, nutrition, and excretion (eliminating wastes). Some cells perform different kinds of work necessary for the body as a whole to function. Some of the various specialized types of cells are:

- Epithelial cells
- Nerve cells
- Muscle cells
- Connective tissue cells

Epithelial cells, which are very close together, form protective coverings and sometimes produce body fluids.

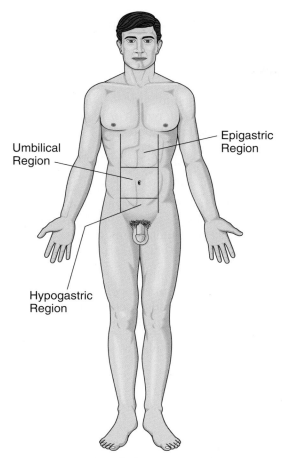

Umbilical Region

Epigastric Region

Hypogastric Region

FIGURE 5-6   The abdomen can also be described as having three medial regions

Nerve cells carry electrical messages to and from the different parts of the body, coordinating activities and making us aware of changes in the environment.

Muscle cells are special in their ability to shorten or lengthen, changing their shape and the position of parts to which they are attached. They also surround body openings, such as the mouth, to control the size of these openings.

Connective tissue cells are present throughout the body in many different types. They support and connect body parts.

TISSUES

Groups of similar cells are organized into tissues. The basic tissue types are:

- Epithelial tissue
- Connective tissue
- Nervous tissue
- Muscle tissue

Epithelial tissue is specialized in its ability to absorb, secrete (produce) fluids, excrete (eliminate) waste products, and protect.

Nervous tissue forms the brain and spinal cord and the nerves throughout the body. This tissue is also found in the special sense organs such as the eyes, ears, and tastebuds. The activities of the rest of the body are directed and coordinated through the nervous tissues.

Three kinds of **muscle tissue** are found in the body:

- **Skeletal muscle** is attached to bones for movement.
- **Cardiac muscle** forms the heart wall.
- **Smooth muscle** (visceral) forms the walls of body organs such as the stomach and intestines.

Connective tissue forms blood, bone, and fibrous and elastic tissues to hold the skin on the body, attach muscles to bones, and support delicate cells throughout the body. Generally, connective tissues support and form connections for other tissue types.

ORGANS

Each organ is made up of more than one kind of tissue and performs special functions that contribute to the function of the body systems. Some organs, like the **kidneys**, are found in pairs. Some single organs contribute to more than one system. For example, the **pancreas** contributes secretions to both the endocrine and digestive systems.

SYSTEMS

The body has 10 major body systems. Figure 5-7 lists the organs that contribute to the function of each system. Notice that some organs are included with more than one system. For example, the ovaries contribute to the endocrine system by producing female hormones and to the reproductive system by producing the female egg.

MEMBRANES

Membranes are sheets of epithelial tissues supported by connective tissues. Membranes:

- Cover the body
- Line body cavities
- Produce some body fluids

FIGURE 5-7 Systems of the body

System	Function	Organs
Cardiovascular (Circulatory)	Transports materials around the body; carries oxygen and nutrients to the cells and carries waste products away; part of the immune system that provides protective cells and chemicals to fight current infections and protect against future infections	Heart, arteries, capillaries, veins, spleen, lymph nodes, lymphatic vessels, blood, lymph, tonsils, thymus, specialized blood cells
Endocrine	Produces hormones that regulate body processes	Pituitary gland, thyroid gland, parathyroid glands, thymus gland, adrenal glands, testes, ovaries, pineal body, islets of Langerhans in pancreas
Gastrointestinal (Digestive)	Digests, transports food, absorbs nutrients, and eliminates solid wastes	Mouth, esophagus, pharynx, stomach, small intestine, large intestine, salivary glands, teeth, tongue, liver, gallbladder, pancreas
Integumentary	Protects the body from injury and against infection, regulates body temperature, eliminates some wastes	Skin, hair, nails, sweat and oil glands
Skeletal	Supports and shapes body, protects internal organs, produces blood cells, acts as levers in movement	Bones, joints, cartilage
Muscular	Protects organs by forming body walls, forms walls of some organs, assists in movement by changing position of bones at joints	*Smooth* muscles—form walls of organs *Skeletal* muscles—attached to bones *Cardiac* muscles—form wall of heart Fascia, tendons
Nervous	Coordinates body functions, coordinates reception of stimuli, transmits messages throughout body	Brain, spinal cord, spinal nerves, cranial nerves, special sense organs such as eyes and ears
Reproductive	Reproduces the species, fulfills sexual needs, develops sexual identity	*Male:* Testes, epididymis, urethra, seminal vesicles, ejaculatory duct, prostate gland, bulbourethral glands, penis, spermatic cord *Female:* Breasts, ovaries, oviducts, uterus, vagina, Bartholin glands, vulva
Respiratory	Brings in oxygen and eliminates carbon dioxide	Sinuses, nose, pharynx, larynx, trachea, bronchi, lungs
Urinary	Manages fluids and electrolytes of body, eliminates liquid wastes	Kidneys, ureters, urinary bladder, urethra

Important membranes include:
- **Mucous membranes**
    - Produce a fluid called **mucus**
    - Line body cavities that open to the outside

Because the respiratory, digestive, and genitourinary systems all open to the outside they are lined with mucous membranes. The eyelids are also lined with a mucous membrane; a mucous membrane covers the eyeballs.

- **Synovial membranes**
    - Produce synovial fluid
    - Line joint cavities

The synovial fluid is a clear fluid resembling the white of an egg. It reduces the friction between the bones of active joints and the tendons.

- **Serous membranes**
    - Produce serous fluid
    - Cover the organs and line the closed cavities of the body

Serous fluid reduces friction as the organs work and move. Important serous membranes are the:

- **Pericardium**—surrounds the heart
- **Pleura**—surrounds the lungs and lines the thoracic cavity

- **Meninges**—cover the brain and spinal cord and line the dorsal cavity
- **Peritoneum**—covers the digestive organs and lines the abdominal cavity
- **Cutaneous membrane (skin)**
    - Protects the body
    - Covers the entire body
    - Helps to control body temperature
    - Eliminates wastes through sweat glands
    - Produces vitamin D when exposed to sunlight

Special epithelial cells in this membrane, called *glands*, secrete perspiration and oils.

CAVITIES

The body seems like a solid structure, but **cavities** (spaces) within it contain the organs. Figure 5-8 lists the two main cavities, the dorsal cavity and the ventral cavity. Each of these cavities is lined by and divided into other cavities by serous membranes. These other cavities are also listed in Figure 5-8, as are the organs contained in each.

Figure 5-9 is a simple drawing of the location of these cavities.

FIGURE 5-8 Body cavities and the organs contained within each cavity		
	Cavity	**Organs**
Dorsal Cavity	Cranial	Brain, pineal body, pituitary gland
	Spinal	Nerves, spinal cord
Ventral Cavity	Thoracic	Lungs, heart, great blood vessels, thymus gland
	Abdominal Peritoneal	Stomach, small intestine, most of large intestine, liver, gallbladder, pancreas, spleen
	Pelvic	*Male* Seminal vesicles, prostate gland, ejaculatory ducts, urinary bladder, urethra, rectum *Female* Uterus, oviducts, ovaries, urinary bladder, urethra, rectum
	Retroperitoneal Space	Kidneys, adrenal glands, ureters

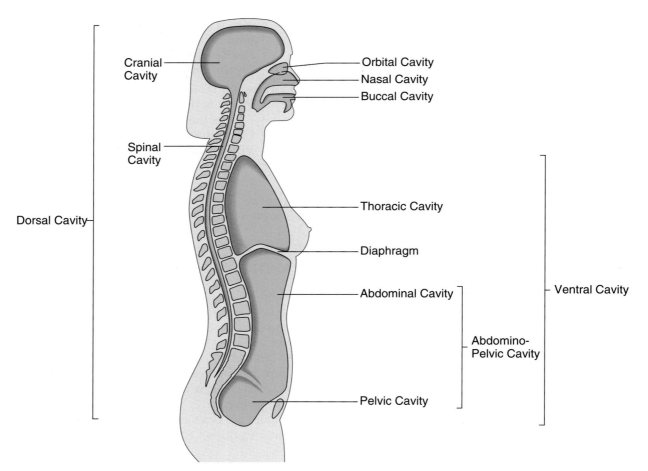

Cranial Cavity

Orbital Cavity

Nasal Cavity

Buccal Cavity

Spinal Cavity

Dorsal Cavity

Thoracic Cavity

Diaphragm

Abdominal Cavity

Ventral Cavity

Abdomino-Pelvic Cavity

Pelvic Cavity

FIGURE 5-9 Lateral view of body cavities

LESSON SYNTHESIS: Putting It All Together

*Y*ou have just completed this lesson. Now go back and review the Clinical Focus. Try to see how the Clinical Focus relates to the concepts presented in the lesson. Then answer the following questions.

1. What health problems has Mrs. England had prior to her present problem?

2. What health problems have made admission to the long-term facility necessary?

3. Which activities would you be performing as part of Mrs. England's care?

4. What value to you, as a nursing assistant, is knowing the language of health care?

REVIEW

A. Complete the definition by crossing out the incorrect term in each sentence.

1. The word part found at the end of a word to change or add to its meaning is the (prefix) (suffix).

2. A word that means the study of aging is (gerontology) (pathology).

3. The term that means the front of the body is (ventral) (dorsal).

4. The term meaning closest to the point of attachment is (distal) (proximal).

5. Cells that are specialized to produce body fluids like mucus are called (nerve cells) (epithelial cells).

B. Based on the prefixes in each of the words, match the correct meaning (items a.–e.) with the word.

a. excessive urine   c. painful urination
b. high blood   d. rapid pulse
   pressure   e. slow pulse

6. _____ bradycardia

7. _____ hypertension

8. _____ dysuria

9. _____ tachycardia

10. _____ polyuria

C. Based on the suffixes in each of the words, match the correct meaning (item a.–e.) with the word.

11. _____ electrocardiogram

12. _____ mastectomy

13. _____ hematology

14. _____ bronchitis

15. _____ anemia

a. excision of a breast
b. record produced by electrocardiography
c. inflammation of the bronchi
d. study of blood
e. insufficient quantity or quality of blood

D. Match the tissue with its function.

Tissue
a. connective   c. muscle
b. epithelial   d. nervous

Function

16. _____ coordinates body activities

17. _____ attached to bones for movement

18. _____ forms the walls of the stomach and intestines

19. _____ connects and supports body parts

20. _____ specialized in its ability to excrete waste products

21. _____ found in the eyes, ears, and tastebuds

22. _____ specialized in its ability to absorb

23. _____ forms the heart wall

24. _____ forms blood and bone

25. _____ forms nerves

E. Match the organ to the system of which it is a part.

System
a. cardiovascular   d. digestive
b. respiratory   e. reproductive
c. endocrine   f. urinary

Organ

26. _____ kidney

27. _____ uterus

28. _____ small intestines

29. _____ heart

30. _____ lungs

31. _____ urinary bladder

32. _____ mouth

33. _____ thyroid gland

34. _____ veins

35. _____ gallbladder

F. **Using your knowledge of combining forms, prefixes, and suffixes, write a medical word that means each of the following. Then check to see if you can find it in the glossary at the back of the book.**

36. without infection

   _____

37. instrument for inspecting the ear

   _____

38. study of the cells

   _____

39. tumor containing fibrous tissue

   _____

40. after surgery

   _____

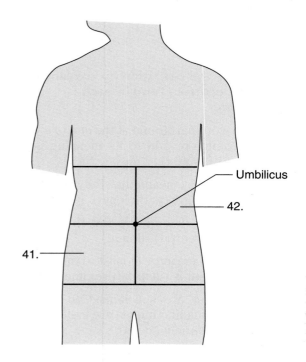

Umbilicus

42.

41.

G. **Name the areas indicated in the diagram. Select from the list provided.**

left lower quadrant   right lower quadrant
left upper quadrant   right upper quadrant

41. _____

42. _____

LESSON 6

Observation, Documentation, and Reporting

Clinical Focus

Think about using your vision, hearing, sense of smell, and your sense of touch to learn about the residents as you study this lesson and meet:

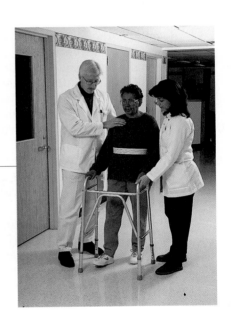

*M*rs. Sara Bass, who was admitted to the facility from the local hospital after having surgery for a fractured hip. She is going to rehabilitation every day in the hope that she will be able to return to her home. The hospital reported that she was disoriented after surgery.

OBJECTIVES
After studying this lesson, you should be able to:

- Define and spell vocabulary words and terms.
- Explain the difference between an objective observation and a subjective observation.
- Explain the difference between signs and symptoms.
- Describe one observation to make for each body system.
- List the information to include when reporting off duty.
- List the guidelines for documentation.
- Name the four components of the interdisciplinary health care team process.
- Describe the responsibilities of the nursing assistant for each component of the interdisciplinary health care team process.

VOCABULARY

approach *(ah-**PROHCH**)*

document *(**DOCK**-you-ment)*

evaluation *(ee-**val**-you-**AY**-shun)*

goal *(gohl)*

implementation *(**im**-plih-men-**TAY**-shun)*

intervention *(**in**-ter-**VEN**-shun)*

Minimum Data Set (MDS 2.0) *(**MIN**-ih-mum **DAY**-tah set)*

nurse's notes *(**NUR**-sez nohts)*

nursing diagnosis *(**NURS**-ing **die**-ag-**NOH**-sis)*

objective observation *(ob-**JECK**-tiv ob-sir-**VAY**-shun)*

observation *(ob-sir-**VAY**-shun)*

resident care plan *(**REZ**-ih-dent kair plan)*

sign *(sighn)*

subjective observation *(sub-**JECK**-tiv ob-sir-**VAY**-shun)*

symptom *(**SIMP**-tum)*

OBSERVATION

One of the most important skills you will develop is the ability to make accurate observations. An **observation** is something you notice about the resident. Some observations must be reported immediately. Other observations may be reported later to the nurse. You must carry a pen and paper with you at all times. You can then make notes of your observations. If you try to rely on your memory, you may forget some vital information when you give your report. You make observations by using your senses:

- You use your eyes to see observations:
  - Blood in the urine
  - Bruises or breaks in the skin
  - The resident crying
  - A change in the way the resident walks
- Your ears to hear observations:
  - Wheezing when the resident breathes
  - Pulse or blood pressure with a stethoscope
  - Comments from the resident such as "I am very tired today"
- Your nose to smell observations:
  - Body odor
  - Stool or urine when the resident is incontinent
- Your hands and fingers to use your sense of touch:
  - A lump under the resident's skin
  - Radial pulse
  - Warmth or coolness of the resident's skin

Signs and Symptoms

The things you notice are called signs and symptoms. A **sign** is objective evidence of disease. These are facts that can be seen or measured by the observer (Figure 6-1). Examples of signs are:

- Rashes, bruises, pressure ulcers
- Elevated temperature
- Vomiting
- Rapid heartbeat

When you observe a sign, you are making an **objective observation**.

Symptoms are subjective evidence of disease. These are facts that need to be relayed from the resident to the observer; that is, the resident tells you either verbally or through body language (Figure 6-2). Examples of symptoms are:

- The resident tells you he has nausea
- Anxiety—may be noted by the resident's behavior such as pacing or the resident may tell you she is nervous

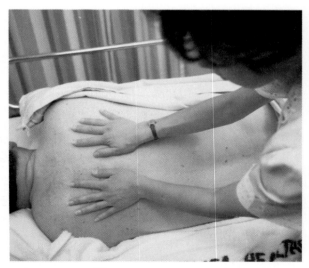

FIGURE 6-1 The nursing assistant observes for bruises, breaks in the skin, rashes, or other skin conditions while giving a backrub.

FIGURE 6-2 The resident's body language and facial expression are examples of subjective observations.

- Pain—may be noted by the resident's position or he may tell you he has pain

When a resident reports a symptom to you, you are making a **subjective observation**.

Observations provide evidence of:

- A change in the resident's physical condition. Example: A resident with diabetes may be having an insulin reaction.
- A new condition that is developing. Example: A pressure ulcer may be noted (Figure 6-3).
- A change in the resident's mental condition. Example: A resident who has shown no signs of disorientation is now wandering about, saying he does not know where he is.
- A change in the resident's emotional condition. Example: A resident is crying and says she "does not want to continue living."

BUILDING CULTURAL AWARENESS

Remember that persons of different cultures may express their symptoms in different ways. It is very important that you closely observe their body language and facial expressions. Report exactly what you observe and do not assume anything.

FIGURE 6-3 The first sign of a pressure ulcer should be reported immediately.

- The effectiveness of a medication or treatment. Example: A resident may be taking an antibiotic for a urinary tract infection. If the signs and symptoms of the infection are not going away, then the medication may not be effective and the physician will need to change the order.
- A change in the resident's ability to function. Example: The resident may not be able to walk as far or may not be able to complete an activity of daily living independently.

Remember that observations:

- Must be accurate and timely
- Are reported to the nurse immediately
- Are documented in the resident's record either by you or the nurse

Making Initial Observations

To make accurate observations, you must first know what is expected or normal for an individual. For this reason, baseline information is collected when the resident is admitted to the facility. If you help admit a resident, make observations while you are completing your assignment. It is especially important to note any signs of injury or skin breakdown. Think of the body systems as an organized way of making observations. This information will provide you with a basis for making future comparisons. For example, one resident may have a blood pressure of 110/68 on admission. If you take the resident's blood pressure later and it is 140/88, you should report this to the nurse, because this is not the usual blood pressure for this person.

Body System Observations

Try to establish a routine way of making observations. Keep in mind the age and known illness of the resident. It may be helpful to think of each body system and note the following observations to report.

TABLE 6-1 General Signs and Symptoms of Illness That Should Be Reported to the RN

Chest pain	Nausea or vomiting	Excessive thirst
Shortness of breath	Diarrhea	Lethargy
Difficulty breathing	Cough	Unusual drainage from a
Weakness or dizziness	Cyanosis or change	wound or body cavity
Headache	in color	Changes in vital signs
Pain	Change in mental status	

System or Problem	Observation to Report
Signs/Symptoms of Infection	Elevated temperature Sweating Chills Skin hot or cold to touch Skin flushed, red, gray, or blue Inflammation of skin as evidenced by redness, edema, heat, or pain Drainage from wounds or body cavities Any unusual body discharge, such as mucus or pus
Evidence of Pain	Chest pain Pain that radiates Pain upon movement Pain during urination Pain when having a bowel movement Pain is not normal; all complaints of pain should be reported to the RN
Cardiovascular (Circulatory) System	Abnormal pulse below 60 or above 100 Blood pressure below 100/60 or above 140/90 (Figure 6-4) Unable to palpate pulse or hear blood pressure Chest pain Chest pain that radiates to neck, jaw, or arm Shortness of breath Headache, dizziness, weakness, vomiting Cold, blue, or gray appearance Cold, blue, painful feet or hands Shortness of breath, dyspnea, or abnormal respirations Blue color of lips, nail beds, or mucous membranes
Respiratory System	Respiratory rate below 12 or above 20 Irregular respirations Noisy, labored respirations Dyspnea Shortness of breath Gasping for breath Wheezing Coughing Retractions Blue color of lips, nail beds, or mucous membranes

(continues)

System or Problem	Observation to Report
TABLE 6-1 General Signs and Symptoms of Illness That Should Be Reported to the RN *(continued)*	
Integumentary System	Rash
	Redness
	Redness in the skin that does not go away within 30 minutes after pressure is relieved
	Pressure sores
	Irritation
	Bruises
	Skin discoloration
	Swelling
	Lumps
	Abnormal sweating
	Excessive heat or coolness to touch
	Open areas/skin breakdown
	Drainage
	Foul odor
	Complaints such as numbness, burning, tingling, itching
	Signs of infection
	Unusual skin color, such as blue or gray color of the skin, lips, nail beds, roof of mouth, or mucous membranes
	Skin growths
	Poor skin turgor/Tenting of skin
	Sunken, dark appearance around eyes
Gastrointestinal (Digestive) System	Sores or ulcers inside the mouth
	Difficulty chewing or swallowing food
	Unusual or abnormal appearance of bowel movement
	Blood, mucus, or other unusual substances in stool
	Unusual color of bowel movement
	Hard stool, difficulty passing stool
	Complaints of pain, constipation, diarrhea, bleeding
	Frequent belching
	Changes in appetite
	Excessive thirst
	Fruity smell to breath
	Complaints of indigestion or excessive gas
	Nausea, vomiting
	Choking
	Abdominal pain
	Abdominal distention
	Coffee-ground appearance of emesis or stool
Genitourinary System	Urinary output too low
	Oral intake too low
	Fluid intake and output not balanced
	Abnormal appearance of urine: dark, concentrated, red, cloudy (Figure 6-5)
	Unusual material in urine: blood, pus, particles
	Complaints of difficulty urinating or inability to urinate
	Complaints of pain, burning, urgency, frequency, pain in lower back
	Urinating frequently in small amounts *(continues)*

TABLE 6-1 General Signs and Symptoms of Illness That Should Be Reported to the RN *(continued)*

System or Problem	Observation to Report
Genitourinary System *continued*	Sudden-onset incontinence Edema Sudden weight loss or gain Respiratory distress Change in mental status
Nervous System	Tremors on one side or of both hands Change in level of consciousness, orientation, awareness, or alertness Increasing mental confusion Progressive lethargy Loss of sensation Numbness, tingling Change in pupil size; unequal pupils Abnormal or involuntary motor function Loss of ability to move a body part Poor coordination
Musculoskeletal System	Pain Obvious deformity Edema Immobility Inability to move arms and legs Inability to move one or more joints (Figure 6-6) Limited/abnormal range of motion Jerking or shaky movements Weakness Sensory changes Changes in ability to sit, stand, move, or walk Pain upon movement
Mental Status	Change in level of consciousness, awareness, or alertness Changes in mood or behavior Change in ability to express self or communicate Mental confusion Excessive drowsiness Sleepiness for no apparent reason Sudden onset of mental confusion Threats of harm to self or others

Observations of Pain and Behavior

You also need to note facts related to the resident's pain and behavior.

- Pain: location, type (sharp, burning, dull, aching), constant or intermittent or related to specific activities
- Behavior: actions, conduct, functioning

It is important that you be very objective in reporting observations of pain and behavior. Never try to judge whether a resident really has pain or how severe it is. Some individuals are expressive about pain and others try not to show their discomfort. Never compare residents. One person may seem to have more pain than another person with the same diagnosis. It is

FIGURE 6-4 Taking blood pressure provides important information about the circulatory system.

FIGURE 6-6 Noting the resident's ability to move the joints is an observation of the musculoskeletal system.

not appropriate to think that they should both respond in the same way.

The nurse may explain to the resident how to describe the intensity of pain on a scale rating from 0 (no pain) to 10 (the worst possible pain). You should report to the nurse the rating that the resident gives you. Figure 6-7 shows an example of a pain assessment guide and an example of a pain intensity scale.

When you report to your supervisor about the resident's behavior, do not use "labels" based on your judgment of the resident. Describe only what you see and hear. Refer to Figure 6-8 for examples of how certain behaviors should be reported.

FIGURE 6-5 Before discarding urine, check the amount, color, clarity, and the presence of blood or sediment.

You will make additional observations that are related to the resident's medical diagnoses. For example, if a resident has a kidney condition, you will look for edema (swelling) of the face, hands, and ankles. You will also monitor the person's fluid intake and output. You will learn more about observations related to medical diagnoses as you study these conditions.

In some situations you may be expected to report "normal" observations. This information tells the nurse and physician whether the resident's condition is improving. For example, if a resident has a respiratory tract infection and the signs and symptoms have decreased, it is important to report that "no coughing or respiratory distress is noted."

REPORTING

When you make observations, you must report your findings to the nurse. Be specific when you describe your observations. If you are relaying a subjective observation (something the resident has told you), repeat it exactly the way the resident told it to you. Here are examples:

- "Mr. Jones in 249 says it hurts every time he urinates."
- "Mrs. Bernetti says her heart is racing and feels like it's skipping beats."
- "Mrs. Goldberg was wandering around in the hall and said she did not know where she was."

When you report off duty at the end of your shift, report to the nurse:

- The condition of each of the residents you cared for

On the Job

The resident's treatment is frequently based on the signs and symptoms that are reported to the physician by the nurse. It is extremely important that you report your findings promptly and accurately.

- The care you gave each resident
- Observations you made while giving care

DOCUMENTATION

In some facilities you may be expected to document your observations on the resident's medical chart. A document is a legal record. The resident's care, response to treatment, and progress are documented (charted) in the resident's chart. To **document** means to write out your findings. Nursing assistants may document on flow sheets in the chart or on the **nurse's notes** (sometimes called nurse's progress notes, Figure 6-9). The charting must:

- Address the problems listed in the resident's care plan

FIGURE 6-7 Examples of a pain assessment guide and a pain intensity scale

A. Pain Assessment Guide

P lace	Point with one finger to site
A mount	0–10 rating: Now? At its worst?
I nteraction	What makes the pain worse?
N eutralizers	What makes the pain better?

B. Pain Intensity Scale

0	1	2	3	4	5	6	7	8	9	10
(no pain)					(moderate pain)				(worst possible pain)	

FIGURE 6-8 When reporting observations of residents' behavior, you will report only what you see and hear (second column). The words in the first column are judgments, opinions, or assumptions.

Resident's Actions	What You Will Report
agitating other residents	0300 Out of bed, talking to roommates, attempting to get them out of bed
confused	0210 States over and over that he "wants to go to Maywood to see his mother."
disoriented	0100 States "I want to go to church today because it is Sunday."
combative	2130 Hit nursing assistant 2x on upper arm with fist when nursing assistant attempted to change incontinent pad.
uncooperative	1300 Refused to get up from chair when nursing assistant tried to take to bathroom.
verbally abusive	1420 Called resident in next bed a "stupid, ignorant idiot."
physically abusive	1000 Scratched nursing assistant on face when bed was being changed.

NURSE'S PROGRESS NOTES

DATE AND TIME	NURSING CARE NOTES	SIGNATURE
3-16-XX	2200 Found lying on floor beside bed. Responds verbally. States was "trying to get to the bathroom." Nurse notified immediately_____	C. Simmons CNA
	2205 ROM satisfactory. Denies having pain. No injuries noted. Assisted back to bed. Call light within reach. Instructed to use call light when having to go to B.R. Pulse 86, strong and regular. B/P 136/84. Oriented to time, place, person. Incontinent after fall. Pajamas chgd._____	
	2300 Sleeping c̄ distress_____	B. Selici RN
3-17-XX	2400-0200 Sleeping soundly. Respirations regular. Pulse 78 strong and regular._____	
	0230 Awake. c/o "arthritis pain" in both hips. Acetaminophen tabs ii given with water. Assisted to bathroom. Voided large amt. clear urine._____	
	0230-0630 Slept soundly. Pulse 72 strong and regular. B/P 128/80. T 98⁶(O). Denies pain anywhere. No other c/o distress._____	P. Hernandez RN
3-17-XX	~~2400 Up to B.R. c̄ assistance~~____Error ES	E. Seldes LPN

FIGURE 6-9   Nursing assistants may document on the nurse's notes in the resident's chart.

- Describe the interventions listed in the care plan and note whether the interventions are effective
- Indicate the progress the resident is making toward meeting the goals on the care plan

Charting Guidelines

A resident's medical record (chart) is a legal document and may be used in court as legal evidence. Everything *must* be correct and legible. All charting and records must be in clear, simple, and accurate language. Entries must be printed or written carefully so that the meaning is not misunderstood. If you follow the established rules of charting, you will avoid problems (Figure 6-10).

Each chart relates only to one resident, so it is unnecessary to use the term *resident* or to use the resident's name. Phrases rather than sentences should be used and there should *never* be erasures or empty spaces on the record. All entries are made in black or blue ink because it is a permanent record; no erasable ink or correction fluid is allowed. If you make an error, draw one line through the error, write "error" above it, and sign your initials.

If you use medical terms in your charting, make sure you are using the correct words and that spelling is correct. Use a medical dictionary if you are not sure. Abbreviations are allowed but they must be on the approved list of your facility. Do not make up your own abbreviations. You must chart only for yourself and only when the procedure or assignment has been completed.

FIGURE 6-10   Guidelines for accurate charting

- Check for: Right resident
  Right chart
  Right room
- Fill out new headings completely.
- Use correct color of ink.
- Date and time each entry.
- Make entries in proper time sequence.
- Make entries brief, objective, and accurate.
- Spell each word correctly.
- Print or write clearly.
- Leave no blank spaces or lines between entries.
- Do not use the term *resident*.
- Do not use ditto marks.
- Sign each entry with first initial, last name, and job title.
- Make corrections by drawing one line through entry; then print the word "error" and your initials above.
- Use quotation marks when directly quoting a resident.

FIGURE 6-11 The 24-hour clock

The time of entry must be noted when the entry is made. Most health care facilities use international (24-hour) time (Figure 6-11) to avoid confusion between AM and PM. With international time, the 24 hours of each day are identified by the numbers 0100 (1:00 AM) through 2400 (12:00 AM, midnight). The last two digits indicate the minutes of each hour, from 01 to 59. Thus, 0101 is 1 minute after 1:00 AM; 1210 is ten minutes after 12 PM (noon); 1658 is 4:58 PM and so on.

THE INTERDISCIPLINARY HEALTH CARE TEAM PROCESS

The interdisciplinary health care team provides the right care for the residents. The members of the team are responsible for completing activities that will result in a care plan for each resident. To do this, the team members must have a foundation of knowledge on which to base their recommendations. The team members and other staff are accountable for implementing the care. Nursing assistants help in each step of this process.

Step 1: Assessment

Assessment means to make an evaluation of the resident's mental, physical, and emotional status. This evaluation is completed by gathering information about the resident's past and present problems. The information is called *data*. Each discipline completes an assessment when the resident is admitted and annually. This assessment is called the **Minimum Data Set**

(MDS 2.0) and is required by law. A less complex assessment is repeated every 3 months. If the resident's condition changes, the assessment is again completed. In addition to the MDS 2.0, the resident may be evaluated for specific risk factors. Examples include:

- Pressure ulcer risk assessment. If data indicate the resident is at risk of developing pressure ulcers, a preventive program is initiated.
- Safety assessment. If the resident is at risk of falling or getting lost, a program to prevent incidents is initiated.
- Mental status examination. This is done to determine the resident's orientation to time and place and mental capabilities.

Data for the MDS 2.0 and the other assessments are collected by the nurse and other members of the team from many sources:

- Interviewing the resident, the family, and nursing staff on all shifts
- Reading the results of the physician's history and physical examination and progress notes
- Reading the results of all diagnostic tests
- Performing a physical assessment (Figure 6-12)
- Performing a functional assessment

When the data are collected, nursing diagnoses are established.

The **nursing diagnosis** is a statement of a problem and its probable cause. Although these are called nursing diagnoses, each member of the interdisciplinary team uses the same system for making problem statements. Here are some examples:

- Impaired physical mobility related to pain and stiffness due to osteoarthritis
- Altered thought processes related to deficits in attention, concentration, and memory resulting from stroke
- Altered family processes related to long-term illness of the resident and the role changes experienced by family members

Nursing Assistant Responsibility: Assessment. The nursing assistant's responsibility for Step 1: Assessment is to:

- Make accurate and thorough observations.
- Report and document observations factually.

Step 2: Planning

After the assessments are completed and the nursing diagnoses have been developed, the care plan is written. The **resident care plan** is the "blueprint" for giving care. Members of the interdisciplinary team attend the care plan conference. The resident is invited to attend. Family members are

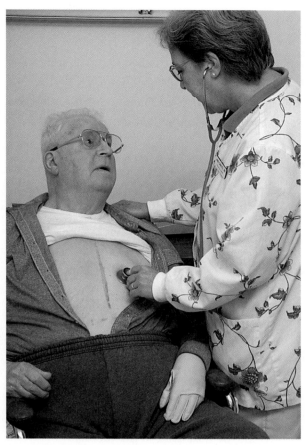

FIGURE 6-12 The registered nurse collects information by doing a physical assessment of the resident.

also invited to participate if the resident agrees. At the care plan conference the team:

- Establishes goals for the resident. A **goal** is an outcome; it states what the team (including the resident) plans for the resident to accomplish or be able to do. The goals are developed by determining the resident's potential. For example, if one of the nursing diagnoses is impaired mobility, the team would set goals to maintain or improve mobility. In some situations goals may come from more than one discipline. A mobility problem may involve goals from both the physical therapist and the nursing staff. The goals must be realistic and measurable. A nursing goal for impaired mobility might be: resident will walk 100 feet with a walker and one assistant two times a day by a certain date. Goals may be restorative (improvement), preventive (prevent complications such as pressure ulcers or infection), or maintenance (the resident's current state will not change).
- Determines the approaches or interventions to use to help the resident meet the goals. The

approach or intervention states exactly which members of the team are responsible for the approach—what they will do, how they will do it, and when. The approach for the impaired mobility goal might be: place transfer belt on resident, assist to standing position, place walker in front of resident, and instruct resident to use three-point gait to walk; to be done by nurse or nursing assistant after breakfast and before supper.

Nursing Assistant Responsibility: Planning. The nursing assistant responsibility for Step 2: Planning is to:

- Give suggestions to the nurse if you think a specific approach may be successful. Example: Mrs. Donetti becomes agitated when you try to give her a shower. You tell the nurse you think Mrs. Donetti might prefer a tub bath instead.
- Attend care plan conference if you have the opportunity to do so.

Step 3: Implementation

Implementation is putting the care plan into practice. Members of the interdisciplinary team carry out the approaches listed on the care plan.

Nursing Assistant Responsibility: Implementation. The nursing assistant responsibility for Step 3: Implementation is to:

- Read the residents' care plans.
- Carry out the approaches assigned to nursing assistants consistently and correctly.

Step 4: Evaluation

The purpose of **evaluation** is to determine whether or not the resident is meeting the goals as set forth in the care plan. If the goals are not met, the problems are not resolved. The resident's condition may be deteriorating; there may be complications or decreasing functional abilities. The team needs to determine why the resident is unable to meet the goals. Then different goals will be written or different approaches will be used.

Nursing Assistant Responsibility: Evaluation. The nursing assistant responsibility for Step 4: Evaluation is to:

- Report to the nurse when you are unable to carry out an approach as stated in the care plan.
- Relay to the nurse any ideas you have about why there is a problem.
- Report to the nurse the resident's progress toward meeting the care plan goals.

LESSON SYNTHESIS: Putting It All Together

You have just completed this lesson. Now go back and review the Clinical Focus. Try to see how the Clinical Focus relates to the concepts presented in the lesson. Then answer the following questions.

1. Which systems would be most important in making observations for Mrs. Bass?

2. Which members of the interdisciplinary health care team would attend Mrs. Bass's care plan conference?

3. Which senses would you use to determine whether Mrs. Bass was disoriented?

4. What information could you gain by observing her facial expressions and body language?

REVIEW

A. Select the one best answer for each of the following.

1. Which of the following examples is a subjective observation?
   (A) Mrs. Pochoski tells you she feels sick to her stomach.
   (B) You take Mr. Johnson's temperature and it is 99.6°.
   (C) Miss Dominick has a reddened area around her tailbone.
   (D) Mr. Flores has a blood pressure of 126/84.

2. Which of the following examples is an objective observation?
   (A) You feel a lump when you are giving Mrs. Smith her bath.
   (B) Mrs. Smith tells you she has a lump in her breast.
   (C) Mr. Johnson tells you he thinks he has a fever.
   (D) Miss Dominick says she has pain in her tailbone.

3. When you make observations, all of the following are recommended practice except
   (A) must be accurate and timely
   (B) reported to the nurse immediately
   (C) documented in the resident's record by you or the nurse
   (D) errors can be erased

4. Initial observations or baseline information is collected when the resident
   (A) is discharged from the facility
   (B) is admitted to the facility
   (C) has a care plan conference
   (D) has a change in condition

5. When observing the integumentary system, you would note the
   (A) resident's ability to move his arms and legs
   (B) resident's blood pressure
   (C) color of the resident's skin
   (D) resident's ability to respond

6. When you observe the resident's breathing, you are observing the resident's
   (A) circulatory system
   (B) digestive system
   (C) respiratory system
   (D) reproductive system

B. Answer each statement true (T) or false (F).

7. T F Charting is done in pencil in case you make a mistake and need to erase.

8. T F Each statement in the chart begins with the word *resident*.

9. T F The resident and the resident's family (if the resident agrees)

are invited to attend the care plan conference.

10. T F The nursing diagnosis is the physician's statement of the resident's problem.

11. T F Goals must be realistic and measurable.

12. T F Residents are quick to report pain when it begins.

13. T F A low urine output should be reported.

14. T F Sudden onset of mental confusion need not be reported, because the resident may just be tired.

15. T F A report of level eight pain indicates a moderate amount of pain being experienced.

C. Fill in the blanks by selecting the correct word or phrase from the list.

approach	intervention
assessment	nurse's notes
baseline	objective
goal	planning
implementation	subjective

16. A sign is a/an _____ observation.

17. A symptom is a/an _____ observation.

18. Making initial observations provides _____ information.

19. The MDS 2.0 is used to make a/an _____ of the resident.

20. The second step of the interdisciplinary health care team process is _____.

21. Carrying out the instructions on the resident's care plan is called _____.

22. Nursing assistants may be expected to document on the _____ in the resident's medical record.

23. A statement of what the interdisciplinary team plans for the resident to be able to accomplish is called a _____.

24. The actions taken by members of the interdisciplinary team to help the resident is called a/an _____ or a/an _____.

25. Change the following times to international time (24-hour clock system).
    a. 6:35 AM
    b. 9:10 AM
    c. 11:25 AM
    d. 1:15 PM
    e. 3:24 PM
    f. 6:42 PM
    g. 9:25 PM
    h. 11:59 PM

SECTION 3

Protecting Residents' Rights and Safety

LESSONS

7 Residents' Rights

8 Safety

9 Emergencies

10 Infection

11 Infection Control

Residents' Rights

Clinical Focus

Think about the basic rights guaranteed to each resident as you study this lesson and meet:

*S*tanley Davidson, who has no close relatives and has chosen you to be a confidant. He has shared many personal facts that he would not want anyone else to know.

OBJECTIVES

After studying this lesson, you should be able to:

- Define and spell vocabulary words and terms.
- Describe the purpose of the Residents' Rights document.
- State the differences between physical abuse, sexual abuse, mental abuse, and verbal abuse.
- Describe the term *involuntary seclusion*.
- Give two examples of neglect.
- List four situations when the nursing assistant should provide privacy for the resident.
- Explain the nursing assistant's responsibilities for meeting (accommodating) the resident's needs.
- List five situations when the resident can make choices.
- Describe four ways the nursing assistant can help residents meet their psychosocial needs.

VOCABULARY

advance directives *(ad-VANS dih-RECK-tivs)*

advocate *(AD-voh-kit)*

artificial nutrition *(are-tih-FISH-al new-TRIH-shun)*

assault *(ass-SALT)*

battery *(BAT-er-ee)*

cardiac arrest *(KAR-dee-ack ah-REST)*

cardiopulmonary resuscitation (CPR) *(kar-dee-oh-PUL-moh-nair-ee ree-sus-ih-TAY-shun)*

chemical restraint *(KEM-ih-kal ree-STRAYNT)*

corporal punishment *(KOR-poh-ral PUN-ish-ment)*

defamation of character *(def-eh-MAY-shun of KAIR-ack-ter)*

ethics *(ETH-icks)*

false imprisonment *(falls im-PRIHS-on-ment)*

financial abuse *(fy-NAN-shul ah-BYOUSE)*

VOCABULARY

grievance *(GREE-vans)*

hospice *(HAHS-piss)*

hot-line number *(hot-line NUM-ber)*

incontinent *(in-KON-tin-ent)*

informed consent *(in-FORMD kon-SENT)*

invasion of privacy *(in-VAY-shun of PRY-vah-see)*

involuntary seclusion *(in-VOL-un-ter-ee sih-KLUE-zhun)*

legal guardian *(LEE-gul GAR-dee-un)*

libel *(LIE-bul)*

living will *(LIV-ing will)*

mental abuse *(MEN-tal ah-BYOUSE)*

neglect *(neh-GLECKT)*

no-code (DNR) (do not resuscitate) *(NO-kohd)*

ombudsman *(OM-buds-man)*

physical abuse *(FIZ-ah-kul ah-BYOUSE)*

physical restraint *(FIZ-ah-kul ree-STRAYNT)*

power of attorney for health care *(POW-er of ah-TUR-nee for helth kair)*

prosthesis *(pros-THEE-siss)*

reprisal *(ree-PRY-zul)*

Self-Determination Act *(self dee-ter-mih-NAY-shun akt)*

sexual abuse *(SEX-you-al ah-BYOUSE)*

sexuality *(sex-you-AL-ih-tee)*

slander *(SLAN-der)*

terminal condition *(TER-mih-nal kon-DIH-shun)*

theft *(theft)*

verbal abuse *(VER-bal ah-BYOUSE)*

PURPOSE OF THE RESIDENTS' RIGHTS DOCUMENT

The Residents' Rights document was legislated by federal and state governments. It is the same as any other law. This document ensures that residents in long-term care facilities are allowed the same rights as any citizen of this country. When these rights are respected by the caregivers, the residents have a higher quality of life.

The resident and family or a court-appointed representative of the resident (**legal guardian**) must be given a copy of this document before admission to the facility. Any questions they have should be discussed with the staff member who is coordinating the admission (Figure 7-1).

The resident has the right to an environment that:

- Promotes quality of life
- Promotes dignity and respect for each resident's individuality
- Is safe, clean, comfortable, and homelike
- Helps the resident maintain the highest practical physical, mental, and psychological well-being

As a nursing assistant, you can assist residents to exercise their rights by:

- Being courteous
- Showing respect at all times

FIGURE 7-1 The resident must receive a full explanation of the Residents' Rights document before admission to the facility.

- Being considerate
- Preserving the resident's dignity
- Giving residents the opportunity to make decisions about matters that relate to their care

BUILDING CULTURAL AWARENESS

There may be major cultural differences among the residents you care for. These differences may be reflected in their beliefs about health and illness and health care practices. These beliefs must always be respected regardless of your own personal feelings.

RESIDENTS' RIGHTS

The Right to Free Choice

The resident has the right to make choices regarding medical treatment, including:

- The right to choose an attending physician. If the attending physician refuses to obey certain federal regulations regarding the resident's care, the facility may replace the physician after notifying the resident.
- The right to full advance information about changes in care or treatment that affect the resident. This includes the right to refuse treatment. Treatment refers to procedures ordered by the physician. The resident must be consistent and persistent in refusing treatment. State laws must

be followed. For example, if a resident cannot take in food and fluids, the resident may refuse to have a feeding tube inserted (**artificial nutrition**). In this case, the specific laws of that state would be obeyed. Whenever a resident refuses treatment, the nurse or physician must explain the possible consequences of the refusal.

- The right to be part of the assessment and care-planning process. This means the resident must be told of the evaluations made by the members of the care team. The resident and the family (if the resident agrees) are invited to the care plan conference so they may help with the planning process (Figure 7-2).
- The resident may self-administer medications if the assessment demonstrates that this is possible and the resident wishes to do so. The nurse is responsible for overseeing this process.
- The right to consent to participate in experimental research. Research that personally affects the resident cannot be done without the resident's consent.

The Right to Freedom from Abuse and Restraints

The term *abuse* refers to mistreatment of a person. Residents may be abused by staff members, family members, other residents, or visitors. The different forms of abuse are physical abuse, sexual abuse, verbal abuse, mental abuse, and financial abuse. Improperly used or applied restraints are another form of abuse.

FIGURE 7-2 The resident and family are invited to participate in the care planning conference.

One of your most important concerns as a nursing assistant is to help the resident maintain dignity. That means that each person must be treated as having worth, no matter what the individual's physical or mental abilities might be. Prevention of abuse is one way to preserve dignity. **Physical abuse** is:

- Hitting, slapping, pinching, or kicking
- Any physical contact that intentionally causes pain or discomfort
- **Corporal punishment**—inflicting pain on residents to force them to follow orders

Sexual abuse is:

- Using physical means or verbal threats to force a resident to perform any sexual act, including fondling, kissing, or sexual intercourse
- Tormenting or teasing a resident with sexual gestures or words

Verbal abuse is:

- Talking to the resident in a sarcastic or rough manner
- Using crude slang or swearing
- Using gestures that are considered demeaning or obscene

Mental abuse is:

- Making verbal threats to hurt or punish a resident (for example, telling a resident you will put him in a restraint if he does not obey you)
- Humiliating a resident (for example, embarrassing a resident who wets her pants)
- Separating a resident from other residents against the resident's will (**involuntary seclusion**), unless this action is part of a therapeutic plan and is documented. Involuntary seclusion may be used if a resident's actions endanger or offend other residents, such as cursing or being physically aggressive.

Financial abuse is:

- Misuse of resident's money or property by family, friends, or staff

Physical and psychosocial neglect may be considered forms of abuse. **Neglect** is the failure to provide safe care. Some examples are:

- Not meeting the resident's physical need for food, fluids, rest, activity, oxygen, cleanliness, shelter, and elimination. This is physical neglect.
- Actions by staff that make the resident agitated or depressed. This is psychosocial neglect.

No resident deserves to be abused or live in fear. Preventing all forms of abuse is everyone's responsibility. If staff members, family members, volunteers, or visitors appear to be abusive or on the verge of becoming so, report this immediately to your supervisor. If you witness abuse and do not report it, you are also guilty. Family members are also under a great deal of stress and may need counseling. Promptly report any bruises or wounds that you observe or any statements of the resident that may possibly be a result of abuse.

Caring for residents requires patience and tolerance. If you feel yourself becoming tense or short-tempered, take action to calm yourself. Take a short break and some deep breaths. If you notice coworkers who appear "uptight," help them to regain their composure. Staff members need to care for each other as well as the residents. Working together with a true team spirit can help prevent abuse.

There are two forms of restraints:

- Chemical restraints
- Physical restraints

Chemical Restraints. At times, medications to alter behavior are needed. These situations must be carefully evaluated by the interdisciplinary team, resident, and family. **Chemical restraints** are medications that affect the resident's behavior so that mental powers such as thinking are changed. Residents receiving such medications are monitored for unusual reactions. The ordering and dispensing of medications is not the responsibility of the nursing assistant. The nursing assistant should report a resident's unusual behavior or a change in behavior.

Physical Restraints. A **physical restraint** (Figure 7-3) is any device that:

- A resident cannot easily remove
- Restricts a resident's movement
- Does not allow resident normal access to his or her own body

Physical restraints are discussed in Lesson 8.

FIGURE 7-3 A physical restraint is a device that inhibits the resident's movements. (Courtesy of J. T. Posey Co., Inc., Arcadia, CA)

FIGURE 7-4 Always knock before you enter a resident's room.

The Right to Privacy

The right to privacy includes:

- Privacy during medical treatment and nursing care
- Receiving and sending unopened mail
- Privacy during telephone calls
- Privacy when visitors are present

Here are some suggestions for ensuring the resident's right to privacy:

- Always knock before entering a resident's room, whether the door is closed or open (Figure 7-4). Wait for a response before entering.
- Close the door, the window curtain, and pull the privacy curtains when you are working with residents in their rooms (Figure 7-5).
- Keep residents covered as much as possible when you perform procedures.
- No other people should be present when you are helping the resident go to the bathroom, to dress, or to complete personal care procedures. The exceptions are times when more than one staff person is required to complete a procedure (for example, to position a dependent person).
- Close the doors to tub rooms, showers, and bathrooms when these areas are in use.

The Right to Confidentiality of Personal and Clinical Records

This means that information about the resident is available only to those who need the information to provide care. This includes information on the resident's chart and care plan. It also includes any information about the resident's personal life and relationship

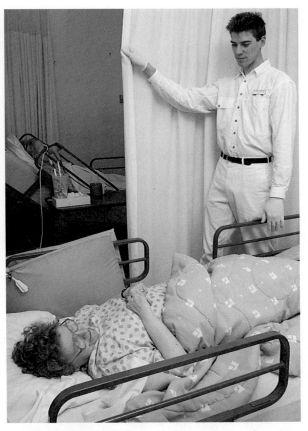

FIGURE 7-5 Pull the privacy curtain when you are working with a resident in her room.

with the family. The caregivers who receive this information must keep the information confidential.

To protect this right:

- Avoid talking about residents or families during breaks or when you are off duty. When you have to discuss a resident with a coworker, do so in private. Family members, other residents, and visitors should not be able to overhear your conversation.
- Shift reports and other conferences should be held in areas of privacy.
- If a resident or family member wishes to see the medical records, relay the request to the nurse.
- Avoid talking about residents to other residents in the facility.

The Right to Accommodation of Needs

This includes the right to make choices about life that are important to the resident. This includes activities, schedules, and health care that are consistent with the resident's interests and care plan.

This right means the resident may make choices about:

- Nutrition and eating
- Times for getting up and going to bed
- Clothing, use of makeup, hair style
- Bath or shower and when to take it
- Use of free time
- Visitors

Accommodation of Needs

The resident has the right to expect the assistance of the staff in meeting both physical needs and psychosocial needs.

Physical Needs. As a nursing assistant, you help residents meet their physical needs when you:

- Assist residents to maintain personal hygiene and cleanliness.
  - Give baths or showers.
  - Clean and trim fingernails and toenails.

- Shave daily.
- Give shampoos and allow residents to wear the hair style of their choice.
- Give regular and thorough oral hygiene.
- Allow residents to choose their own clothing (Figure 7-6).
- Provide clothing that is:
  - Clean
  - In good repair and fits properly
  - Appropriate for the season and the weather
  - Appropriate for the resident's age and sex
- Assist residents with toileting needs as necessary.
  - Take residents to the bathroom as needed or at regularly scheduled times. The bathroom is designed to meet the physical needs of the residents, with grab bars and elevated toilet seats (Figure 7-7).
  - Attend to **incontinent** residents (those unable to control bladder or bowel) immediately.
- Assist residents to remain adequately nourished.
  - Consider the residents' food choices as much as possible.
  - Give residents the assistance necessary to eat independently.
  - Feed residents who cannot feed themselves in a dignified manner.

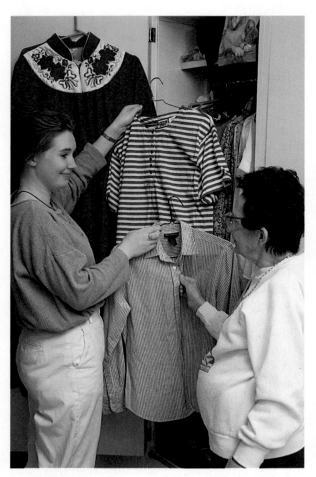

FIGURE 7-6 Allow residents to choose their own clothing.

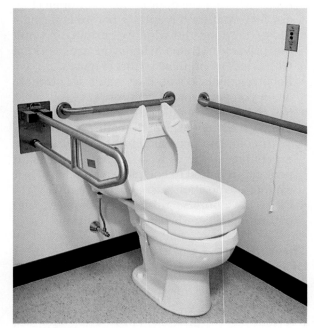

FIGURE 7-7 Raised toilet seats and grab bars assist residents to be more independent.

FIGURE 7-9   Facilities must offer an activity program to all residents.

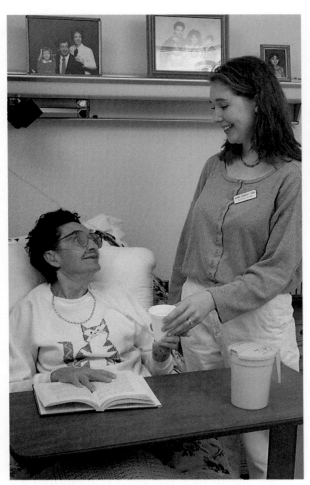

FIGURE 7-8   Residents should always have access to fresh drinking water.

- Never force residents to eat.
- Provide access to fresh drinking water throughout the day (Figure 7-8).
- Give dependent residents drinks of fresh water regularly.
- Assist residents with the use of devices to meet their needs.
  - Make sure they have their eyeglasses and that the glasses are clean and in good repair.
  - Assist residents with insertion of hearing aids and report improperly functioning hearing aids to the proper person.
  - Assist with the use of canes and walkers.
  - Help residents with a **prosthesis** (artificial body part) or other devices.

Psychosocial Needs.   Residents have the right to expect the staff to help them meet their psychosocial needs as much as possible. This

may require the attention of various members of the interdisciplinary team. The staff needs to remember:

- The medical condition of a resident when providing these rights
- That the rights of all residents are equal
- That no resident has the right to infringe on the right or safety of other residents

  The team works together to:

- Allow residents to:
  - Spend their free time as they wish
  - Move about the facility (if their medical condition permits) as long as they respect the privacy of other residents and staff members
  - Participate, if desired, in structured activities offered by the facility (Figure 7-9)
  - Visit other residents in the facility
- Allow married couples who both reside in the facility to share a room, if they both so desire and if it is medically appropriate.
- Respect the **sexuality** and sexual needs of the resident. Sexuality is one aspect of human

Clinical Focus
Family members frequently assist residents and do things for them to increase the resident's enjoyment. Since Mr. Davidson has no close relatives, what are some issues that the staff may need to think about?

psychosocial needs. Whether married to each other or not, residents have the right to express their needs and to experience satisfaction as long as this is mutually agreeable. Residents must be mentally and physically able to agree to the relationship.

Environmental Needs

The resident has the right to expect that the environment will be adapted to meet the needs of individuals with disabilities. This means:

- The residents must be able to safely move about and function within the facility. This requires:
  - Handrails attached to corridor walls (Figure 7-10)
  - Elevators for resident use
  - Ramps that allow wheelchair access into and out of the facility
  - Permanent grab bars in bathrooms and elevated toilet seats
  - Signal lights in the residents' rooms and in the bathrooms and showers

FIGURE 7-11 Calendars with large numbers help residents remain oriented.

- Safety measures for residents who wander
- Clocks and calendars with large numerals located throughout the building to help residents remain oriented (Figure 7-11)
- The facility environment is expected to be homelike and to allow social interaction, including:
  - Furniture arrangements in public areas that allow for visiting (Figure 7-12)
  - The use of color, plants, and artwork to create a cheerful environment

FIGURE 7-10 Handrails attached to the wall allow residents more independence.

FIGURE 7-12 Facilities should have comfortable visiting areas.

Advance Directives

Residents also have the right to make **advance directives**. In 1990, the federal government passed a law called the **Self-Determination Act**. This law states that all competent adults have the right to:

- Accept or refuse any medical treatment, including life-sustaining treatments
- Be adequately informed about:
  - Their medical condition
  - Treatment alternatives
  - Likely risks of each treatment alternative
  - Benefits of each alternative
  - Possible consequences of each alternative

The law applies to competent adults entering hospitals, nursing homes, home health care, or **hospice** (an agency that provides care for terminally ill persons). The law requires that residents:

- Be informed of what kinds of advance directives are available to ensure that their wishes are carried out when they are no longer able to make or communicate their decisions
- Be informed that it is the right of every competent adult to choose whether he or she wants to execute an advance directive

There are two types of advance directives:

- **living will** (Figure 7-13)
- **power of attorney for health care** (Figure 7-14)

A living will:

- Allows individuals to describe their wishes about discontinuing procedures that delay death if they have a **terminal condition**. This means that death is expected soon and the person's condition is incurable and irreversible.
- Is legal in most states
- Must be witnessed by two people who will not benefit from the resident's death. (In most facilities, the nursing assistant should not be a witness for the signing of legal forms.)

A durable power of attorney for health care:

- Permits a person (called the *principal*) to delegate to another person (called the *agent*) the power to make any health care decision that the principal is unable to make

Even though these advance directives have been completed, the resident must still make decisions regarding other support measures.

Cardiopulmonary Resuscitation (CPR)

- The resident must inform the physician whether **cardiopulmonary resuscitation** is to be administered if **cardiac arrest** occurs. In most states, the law requires that all persons be resuscitated unless they have previously made their wishes known.
- The physician must write the order on the resident's chart if a resident or the person with a power of attorney for health care determines that CPR should not be administered. This is called **no-code** or **DNR (do not resuscitate)**.

When there is a DNR order, resuscitation is not performed when the resident stops breathing. The resident is allowed to die with peace and dignity. All personnel should be aware when a DNR order is written. It is often difficult to carry out a DNR order when you have come to know and love the resident. Try to remember that life needs to be meaningful and that quality of life is limited for a person on life support systems.

If a resident has chosen to be resuscitated in the event that cardiac arrest occurs, then every effort is made to keep the resident alive. A "code" is called and CPR is initiated. An ambulance is called to transport the resident to the hospital for additional life support measures.

Hospitalization

- Some technical procedures cannot be performed in the long-term care facility.
- When residents become acutely ill, hospitalization may be necessary if lifesaving measures are to be taken.
- Residents may choose not to go to the hospital, but to remain in the facility for supportive care only.

Feeding Restrictions

- Residents who are terminally ill frequently do not wish to eat or drink.
- The physician may suggest inserting a feeding tube into the stomach.
- In most states this procedure will not be done if the resident has made his wishes clear in the advance directives.

In an advance directive, the resident may state that this procedure is not to be performed. Most states will honor this statement and not insert a feeding tube.

FLORIDA LIVING WILL

Declaration made this _____ day of _____, _____,
(day)   (month)   (year)

I, _____, willfully and voluntarily make known my desire that my dying not be artificially prolonged under the circumstances set forth below, and I do hereby declare that:

If at any time I am both mentally and physically incapacitated
_____ and I have a terminal condition, or
_____ and I have an end-stage condition, or
_____ and I am in a persistent vegetative state

and if my attending or treating physician and another consulting physician have determined that there is no reasonable medical probability of my recovery from such condition, I direct that life-prolonging procedures be withheld or withdrawn when the application of such procedures would serve only to prolong artificially the process of dying, and that I be permitted to die naturally with only the administration of medication or the performance of any medical procedure deemed necessary to provide me with comfort care or to alleviate pain.

It is my intention that this declaration be honored by my family and physician as the final expression of my legal right to refuse medical or surgical treatment and to accept the consequences for such refusal.

In the event that I have been determined to be unable to provide express and informed consent regarding the withholding, withdrawal, or continuation of life-prolonging procedures, I wish to designate, as my surrogate to carry out the provisions of this declaration:

Name: _____

Address: _____

_____ Zip Code: _____

Phone: _____

FIGURE 7-13 A living will allows individuals to describe their choices if they become terminally ill. (Reprinted by permission of Partnership for Caring, 1035 30th Street, NW, Washington, DC 20007; 800-989-9455)

FLORIDA LIVING WILL — PAGE 2 OF 2

PRINT NAME, HOME ADDRESS AND TELEPHONE NUMBER OF YOUR ALTERNATE SURROGATE

I wish to designate the following person as my alternate surrogate, to carry out the provisions of this declaration should my surrogate be unwilling or unable to act on my behalf:

Name: _____

Address: _____

_____ Zip Code: _____

Phone: _____

ADD PERSONAL INSTRUCTIONS (IF ANY)

Additional instructions (optional):

I understand the full import of this declaration, and I am emotionally and mentally competent to make this declaration.

SIGN THE DOCUMENT

Signed: _____

WITNESSING PROCEDURE

Witness 1:

    Signed: _____

    Address: _____

TWO WITNESSES MUST SIGN AND PRINT THEIR ADDRESSES

Witness 2:

    Signed: _____

    Address: _____

© 2000
PARTNERSHIP FOR
CARING, INC.

Courtesy of **Partnership for Caring, Inc.**   10/99
1035 30th Street, NW Washington, DC 20007 800-989-9455

FIGURE 7-13 *(continued)*

INSTRUCTIONS

FLORIDA DESIGNATION OF HEALTH CARE SURROGATE

PRINT YOUR NAME

Name:_____

　　　　　　(Last)　　　　　　(First)　　　　(Middle Initial)

In the event that I have been determined to be incapacitated to provide informed consent for medical treatment and surgical and diagnostic procedures, I wish to designate as my surrogate for health care decisions:

PRINT THE NAME, HOME ADDRESS AND TELEPHONE NUMBER OF YOUR SURROGATE

Name:_____

Address: _____

_____ Zip Code: _____

Phone: _____

If my surrogate is unwilling or unable to perform his or her duties, I wish to designate as my alternate surrogate:

PRINT THE NAME, HOME ADDRESS AND TELEPHONE NUMBER OF YOUR ALTERNATE SURROGATE

Name: _____

Address: _____

_____ Zip Code: _____

Phone: _____

I fully understand that this designation will permit my designee to make health care decisions and to provide, withhold, or withdraw consent on my behalf; to apply for public benefits to defray the cost of health care; and to authorize my admission to or transfer from a health care facility.

ADD PERSONAL INSTRUCTIONS (IF ANY)

Additional instructions (optional):

© 2000
PARTNERSHIP FOR
CARING, INC.

FIGURE 7-14 The power of attorney for health care is a document that appoints another person to make decisions for the resident. (Reprinted by permission of Partnership for Caring, 1035 30th Street, NW, Washington, DC 20007; 800-989-9455)

FLORIDA DESIGNATION OF HEALTH CARE SURROGATE — PAGE 2 OF 2

I further affirm that this designation is not being made as a condition of treatment or admission to a health care facility. I will notify and send a copy of this document to the following persons other than my surrogate, so they may know who my surrogate is:

PRINT THE NAMES AND ADDRESSES OF THOSE WHO YOU WANT TO KEEP COPIES OF THIS DOCUMENT

Name: _____

Address: _____

Name: _____

Address: _____

SIGN AND DATE THE DOCUMENT

Signed: _____

Date: _____

WITNESSING PROCEDURE

TWO WITNESSES MUST SIGN AND PRINT THEIR ADDRESSES

Witness 1:

　　　Signed: _____

　　　Address: _____

Witness 2:

　　　Signed: _____

　　　Address: _____

© 2000
PARTNERSHIP FOR CARING, INC.

Courtesy of **Partnership for Caring, Inc.**   10/99
1035 30th Street, NW Washington, DC 20007 800-989-9455

FIGURE 7-14 *(continued)*

Medication and Treatment Restrictions

The resident has the right to refuse:

- Life-sustaining medications such as chemotherapy or antibiotics
- Blood transfusions
- Surgery
- Being placed on a ventilator
- Any medical treatment

Residents always have the right to change their minds. For example, if the advance directives state that a feeding tube is not to be inserted, the resident may change this directive if the time comes.

The Right to Voice Grievances

This means the resident may voice **grievances** (complaints) to the facility without fear of retaliation (**reprisal**) or discrimination. The facility must take prompt action to resolve the grievances (Figure 7-15).

The resident may have a grievance about:

- The way in which care is given
- Treatment or care that is not given

As a nursing assistant, you can help avoid problems by following these guidelines.

1. Relay concerns of the resident to the nurse in charge.
2. Carry out all instructions you may be given for solving the problem.
3. Never withhold care or attention from a resident because of grievances or complaints voiced by the resident.

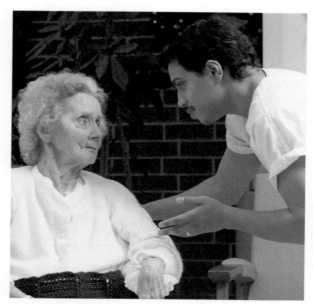

FIGURE 7-15 Residents have the right to voice grievances.

4. Avoid discussing grievances with other staff members unless there is a valid need for such discussion. You may, for example, discuss a grievance at a care plan conference as a way of trying to solve the problem.

The Right to Organize and Participate in Family and Resident Groups

This means:

- The facility must provide space for meetings.
- A staff member from the facility will attend if invited.
- The staff will address written recommendations from the meetings that concern decisions affecting the resident's care and life in the facility.

Most long-term care facilities have resident councils. These councils meet regularly and all residents are invited to participate in the meetings. The councils give the residents a way to communicate with each other and with staff in a constructive and organized manner.

To assist in providing these residents' rights, you can:

1. Cooperate in assisting residents to attend council meetings.
   - Help residents to get dressed to attend the meeting.
   - Arrange residents' care so it does not interfere with their attendance at the meetings.
   - Toilet residents if necessary before they go to the meeting.
   - Help transport residents to the meeting if necessary.
2. Cooperate in carrying out recommendations of the council that are implemented by the facility administration.

The Right to Participate in Social, Religious, and Community Activities

Social Activities. Someone from the activities staff meets with each resident shortly after admission to the facility. Residents are given an opportunity to express their choices for activities. Activities must include:

1. Empowerment activities
   - Activities that increase self-respect by providing opportunities for self-expression such as doing artwork or creative crafts
   - Activities that require personal responsibility and choices. Voting is an example of this type of activity. Residents have the right to vote in all local, state, and federal elections. Residents are given the opportunity to vote by absentee ballot or they are taken to the polls.

2. Maintenance activities
   - Maintenance activities promote physical, mental, social, and emotional health.
   - Maintenance activities include physical exercise, current events discussion groups, picnics, and musical or dramatic presentations.
3. Supportive activities
   - Supportive activities provide stimulation to residents with severe mental or physical disabilities who cannot participate in other types of programs.

As a nursing assistant, follow these guidelines for supporting the residents' participation in activities.

1. Cooperate with the activities staff schedule of events. Schedule resident care so it does not interfere with the residents' attendance.
2. Be aware of the activities that are scheduled. Give residents information if they ask about the nature and time of the activities being offered.

Residents also have the right to refuse to participate in any of these activities. They can develop their own individual activities, for example, reading or doing needlework or crossword puzzles.

Religious Activities. Worship and religious activities are an important aspect of living in a long-term care facility. Freedom of worship must be allowed for each resident.

1. Respect the residents' religious beliefs and practices.
2. Assist residents to attend church services and other religious activities within the facility.
3. Treat religious articles such as Bibles, crucifixes, and rosaries with respect (Figure 7-16).
4. Provide privacy for residents' visits with the clergy (such as priest, pastor, or rabbi).
5. Allow residents privacy for prayer and meditation.
6. Remember that the resident also has the right to not have religious beliefs or practices.

Community Activities. Involvement with the community can be important for the residents' interest and enthusiasm. Many long-term care facilities have large vans or buses with wheelchair access that enable residents to attend community events. These activities might include entertainment, educational, religious, or recreational programs. Groups from the community visit the long-term care facility to provide these events for residents who cannot leave the facility.

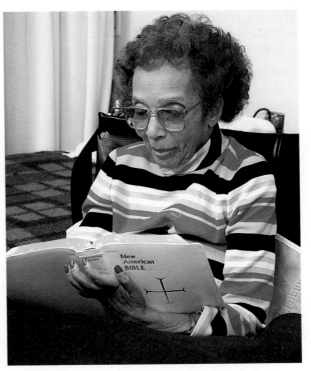

FIGURE 7-16   The resident has the right to keep religious items in the room.

The Right to Examine Survey Results and Correction Plans

Surveys of all facilities are completed on a regular basis by regulatory agencies. The surveyors write up their findings from the survey. If any problems are found, the facility must write a plan of correction that states how the problems will be solved. The resident (or family, if resident wishes) may inspect these records during normal business hours or by special appointment.

The Right to Manage Personal Funds

This means:

- The resident may request the facility to manage the funds. The resident must give written authorization.
- If the account exceeds $50, it must earn interest, which is given to the resident.

The Right to Information About Eligibility for Medicare/Medicaid Benefits

This means:

- The resident has the right to receive these benefits if the resident is eligible for the benefits, and the facility participates in the programs.

The Right to File Complaints About Abuse, Neglect, or Misappropriation of Property

This means:

- If the resident believes there has been abuse, neglect, or property stolen, the resident can file a complaint with the state agency that inspects the facility.

The Right to Information About Advocacy Groups

This means:

- Each state has an **ombudsman** program. An ombudsman may visit facilities to question residents about the care they are receiving. This person is trained by a state agency to perform this responsibility.
- Each facility also has agencies in the area that serve as **advocates** (spokespersons) for the residents to ensure that they receive appropriate care.
- The telephone numbers of these groups must be available to residents. Each facility must also post a **hot-line number** that can be used to register complaints about a facility or caregiver (Figure 7-17).

The Right to Immediate and Unlimited Access to Immediate Family or Relatives

This also includes:

- The long-term care ombudsman
- Government agency representatives
- The attending physician

   The resident may also withdraw consent to visit with any of these people.

The Right to Share a Room with Spouse

If spouses are residents in the facility, they may share a room. This may not be possible if there are medical reasons to keep one of the couple in a special unit.

The Right to Perform or Not Perform Work for the Facility

The resident may perform work at the facility if it is medically appropriate for the resident to do so. In addition:

- The resident must formally agree to any work arrangement.
- If the work is for pay, the resident earns the prevailing rate for the services.

NURSING HOME
HOTLINE
CALL TOLL FREE 24 HOURS
1-800-252-4343

If you have a complaint concerning this long-term care facility, you may discuss it with the administrator or a person designated by the administrator to discuss complaints. If this does not resolve your complaint, you have the right to contact the Illinois Department of Public Health's Nursing Home Hotline, 1-800-252-4343, or you may write

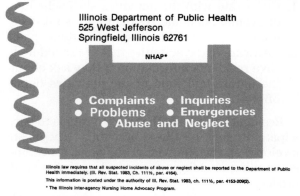

Illinois Department of Public Health
525 West Jefferson
Springfield, Illinois 62761

NHAP*

- Complaints   - Inquiries
- Problems   - Emergencies
- Abuse and Neglect

Illinois law requires that all suspected incidents of abuse or neglect shall be reported to the Department of Public Health immediately. (Ill. Rev. Stat. 1983, Ch. 111½, par. 4164).

This information is posted under the authority of Ill. Rev. Stat. 1983, ch. 111½, par. 4153-209(2).

* The Illinois inter-agency Nursing Home Advocacy Program.

FIGURE 7-17 Each resident must have access to the hot-line number. (Courtesy of Illinois Department of Public Health)

The Right to Remain in the Facility

The resident can remain in the facility unless one or more of the following items applies:

- The resident no longer needs the care.
- The resident's welfare requires transfer.
- The facility no longer meets the resident's needs.
- The health or safety of others in the facility is endangered.
- The resident fails to pay for services.
- The facility ceases to operate.
- In these cases, 30 days notice must be given except when health is improved, there is an emergency, or there is danger to the health or safety of individuals in the facility.

The Right to Use Personal Possessions

Personal possessions means:

- Personal clothing and jewelry (Figure 7-18)
- Personal furnishings when these can be used in accordance with health and safety regulations

FIGURE 7-18 Residents can wear their own jewelry and clothing.

The residents' right to retain and use personal possessions ensures that the residents' environment is homelike. Using personal possessions gives residents some control over their lives. The facility is responsible for taking reasonable measures to safeguard residents' belongings. Each resident's record contains a personal possession list. It must be noted on this list any time an item is brought into the facility or any time an item is removed from the facility. Nursing assistant responsibilities include the following:

1. Encourage residents to display pictures and family photos in their rooms.
2. Assist residents to arrange their personal items if they need help.
3. Report any lost items immediately and take measures to find the items.
4. Do not rearrange furniture in a resident's room without the person's permission, unless there is a valid health or safety reason.
5. Do not go through dresser drawers, closets, lockers, or purses without the resident's permission.
6. Be careful what you throw out when tidying the room.

The Right to Notification of Change in Condition

This means the facility will notify the resident's attending physician, legal representative, and family member of:

- An accident involving the resident
- A significant change in the resident's condition
- A need to alter treatment significantly
- A decision for transfer or discharge

The members of the interdisciplinary team work together to provide the residents with the rights expressed in this document.

LEGAL ASPECTS OF HEALTH CARE

The Residents' Rights document has a legal foundation. Contained within the document are several rights which, if violated, could result in legal action against the facility or care provider. This action may be a fine or imprisonment for the offender. Each employee is responsible for personal actions. The OBRA legislation requires that a facility report any case of abuse and the names of the persons involved. Each state has a designated agency that investigates such reports.

Assault and Battery

Assault and battery are examples of actions that violate the residents' rights and are criminal offenses. Any type of abuse of a resident may be a form of assault or battery. **Assault** is a threat or an attempt to harm another person. Threatening to restrain a resident if he does not stay in bed is an example of assault. **Battery** is touching another person without that person's consent. Grabbing a resident to give him a bath when he does not want one is battery. To protect the caregivers, legal permission is required from the resident, family, or legal guardian for certain procedures. This permission must be obtained with the **informed consent** of the resident. This means the resident fully understands the procedure. This formal consent is not required for routine personal care and procedures. However, you must explain what you are going to do to the resident before you do it. If the resident objects, discuss the situation with the nurse.

False Imprisonment

The unauthorized use of restraints can be considered **false imprisonment** (detaining an individual without a reason and against that individual's will).

Invasion of Privacy

Violating a resident's right to privacy and confidentiality of personal and medical records is an example of **invasion of privacy.**

Defamation of Character

If a person spreads false information about a resident, then that person may be guilty of **defamation of character**. If the false information is verbal or spoken, it is called **slander**. If it is written, it is called **libel**.

Neglect

Neglect may also be considered a criminal offense. Neglect was discussed earlier in this lesson.

Theft

The resident has the right to use personal possessions. To take anyone's personal possessions is **theft**.

You will avoid problems as a health care provider if you:

• Always do the very best job possible.
• Treat the resident with respect.
• Remember the rights of the resident.
• Do only those tasks that you are legally qualified to perform.

ETHICS AND THE HEALTH CARE PROVIDER

The term **ethics** refers to conduct or behavior. Every profession has a code of ethics for its members. These codes are especially important in health care. Persons receiving care are dependent on caregivers to meet many of their physical, mental, and emotional needs. Whether you are following the ethics of your profession is determined by the behavior you exhibit while you are working. For example:

• Report for work when scheduled, unless you have a truly justifiable reason for being absent. Your absence may mean that residents will not be given the care they deserve. If you cannot report for work, call in well in advance so a substitute can be found or assignments can be rearranged.

• Report to work on time. When you are late, it can upset the resident's schedule for the rest of the day.
• Health care providers do not accept tips in the form of money or gifts. If these are offered, thank the resident and explain that you are not allowed to accept them.
• Do not take supplies or items that belong to the facility, to residents, or to other staff members.
• Accept your assignments willingly and help others as needed.
• Always be honest. If you make a mistake, report it to your supervisor immediately. If you do not know how to perform a task, ask for help so that you do not harm anyone.
• Avoid horseplay, joking around, and loud laughter when you are working. Humor is necessary but should be appropriate. Never make fun of a resident.
• Do not discuss your personal problems at work. If you have problems that may affect your work, discuss them with your supervisor.
• Avoid gossiping and griping. A negative attitude from one person can affect the morale of everyone else.
• Use only language that the resident understands.
• Your physical appearance reflects your attitude. Follow the dress code of your employer and follow the rules of personal hygiene and grooming.

On the Job

You may be assigned to work with employees who do not follow the rules of ethical behavior. For instance, if you work with someone who continually complains, you may need to avoid that employee or explain that you do not wish to listen to the complaints. In some situations, you may have to go to your supervisor for guidance.

LESSON SYNTHESIS: Putting It All Together

You have just completed this lesson. Now go back and review the Clinical Focus. Try to see how the Clinical Focus relates to the concepts presented in the lesson. Then answer the following questions.

1. Why is it necessary to know and actively protect Mr. Davidson's rights?

2. How do the rights of Mr. Davidson differ from those that every citizen enjoys?

3. What nursing assistant actions would interfere with the rights of a resident?

4. When a resident is unable to make decisions, how may his or her rights be protected?

5. How could you protect Mr. Davidson's right of privacy?

REVIEW

A. Select the one best answer for each of the following.

1. The purpose of the Residents' Rights document is to
   (A) separate the resident from the community
   (B) provide a moderately comfortable environment
   (C) help the resident maintain the highest level of well-being possible
   (D) restrict some resident choices

2. The right to free choice means the resident
   (A) will be assigned a room by the facility
   (B) must use the facility physician
   (C) can choose which nursing assistants will provide his or her care
   (D) will be able to read the evaluation report but not participate in care planning

3. An example of mental abuse is
   (A) not taking the resident to the bathroom when she needs to go
   (B) swearing at the resident
   (C) slapping the resident when she refuses to eat
   (D) fondling the resident's breasts

4. Corporal punishment means
   (A) isolating the resident without providing care
   (B) using chemical restraints
   (C) using painful treatment for correction of behavior
   (D) using physical restraints

5. Involuntary seclusion is
   (A) helping the resident to his room and closing the door when the resident wants to lie down
   (B) isolating the resident when it is not part of a therapeutic plan
   (C) placing a resident with a communicable disease in isolation
   (D) giving the resident medication to put him to sleep

6. A chemical restraint
   (A) is a medication that influences behavior
   (B) is any device that enhances the resident's mobility
   (C) has no effect on the resident's behavior
   (D) is administered by the nursing assistant

7. The resident has the right to privacy when
   (A) walking down the hall
   (B) receiving nursing care or medical treatment

(C) talking to the housekeeper

(D) being served a meal tray

8. The right to confidentiality means
   (A) the resident cannot see her chart or medical record
   (B) that only the physician can read the chart
   (C) information about the resident is available only to those who need it to provide care
   (D) that nursing assistants cannot read the chart

9. Accommodation of needs means that the staff must
   (A) provide the resident with fresh fruit at every meal
   (B) escort the resident to the church of his or her choice
   (C) give every resident a private room with bath
   (D) assist the resident to maintain personal hygiene and cleanliness

10. Residents are not allowed to
    (A) move about the facility
    (B) visit other residents
    (C) enter another resident's room without permission of that resident
    (D) have visitors in their rooms

11. If a husband and wife are both admitted to the facility, they are
    (A) not allowed to have sexual activity
    (B) allowed to share the same room if their medical conditions permit
    (C) expected to help take care of each other
    (D) not allowed to have the same physician

12. Providing an environment to meet the needs of the residents means that
    (A) the resident can choose the color of his room and drapes
    (B) there are permanent grab bars in the bathrooms
    (C) there must be wall-to-wall carpeting throughout the facility
    (D) the residents' personal furnishings are not allowed

13. A living will provides instructions for
    (A) who will inherit the resident's money
    (B) how the resident will pay her bill
    (C) carrying out the resident's wishes if she has a terminal illness

(D) the resident's funeral in the event of her death

14. A person who has power of attorney for health care
    (A) must be a lawyer
    (B) makes decisions for the resident even if he is able to do so himself
    (C) can make health care decisions if the resident is unable to do so
    (D) can decide how the resident's money is spent

15. A grievance is a
    (A) complaint
    (B) sad feeling
    (C) lawsuit
    (D) casual remark

16. An ombudsman
    (A) is the person who has power of attorney for health care
    (B) visits facilities to make sure residents are receiving adequate care
    (C) is the administrator
    (D) has an office in the facility

17. The hot-line number is used
    (A) by a resident or family member to call a state agency to register a complaint about the facility
    (B) to call the fire department in the event of fire
    (C) to order meals to be sent in to the resident
    (D) by staff members to register complaints about their supervisors

18. Assault is the legal term for
    (A) touching another person without consent
    (B) a threat or an attempt to harm another person
    (C) placing a restraint on a resident
    (D) invasion of privacy

19. The term *slander* means
    (A) spreading false information about a resident verbally
    (B) writing false information about a resident
    (C) mental abuse
    (D) false imprisonment

20. Which situation would be considered unethical?
    (A) accepting a tip from a resident
    (B) accepting a homemade cookie from the resident's daughter

(C) calling in sick when you have an elevated temperature and the flu

(D) asking another nursing assistant to help you get a heavy resident out of bed

B. Match the resident right (items a.–e.) with the nursing assistant actions that protect that right.

a. freedom from abuse
b. providing privacy
c. ensuring confidentiality
d. accommodating individual needs
e. participation in religious activities

21. _____ encouraging the resident to feed himself

22. _____ frequently visiting a disoriented resident

23. _____ informing the nurse that the resident wishes a visit from a clergy-person

24. _____ knocking before entering a room

25. _____ refusing to discuss one resident's condition with another

26. _____ assisting the resident to the telephone

27. _____ gently handling the resident when turning him

28. _____ leaving all written notes regarding residents in the facility

29. _____ drawing the curtains during a bedbath

30. _____ encouraging residents to choose their own clothing

C. Fill in the blanks by selecting the correct word or phrase from the list.

chemical restraints   physical restraint
empowerment   supportive care
maintenance

31. Medications that affect the resident's behavior and alter thinking are called _____.

32. A device that restricts a resident's movement and does not allow normal access to the body is called a _____.

33. An activity that promotes self-respect by providing opportunities for self-expression is a/an _____ activity.

34. _____ activities promote physical, mental, social, and emotional health.

35. Providing comfort measures to a person who is dying is called giving _____.

LESSON 8

Safety

Clinical Focus

Think about the role the nursing assistant can play in ensuring a safe environment for each resident as you study this lesson and meet:

*D*ebra, who is a nursing assistant at the Great Neck Nursing Center. Each month, Debra and members of the staff carry out a fire drill. This practice means that they will all be prepared to act promptly in case of a real emergency.

OBJECTIVES

After studying this lesson, you should be able to:

- Define and spell vocabulary words and terms.
- List the ergonomic factors that may lead to work-related musculoskeletal disorders.
- List the ergonomics techniques you can use to prevent incidents on the job.
- Demonstrate the correct use of body mechanics.
- Describe the types of information contained in Material Safety Data Sheets (MSDS).
- Use equipment safely.
- Describe three safety rules for when oxygen is in use.
- Identify residents who are at risk of having incidents.
- Describe four precautions to take when the side rails of the bed are down.
- List three alternatives to the use of physical restraints.
- Describe the guidelines for the use of restraints.
- Demonstrate the correct application of restraints.
- Describe three measures for preventing resident incidents: accidental poisoning, thermal injuries, skin injuries, falls, and choking.
- List four measures to follow for safe wheelchair use.
- Describe three procedures to follow in the event of fire.

VOCABULARY

aspiration   *(ass-pih-**RAY**-shun)*

body mechanics   *(**BAH**-dee mih-**KAN**-icks)*

ergonomics   *(er-goh-**NOM**-icks)*

incident   *(**IN**-sih-dent)*

laceration   *(lass-er-**AY**-shun)*

Material Safety Data Sheet (MSDS)   *(mah-**TEER**-ee-al **SAYF**-tee **DAY**-tah sheet)*

Occupational Safety and Health Administration (OSHA)   *(ock-you-**PAY**-shun-al **SAYF**-tee and helth ad-**min**-iss-**TRAY**-shun)*

SAFETY IN HEALTH CARE FACILITIES

A major concern in health care facilities is the prevention of injuries to residents, employees, volunteers, and visitors. An **incident** (accident) is any unexpected situation that can cause a resident, employee, or any other person harm. Prevention of incidents depends on:

- Employees knowing their jobs and all policies and procedures related to safety
- Maintaining a safe environment
- Knowing the residents and using safety measures to decrease their risk of injury

When an incident occurs, it must be reported immediately. Report to your supervisor and follow the policy of your facility.

EMPLOYEE SAFETY

Health care workers are required to perform many physical tasks. You must learn how to use your body correctly while you are completing your assignments. This is called using good **body mechanics**. This means you are using your muscles correctly when you lift or move residents or heavy objects. If you always apply the rules of body mechanics, you will avoid injury to yourself and to the residents.

Ergonomics

The word **ergonomics** means adapting the environment and using techniques and equipment to prevent injury to the body. The **Occupational Safety and Health Administration (OSHA)** is a part of the federal government under the Department of Labor. This agency is responsible for overseeing the health and safety of all employees in the country. For health care employees, work-related disorders of the musculoskeletal system are a major concern. These types of injuries can result in permanent disability, preventing the individual from performing job duties and personal responsibilities. Ergonomic programs are designed to prevent injuries by educating employees about potential hazards of the job, risk factors that may result in injury, techniques to use to prevent injuries, and reporting procedures.

If certain risk factors are present, it is likely that an ergonomic (work-related) problem will occur. These risk factors include:

1. Performance of the same motion or motion pattern every few seconds for more than 2 to 4 hours at a time
2. Being in a fixed or awkward posture for more than 2 to 4 hours
3. Using forceful hand movements for more than 2 to 4 hours at a time
4. Doing heavy lifting, unassisted, for more than 1 to 2 hours

Body Mechanics

The use of proper body mechanics at all times can prevent fatigue and body injury. Good body mechanics means to:

1. Maintain good standing posture.
   - Stand with your feet flat on the floor.
   - Separate your feet about 12 inches (shoulder width apart).
   - Bend your knees slightly.
   - Keep your back straight.
   - Tighten your abdominal muscles.
2. Use the weight of your body to help to push or pull an object.
3. Use the strongest muscles to do the job.
   - It is easier to bring the resident or object toward you than to lift the resident or object away from you.
   - Use stronger muscles (leg muscles) rather than weaker muscles (back muscles) when lifting, pushing, or pulling.
4. Avoid twisting your body and overreaching as you work.
5. Avoid bending for long periods of time.

*G*uidelines for

Using Ergonomic Techniques to Reduce the Risk of Having an Incident

1. Use correct body mechanics at all times, at work and when you are off duty.
2. Raise the beds to a comfortable working height (remember to lower the beds when you finish your task).
3. Use a mechanical lift when you need to transfer very heavy or dependent residents into or out of bed.
4. Use a back support if your employer requires it. The use of a back support is controversial because it does not really prevent injury, but it does remind the wearer to use good body mechanics. Many nursing assistants find them helpful (Figure 8-1).

5. Get another person to help when you need to transfer a resident who is not full weight bearing. Use a transfer belt when ordered.
6. Use a cart to move heavy items (Figure 8-2).

FIGURE 8-2 Use a cart to move heavy items.

FIGURE 8-1 Your employer may require you to wear a back support while you work.

6. Use the method that has been ordered to move a resident. For example, if the care plan states that two people are needed to transfer a resident from bed to chair, always get another person to help you.

7. Follow the eight commandments of lifting to greatly decrease the risk of injuring yourself:

   • Plan your lift and test the load (Figure 8-3A).
   • Ask for help (Figure 8-3B).

- Get a firm footing (Figure 8-3C).
- Bend your knees (Figure 8-3D).
- Tighten your stomach muscles (Figure 8-3E).
- Lift with your legs (Figure 8-3F).
- Keep the load close (Figure 8-3G).
- Keep your back straight (Figure 8-3H).

8. Ask your physician or a physical therapist for specific exercises for the back that can help prevent injuries.

9. Warm up before working to help prevent strains. Perform the exercises shown in Figures 8-4A–J before each work shift. Remember that you can avoid many problems if you also:

- Exercise every day. Get outside if possible and take several deep breaths.
- Eat a nourishing, well-balanced diet.
- Get adequate sleep.
- Avoid alcohol, tobacco, and drug use and too much caffeine.

- Wear comfortable shoes with good support and nonskid soles.

10. Remember that most back injuries can be prevented if you follow the rules for good body mechanics and if you complete all lifting procedures correctly.

On the Job

It is possible that you will be assigned to work with someone who does not always follow the precautions for preventing work-related injuries. For example, the person may want to take shortcuts in an effort to save time. Remember that in the end, what little time is saved may result in painful injuries.

A. Plan your lift and test the load.
Before you lift, think about the item you are going to move and ask yourself: "Can I lift this alone?" "Is it too awkward for one person?" "Is the path clear?" Also, test the load to see approximately how heavy it is before lifting.

B. Ask for help.
If the load is too heavy or too awkward for you to lift ask for assistance.

C. Get a firm footing.
Keep your feet apart for a stable base and point your toes out.

D. Bend your knees.
Don't bend at the waist. Keep the principles of leverage in mind at all times. Don't do more work than you have to.

E. Tighten your stomach muscles.
Use intra-abdominal pressure to support your spine when you lift, offsetting the force of the load. Train your muscles to work together.

F. Lift with your legs.
Let your leg muscles do the work of lifting. Don't rely on your weaker back muscles.

G. Keep the load close.
Don't hold the load away from your body. The closer it is to your spine, the less force it exerts on your back.

H. Keep your back upright.
Whether lifting or putting down the load, don't add weight of your body to the load. Avoid twisting.

FIGURE 8-3 Eight rules for lifting (Reprinted with permission from Ergodyne Corporation, St. Paul, MN)

FIGURE 8-4 Warm-up exercises (Reprinted with permission from Ergodyne Corporation, St. Paul, MN)

The student should check with a physician before beginning any exercise program.

A.

Neck Flexion and Extension:
SLOWLY tip your head forward and touch your chin to your chest. Then SLOWLY tip head back as far as possible. Repeat five times.

B.

Neck Rotation:
Keep your chin tucked down and look over your right shoulder as far as possible, then look over your left shoulder as far as possible. Repeat five times in each direction.

C.

Shoulder Flexion:
Clasp your hands together and inhale as you raise your arms over your head as far as possible with palms pointing up. Exhale as you bring your hands down behind your back. Repeat five times.

D.

Shoulder Extension:
Stand erect. Clasp hands behind your back and push them out as far as possible. Hold for a count of three. Repeat five times.

E.

Shoulder Circles:
Place your hands on top of your shoulders and make circles as big as possible with your elbow. Circle five times forward and then five times backward.

F.

Back Extension:
Standing, put your hands on your hips and lean back, slowly arching your back. Repeat five times.

G.

Low Back Flexion:
Sit in a chair with your knees shoulder width apart. Tip your chin to your chest and place your arms between your knees. SLOWLY lean forward and touch the floor. Repeat five times.

IF CHAIRS ARE ABSENT: Stand with feet shoulder width apart. Move into a squat position with your arms between your knees and your feet flat on the floor. Hold the position for a count of ten.

H.

Heel Cord Stretching:
Place one foot forward and one foot in back, keep your back heel on the floor and back foot pointing forward. SLOWLY lean forward until you feel stretching in your calf muscles. Hold this position for five counts, then repeat with the opposite leg.

I.

Hamstring Stretching:
Place your heel on a stool or chair and pull your toes toward your head. Keep your chin up and your back straight as you SLOWLY lean forward until you feel a stretch in the hamstring and calf muscles. Hold this position for ten counts, then repeat with opposite leg.

J.

Hip Flexor and Quad Stretching:
While standing, hold on to the back of a chair, grab your right ankle with your left hand and pull your heel towards your right buttock. Do not bend forward and do not arch your back. Hold this position for ten counts, then repeat with the opposite leg.

HAZARDS IN THE WORK ENVIRONMENT

Chemical Hazards

All health care facilities have hazards that may injure employees. Many of these items are chemicals that you may have in your own home (for example, chlorine bleach). A nursing unit may contain cleaning supplies, disinfectants, and other hazardous products. Injuries can be pre-vented if you know what the hazards are and how to protect yourself and others. OSHA requires that all manufacturers of these items supply **Material Safety Data Sheets** or **MSDS** with all hazardous products they sell. The MSDS provide hazard information that explains:

- What precautions to take in the presence of a hazard (for example, wearing personal protective equipment)
- Instructions for safe use of the potentially dangerous substance

- How to clean up and dispose of the hazardous product
- First aid measures to use if exposure occurs

OSHA has established other rules for a safe environment. Employers are required to inform employees of:

- The location of the MSDS
- The hazards in the work environment and where they are in the building
- The location of information related to the hazards
- How to read and understand chemical labels and hazard signs
- What type of personal protective equipment should be worn if working with these hazards and where the personal protective equipment is stored
- How to manage spills and where cleaning equipment is stored

All hazardous products must be kept in the original container with the original label intact and legible. Long-term care facilities must keep all chemicals in locked cabinets.

Equipment Safety

Learn to use equipment correctly. Report equipment that is broken or needs repair. Your facility may have a system of tagging equipment that needs repair. The tag will have the words "DO NOT OPERATE." NEVER attempt to use equipment that has been tagged. Your facility designates who is responsible for removing the tag. The equipment is returned to service only after it has been repaired and tested.

1. Beds
   - The wheels of the bed should always be locked, unless you need to move the bed.
   - Raise the bed to a comfortable working height when giving resident care.
   - Put the bed in the lowest horizontal position when you are finished giving care.
   - Make sure gatch handles on manually operated beds do not stick out.
   - Raise side rails if ordered, and check for security.
   - Do not attach restraints, supports, drainage bags, or tubing to side rails.
   - Ensure that all therapeutic, support, and protective devices are attached securely and properly to the bed. These devices include bed cradles, side rail pads, restraints, wandering alerts, special mattresses, and pads.

2. Signal cords (call lights)
   - Check call lights to make sure they are in working order.
   - Residents must always have access to caregivers. If a resident is physically or mentally unable to use a signal cord, the resident must be monitored frequently. The call light must still be within reach.
   - Answer call lights promptly.

3. Other equipment
   - Use equipment only if you know how to use it correctly.
   - Report needed repairs promptly.
        Lost screws
        Frayed straps or cords
        Loose wheels
        Broken control knobs
        Latches that do not hook
        Side rails that do not fasten
            correctly

4. Avoid injury from "sharps." These are needles, blades, disposable razors, or instruments that can puncture your skin.
   - Dispose of needles and blades in puncture-resistant, leakproof containers that are labeled or color coded. (This is described further in Lesson 11.)

FIGURE 8-5   Small pieces of glass may be swept into a dustpan using a small brush.

- Never handle broken bits of glass with your bare hands. Before cleaning up broken glass, put on disposable gloves or utility gloves. Use a brush and dustpan to sweep up the broken glass. Discard the glass according to facility policy (Figure 8-5).

Oxygen Safety

All health care facilities have oxygen in the building. Oxygen is provided through a system installed in the walls of the facility with outlets in the residents' rooms (Figure 8-6A) or by portable oxygen tanks (Figure 8-6B). Oxygen concentrators are used in many long-term care facilities. These devices use room air to deliver oxygen to residents (Figure 8-7).

Oxygen is flammable in the presence of a spark or open flame. For safety when a resident is using oxygen, remember:

- Do not allow smoking.
- Do not use woolen blankets.
- Do not allow an open flame such as matches, lighters, or candles.
- Disconnect oxygen before using electrical equipment.
- Do not adjust the liter flow.
- Be sure the oxygen source (if a tank) is secure.
- Post oxygen safety signs.

FIGURE 8-6B Small portable tanks of oxygen are kept on hand.

FIGURE 8-7 Oxygen concentrators extract oxygen from room air for delivery to a resident.

FIGURE 8-6A Oxygen is piped into the resident's room and attached to a flow meter.

RESIDENT SAFETY

You can contribute to resident safety by performing procedures as taught and correctly following orders. Review the care plans for the residents in your care as soon as you receive your assignments after the shift report. This will allow you to see any changes in the orders for the residents. For example, on your previous shift, a resident was up and about with minimal supervision; now the resident is anxious and disoriented because of a slight stroke during the night.

All staff members in long-term care facilities are responsible for monitoring residents as they move about the building.

Risk Factors for Incidents

Residents in long-term care facilities are at risk for incidents. There are several reasons why residents may have incidents:

- The changes in vision and hearing that most older people experience cause a loss of "warning systems." They are unaware of dangerous situations.
- Problems with mobility result from arthritic changes. These changes cause the joints to be less flexible.
- Dehydration may weaken the resident and lead to confusion that can affect perception.
- Residents may tire more easily. This increases the risk of an incident.
- Inner ear changes can cause a loss of balance and coordination.
- Frequency of urination often leads to fear of incontinence. This can result in unsafe toileting habits.
- Disorientation can cause residents to have poor judgment and an inability to recognize unsafe conditions.
- Some elderly persons experience dizziness when they stand up too quickly. This can cause them to fall.
- Certain medications can affect mental status, balance, and coordination.
- Residents may use assistive mobility devices (canes, walkers) unsafely.

Restraints

A *physical restraint* is any device or equipment that:

- A resident cannot easily remove
- Restricts a resident's movement
- Does not allow normal access to one's own body

FIGURE 8-8 Any device that restricts movement (including side rails) is considered a restraint.

Restraints include wrist or arm and ankle or leg restraints, vests, jackets, hand mitts, geriatric and cardiac chairs, and wheelchair safety belts and bars. Side rails may be considered restraints.

The term *safety device* is often used when referring to a physical restraint. However, if a device meets the definition given above, it is still a physical restraint (Figure 8-8). Postural supports used to maintain a resident's position are not considered restraints unless they fit the description of a restraint.

Alternatives to restraints should be tried before restraints are applied. Restraints are used only as a last resort in situations where the resident may harm himself or others. Nursing assistants can take a number of actions to help reduce the resident's need for restraints:

1. Care for residents' personal needs promptly.
   - Take residents to the bathroom regularly.
   - Meet their needs if they are hungry or thirsty.
   - Report signs and symptoms of pain or illness promptly.
   - Follow all instructions for assisting residents with exercise.
   - Be sure that residents have their eyeglasses and hearing aids if they need them.
   - Answer call signals promptly.
   - Check residents often to see if they need anything.
2. Know which residents are at risk of falling. Monitor these residents during your shift. All staff members should help with monitoring.
3. Check with the nurse to see if a resident can be instructed on safe mobility skills.

4. Observe residents who walk and transfer independently. Sometimes falls occur because they use incorrect and unsafe methods. Report these situations and learn how to teach residents the correct way.
5. Report immediately any physical or mental changes that can increase the resident's risk for an incident, such as:
   • Disorientation (the resident does not know time, place, or self)
   • A resident's complaints of dizziness
   • A resident's problems with balance and coordination
6. Maintain a calm, quiet, consistent environment. Too much noise and too many distractions can agitate residents.
7. Help maintain a homelike environment. Small, cozy seating areas located throughout the building give residents the opportunity to sit down if they become tired.
8. Provide comfortable chairs for residents. Position residents for comfort and to prevent slumping to the side and sliding. Use supportive devices and pillows as necessary.
9. Work with the activities personnel to provide residents with activities that prevent boredom (Figure 8-9).

FIGURE 8-10   A special sensor may be attached to the leg of a wandering, disoriented resident. Some manufacturers recommend that the sensor be worn on the wrist.

10. Make sure residents have access to signal lights at all times.
11. Use side rails only if necessary.
12. Wandering residents should be allowed to wander. Security devices are available that alert staff to residents who try to wander into unsafe areas (Figure 8-10).

The inappropriate use of restraints or safety devices can lead to physical and psychosocial complications. Restraints reduce physical mobility. This can lead to contractures, pressure ulcers, and other complications that result from inactivity. Restraints can cause disorientation, depression, hostility, and agitation in residents.

Preventing Accidental Poisoning

Residents who are disoriented may eat poisonous substances. Persons with dementia may eat or drink items that other residents have in their rooms, such as shaving lotion, cologne, nail polish, denture cleaning tablets, and plants. Residents may store food in their rooms until it spoils. Because of poor vision and reduced ability to taste and smell, they are unaware of spoilage. To prevent accidental poisonings:

• Keep all chemicals and cleaning solutions in locked cupboards (OSHA requirement).
• Use only nonpoisonous plants in the facility.
• The facility may provide residents with refrigerator space for perishable food items. Label containers with the residents' names, room numbers, and date. Remind residents that food is being kept for them in the refrigerator.

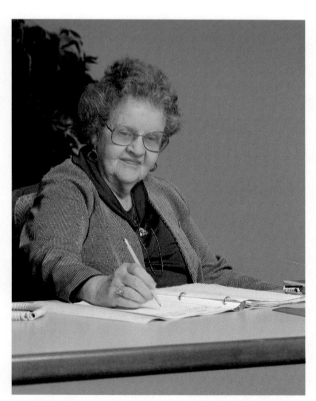

FIGURE 8-9   Providing appropriate activities can reduce the need for restraints.

Guidelines for

The Use of Restraints

Restraints may be needed in life-threatening situations. They are never used for staff convenience or as a substitute for good nursing care. The need for a restraint or safety device must be continually evaluated. If physical restraints are necessary, follow these guidelines.

1. The reasons for the restraint and all actions taken to avoid restraints must be carefully documented.

   - The resident, resident's family, or legal guardian must give written consent to the use of the restraint.
   - The charge nurse is responsible for the documentation and obtaining approval.

2. The physician must write an order for the restraint. The order must include:

   - The reason for the restraint or safety device
   - The type of device
   - The length of time it can be used
   - Where it can be used (chair, bed, or both)

3. The least restrictive device is always tried first. The restraint or safety device should be clean and in good repair.

4. Always apply restraints or safety devices according to the manufacturer's directions.

   - Make sure the restraint or safety device is the right size for the resident.
   - Apply restraints over clothing; never apply them next to the resident's skin.
   - Use only the type of restraint or safety device that is ordered (Figures 8-11 through 8-14).
   - Tie the device in a slip knot so that it can be released immediately in an emergency (Figure 8-15).
   - Restraints applied to a resident sitting in a chair must be tied correctly and not too tightly. You should be able to insert three fingers between the restraint and the resident.

FIGURE 8-11 Example of a jacket restraint (Courtesy of the Posey Company, Arcadia, CA)

FIGURE 8-12 A soft belt may be used when the resident is in a wheelchair. (Courtesy of the Posey Company, Arcadia, CA)

(continues)

*G*uidelines *(continued)*

FIGURE 8-13   A safety vest is always applied so the straps criss-cross in front. (Courtesy of the Posey Company, Arcadia, CA)

FIGURE 8-14   Always read the manufacturer's directions for the correct application of safety devices. (Courtesy of the Posey Company, Arcadia, CA)

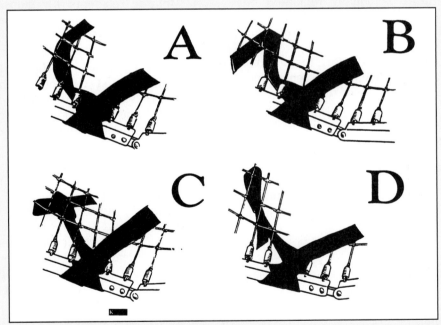

FIGURE 8-15   Use a quick-release tie for securing the restraint. (Courtesy of the Posey Company, Arcadia, CA)

- Do not tie restraints to the stationary bed frame or side rails. Tie restraints to the mattress frame, so that the restraint will move with the resident if the bed is raised.

- The side rails should always be up when a resident is wearing a restraint in bed.

5. Check residents who are in restraints at 15-minute intervals and document this action.

(continues)

> ### *G*uidelines *(continued)*
>
> 6. Release the restraints every 2 hours and document this action.
>
>   - Assist the resident to stand and walk if possible.
>   - If the resident cannot stand, do passive range of motion exercises on all extremities.
>   - Take the resident to the bathroom.
>
> - If the resident is incontinent, clean the resident; change clothing, chair pads, or bedding; and provide skin care.
> - Check the resident for any signs of skin breakdown or irritation and report these to the nurse.
> - Give the resident fluids and food.
> - Always place the signal light within the resident's reach.

Preventing Thermal Injuries

Thermal injuries (those caused by heat or cold) occur less frequently than other injuries but are still a source of concern.

- Follow procedures accurately when administering warm or cold treatments.
- Water temperature is usually regulated but check it before placing a resident in the tub or shower. Turn the hot water on last and turn it off first.
- Check food temperatures before feeding residents. Using a microwave oven to reheat food can be dangerous because of the uneven temperatures.
- Store smoking materials in a safe place and supervise residents while they smoke.

Preventing Skin Injuries

Residents may receive **lacerations** (cuts or breaks in the skin) or skin punctures. To prevent these injuries:

- Store knives, scissors, razors, and tools in locked cupboards.
- Store needles and syringes in locked cupboards. Syringes and needles should be disposed of immediately after use in the proper sharps container.
- Clean up broken glass immediately, using the methods described earlier.

Preventing Falls

It is estimated that each year 30% to 40% of all residents in long-term care facilities fall. To reduce falls, the environment can be altered to meet the needs of elderly persons. In Section 4 you will learn more about the changes of aging and how to adapt the environment to these changes.

1. Do not obstruct open areas with supplies and equipment. Place equipment on one side only of the hallway so residents do not have to navigate through an obstacle course.
2. Wipe up spills immediately.
3. Encourage residents to use rails along corridor walls when walking.
4. Monitor residents for signs of weakness, fatigue, dizziness, and loss of balance. Observe their actions to detect unsafe habits. Give instructions when necessary:
   - Residents who self-propel their wheelchairs need instructions on how to enter and leave elevators, how to use ramps, and reminders to use the brakes.
   - Dependent residents may benefit by learning some techniques of self-transfer. Check with the nurse to see if this is possible.
5. Provide adequate lighting in all resident areas. Avoid glare.
6. Eliminate noise and other environmental distractions. Noise can increase confusion and create anxiety even in alert individuals.
7. Do not leave residents alone in the tub or shower. All tubs and showers should have chairs so residents can remain seated throughout the procedure. Lifts for tubs minimize the risk of injuries in getting in and out of the tub. Avoid using oils that make the tub bottom slippery.
8. Check residents' clothing for fit. Loose shoes and laces, long robes, and slacks increase the risk of falling. Residents should always wear properly fitted, nonskid shoes when walking and during standing transfers.
9. Side rails are a frequent cause of falls. Many facilities leave side rails down on one side for residents who can safely transfer without help. In some situations, half-rails are more effective.

10. Care for residents' personal needs promptly. This may prevent residents from attempting unsafe transfers or ambulation.

11. Always use the correct techniques for transferring residents. Use a gait belt (transfer belt) when it is ordered. Use lift sheets when moving residents in bed to prevent skin tears from friction.

Preventing Choking

Aspiration is the accidental entry of food or a foreign object into the trachea (windpipe). This causes the resident to choke. Because swallowing becomes less efficient as people age, choking occurs more often in the elderly. Residents with dementia have an increased risk of choking. To prevent incidents of choking or aspiration:

1. Be aware of residents who have problems with swallowing. Follow all instructions for giving feeding assistance to these residents.
   - Cut food into small pieces.
   - Feed slowly.
   - Offer fluids carefully between solid foods.
   - If the resident has had a stroke, place the food in the unaffected side of the mouth.
   - Make sure dentures fit well.

2. Place residents upright in good position before meals. Have them remain in this position for at least 30 minutes after eating.

3. At the end of the meal, give oral care to residents who are known to keep food in their mouths. Food may remain in the mouth for several minutes after a meal and be accidentally aspirated if the resident coughs.

4. Monitor disoriented residents for placing nonedible items in their mouths. Remove such items from the environment.

5. Know how to administer the procedure for obstructed airway (see Lesson 9).

WHEELCHAIR SAFETY

Many residents can propel their own wheelchairs. This increases their independence and allows them to move from one part of the facility to another. Whether a resident can propel a wheelchair or a care provider does it, safety measures must be followed.

1. Place the casters (smaller front wheels) in forward position for balance and stability.
   - To do this, go forward and then back up so the casters swing to the forward position.

- Remind the resident to keep the wheelchair locked when it is not moving and when the resident wishes to get up or sit down.
- The footrests must be lifted out of the way when the resident is getting in or out of the wheelchair. Footrests are usually removed if the resident can propel the wheelchair independently with his or her feet.

2. It is not safe for the resident in a wheelchair to attempt to pick up an object from the floor. If the resident has a reaching aid or "grabber," then small items can be picked up. The wheelchair should be moved next to the object to be picked up and the small front wheels turned forward and the large wheels locked. The resident should not attempt to pick up an item using a reaching aid by leaning over and reaching between the knees. If the resident does not have a reaching aid, the resident should be instructed to ask for assistance in picking up an object from the floor.

3. A wheelchair should never be used as a seat in a motor vehicle unless the vehicle is equipped for wheelchairs.

Procedures for manipulating curbs, ramps, and steps are not generally needed in long-term care facilities because the facilities are designed for wheelchair use. However, you must be instructed in these procedures if you will be expected to perform them.

FIRE SAFETY

Three things are needed to start a fire: heat, fuel, and oxygen (Figure 8-16). Every staff member must know and practice the fire and evacuation procedures for the facility.

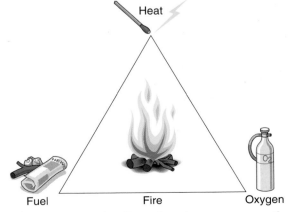

FIGURE 8-16 The fire triangle represents the elements needed for combustion (burning).

1. You must know:
   - The facility fire procedure
   - Evacuation routes
   - Locations of extinguishers, fire alarms (call boxes), fire doors, and fire escapes
   - How to use fire extinguishers
2. Participate in facility fire drills.
3. Be alert to fire hazards and report:
   - Frayed electrical wires
   - Overloaded circuits
   - Improperly grounded plugs
   - Accumulated clutter
   - Inadequate steps to prevent fire during oxygen therapy
   - Uncontrolled smoking
   - Matches and cigarette lighters
   - Unsafe smoking habits of staff, residents, or visitors
   - Oily rags and paint rags
4. Remember the *RACE* steps if fire occurs (Figure 8-17):
   - *Remove* all residents, staff, and other people in the immediate vicinity of the fire.
   - *Activate* the alarm and notify other staff members that a fire exists.
   - *Contain* the fire and smoke by closing all doors in the area.
   - *Extinguish* the fire, if it is very small, or allow fire department to extinguish fire.
5. Be sure that you know evacuation procedures:
   - Read evacuation plan.
   - Know the whereabouts of residents in your care.
   - Know the method of transport for residents in your care.
   - Know emergency exit routes.

Safety in the long-term care facility is the responsibility of all staff members. Teamwork prevents injuries to employees and residents.

Fire Extinguishers

There are many different types of fire extinguishers. Each is used for a different type of fire:

- Type A extinguishers are filled with water and are used to put out paper and wood fires.
- Type B extinguishers are used for grease and oil fires.
- Type C extinguishers are used for electrical fires.
- Extinguishers marked ABC may be used on all three types of fires.

It is important that you learn:

- The location of the extinguishers
- The type of fire for which they are used
- How to use them properly. Always carefully follow the manufacturer's instructions for the use of a fire extinguisher.

Many emergency situations require rapid and effective responses from the staff. Tornadoes, hurricanes, earthquakes, floods, and bomb threats are examples of disasters that are possibilities in various parts of the country. Each facility should have its own procedures for dealing with these emergencies. You should become familiar with the procedures as quickly as possible.

FIGURE 8-17 Remember the sequence of critical actions in case of a fire.

R	Remove resident
A	Activate alarm
C	Contain fire
E	Extinguish (put out) fire

LESSON SYNTHESIS: Putting It All Together

*Y*ou have just completed this lesson. Now go back and review the *Clinical Focus. Try to see how the Clinical Focus relates to the concepts presented in the lesson. Then answer the following questions.*

1. Why are residents in long-term care particularly at risk for injury due to accidents such as falls?

2. Why are fire drills carried out routinely in long-term care facilities?

3. Explain how the principles of safety applied to resident care also apply to the protection of the nursing assistant.

4. What actions can the nursing assistant take to avoid the need for restraints?

REVIEW

A. Select the one best answer for each of the following.

1. The word that means adapting the environment to prevent body injury is
   (A) body mechanics
   (B) incident
   (C) ergonomics
   (D) RACE

2. One principle of body mechanics is to
   (A) bend from the waist when lifting
   (B) keep your feet close together when lifting
   (C) use the muscles of your arms and legs for lifting
   (D) keep the load as far from your body as possible

3. Material Safety Data Sheets (MSDS)
   (A) explain whether you need personal protective equipment when using the product
   (B) require that all spills be cleaned up by housekeeping staff
   (C) describe a system of tagging all chemical agents
   (D) require that hazardous materials be kept in unlocked cabinets

4. Which of the following residents is not at risk for having an incident?
   (A) Mrs. Smith who has frequency of urination because of a bladder infection

   (B) Mr. James who has terminal cancer and is on bed rest
   (C) Mr. Edwards who is ambulatory and has stable diabetes
   (D) Mrs. Porter who has a fractured leg and is in bed in traction

5. Which of the following contributes to unsafe conditions in the facility?
   (A) equipment sitting in the halls
   (B) chemicals in locked cupboards
   (C) allowing residents to smoke only with supervision
   (D) teaching residents how to use assistive devices such as canes and walkers

6. When oxygen is in use, you should
   (A) use woolen blankets on the resident's bed
   (B) allow smoking in the room
   (C) adjust the liter flow
   (D) be sure the oxygen source is secure

7. Which of the following could cause a resident to fall?
   (A) taking residents to the bathroom promptly
   (B) answering call lights promptly
   (C) pulling the side rails up on every resident's bed
   (D) monitoring residents' ambulation abilities

8. Alternatives to the use of physical restraints include
   - (A) always putting up side rails
   - (B) maintaining a stimulating environment
   - (C) preventing residents from wandering
   - (D) maintaining a calm, quiet environment

9. Physical restraints may be used for residents who
   - (A) wander about the building
   - (B) are disoriented
   - (C) refuse to eat or take medication
   - (D) may harm other residents

10. Fire safety in the facility means that
   - (A) only the administrative staff needs to know the evacuation plan
   - (B) knowing how to operate the fire extinguishers is optional
   - (C) every staff member must take part in fire drills
   - (D) the fire alarm is activated by a supervisor only

B. Fill in the blanks by selecting the correct word or phrase from the list.

ABC	laceration
aspiration	mechanical lift
body mechanics	Material Safety
call light	Data Sheets
earthquake	(MSDS)
ergonomics	OSHA
hips and knees	physical restraint
incident	RACE

11. Using your body correctly while you are working is called _____.

12. Basic rules for lifting include bending from the _____ and not from the waist.

13. An unexpected situation that can cause harm to an employee, a resident, or a visitor is called a/an _____.

14. Adapting the environment and using techniques and equipment to prevent body injury is called _____.

15. You should use a _____ when you need to transfer very heavy or dependent residents.

16. All residents must have access to a _____ because it may be the only way they have to summon help.

17. All manufacturers must supply _____ with the hazardous products they sell.

18. The section of the federal government that oversees employee safety is called _____.

19. A cut or break in the skin is called a/an _____.

20. Any device that restricts a resident's movement is called a/an _____.

21. _____ is the accidental entry of food or a foreign object into the trachea (windpipe).

22. The acronym used to remember the sequence of critical actions in case of fire is _____.

23. The type of extinguisher that can be used on all types of fires is the _____ extinguisher.

24. An example of a disaster involving a long-term care facility would be a/an _____.

LESSON 9

Emergencies

Clinical Focus

Think about ways you can help prevent incidents to residents as you study this lesson and meet:

*S*elina Lattini, who lives at the Community Nursing and Rehabilitation Center. Selina had a stroke but is able to walk with a cane. Since the stroke she receives medication for seizures but still occasionally has a seizure. She is disoriented at times and is not always able to remember recent events.

OBJECTIVES

After studying this lesson, you should be able to:

- Define and spell vocabulary words and terms.
- List general measures to take in the event of an emergency.
- Describe the actions to take for the emergencies discussed in the lesson: cardiac arrest, obstructed airway, hemorrhage, falls, seizures, burns, orthopedic injuries, accidental poisoning, and fainting.
- Demonstrate the following:
  - Procedure 1   Assisting the Conscious Person with Obstructed Airway—Heimlich Maneuver
  - Procedure 2   Obstructed Airway, Unconscious Person
  - Procedure 3   One-Rescuer CPR, Adult
  - Procedure 4   Positioning the Resident in the Recovery Position
  - Procedure 5   Hemorrhage
  - Procedure 6   Care of Falling Resident

VOCABULARY

aspiration *(ass-pih-**RAY**-shun)*

aura *(**AWE**-rah)*

automatic external defibrillator *(awe-tuh-**MAT**-ik eks-**TURN**-uhl dee-**FIB**-rill-ay-tur)*

cardiac arrest *(**KAR**-dee ack ah-**REST**)*

cardiopulmonary resuscitation (CPR) *(kar-dee-oh-**PUL**-moh-nair-ee ree-**sus**-ih-**TAY**-shun)*

defibrillation *(dee-**fih**-bryl-**AY**-shun)*

dislocation *(**dis**-loh-**KAY**-shun)*

do not resuscitate (DNR) *(do not ree-**SUS**-ih-tayt)*

emergency *(ee-**MER**-jen-see)*

Emergency Medical Services (EMS) *(ee-**MER**-jen-see **MED**-ih-kul **SIR**-vih-sez)*

VOCABULARY

fracture   (*FRACK-shur*)

Heimlich maneuver   (*HIGHM-lick mah-NEW-ver*)

hemorrhage   (*HEM-or-ij*)

recovery position   (*rih-KUV-er-ee puh-zih-shun*)

respiratory arrest   (*RES-pih-rah-tor-ee ah-REST*)

seizure   (*SEE-zhur*)

sprain   (*sprayn*)

strain   (*strayn*)

syncope   (*SIN-koh-pee*)

GENERAL MEASURES TO FOLLOW FOR EMERGENCIES

An **emergency** is any unexpected situation that requires immediate action. In a true emergency, prompt action is needed to prevent further complications and injuries and to save the victim's life. It is important that you know the signs and symptoms of an emergency and that you are able to initiate immediate actions.

The instructions here are for emergencies in the long-term care facility. In some emergency situations the resident may be transferred by ambulance to a hospital. In other cases, the nurses will handle the emergency and the resident will remain in the facility. The following guidelines are basic actions to follow in any emergency.

On the Job

Emergencies require prompt action. Do not be tempted to overstep your knowledge base or authority.

Guidelines for
Responding to an Emergency

- Always remember the priorities of any emergency—the ABCs:
    - **A**irway (obstructed or unobstructed?)
    - **B**reathing (is the resident breathing?)
    - **C**irculation (is the heart beating, is there hemorrhage?)
- Stay calm. Nothing is accomplished and more problems can result if the people at the scene of an incident become flustered and agitated. If you are calm, you will be a calming influence on the resident.
- Know what to do to summon immediate help; you need to get the nurse to the scene as soon as possible. Stay with the resident and call out for help.
- Stay with the resident until the person in charge gives you permission to leave.
- Know your limitations. Be aware of what procedures nursing assistants are qualified

to perform in an emergency. Never attempt a procedure unless you have received the appropriate training.
- Do not move the resident involved unless the resident is clearly in danger by staying where he or she is.
- Know the procedures to follow for emergencies. Most health care facilities have code names for various emergencies. Know what these are and how to announce a code.
- Know the procedures for activating the **Emergency Medical Services (EMS)** system. In most parts of the country this is done by dialing 911 (Figure 9-1). You will need to give the address and be able to describe what has happened (e.g., a resident was burned or has had cardiac arrest).

(continues)

Guidelines *(continued)*

FIGURE 9-1 In most communities, the number for contacting EMS is 911.

- Keep the person warm. Cover with blankets.
- Do not give the person any fluids or food.
- If the person starts to vomit, turn his or her head to one side to avoid aspiration.
- If the person is conscious, assure him or her that help has been called and is on the way.
- Protect the person's privacy. Keep other residents and visitors away from the scene.

CARDIAC ARREST

A person may stop breathing but still have a heartbeat. This is called **respiratory arrest**. If the situation is not reversed, the heart will stop beating. **Cardiac arrest** is the term used when the heart has stopped beating. When the heart and lungs are not functioning, blood and oxygen are not circulated to the brain and the rest of the body. The person is clinically dead. Permanent damage to the brain and other organs occurs within 4 to 6 minutes. Indications of cardiac arrest are:

- No response from the victim
- No breathing noted
- No pulse

Cardiac Chain of Survival

There are four steps to the cardiac chain of survival, which is designed to assist a victim of cardiac arrest. These steps include:

1. Early recognition of the emergency and use of 911 or the local emergency number
2. Cardiopulmonary resuscitation by a trained person
3. Defibrillation with an automated external defibrillator (AED) by a qualified person
4. Advanced life support by trained professional health personnel

The *first step* in the chain is to identify the resident in cardiac arrest and activate the emergency number (911 or local). The *second step* is cardiopulmonary resuscitation (CPR), a procedure designed to rescue a resident in cardiac arrest. The *third step* in the chain of survival is the use of the automated external defibrillator (AED). If this device is available in the facility, someone must bring it to the room and prepare it for use while step two is being performed. This device has been proven to increase survival. It is operated by someone specially trained in this function.

The instrument is designed to automatically administer an electrical shock to the resident's heart after proper placement of the conduction patches. The machine analyzes the resident's heart rhythm and determines if a shock is needed. The machine will announce "stand clear" if a shock will be delivered. Make sure your body and uniform are not in contact with the resident or equipment attached to the resident's body when the shock is delivered. If the shock is successful, the resident's heart beat is reestablished, although ventilation assistance may be required.

Many communities have recognized the value of placing AEDs in areas where many people gather, such as airports, schools, and sports facilities. This is an important and growing trend.

The *fourth step* is intervention by trained health care personnel, who provide advanced respiratory support, medications, and other services during transport to the hospital.

FIGURE 9-2 CPR is an emergency procedure that is performed only by persons who have completed an approved course.

CPR

Cardiopulmonary resuscitation or **CPR** (Figure 9-2) is a procedure used to maintain blood circulation throughout the body until the EMS can respond to the emergency. *You must never perform CPR unless you have completed an*

On the Job

Be aware that not all attempts at resuscitation are successful, especially if the resident is advanced in years. A resident may die even though vigorous efforts are made to maintain life.

FIGURE 9-3 DNR on a resident's chart means that the resident does not wish to be resuscitated in the event of cardiac arrest.

approved course. A CPR course may be offered by your facility or the local hospital. These courses are usually sponsored through the American Heart Association or the American Red Cross. You must also know whether CPR is to be initiated. Many residents in long-term care facilities are very elderly and have been ill for a long time. They are ready for death. These residents may have indicated that they do not wish to be resuscitated. The physician must write the order "**do not resuscitate (DNR)**" or "no codes" (Figure 9-3). Other residents may indicate that they wish full life support measures in the event of cardiac arrest. For these individuals, the EMS system is activated and CPR is started immediately.

FOREIGN BODY AIRWAY OBSTRUCTION (CHOKING)

NOTE: If time permits, gloves should be worn for emergency procedures. Other personal protective equipment may also be needed.

Aspiration means the accidental entry of food or a foreign object into the trachea (windpipe). This causes the resident to choke. Choking occurs more readily in the elderly because the swallowing mechanism is less efficient. Aspiration can occur during vomiting. When a resident begins to vomit, it is important to:

• Stay with the resident until the vomiting has ceased and you are sure the resident is out of danger.

- If the resident is in bed, turn the head to one side to allow the vomitus to drain out of the mouth instead of going into the trachea. Wipe the mouth as necessary.
- If the resident is in a chair, help the resident flex the neck to allow the vomitus to drain out of the mouth. Wipe the mouth as necessary.

When choking occurs, immediate action is necessary. There are two procedures you must know. The **Heimlich maneuver** is used for persons who are choking but are still conscious. The other procedure is cardiopulmonary resuscitation. You should be instructed and approved for performing these procedures.

THE RECOVERY POSITION

If the resident is unresponsive, but is breathing and has a pulse, he or she should be positioned in the **recovery position** to prevent complications. The recovery position is a modified lateral position. Avoid pressure on the lower arm. The resident's position must be stable, and must avoid pressure on the chest. The airway must remain open. Continue to monitor the resident according to facility policy to ensure that the pulse and respirations remain adequate.

EARLY DEFIBRILLATION

Early **defibrillation** has proven to be critical to survival in cardiac arrest. Defibrillators are placed in various locations in the community and are used by trained rescuers in the event of cardiac arrest. Some studies have shown that the chance of survival doubles when early access to defibrillation is available. The speed

---

PROCEDURE 1

Assisting the Conscious Person with Obstructed Airway— Heimlich Maneuver

1. Ask the resident if he or she can speak.
2. Call for help.
3. Do not attempt to interfere if the resident is coughing or is able to speak.
4. If the resident cannot speak, is not coughing, or shows the universal distress sign (both hands clutching throat) (Figure 9-4), take immediate action. Tell the resident you are going to help.
5. Stand behind the resident. Wrap your arms around the resident's waist. Avoid placing pressure on the resident's ribs with your forearms.
6. Clench your fist. Tuck the tip of your thumb inside your fist. (Figure 9-5).
7. Place your fist, thumb side in, against the resident's abdomen between the navel and the tip of the sternum (Figure 9-6).
8. Grasp your fist with your other hand and press your fist into the resident's abdomen with quick inward and upward thrusts (Figure 9-7).

FIGURE 9-4 Immediate action is required if the resident cannot cough or speak, or if she shows the universal distress sign.

(continues)

PROCEDURE 1 *(continued)*

FIGURE 9-5 Clench your fist, keeping your thumb straight.

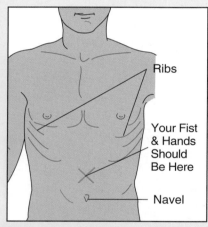

FIGURE 9-6 Place your fist, thumb side in, against the resident's abdomen between the navel and the tip of the sternum.

Ribs

Your Fist & Hands Should Be Here

Navel

FIGURE 9-7 Grasp your fist with your other hand and press your fist into the resident's abdomen with quick inward and upward thrusts.

9. Repeat the abdominal thrusts until the food or foreign object is expelled.

If the object remains in the airway, the resident will eventually lose consciousness. If this happens, you must proceed with the procedure for Obstructed Airway, Unconscious Person.

with which defibrillation is performed is the key to success. Early defibrillation (within 5 minutes) is a high-priority goal in the community. In health care facilities, the goal is to defibrillate within 3 minutes.

Automatic external defibrillators (AEDs) are computerized devices that are simple to learn and operate. The AED is used *only* when a resident is unresponsive, not breathing, and pulseless. When the device is attached to the vic-

tim's chest, the unit determines if an electrical shock is necessary to reestablish or regulate the heartbeat. Several different models are available, and the operating instructions are slightly different for each. The four basic steps to using an AED are:

1. Turn the power on to the unit.
2. Apply the electrode pads to the resident's chest.

PROCEDURE 2 · Obstructed Airway, Unconscious Person

1. If the resident loses consciousness, place her on the back with face up and arms at sides.
2. Open the mouth with tongue-jaw lift method and sweep deeply into the mouth to remove the foreign body, if possible (Figure 9-8). To perform a tongue-jaw lift, grasp the tongue and lower jaw between your thumb and fingers and lift the jaw. To sweep, insert the index finger of your other hand deep into the resident's throat at the base of the tongue. With a hooking motion, attempt to remove the obstruction. Take care not to push the obstruction further into the throat.
3. If the foreign body cannot be removed, open the resident's airway with head-tilt/ chin-lift method. First, extend the neck (Figure 9-9). Then, place your upper hand on the resident's forehead. Apply pressure to tilt the head back. Place the fingertips of your other hand under the bony part of the resident's lower jaw near the chin. Lift the chin while keeping the mouth partially open. Apply the barrier device to the face, covering both the nose and mouth. Seal the device tightly by placing the thumb and index finger of your top hand on the top of the mask. Place the thumb of your other hand on the lower part of the mask. Place the remaining fingers of your hand on the jaw to keep it in position. Sealing the mask is an important step that prevents air from leaking around the sides.

FIGURE 9-8 Open the resident's mouth with tongue-jaw lift method and sweep deeply into the mouth with your finger to remove the foreign body, if possible.

FIGURE 9-9 If the foreign body cannot be removed, open the resident's airway with head-tilt/chin-lift method. Extend the neck first.

(continues)

PROCEDURE 2 *(continued)*

4. Attempt to ventilate through the mask. If the resident's chest does not rise, reposition the head and attempt to ventilate a second time.
5. Straddle the resident's thighs. Place the heel of one hand against the resident's abdomen midway between navel and xiphoid process (bottom of sternum) as in Figure 9-10.
6. Place your second hand on top of first hand (Figure 9-11). Press into abdomen with quick, upward thrusts. Perform five thrusts.
7. If the foreign body is still not expelled, repeat steps 2 through 6 until the foreign body is expelled or until help arrives.

NOTE: If the foreign body is not expelled and breathing does not resume, the resident will probably go into cardiac arrest.

The obstruction must be removed for further emergency procedures to be effective. If the obstruction is removed, immediately evaluate the resident for breathing and pulse. Your facility will have an established procedure for this type of emergency. Follow your facility policy and practices. If permitted, it may be necessary for you to begin the steps of the CPR procedure. To be effective, the resident's upper torso must be on a firm surface during CPR. *This information is presented for your information and understanding. Do not perform this procedure unless you have been properly trained to do so.*

FIGURE 9-10 Straddle the resident's thighs. Place heel of one hand against the resident's abdomen midway between the navel and the xiphoid process.

FIGURE 9-11 Place second hand on top of first hand.

PROCEDURE
3
One-Rescuer CPR, Adult

Supplies needed:
- Disposable exam gloves
- Ventilation device

1. Gently shake or tap the resident and ask, "Are you okay?" If the resident does not respond, you must get help immediately.

2. If other personnel are available in the vicinity, call out for help. If it is not likely that others will hear your call, go immediately to the phone to call for help, according to your facility policy. Return to the resident as quickly as possible. If a second person responds to your call, advise him or her to go for help, according to facility policy. Stay with the resident and perform emergency procedures you are trained and qualified to perform.

3. Position the resident on his back with the torso on a firm surface. Open the airway using the head-tilt/chin-lift procedure. If the dentures are loose, remove them.

4. Place your ear next to the resident's nose and mouth. Look at the resident's chest to see if it is rising and falling. Feel and listen for breathing on your ear. Ineffective, gasping breaths may be present. Do not confuse these with normal respirations. If you are not *confident* that the respirations are adequate, proceed with rescue breathing.

5. If the resident is not breathing, give two slow breaths through the ventilation device. Take a deep breath before each ventilation. Allow time for exhalation between breaths.

6. Locate the carotid pulse on the side of the neck; palpate lightly for 5–10 seconds. If the resident is not breathing, but has a pulse, give one breath every 4 to 5 seconds. Do not perform chest compressions if the resident has a pulse. If you are not *confident* that the pulse is present, proceed to the next step.

7. If you cannot feel the pulse, locate the "landmark" on the tip of the sternum. Move your fingers up the lower margins of the ribs. The landmark, or xiphoid process, is where the margins meet, in the center of the chest. Hold your index and middle fingers over the xiphoid process. This is a key step to prevent injury.

8. Place the heel of the opposite hand on the chest next to your fingers. Place the landmark hand on top of the other hand, interlacing the fingers. Lock your elbows.

9. Using the heels of your hands, press the sternum straight down 1½ to 2 inches at an approximate rate of 100 compressions a minute. Press only on the sternum. Avoid pressure on the ribs with your fingers. Keep your fingers interlaced and slightly elevated. Compressions should be smooth and even. Completely release pressure to allow the heart to refill with blood at the end of each compression. However, your hands must remain in contact with the chest.

10. At the end of each 15 compressions, deliver two full breaths.

11. Upon completion of 4 cycles of 15 compressions and 2 ventilations, reevaluate the resident for return of the carotid pulse. If present, monitor for spontaneous breathing. If absent, continue. If present, perform rescue breathing, using the airway adjunct, once every 5 seconds.

PROCEDURE 4 — Positioning the Resident in the Recovery Position

1. Kneel beside the resident and straighten the legs.
2. Place the arm nearest you above the resident's head with the palm up and the elbow bent slightly.
3. Position the opposite arm across the chest.
4. Place your lower hand on the resident's thigh on the far side of the body. Pull the thigh up slightly, closer to the center of the resident's body.
5. Place your upper hand on the resident's shoulder on the opposite side of the body.
6. With one hand on the thigh and the other on the shoulder, roll the resident on the side facing you.
7. Move the resident's upper hand close to the cheek, bending the elbow. This hand should be close to the face, but not under the body. Adjust the upper body so that the hip and knee are at right angles.
8. Tilt the resident's head back slightly to keep the airway open. Now place the upper hand, palm facing down, under the cheek to maintain the head position.
9. Continue to monitor the resident closely for adequate breathing.

3. All rescuers stand back to allow the machine to analyze the heart rhythm.
4. All rescuers continue to stand back; the operator of the unit presses the shock button and/or follows the unit's instructions, which are usually audible through a voice-synthesized message.

If your facility purchases an AED, employees will be trained in its use. Although the AED is simple to operate, only those who are properly trained may use it. CPR and use of the AED are included in basic life support classes for health care professionals.

HEMORRHAGE

Hemorrhage is the rapid loss of a large amount of blood from the body. Death will occur if the hemorrhage is not stopped. Hemorrhage may be internal or external. Internal hemorrhage is suspected when the resident's:

- Pulse becomes weak, rapid, and irregular
- Blood pressure is falling
- Skin is dusky gray, cold, and clammy

Call the nurse immediately if these signs are present. Internal hemorrhage requires immediate action by the physician.

External hemorrhage is more obvious and is noted by the obvious loss of blood. Bleeding may be from an artery or from a vein. Blood coming from an artery will spurt and be bright red. A large amount of blood can be lost in a very short time from an artery. Blood coming from a vein will ooze out and have a bluish tinge.

RESIDENT FALLS

Lesson 8 described measures for preventing falls. If a resident falls, you must protect both the resident and yourself.

SEIZURES

A **seizure** or convulsion involves sudden, involuntary contractions of a group of muscles. A disturbance in consciousness and changes in behavior occur. The two categories of seizures are:

- Partial seizure
  - The seizures begin in one part of the body. They may be considered simple (without disturbance in consciousness) or complex (with impairment of consciousness).

PROCEDURE 5

Hemorrhage

Gloves should be readily available throughout the facility. Apply gloves before contacting blood.

1. Call for help.
2. Find out where the bleeding area is.
3. Apply continuous, firm, direct pressure over the bleeding area with a pad or towel or whatever is available (Figure 9-12). Elevate the area (arm or leg) above the level of the heart, if possible.
4. If seepage occurs, increase the padding and the pressure. Do not remove the saturated dressings.
5. If bleeding continues, maintain firm, direct pressure over the site, continue to elevate the extremity, and apply pressure to pulse points proximal to the injury (Figure 9-13). NEVER USE A TOURNIQUET.
6. Keep the resident warm and quiet until help arrives.

FIGURE 9-12 Apply continuous, firm, direct pressure over the bleeding area.

Temporal Artery

Temporal Artery

Carotid Artery

Carotid Artery

Brachial Artery

Brachial Artery

Radial Artery

Radial Artery

Femoral Artery

Femoral Artery

Popliteal Artery (Behind the Knee)

Popliteal Artery (Behind the Knee)

Dorsalis Pedis Artery (Pedal Pulse)

Dorsalis Pedis Artery (Pedal Pulse)

FIGURE 9-13 If bleeding continues, maintain direct pressure, continue to elevate the extremity, and apply pressure to pulse points proximal to the injury.

PROCEDURE
6

Care of Falling Resident

1. Keep your back straight, bend from the hips and knees, and maintain a broad base of support as you assist the falling resident.
2. Ease the resident to the floor, using your leg to let the person slide down gently to the floor. Protect the resident's head.
3. As you ease the resident to the floor, bend your knees and go down with the resident (Figure 9-14).
4. Call for help. *Do not attempt to move the resident until the nurse or physician has examined the resident and has given you instructions.*
5. Assist in returning the resident to bed or chair. Be sure you have adequate help.
6. Carry out procedure completion actions.
7. Record according to facility policy.

FIGURE 9-14 Ease the resident to the floor as you bend your knees and go down with the resident.

- Generalized seizure
  - Generalized seizures involve the entire body (Figures 9-15A and B).

Adult-onset seizures may occur after a brain injury, along with a brain tumor, after a stroke, and along with dementia.

Side rails on the bed should be padded if the resident may have a seizure.

Emergency Treatment for Seizures

Seizures can occur suddenly and without warning. Some people have an aura before a seizure. An **aura** is a sensory disturbance; the person may hear a noise, smell something, or see a certain pattern. If the resident is aware of this, he or she may have time to get to a chair or to lie down. When a seizure occurs:

1. Do not leave the resident alone. Call for help.
2. Do not restrain movements. Do not force anything into the resident's mouth. Provide privacy and keep onlookers away.
3. Protect the resident from injury. Move any objects that might cause injury.
4. Place a small pillow, folded towel, or blanket under the resident's head if the resident is on the floor.
5. Loosen clothing around the resident's head.
6. Maintain open airway. Turn the resident's head to the side, if possible.
7. Observe the seizure. Include time started and stopped and what occurred during the seizure. Most seizures stop on their own.
8. After movements subside, turn the resident to the recovery position so fluid or vomitus can drain freely from mouth.
9. Incontinence is common during or after a seizure. Provide perineal care and assist the resident to apply clean clothing.
10. Allow the resident to rest.
11. Check for breathing and pulse. Initiate appropriate actions if either is absent.
12. Comfort and reassure the resident and assist him or her in becoming reoriented.
13. Allow the resident to sleep after seizure has subsided. Position the resident on the side and observe closely while resident sleeps.

FIGURE 9-15   Generalized seizures involve the entire body. Note that side rails should be padded and up during a seizure. The side rails are down in the figure for clarity of the view. A. Rigid posturing. B. Uncontrolled movements.

BURNS

Burns result in loss of skin integrity and may be caused by hot liquids or other substances, chemicals, or radiation. There is a high risk of infection with any burn. Burns may occur in the long-term care facility from:

- Spilling hot coffee, tea, or soup
- Hot water
- Careless use of smoking materials

Burns are classified as partial thickness or full thickness depending on the degree of injury. Partial thickness burns are:

- First-degree burns—involve only the top layer (epidermis) of skin. There is redness, temporary swelling and pain. There is usually no permanent scarring.
- Second-degree burns—involve both epidermis and dermis. The skin color may vary from pink or red to white or tan. Blistering, pain, and some scarring occur.
- Third-degree burns (also called full thickness burns)—involve epidermis, dermis, and subcutaneous tissue. The tissue is bright red to tan and brown. There may be no pain initially because nerve endings have been destroyed. Later, pain and scarring will result.

Emergency Treatment for Burns

1. Call the nurse immediately.
2. If the resident's clothing is on fire, use a coat or blanket to smother the flames.
3. Cool water may be applied to lower the skin temperature and stop further tissue damage. Remove wet clothing. (Follow the nurse's instructions.)
4. Second-degree burns may require treatment at the hospital emergency room. Third-degree

burns will probably require hospitalization for special treatment.

ORTHOPEDIC INJURIES

Orthopedic injuries include injuries to bones, joints, muscles, and ligaments. These include fractures, sprains, strains, and dislocations.

Treatment for Orthopedic Injuries

A **fracture** is a break in a bone. If you suspect a resident has suffered a fracture:

- Stay with the resident.
- Do not attempt to move the resident.
- Call the nurse immediately.

If a fracture is suspected, the EMS will be called and the resident will be transported by ambulance to the hospital for x-rays. If a fracture is present, the physician will put a cast on the affected extremity or place the resident in traction or do surgery. (This is explained further in Lesson 28.)

A **sprain** is an injury to a ligament caused by sudden overstretching. A sprained ankle may occur, for example, if a person falls and turns the ankle quickly while falling. Swelling may be noted shortly afterward.

A **strain** is excessive stretching of a muscle resulting in pain and swelling of the muscle. You may strain the muscles in your back if you use incorrect lifting and moving techniques.

A **dislocation** occurs in a joint, when one bone is displaced from the other bone. This can occur in a paralyzed arm that is allowed to hang without support. The weight of the arm pulls the upper arm bone out of position in the shoulder joint. A dislocation can also be caused by improperly lifting the resident under the arms.

If you suspect that a resident has suffered a sprain, strain, or dislocation:

- Notify the nurse at once.

You may be instructed to:

- Elevate the injured extremity.
- Apply ice packs to the area. (See Lesson 21 for instructions on application of ice packs.)

After 24 hours, you may be instructed to apply warm packs to the area.

ACCIDENTAL POISONING

Immediate attention is needed if a resident is the victim of accidental poisoning. All potentially harmful substances must be kept in locked cupboards. However, a confused resident may obtain and ingest a harmful substance. If you suspect that this has happened:

- Call the nurse immediately.
- Try to determine what the resident has taken; save the container.
- The nurse may administer a substance that will cause vomiting. (Not all ingested poisons can be safely removed from the resident's body by vomiting.)
- Know where to find the telephone number for the regional poison control center.
- The resident may need to be transported to a hospital by ambulance.

FAINTING

Fainting (**syncope**) is a loss of consciousness due to temporary insufficient blood flow to the brain. The attack comes on gradually with lightheadedness, perspiring, and blurred vision. Fainting can occur in otherwise healthy people and may be related to emotional shock or standing in one place for a long time. Residents experiencing these symptoms should sit down in a chair, bend forward, and lower the head between the knees, or lie down before they lose consciousness. Elevate the legs so there is adequate blood flow to the brain. If they faint and fall, allow them to lie still unless they are in immediate danger. Elevate feet and legs 10–12 inches to encourage blood flow back to the brain. Recovery is usually prompt and without complications or aftereffects. Call for the nurse immediately. A person who has fainted should lie down and rest for several minutes. Provide reassurance and emotional support.

LESSON SYNTHESIS: Putting It All Together

*Y*ou have just completed this lesson. Now go back and review the *Clinical Focus. Try to see how the Clinical Focus relates to the concepts presented in the lesson. Then answer the following questions.*

1. Mrs. Lattini is at high risk for falling. Her use of a cane is one risk factor. What observations should you make in regard to ambulation with a cane?

2. What steps can you take in an effort to prevent Mrs. Lattini from falling?

3. Describe what you would do in the event that Mrs. Lattini falls.

4. What can you do as a nursing assistant to ensure that you will know how to respond in the event of an emergency?

REVIEW

A. Select the one best answer for each of the following.

1. If an emergency occurs in the long-term care facility, you should
   (A) leave the resident where he or she is and get the nurse as quickly as possible
   (B) do as much as you can and then call for the nurse
   (C) call the EMS right away
   (D) know your limitations

2. Indications of cardiac arrest include
   (A) no pulse
   (B) rapid breathing
   (C) confusion
   (D) incontinence

3. When a resident makes an advance directive indicating that the resident does not wish to be resuscitated, the physician writes the order referred to as
   (A) CPR
   (B) ABC
   (C) DNR
   (D) EMS

4. The Heimlich maneuver should be initiated when the resident
   (A) is coughing
   (B) suffers cardiac arrest
   (C) vomits
   (D) cannot speak, is not coughing, and is conscious, or clutches the throat

5. If a resident is hemorrhaging externally, you should first
   (A) apply pressure directly over the wound
   (B) apply pressure over the closest pressure points
   (C) apply a tourniquet
   (D) run for help

6. When a resident falls, you should
   (A) try to hold the resident in an upright position
   (B) let go of the resident immediately to avoid injuring yourself
   (C) ease the resident to the floor, protecting the resident's head
   (D) scream for help

7. If a resident has a seizure, you should first
   (A) place something between the resident's teeth
   (B) begin CPR
   (C) restrain the resident's arms and legs
   (D) protect the resident from injury and allow the seizure to run its course

8. If a resident suffers a burn from hot coffee, the nurse may instruct you to
   (A) apply cool water to the area
   (B) apply butter or some other greasy substance
   (C) hold ice cubes against the area
   (D) apply a warm water bottle

B. Answer each statement true (T) or false (F).

9. T   F   The first thing to consider in an emergency are the ABCs.

10. T   F   Cardiopulmonary resuscitation is always administered when a resident has cardiac arrest.

11. T   F   If applying direct pressure to hemorrhage is not successful, you should apply a tourniquet.

12. T   F   It is common for incontinence to occur during or after a seizure.

13. T   F   If a resident ingests a poisonous substance, you should immediately force the resident to vomit.

14. T   F   You should not move a resident who has fallen until the nurse has examined the resident and given instructions.

15. T   F   Recovery from fainting is usually quick and without complications.

16. T   F   When a person is in cardiac arrest, the heart continues to beat although respirations cease.

17. T   F   The chain of survival refers to the immediate care given to assist a person in cardiac arrest.

18. T   F   The first step in the chain of survival is to use the AED.

19. T   F   When providing CPR, chest compressions are given at a rate of 100 per minute.

20. T   F   If a resident falls you must protect both the resident and yourself.

LESSON 10

Infection

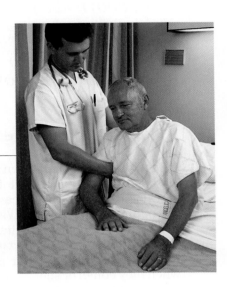

Clinical Focus

Think about the causes of infections as you study this lesson and meet:

*F*ranklin Dwyer, who is 66. He is HIV positive and has a history of repeated pneumonia. He also had hepatitis A and tuberculosis in his youth. Each infection was treated aggressively with medication. Now Mr. Dwyer's CD4 count has dropped significantly and he has been diagnosed with AIDS.

OBJECTIVES

After studying this lesson, you should be able to:

- Define and spell vocabulary words and terms.
- Describe how infections can be introduced to the long-term care facility.
- Recognize the causes of several important infectious diseases.
- List the ways that infectious diseases are spread.
- List the parts of the chain of infection.
- List natural body defenses against infections.
- Name five serious infectious diseases.
- Explain why residents are at risk for infections.

VOCABULARY

antibiotic *(an-tih-buy-OT-ick)*

antibody *(AN-tih-bah-dee)*

antigen *(AN-ti-jen)*

bacteremia *(back-ter-EE-mee-ah)*

carrier *(KAIR-ee-er)*

contagious *(kon-TAY-jus)*

culture and sensitivity *(KUL-tyour and sen-sih-TIV-ih-tee)*

flora *(FLOOR-ah)*

fomite *(FOH-myt)*

hemoptysis *(he-MOP-tih-sis)*

hepatitis *(hep-ah-TYE-tis)*

human immunodeficiency virus (HIV) *(HYOU-man im-MYOUN-oh-dih-fish-en-see VYE-rus)*

immunity *(im-MYOUN-ih-tee)*

immunization *(IM-myou-nigh-zay-shun)*

immunosuppression *(im-myoun-oh-suh-PREH-shun)*

infection *(in-FECK-shun)*

VOCABULARY

inflammation   (*in-flah-MAY-shun*)

methicillin-resistant *Staphylococcus aureus* (MRSA)   (*meth-ih-SILL-in ree-SIS-tant staff-ill-oh-KOCK-us AWE-ree-us*)

microbe   (*MY-krohb*)

NIOSH-approved respirator   (*NEYE-osh ah-PROOVD RES-pir-ay-tor*)

nosocomial infection   (*noh-soh-KOH-mee-al in-FECK-shun*)

pathogen   (*PATH-oh-jen*)

seropositive   (*see-roh-POZ-ih-tiv*)

transmission   (*trans-MISH-un*)

tubercle   (*TOO-ber-kul*)

tuberculosis disease   (*too-ber-kyou-LOH-sis dih-ZEEZ*)

tuberculosis infection   (*too-ber-kyou-LOH-sis in-FECK-shun*)

vaccine   (*VACK-seen*)

vancomycin-resistant enterococci (VRE)   (*van-koh-MY-sin ree-SIS-tant en-ter-oh-KOCK-ee*)

INFECTIOUS DISEASE

Infections can occur when disease-producing organisms enter the body. Infections that occur in residents who are in the care facility are called **nosocomial infections**. Visitors, staff members, and residents can introduce infections through the spread of **microbes** (germs). Visitors and staff can transfer germs to residents when they cough or sneeze or even touch the resident with improperly washed hands. This is one reason why it is so important to carry out proper handwashing techniques and to discourage visiting when infections are present.

MICROBES

Some microbes are useful and necessary to life. For example, the lower digestive tract is filled with bacteria that help in the breakdown of food and the elimination of feces. Other microbes cause disease and are called **pathogens**. They are tiny forms of life that can only be seen with a microscope. Some of the most common pathogens are:

- Bacteria
- Viruses
- Fungi (yeast and molds)
- Parasites

On the Job

Only you and your conscience will ever know if you are the one who caused contamination because you did not wash your hands.

Bacteria

There are many forms of bacteria (Figure 10-1). They can cause infections in the skin, respiratory tract, urinary tract, and bloodstream. Boils and strep throat are common bacterial infections.

Antibiotics are often effective against bacterial infections. However, over the years, some bacteria, such as *Staphylococcus aureus*, have become very resistant to most antibiotics.

Viruses

Viruses are smaller than bacteria. Viruses cause the common cold, flu, and many childhood diseases such as mumps, chickenpox, measles, and

FIGURE 10-1 This is the way the organisms (bacteria) look under the microscope. This organism causes scarlet fever and strep sore throat. (Courtesy of the Centers for Disease Control and Prevention, Atlanta, GA)

FIGURE 10-2   The white patches on the tongue are the result of a yeast (fungus) infection. This condition is called thrush.

polio. Viruses also cause some forms of pneumonia, herpes simplex, herpes zoster (shingles), acquired immune deficiency syndrome (AIDS), and hepatitis. Antibiotics are not effective in controlling infections caused by viruses.

Fungi

Fungi cause skin and mucous membrane infections like yeast vaginitis, athlete's foot, ringworm, and thrush (Figure 10-2).

Parasites

Infections due to parasites are more rare but can affect the blood, lungs, and intestines when they occur.

Parasites are organisms that live within or upon another organism (the host). Examples of parasites are worms that live in the digestive tract and fleas, lice, mites, and ticks that live on the outer surface of the host.

THE CHAIN OF INFECTION

Infections occur when certain conditions are met. These conditions are called the *chain of infection* (Figure 10-3) and include:

- Causative agent or microbe—pathogen germ that causes the disease
- Source—human body in which the microbe can live
- Portal of exit—manner in which the microbe leaves the body
- Method of transmission—manner in which the microbe is carried to another person. Trans-

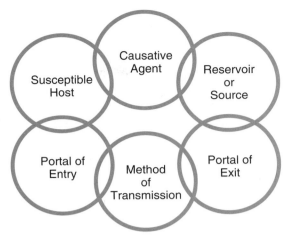

FIGURE 10-3   The chain of infection

mission may be from person to person or from insects and animals to people.
- Portal of entry—manner in which the microbe enters another person
- Susceptible host—a person who will become ill from the entry of microbes into the body

Microbes cause disease by entering the body through a portal of entry. They spread disease by leaving the body through a portal of exit and being transmitted to another person. They enter that person's body and can again cause disease.

Microbes enter and leave the body through body openings such as:

- Eyes, ears, nose, or mouth
- Breaks in the skin
- Penis, vagina, urinary meatus (bladder opening), or rectum

Transmission (spread) of infectious organisms may occur in one of three ways (Figure 10-4):

- Airborne transmission. Small particles remain suspended in the air and move with air currents or become trapped in dust, which is also carried in air currents. The resident breathes in the pathogens carried in this manner.
- Droplet transmission. Droplets are moist particles from coughing, sneezing, or talking. Pathogens are transmitted into the air with the droplets. Droplets usually travel only 3 feet from the source.
- Contact transmission. Direct contact occurs by touching the source of the pathogens. Indirect contact occurs when a person touches an item contaminated with pathogens, such as soiled linen or environmental surfaces. These items are known as **fomites**.

Not all organisms are transmitted in the same way and some organisms may be transmitted in

FIGURE 10-4 Ways in which microbes are spread from one person to another

Airborne Transmission

- Pathogens carried by moisture or dust particles in air; can be carried long distances

Droplet Transmission
Droplet Spread Within Approximately 3 Feet (No Personal Contact) of Infected Person by:

- Coughing
- Sneezing
- Talking
- Laughing
- Singing

Contact Transmission
Direct Contact with Infected Person:

- Touching
- Sexual contact
- Blood
- Body fluids (drainage, urine, feces, sputum, saliva, vomitus)

Indirect Contact with Infected Person:

- Clothing
- Dressings
- Equipment used in care and treatment
- Bed linens
- Personal belongings
- Specimen containers
- Instruments used in treatment
- Food
- Water

Vectors
Pathogens can also be carried by insects and animals and passed to humans. These carriers are called vectors.

more than one way. Figure 10-5 shows how health care providers can interrupt the chain of infection at various points and thus prevent the spread of infection.

Types of Infections

Infections can be:

- Local (confined to one area)—such as a boil or skin abscess
- Generalized—such as pneumonia (in the lungs)
- Systemic—widespread through the bloodstream (**bacteremia**)

People who have pathogens in their bodies, but do not show signs of disease, are called **carriers**. Carriers can transmit diseases to others. The pathogens in their bodies are not harmful to the carriers, but they may be harmful to other people.

BODY FLORA

Different microbes live on our body surfaces. These microbes are called the normal body **flora**. The flora are not the same in all body areas. For example, the organisms making up the flora of the intestinal tract are different from those of the respiratory tract. Healthy individuals live in harmony with the normal body flora. However, the balance may be disturbed by:

- Pathogenic organisms
- Normal flora organisms that become pathogenic
- Organisms from one flora that are transferred into a different body flora
- Drugs such as antibiotics that upset the normal balance of organisms within a flora, allowing one group to flourish

You can help avoid infections in yourself by:

- Eating a healthy diet
- Getting an adequate amount of sleep daily
- Keeping your body clean and living in a clean environment
- Avoiding unhealthy habits such as smoking, drinking alcohol, or using drugs
- Learning how to cope with stress
- Washing your hands
- Following standard precautions faithfully

NATURAL BODY DEFENSES AGAINST DISEASE

Natural body defenses that can help prevent infectious diseases include:

- Tears
- Mucous membranes (the lining) of the respiratory, reproductive, and genitourinary tracts
- Intact skin
- Hydrochloric acid in the stomach
- Hair in the nose and eyelashes
- White blood cells (leukocytes) that multiply and attempt to destroy pathogenic microbes in the body
- Enzymes in saliva

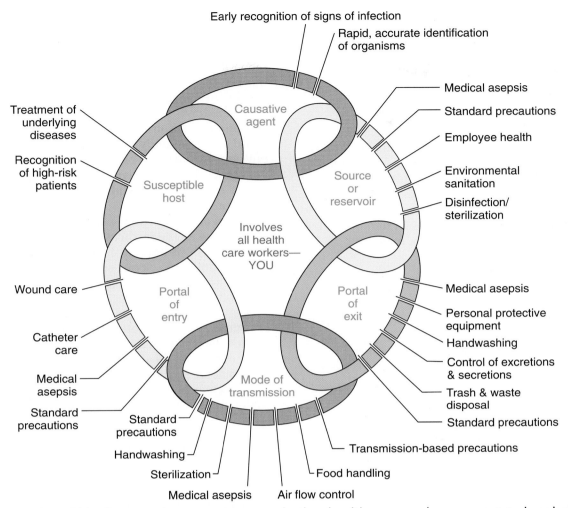

Early recognition of signs of infection

Rapid, accurate identification of organisms

Treatment of underlying diseases

Recognition of high-risk patients

Medical asepsis

Standard precautions

Employee health

Environmental sanitation

Disinfection/ sterilization

Causative agent

Susceptible host

Source or reservoir

Involves all health care workers— YOU

Portal of entry

Portal of exit

Mode of transmission

Wound care

Catheter care

Medical asepsis

Standard precautions

Standard precautions

Handwashing

Sterilization

Medical asepsis

Air flow control

Food handling

Transmission-based precautions

Standard precautions

Trash & waste disposal

Control of excretions & secretions

Handwashing

Personal protective equipment

Medical asepsis

FIGURE 10-5 This diagram shows ways you and other health care workers can act to break the chain of infection and block the transmission of disease.

- Antibodies that develop in the blood after a person has had an infectious disease
- **Inflammation**—a process that brings blood and white blood cells to the area of infection; a skin infection, for example, generally becomes swollen, hot, and painful, signs that inflammation is occurring (Figure 10-6).
- Temperature—an elevated temperature is believed to increase the body's ability to fight infection.

IMMUNITY

Immunity is the ability to fight off disease caused by microbes. A pathogenic microbe that enters the body is an **antigen**. In response to this, the blood develops substances called **antibodies**.

FIGURE 10-6 Redness, swelling, heat, pain, and loss of function are signs of the inflammatory process.

These antibodies provide immunity to the disease caused by that particular antigen. For example, if an individual has antigens in the bloodstream from having had measles, he or she will form antibodies in the blood that prevent the occurrence of measles a second time.

Immunosuppression

Immunosuppression occurs when the body's immune system is inadequate and fails to respond to the challenge of infectious disease organisms that it normally would fight successfully. The individual becomes more likely to develop a variety of infections. A number of factors can lead to this condition, including:

- Diseases such as leukemia
- Advanced age
- Frailty
- Drug therapy
- Infection with human immunodeficiency virus (HIV)
- Injury or removal of the spleen
- Radiation therapy

IMMUNIZATIONS

Artificial defenses called **immunizations** protect against specific pathogens. Immunization is provided by **vaccines**. These are artificial or weakened antigens that help the body develop protective antibodies before the need arises. Vaccines are available to prevent most childhood diseases such as measles, rubella (German measles), mumps, polio, diphtheria, chickenpox, whooping cough, and tetanus. Pneumonia vaccine and influenza vaccine are frequently given to elderly people. Health workers who have direct contact with residents are advised to take hepatitis B vaccine. Federal legislation requires that employers provide this vaccine without charge to employees who are considered at risk.

SERIOUS INFECTIONS IN HEALTH CARE FACILITIES

Serious bacterial and viral infections are increasing in health care facilities as well as in the general public. Elderly and frail people are particularly susceptible to infectious diseases, as are the very young and those with autoimmune disease or compromised (poorly functioning) immune systems.

BACTERIAL INFECTIONS

Bacteria are often the cause of serious skin, respiratory, urinary, and gastrointestinal infections in residents. If the physician suspects that a resident has a bacterial infection, a **culture and sensitivity** test may be ordered. This test can be done on urine, drainage from a wound, blood, or other body fluid. The culture tells the physician what type of microbe is causing the infection. The sensitivity tells the physician which **antibiotic** should be used to treat the infection.

When an antibiotic is prescribed, it is important to take all the medication prescribed for the stated length of time. If the person stops taking the antibiotic too soon, some of the microbes may remain and develop a resistance to the antibiotic.

Certain infectious microbes have become resistant to the antibiotics most commonly used against them. This is a serious problem in controlling infections in health care facilities. The antibiotics that are still effective often are more expensive and may have serious side effects compared to the previously preferred antibiotics. It is possible that, in time, these infectious microbes may also become resistant to these antibiotics.

MRSA and VRE

Two groups of organisms have become resistant to two powerful antibiotics, methicillin and vancomycin. Both organisms are part of the normal flora of the human body. These organisms are:

- **Methicillin-resistant *Staphylococcus aureus* (MRSA)**
  Staphylococci are normally found on skin and mucous membranes. MRSA is now found almost everywhere (endemic) in health care facilities. It can be spread by direct or indirect contact. It causes life-threatening infections involving the respiratory and urinary systems and the skin. MRSA is most often spread through direct contact with the hands of health care providers. The infection control precautions used depend on the type of tissue infection. For example, standard precautions are required if there is a skin infection. Figure 10-7 shows *Staphylococcus aureus* organisms.
- **Vancomycin-resistant enterococci (VRE)**
  Enterococci are found in the gastrointestinal tract. They are a major cause of nosocomial infections in health care facilities. Most strains are highly resistant to many antibiotics. VRE is spread directly from the resident or caregiver

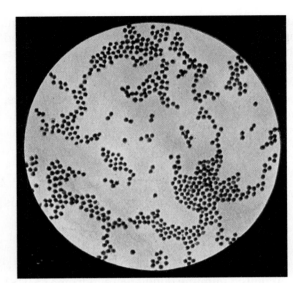

FIGURE 10-7 Methicillin-resistant *Staphylococcus aureus* (MRSA) has developed a resistance to the antibiotic of choice for treating the infection. (Courtesy of the Centers for Disease Control and Prevention, Atlanta, GA)

to another resident. It may also be spread from contaminated surfaces or objects such as side rails or bed linens. Standard precautions are required. Newer strains are resistant to vancomycin.

Other Bacterial Infective Agents

Serious infections are also caused by the following types of bacteria:

- *Streptococcus pyogenes* (*streptococcus A*)—this pathogen is known as the "flesh-eating" bacterium. This organism is frequently involved in soft tissue destruction because it produces powerful toxins and enzymes. Without early diagnosis, treatment to remove the diseased tissue, and aggressive treatment with antibiotics, the mortality rate can be very high.
- *Pseudomonas aeruginosa*—this organism is found in water and on other environmental surfaces. It causes urinary tract infections.
- *Escherichia coli*—bacterium commonly found in the intestinal tract where it is normally nonpathogenic. Outside the intestinal tract, however, it can cause urinary tract infections or infections in pressure ulcers. There are many strains of *E. coli*. One strain produces powerful toxins that can cause severe, bloody diarrhea and kidney complications. The organisms can live in the intestines of healthy cattle. Meat can become contaminated during the slaughtering process and when it is ground.

Udders of cows can become contaminated and the organisms transferred through unpasteurized milk. Thorough cooking of ground meat, drinking only pasteurized milk, and careful handwashing are important steps in controlling this foodborne disease.

- Salmonella—a group of bacteria that cause mild to life-threatening intestinal infections, including "food poisoning"
- *Mycobacterium tuberculosis*—the bacterium that causes tuberculosis
- *Clostridium difficile*—a bacterium that is part of the normal bowel flora but can cause serious diarrhea in residents who are receiving antibiotics. It is common in long-term care facilities. One-third of residents infected with this bacterium die.

Tuberculosis

Prior to 1950 and the development of antibiotics to target tuberculosis, it was a widespread disease with a high fatality rate. The number of cases dropped over the next 30 years. However, from 1985 to 1992, the number of tuberculosis cases once more increased. The increase was due to less public effort to combat the disease and the development of forms of the organism that are resistant to the antibiotics commonly used in treatment. By 1996 the number of cases again began to decline as resistant strains were better identified, diagnostic techniques were improved, and a program of direct observation therapy was introduced. Direct observation involves delivery of the medication to the patient at home, school, or work and watching as it is taken, to ensure compliance with the prescribed drug therapy.

Today more people are at risk for infection, including those who:

- Are HIV positive
- Are infected but fail to take their medication for the full treatment period
- Live in poverty and are malnourished
- Have immigrated to the United States from countries where tuberculosis is still common
- Have inactive tuberculosis but have grown older and experience increased disability

Tuberculosis Infection. **Tuberculosis infection** occurs when the bacterium that causes the disease enters the body. The lungs are the most common site of involvement. The body usually responds to the infection by creating a barrier that prevents the spread of the pathogens to other parts of the body. This barrier is called a **tubercle**. As long as the tubercle remains intact and no other tuberculosis bacteria enter the body, the infection is called inactive or controlled. In this state the person is not **contagious** (capable of passing the infection to others). If the person is immunocompromised, the tubercle may not form and the person develops active tuberculosis disease (primary tuberculosis).

Tuberculosis Disease. **Tuberculosis disease** develops if the tubercle breaks down or more tuberculosis bacteria enter the body. The bacteria multiply, tissue damage increases, and the bacteria may spread to other parts of the body. As the disease progresses, the person will show one or more of the following signs and symptoms:

- Fatigue
- Loss of appetite and weight
- Weakness
- Elevated temperature in the afternoon and evening
- Night sweats
- Spitting up blood **(hemoptysis)**
- Coughing

The person with tuberculosis in the lungs can spread the bacteria to others through droplets in respiratory secretions.

Diagnosis. The presence of tuberculosis bacteria in the body can be shown by:

- A sputum culture—grows the organisms from the person's lungs
- Chest x-rays—show the extent of the disease process in the lungs
- A positive skin test (Mantoux test)—shows the presence of antibodies to the tuberculosis organisms in the body

Health care providers in long-term care must undergo a skin test for tuberculosis before employment. They are then tested regularly (usually every 6–12 months) according to the degree of risk of exposure to ensure that they remain disease-free.

Residents usually are skin tested once a year. Because the immune response may be weaker in the elderly, a two-step procedure of skin testing is recommended for those over 50 years of age. If the first skin test is negative, the test is repeated in 1 to 2 weeks. The second test acts as a "booster" to the test stimulus. A negative response after the second test usually indicates the person is free from infection.

Treatment. A person with tuberculosis is treated with a selected antibiotic or combination of antibiotics. Because many disease organisms have become more resistant to specific drugs, a combination of drugs must be used to control them. Once

antitubercular drug therapy starts, the resident usually becomes noncontagious (cannot spread the disease organism) within 2 to 3 weeks. The therapy, however, continues for 6 months to 2 years. While the resident is contagious, however, airborne precautions, negative pressure ventilators, and **NIOSH-approved respirators** are needed.

VIRAL INFECTIONS

Several viral infections are described in this section:

- Shingles (herpes zoster)
- Influenza
- Hepatitis
- Acquired immune deficiency syndrome (AIDS)

The viral infection herpes venereum is covered in Lesson 27.

Shingles

Shingles (herpes zoster) occurs in people who were infected by the virus that causes chickenpox. Although the person recovered from chickenpox, the organisms did not leave the body. They remained in the body's nervous system in a nonactive state.

Years later, when the person is in a weakened condition, the organisms become active. Painful blister-like lesions develop in the skin along the paths of sensitive nerves. Eventually the lesions heal on their own. They contain infectious organisms and contact and airborne precautions should be used.

Influenza

Influenza (or flu) is caused by a family of viruses. The infection can lead to serious consequences for elderly or frail residents. Each year new types of viruses spread rapidly by way of respiratory secretions from person to person, causing many people to become ill.

Vaccines offer some protection against influenza viruses and are often given to residents in long-term care.

Someone with the flu may experience:

- Malaise (general unwell feeling)
- Chills
- Fever
- Muscle aches and pains
- Coldlike symptoms

In addition to making the person feel ill, the viruses may lower the resident's resistance to other infectious organisms. These other organisms can cause pneumonia and other life-threatening infections. Medicines may be given that limit the effects of the viruses and antibiotics are given to combat bacterial infections that may develop. Droplet precautions should be applied.

You can help protect the residents in your care against influenza by:

- Staying healthy
- Not reporting for duty when you are ill
- Carrying out standard precautions faithfully
- Following the facility's policies regarding special precautions when a resident has a respiratory infection
- Encouraging the resident to drink fluids
- Reporting to the charge nurse when a visitor seems to be ill

Hepatitis

Hepatitis is an inflammation of the liver caused by several viruses, including:

- Hepatitis A virus
- Hepatitis B virus
- Hepatitis C virus

Characteristics of these viruses are:

- Hepatitis A virus (HAV)
  - Most common
  - Transmitted by fecal-oral route
  - Vaccine is available
  - Many people become infected with only minimal signs or symptoms
  - Does not lead to sclerosis of the liver or chronic hepatitis
- Hepatitis B virus (HBV) (Figure 10-8)
  - Can survive on environmental surfaces
  - Most serious
  - Transmitted by way of blood, sexual secretions, and fecal-oral route
  - Vaccine available for protection
  - Tends to cause a severe, acute infection
  - May progress to chronic infection and permanent liver damage
- Hepatitis C virus (HCV)
  - Transmitted mainly through blood, blood products, body fluids, and sexual contact
  - Can lead to sclerosis of the liver, liver cancer, chronic hepatitis, and death
  - 50% of persons infected develop chronic infection of the liver; 10% may develop cirrhosis
  - Treated with alpha interferon

Any infection of the liver is serious because the liver is a vital organ. You can best protect yourself by:

FIGURE 10-8   Hepatitis B virus (Courtesy of the Centers for Disease Control and Prevention, Atlanta, GA)

- Using standard precautions (discussed in Lesson 11)
- Taking the vaccine, if available
- Practicing safe sex (using condoms)
- Not using illegal drugs
- Giving your full attention to the handling of sharps such as needles or razors
- Maintaining your own proper nutrition

Acquired Immune Deficiency Syndrome (AIDS)

AIDS is a viral disease. It is transmitted primarily through direct contact with the bodily secretions of an infected person. The virus that causes AIDS is the **human immunodeficiency virus (HIV)**.

The ways in which HIV is transmitted include:

- Blood to blood through:
  - Transfusion of infected blood. Note that federal regulations prohibit the use of untested and unregulated blood in the United States.
  - Treatment of hemophilia with clotting factor from infected blood
  - Needle sharing among drug users
  - Prick from a contaminated needle or sharp
  - Unsterile instruments used for procedures such as body piercing or tattooing
  - Shaving razors
  - Toothbrushes
- Unprotected vaginal or anal intercourse when one partner is infected
- Infected mother to infant during:
  - Pregnancy
  - Birth process
  - Nursing

FIGURE 10-9 HIV infection predisposes the person with AIDS to develop Kaposi sarcoma. (A) Typical purple lesions caused by Kaposi sarcoma. (B) Raised Kaposi sarcoma lesions. (Courtesy of Daniel J. Barbaro, MD, Fort Worth, Texas)

The AIDS Virus. The AIDS virus (HIV):

- Has no known cure
- Has many variants
- Does not live for long outside the body
- Is affected by common chemicals
- Depresses the body's immune system
- Makes the infected person more susceptible to infections
- Makes the infected person more likely to experience complications such as:
  - *Pneumocystis carinii* pneumonia—a serious lung infection
  - Kaposi sarcoma—a serious malignancy affecting many body organs. Figure 10-9 shows skin lesions of Kaposi sarcoma.
  - Brain involvement leading to dementia
  - Eye involvement leading to blindness
  - Tuberculosis
  - Other opportunistic infections

Incubation Period. Not everyone who comes in contact with the HIV virus becomes infected. For those who are infected, there is always a period of time between contact and the start of the signs and symptoms of the infection.

- During this period the virus is in infected cells but is not active in making RNA and proteins. The body does not make antibodies to the virus.
- Most people become **seropositive** or HIV positive (show antibodies to HIV in the bloodstream) approximately 3 months after infection. The person has HIV disease, which may progress to AIDS.

- The asymptomatic period (when no signs and symptoms are present) following infection may last months to years. AIDS does not always develop, but the person is an HIV carrier for life.

Disease Progression. Progression of the disease process is determined by the effect of the viruses on special protective white blood cells known as CD4 cells (T cells). Over time the number of the protective white blood cells drops. As a result, the immune system of the infected person becomes more suppressed and less able to fight infection. When the number of CD4 cells drops to a critical level (below 200 cells/mm^3), the person is diagnosed with AIDS.

- Symptoms of HIV infection, when they do appear, consist of:
  - Acute flulike symptoms
  - Fever
  - Night sweats
  - Fatigue
  - Swollen lymph nodes
  - Sore throat
  - Gastrointestinal problems
  - Headache
- One-fourth to one-half of people exposed to HIV show evidence of disease within 5 to 10 years of antibody development (becoming seropositive).

More older persons are developing AIDS because they contracted HIV when young or in their middle years. Physicians often fail to consider them as possible AIDS patients when treating possible AIDS-related illnesses. This is especially true of women.

- Even though the incidence of age-related illness is higher among younger age groups (under 50 years), the proportion of AIDS-related illnesses in those over 50 years of age is substantial.
- HIV-related illnesses often mimic other diseases associated with aging, such as Alzheimer's disease, depression, and malignancies. This may delay the correct diagnosis of AIDS.
- HIV infection progresses more rapidly in people over 50 years of age.

Testing. Several tests have been developed to confirm the presence of antibodies to HIV (positive for HIV infection) and to confirm the presence of AIDS.

The test for antibodies is also used to check the national blood supply. When people donate blood, it is tested to be sure that it is free of HIV antibodies. This protects the people who receive blood transfusions and other blood products.

Treatment.   No specific treatment is able to cure AIDS at the present time.

- No vaccine prevents the infection from developing. However, millions of dollars are being spent on research to develop a vaccine.
- Therapy is directed toward vigorously treating each infection as it appears.
- Nutritional and other forms of preventive therapy are aimed at maintaining a person with AIDS in the best health possible.
- The drug industry continues to develop drugs that slow down the disease process or reinforce the immune system. These drugs, however, do not cure the disease. At the present time there is *no* evidence that AIDS is transmitted:
    - Through touching or hugging an HIV-infected person
    - By eating at the same table with an infected person
    - By using the same toilet seat

Nursing facilities are admitting more people in their thirties and forties who are seriously ill with AIDS. Many of these people have wasting or dementia (irreversible brain disease). This is stressful to the health care providers because it is easy to identify with the age group. It takes maturity to offer the support and care needed.

OTHER IMPORTANT INFECTIONS

Infection Caused by Fungi

Coccidioidomycosis (valley fever) is caused by *Coccidioides immitis*. It occurs primarily as a respiratory infection. It is seldom fatal in otherwise healthy people. In people with immunosuppression, however, the death rate is high. It is treated with antibiotics.

Infection Caused by Parasites

Two diseases caused by parasites are becoming more common in the general public and in health facilities. Giardiasis is caused by *Giardia lamblia*, which is found in the water supplies of many communities. It causes severe diarrhea but responds to medication. Cryptosporidiosis is caused by the *Cryptosporidium* protozoa, which is found in the digestive tract of domestic animals and is transferred by contact. It causes severe diarrhea, especially in immunosuppressed people. There is no specific treatment.

External Parasites

External parasites (ectoparasites) that can live on the body are head lice and mites.

Lice (Pediculosis).   These parasites are easily spread from person to person through contact with personal articles such as combs or bedding. The small eggs (nits) of lice cling to hair follicles. Contact precautions are needed. Medicated shampoos and baths are ordered and the clothing and bedding are bagged and sent to the laundry. The environment is vacuumed and then wiped with a disinfectant. At times it may be necessary to cut the hair to remove the nits. Lice can be removed by hand using a fine-toothed comb, double-sided tape, or tweezers. Your supervisor will tell you how to proceed.

Scabies

Tiny mites carry scabies, which burrow into the skin and cause a rash. Scabies is spread by skin-to-skin contact. The resident is bathed and lotion is applied to the entire body for the designated time. The mattress and furniture are checked for cracks and treated. Scabies are a serious problem in some facilities and the facility protocol must be carefully and conscientiously followed.

WHY THE ELDERLY IN LONG-TERM CARE ARE AT RISK FOR INFECTIONS

There are several reasons why elderly people are at risk for infections.

- Residents usually have several chronic health problems. This lowers their resistance to disease.
- Body changes caused by aging make older people more susceptible to infections. They have less ability to fight disease.
- Residents may have colds or flu and spread the microbes to other residents.
- The skin of the elderly offers less protection because it is fragile and easily broken. Any break in the skin, such as a pressure sore or skin tear, can quickly become infected.
- Poor bladder emptying and indwelling catheters increase the risk of bladder infections.
- Bowel-incontinent residents are at risk for infections through accidental ingestion of feces or by contact of feces with nonintact skin (skin tears, rashes, pressure sores and ulcers).
- The ability to cough and raise secretions is reduced, so the elderly have less ability to get rid of pathogens from the lungs.

The elderly are also more likely to develop serious complications from infections. A simple urinary tract infection can result in bacteremia (blood infection), causing the resident to be acutely ill. This can be fatal to the resident who has little ability to cope with additional health problems.

Infections may not be readily detected in older adults for the following reasons:

- The elderly are less likely to have an elevated temperature as a result of an infection.
- The elderly do not readily develop signs of inflammatory response, which may include pain, heat, and swelling at the site of the infection. These signs may be missing or delayed in the elderly person.
- Some elderly people do not feel pain as acutely as younger people. For example, they may feel no discomfort with a bladder infection.

Because of these factors an infection may be present in the body for several days before it is detected.

GENERAL MEASURES TO PREVENT INFECTIONS

1. Assist residents to maintain an adequate fluid intake. This helps prevent urinary tract and respiratory tract infections and keeps the skin healthier.
2. Assist residents to maintain adequate nutritional intake. Report to the nurse when residents eat less or refuse food.
3. Assist residents to carry out exercise programs established by the nurse or physical therapist. Follow positioning schedules and orders for range of motion exercises and ambulation. This increases circulation, thus lowering the risk for pressure ulcers (a frequent source of infection). Exercise improves breathing, thereby decreasing the risk of respiratory infections.
4. Encourage residents to be outdoors to enjoy the fresh air whenever possible.
5. Regularly toilet residents who need assistance. This keeps the bladder empty and also assures residents that they will receive help when they need to urinate. Some residents hesitate to drink fluids for fear they will be incontinent.
6. When cleaning the perineal area of residents, be sure to wipe women from front to back. This prevents contaminating the urethra (bladder opening) with stool or vaginal excretions.
7. Perform catheter care as directed. Avoid opening the drainage system.

On the Job

Long artificial nails can accumulate organisms that cause serious infections.

8. Observe residents carefully and report any unusual signs or changes, such as:
   - Changes in frequency of urination or amount of urine voided
   - Complaints of pain or burning on urination
   - Changes in character of urine
   - Coughing or respiratory problems
   - Confusion/disorientation that was not present before or that has increased
   - Drainage or discharge from any body opening or skin wound
   - Changes in skin color
   - Complaints of pain, discomfort, or nausea
   - Elevated temperature
   - Red, swollen areas on body
9. Keep residents clean (Figure 10-10).
10. Staff members who have an infectious disease should not be on duty. Caring for your own health is vital in preventing illness in residents. Friends and family of residents should be advised not to visit when they do not feel well. If you notice a visitor coughing and sneezing, or otherwise obviously sick, inform your supervisor.
11. Encourage all residents to practice good hygiene, such as proper handwashing.

FIGURE 10-10 Maintaining the resident's cleanliness helps prevent infectious disease.

OUTBREAK OF INFECTIOUS DISEASE IN A LONG-TERM CARE FACILITY

An outbreak of an infection in the facility can be serious for all residents. Unless steps are taken immediately, the infection can spread rapidly. Examples of outbreaks include:

- Influenza
- Gastroenteritis
- Hepatitis
- MRSA
- Tuberculosis
- Foodborne illnesses
- Scabies (parasites that invade the skin)

Most facilities have an action plan that is used in response to an outbreak of infection. The local health department is notified of the outbreak. The health department will assist the facility in determining the type of outbreak and its cause. All staff are informed of the characteristics of the disease and are trained in the precautions to be followed until the outbreak is over. If necessary, notices will be posted to advise visitors that the facility is closed to them for a specific length of time.

LESSON SYNTHESIS: Putting It All Together

*Y*ou have just completed this lesson. Now go back and review the *Clinical Focus. Try to see how the Clinical Focus relates to the concepts presented in the lesson. Then answer the following questions.*

1. Why should Mr. Dwyer be monitored for the possibility that his tuberculosis infection will become active again?

2. Why is Mr. Dwyer's drop in white blood cell count so important?

3. What condition did Mr. Dwyer have that might have injured his liver?

4. What effect does HIV have on Mr. Dwyer's immune system?

REVIEW

A. Match each term (items a.–e.) with the proper definition.

   a. antigen   d. pathogen
   b. antibody   e. vaccine
   c. inflammation

   1. _____ a body response to infection

   2. _____ term meaning a pathogenic microbe that enters the body

   3. _____ provides immunization

   4. _____ develops in the body after an infection

   5. _____ disease-producing microbe

B. Fill in the blanks by selecting the correct word or phrase from the list.

insects   reservoir
method of   sexual contact
  transmission   sneezing
portal of entry   susceptible host
portal of exit   water

   6. Complete the chain of infection by naming the missing parts.
     a. _____
     b. _____
     c. _____
     d. _____

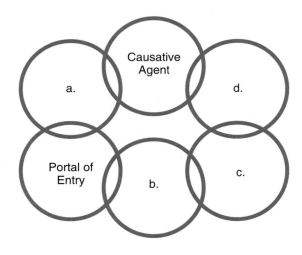

7. An example of transmission by direct contact is _____.

8. An example of direct transmission is through _____.

9. A common vehicle for the transmission of microbes is _____.

10. Vectors, such as animals and _____ also transmit disease organisms.

C. Match the organism (items a.–e.) with the specific disease it causes.

a. *Mycobacterium tuberculosis*   c. HBV
b. *Coccidioidomycosis*   d. HIV
                                     e. MRSA

11. _____ AIDS

12. _____ valley fever

13. _____ tuberculosis

14. _____ skin and wound infections by resistant *Staphylococcus aureus*

15. _____ hepatitis

D. Select the one best answer for each of the following.

16. A person who is infected with a pathogenic organism but does not show any signs of an infection is a (an)
   (A) transporter
   (B) harborer
   (C) infector
   (D) carrier

17. White blood cells that multiply and attempt to destroy pathogens are
   (A) antigens
   (B) phagocytes
   (C) antibodies
   (D) red blood cells

18. Which of the following is not a natural body defense?
   (A) antibiotic
   (B) hydrochloric acid in the stomach
   (C) hair in the nose
   (D) tears

19. Which is an example of a local infection?
   (A) pneumonia
   (B) septicemia
   (C) boil
   (D) AIDS

20. A parasite is
   (A) a type of virus
   (B) an organism that lives in or on other organisms
   (C) cured with antibiotics
   (D) not contagious

21. When a microbe can no longer be controlled or destroyed by a drug, it is said to be
   (A) difficult
   (B) resistant
   (C) untreatable
   (D) noncompliant

22. A major reason residents are at risk for infection is
   (A) they have new chronic problems
   (B) aging makes them more susceptible
   (C) their ability to cough is strong
   (D) their skin is thicker and less likely to tear

23. Sonny, a nursing assistant, notices that the daughter of one of the residents is coughing and looks flushed. His best action is to
   (A) ask the visitor to leave
   (B) put a mask on the visitor
   (C) put a mask on the resident
   (D) refer the matter to the nurse

24. Juan is not feeling well this morning when he wakes up. He has an elevated temperature and is sneezing. He is due on duty at 1500. His best action is to
   (A) call in sick
   (B) go to work
   (C) stay home without notifying the facility
   (D) call a friend to go to work for him

25. Scabies
   (A) are spread via the respiratory route
   (B) can be spread person to person through contact
   (C) can be controlled with a simple bath
   (D) have small eggs, which burrow into the skin crevices

LESSON 11

Infection Control

Clinical Focus

Think about ways you can help residents avoid infections as you study this lesson and meet:

*O*scar Uritz, who is a resident in your care. He was transferred from home with a large, stage three pressure ulcer on his right ankle. He lost the use of his left side from an earlier stroke. He shared a room at the facility with Mr. Jules, who also had a stroke but is ambulatory. Mr. Uritz has an MRSA infection and is now in a single room on contact isolation. The nursing assistant should wear personal protective equipment when providing care for Mr. Uritz.

OBJECTIVES

After studying this lesson, you should be able to:

- Define and spell vocabulary words and terms.
- Explain the principles of medical asepsis.
- Explain the components of standard precautions.
- List the types of personal protective equipment.
- Describe nursing assistant actions related to standard precautions.
- Describe airborne precautions.
- Describe droplet precautions.
- Describe contact precautions.
- Demonstrate the following:
  Procedure 7 Handwashing
  Procedure 8 Putting on a Mask and Gloves
  Procedure 9 Removing Contaminated Gloves
  Procedure 10 Putting on a Gown
  Procedure 11 Removing Contaminated Gloves, Mask, and Gown
  Procedure 12 Caring for Linens in Isolation Unit
  Procedure 13 Measuring Vital Signs in Isolation Unit
  Procedure 14 Serving a Meal Tray in Isolation Unit
  Procedure 15 Specimen Collection from Resident in Isolation Unit
  Procedure 16 Transferring Nondisposable Equipment Outside of Isolation Unit
  Procedure 17 Transporting Resident to and from Isolation Unit
  Procedure 18 Opening a Sterile Package

VOCABULARY

airborne precautions   (*AIR*-born pree-*KAW*-shuns)

asepsis   (ah-*SEP*-sis)

autoclave   (*AWE*-toh-klayv)

biohazard   (*bye*-oh-*HAZ*-ard)

communicable   (kom-*MYOU*-nih-kah-bul)

contact precautions   (*KON*-tact pree-*KAW*-shuns)

contagious   (kon-*TAY*-jus)

contaminated   (kon-*TAM*-ih-nay-ted)

dirty   (*DER*-tee)

disinfection   (*dis*-in-*FECK*-shun)

droplet precautions   (*DROP*-let pree-*KAW*-shuns)

exposure incident   (ecks-*POH*-zhur *IN*-sih-dent)

isolation   (*eye*-soh-*LAY*-shun)

medical asepsis   (*MED*-ih-kul ah-*SEP*-sis)

occupational exposure   (*ock*-you-*PAY*-shun-al ecks-*POH*-zhur)

personal protective equipment (PPE)   (*PER*-son-al proh-*TECH*-tiv ee-*KWIP*-ment)

potentially infectious material   (poh-*TEN*-shal-lee in-*FECK*-shus mah-*TEER*-ee-al)

sharps   (sharps)

standard precautions   (*STAN*-dard pree-*KAW*-shuns)

sterile   (*STER*-ill)

sterilization   (ster-ih-lie-*ZAY*-shun)

work practice controls   (werk *PRACK*-tis kon-*TROLS*)

In the last lesson you learned what infections are, some of their causes, and why residents are at risk for infections. In this lesson, you will be introduced to actions and procedures that can help prevent the transmission (spread) of infection to protect yourself, your coworkers, and those in your care.

MEDICAL ASEPSIS

The term **asepsis** means that disease-causing pathogens and infection are not present. **Medical asepsis** means the methods by which cleanliness and freedom from pathogens are maintained:

- In your own personal hygiene
- With residents
- With equipment and supplies
- Throughout the facility

You will hear the terms "clean" and contaminated ("dirty") applied to equipment and supplies used in the facility. For example, the linen you take from the linen cart is "clean." After it is carried into the resident's room, it is considered to be contaminated. If it is not used, it cannot be returned to the clean linen cart but must be placed in the laundry hamper. Once linen is in the resident's room, it is exposed to the resident's pathogens. To prevent the spread

of these pathogens to other residents, the linen must be laundered. Keeping each resident's equipment and supplies separate from those for other residents is part of an action called medical aseptic technique. Articles that have come into contact with known pathogens or are exposed to potential pathogens are called **dirty** or **contaminated**. Articles that are free of pathogens are considered clean or uncontaminated.

Maintaining Medical Asepsis

Nursing assistant actions to maintain medical asepsis include:

1. Wash your hands thoroughly and at appropriate times. (See Procedure 7.) Protect the skin on the hands by using warm water, drying thoroughly, and applying lotion if needed.
2. Treat breaks in the skin immediately by washing thoroughly, cleaning with an antiseptic, and covering. Report any breaks in the skin to your supervisor.
3. Use gloves when required.
4. Bathe or shower daily. Daily changes of clothing are necessary. Keep your hair clean and away from your face and shoulders. Keep fingernails short and clean. Do not wear rings, other than a plain wedding band.

FIGURE 11-1 Personal care items should be labeled with the resident's name and used by that resident only.

5. Personal hygiene for residents is maintained by following bathing schedules and giving AM and PM care as required. Change clothing daily or as needed.

6. Items used for one resident are *never* used for another resident.

7. The following items should be placed in the top two drawers of each resident's bedside table and labeled with the resident's name:
   - Toothbrush and toothpaste
   - Comb and hairbrush (Figure 11-1)
   - Denture cup if resident wears dentures

8. The following items are located in the second drawer or shelf of the bedside table or in the bathroom. They are used for one resident only and are disinfected (cleaned to remove pathogens) at least once a week.
   In the second drawer you will find:
   - Emesis basin
   - Wash basin
   - Soap and soap dish

   On the lower shelf you will find:
   - Bedpan
   - Urinal for male residents

   Items such as a toothbrush, denture cup, wash basin, and emesis basin should always be placed on a separate shelf from items such as a bedpan and a urinal.

FIGURE 11-2 Equipment should be disinfected between use by different residents.

9. Disinfect bathtubs and shower chairs after each use according to facility policy (Figure 11-2). Clean items used by more than one resident, such as wheelchairs, before each use. Other equipment is cleaned regularly by the housekeeping department or as indicated by facility policy.

10. Disinfect equipment, such as a stethoscope, that is used by more than one health care provider or resident before and after each use.

11. Disinfect personal care equipment, such as bedpans, urinals, and commodes according to facility policy.

12. Be careful when handling bedpans and urinals after use to prevent spills and splashes. Use a cover when transporting.

13. Keep food and water supplies clean. Food trays are to remain covered until they reach their destination. Remove food dishes immediately after use. Do not place used trays on cart until all clean trays have been delivered to residents.

14. Do not allow the residents to keep puddings or custards from meal trays. Bacteria multiply rapidly in these foods when they are not refrigerated.
15. Carry soiled equipment, supplies, and linens away from your uniform so that you do not spread microorganisms from resident to resident. Dispose of items according to facility policy.
16. The floor is heavily contaminated with pathogens. Do not use anything that has touched the floor without recleaning or sterilizing it first. If you are in doubt about whether an item is clean, do not use it. Any personal items that touch the floor should be disinfected before use.
17. Avoid raising dust. Vacuum cleaners, wet mops, and damp cloths are used for cleaning.
18. Do not shake linens. This scatters contaminated dust and lint. Gather or fold linens inward with the dirtiest area toward the center. Keep soiled linen hampers covered. Keep linens (even if soiled) off the floor.
19. Clean least soiled areas first and the most soiled last.
20. Keep residents' rooms as clean, bright, and dry as possible.
21. Keep work areas such as utility rooms clean. Return clean equipment to the proper storage areas after use.

HANDWASHING

The importance of handwashing can never be overemphasized.

Handwashing is the most important procedure you will carry out to prevent the spread of infection. It is the foundation of all preventive techniques. (Refer to Procedure 7.)

Whenever you prepare for resident care, you must wash your hands before you start. For routine care, it may not be necessary to wear gloves. For many procedures, gloves must be worn. It may be necessary to change gloves several times during the procedures for one resident. Each time gloves are removed, your hands must be washed before you touch any noncontaminated items or environmental surfaces. Hands are also washed just before you leave the room to go to another resident. When you enter the room of another resident, do not assume that your hands are still clean after being with the last resident. Wash your hands before providing care to the next resident.

On the Job

It may be tempting to take shortcuts when using precautions to prevent the spread of disease. Remember that as a caregiver you are responsible for protecting the well-being of the residents and of yourself.

PROCEDURE 7 Handwashing

1. Check that there is an adequate supply of soap and paper towels. A waste container lined with a plastic bag should be in the area near you.
2. Turn on the faucet with a dry paper towel held between your hand and the faucet (Figure 11-3). Drop the towel in the waste container. Stand back from the sink so you do not contaminate your uniform.
3. Adjust water to a warm temperature. Wet your hands with the fingertips pointed downward (Figure 11-4).

(continues)

PROCEDURE 7 *(continued)*

FIGURE 11-3 A dry, clean paper towel should be used to turn faucets on and off.

FIGURE 11-5 Interlace the fingers to clean between them.

FIGURE 11-4 Fingertips should be pointed down while washing hands.

FIGURE 11-6 Rub nails against the palms of the hands to clean under the nails.

4. Apply soap and lather over your hands and wrists and between fingers. Use friction and interlace your fingers (Figure 11-5). Work lather over every part of your hands and wrists. Clean your fingernails by rubbing them against the palm of the other hand to force soap under the nails for 10 to 15 seconds (Figure 11-6).

5. Rinse hands with your fingertips pointed down. Do not shake water from hands.
6. Dry hands thoroughly with a clean paper towel.
7. Turn off the faucet with another paper towel; drop the towel in the waste container.
8. Apply lotion to your hands.

PROTECTING YOURSELF

As you perform your duties you may contact **potentially infectious material,** such as blood or other body fluids that may contain pathogens (Figure 11-7). This is called **occupational exposure.**

Using proper medical asepsis technique and following standard precautions according to your facility policy are the best ways to limit the potential for being infected.

An **exposure incident** means that your eyes, mouth, or nonintact skin had contact with blood or other potentially infectious material. Rinse immediately with clear water. Report this at once to your supervisor and follow facility procedure.

Exposure Control

Exposure control training programs are required by OSHA. The programs must be given upon employment, yearly during employment, and whenever new tasks must be carried out that may involve exposure to bloodborne pathogens.

The training program must include information about:

- Bloodborne pathogens and their transmission
- The facility's Exposure Control Plan (where and how to obtain a copy)
- How to know which tasks may cause occupational exposure
- Use and limitations of safe work practices, engineering controls, and personal protective equipment
- Warning labels and color coding
- Who to contact and what to do in an emergency
- How to report an exposure incident, postexposure evaluation, and follow-up

If an exposure occurs, immediately:

- Wash the area thoroughly
- Report the incident to the proper authority

FIGURE 11-7 Common bloodborne pathogens that can be transmitted person to person through blood and body fluid contact	
HIV	Human Immunodeficiency Virus
HBV	Hepatitis B Virus
HCV	Hepatitis C Virus

STANDARD PRECAUTIONS

Standard precautions (Figure 11-8) are the infection control actions used for all people receiving care, without regard for their condition or diagnosis. Standard precautions apply to situations in which care providers may contact:

- Blood, body fluids (except sweat), secretions, and excretions

STANDARD PRECAUTIONS

Visitors - Report to Nurses' Station Before Entering Room

BEFORE CARE

1. Wash hands.

2. Wear gown if soiling is likely.

DURING CARE

1. Wear gloves when touching body substances, mucous membranes, nonintact skin, and contaminated items. Change frequently after contact with infected material.

2. Mask/face shield is indicated if splashing of body substances is likely.

AFTER CARE

1. Place needles in sharps container. Do not recap.

2. Wash hands.

FIGURE 11-8 Standard precautions are used in the care of all residents, regardless of disease or diagnosis. (Courtesy of Briggs Corporation, Des Moines, IA (800) 247-2343)

*G*uidelines for

Standard Precautions

1. Wash hands
   - When arriving for work and just before leaving for home
   - Immediately after touching blood, body fluids, mucous membranes, or contaminated articles, whether or not gloves are worn
   - Before putting on gloves and after taking them off
   - Before caring for a resident and after completing care for that resident
   - Before care procedures that may transfer pathogens from one part of the resident's body to another
   - After personal use of the bathroom
   - Before handling food
   - Using soap provided by the facility
   - Before touching your mouth, eyes, or eyeglasses
   - Before and after touching your contact lenses
   - After touching any soiled linen, clothing, equipment, or supplies
2. Wear gloves for any contact with blood, body fluids, mucous membranes, or nonintact skin, such as when:
   - Hands are cut, scratched, or have a rash
   - Cleaning up body fluid spills
   - Cleaning potentially contaminated equipment
3. Gloves are provided in resident rooms or on supply carts.
4. Carry gloves with you so they will always be available as you need them.
5. If you have an allergy to latex gloves, follow your physician's advice. Three possible options are:
   - Change to nonlatex gloves (facilities must supply them because latex allergies are not uncommon).
   - Apply a skin barrier cream to your hands before putting on latex gloves; the cream protects hands against most irritants, including latex.
   - Put on glove liners that prevent direct contact between the skin of the hands and the latex gloves.
6. Change gloves:
   - After contacting each resident
   - Before touching noncontaminated articles or environmental surfaces
   - Between tasks with the same resident if there is contact with infectious materials
7. Dispose of gloves according to facility policy.
8. Wear a waterproof gown for procedures likely to produce splashes of blood or other body fluids.
   - Remove soiled gown as soon as possible and dispose of it properly according to facility policy.
   - Wash your hands.
9. Wear a mask and protective eyewear or face shield for procedures likely to produce splashes of blood or other moist body fluids. This is to prevent contact with pathogens by your mucous membranes.

   The surgical mask covers both the nose and mouth. Masks are effective for only 30 minutes, then must be changed and hands washed. The mask is used once and discarded. When a mask is required, a new one is put on for each resident receiving care. If the mask becomes wet, a new one must be put on because the mask loses its effectiveness when moist.
10. Goggles or a face shield helps protect the mucous membranes of the eyes from splashes or sprays of blood and other body fluids. A surgical mask must be worn with goggles and with a face shield to protect the nose and mouth.
11. When using personal protective equipment (PPE), you should:
    - Know where to obtain these items in your work area.
    - Always remove the items before leaving the work area, whether it is the resident's room, an isolation unit, or the utility room.
    - Place these items in the proper container for laundering, decontamination, or disposal, according to facility policy.

*G*uidelines for

Environmental Procedures

1. Handle all patient care items so that infectious organisms will not be transferred to skin, mucous membranes, clothing, or the environment. Reusable equipment must be cleaned and decontaminated according to facility policy before it can be used with another resident. Dispose of single-use items according to facility policy.
2. Follow facility procedures for routine care and cleaning of environmental surfaces such as beds, bedside equipment, and other frequently touched surfaces.
3. Dispose of **sharps**—needles with syringes, razors, and other sharp items—in a puncture-resistant, leakproof container near the point of use (Figure 11-9). The container should be labeled with the **biohazard** symbol (Figure 11-10) and color-coded red.
4. Do not recap needles or otherwise handle them before disposal.
5. Mouthpieces or resuscitator bags should be available to minimize the need for

mouth-to-mouth resuscitation. You must be trained to use them.
6. Waste and soiled linen are handled as if infectious and should be placed in plastic bags and handled according to facility policy. There are separate containers for regular waste and for biohazardous waste (waste that has contacted blood or body fluids). Containers for biohazardous waste should have the biohazard symbol (Figure 11-10), or be color-coded in red (Figure 11-11). Learn your facility policy for what is biohazardous waste and follow the guidelines.
7. Wipe up blood spills immediately. Disinfect the floor according to facility policy.

   - Use disposable gloves.
   - For small spills, use 1:10 dilution of bleach or disinfectant required by facility policy. Fresh bleach solution must be made daily and dated.
   - For larger spills, use a commercial blood cleanup kit. This contains an absorbent powder that is sprinkled over the blood to absorb the spill. The blood and powder are then scooped up with the scoop provided in the kit. The material and scoop are placed in a biohazard bag for disposal (Figure 11-12).
   - Use disposable cleaning cloths.
   - Dispose of gloves and cleaning cloths in appropriate infectious waste receptacles.

FIGURE 11-9 Sharps must be disposed of carefully in a safety container designed specifically for this use.

FIGURE 11-10 This is a universal biohazard symbol used to indicate potentially infectious waste.

(continues)

Guidelines *(continued)*

FIGURE 11-11 All potentially infectious materials should be disposed of in the correct waste container.

8. Dispose of body fluids and contaminated articles according to facility policy. This includes the contents of:
   - Urinary drainage bags
   - Bedpans
   - Urinals
   - Emesis basins
   - Drainage receptacles from tracheal and gastric suction
   - Solutions returned from vaginal douches, enemas, and bladder irrigations
   - Soiled dressings
   - Incontinent pads (Chux®)
   - Vaginal pads
   - Incontinent briefs
   - Bedside wastebasket
9. Eating, drinking, smoking, applying cosmetics or lip balm, and handling contact lenses

FIGURE 11-12 Clean all blood spills immediately using a 1:10 solution of bleach or the disinfectant approved by your facility. For larger spills, use a blood spill kit. The powder absorbs the blood quickly and can be scooped up for disposal in the biohazard bag.

are prohibited in work areas where there may be exposure to infectious material.
10. Food and drink should not be kept in refrigerators, freezers, shelves, cabinets, or on countertops or benchtops where they may be exposed to blood or other materials that may be contaminated.
11. Do not pick up potentially contaminated broken glassware with your bare hands. Wear gloves and use a brush and dust pan, tongs, or forceps. Clean and disinfect properly. Discard according to facility policy.

- Mucous membranes
- Nonintact skin

Some examples of secretions and excretions are:

- Respiratory mucus (phlegm)
- Cerebrospinal fluid

- Urine
- Feces
- Vaginal secretions
- Semen
- Vomitus

This means that all health care workers follow specific procedures called **work practice controls** to prevent the spread of infections.

Standard precautions stress handwashing and the use of **personal protective equipment (PPE)**: gloves, gown, mask, and goggles or face shield.

TRANSMISSION-BASED PRECAUTIONS

Isolation means to separate or set apart. The purpose of isolation is to separate the resident with a **communicable** or **contagious** disease (one that is readily spread to other people) to help prevent the spread of the infectious pathogens.

For residents in isolation, the proper use of precautions, known as transmission precautions, requires extra effort by all care providers, but especially nursing assistants, and is more time-consuming. The fear of infection also makes working with these precautions more stressful for the care providers. Residents in isolation and their families and other visitors also feel stress.

Psychological Aspects of Isolation

The resident in isolation fears both the disease condition requiring the isolation precautions and the practices that must be followed for these precautions to be effective. These include:

- PPE worn by all who enter the isolation unit
- Special procedures for handling waste, specimens, food, linens, and personal effects of the resident
- Restrictions on the resident's movement in the facility
- Procedures to be followed when resident is moved outside of the isolation unit
- Possible restrictions on visiting hours or number of visitors
- Need for visitors to use PPE
- Likelihood that close personal contact, such as kissing of family members, is not permitted

The resident may fear passing the infection to family and friends. If the resident does not understand the infectious process, this fear is increased. If the resident is confused, he or she may be very fearful of the PPE.

Because of the resident's fears and the possibility of decreased contact with other residents, family, and friends, the resident in isolation requires more emotional support and care. The increased time required to follow the isolation

BUILDING CULTURAL AWARENESS

Keep in mind that residents of different cultures may be offended or frightened by the isolation procedures used in American health care facilities.

precautions, such as putting on PPE, could easily decrease the time the care providers spend with the resident at a time when the emotional attention is most needed. Nursing assistants are mindful of the resident's needs and will plan their schedules to spend the necessary time with a resident in isolation.

Transmission-Based Isolation Precautions

Standard precautions are used with all residents, regardless of their condition. When residents are known to have or are suspected of having an infectious disease, isolation precautions are used *in addition to* standard precautions. The isolation precautions used depend on the way in which the infectious pathogens are transmitted. Guidelines from the Centers for Disease Control and Prevention (CDC) indicate the specific precautions and personal protective equipment to be used based on how the disease is transmitted. The three transmission precautions are:

- Airborne precautions
- Droplet precautions
- Contact precautions

Airborne Precautions. Airborne precautions are used for diseases that are transmitted by air currents. The pathogens are suspended in the air or on dust particles in the air. They can

FIGURE 11-13 Infections requiring airborne precautions
• Tuberculosis
• Varicella (chicken pox)
• Disseminated Zoster
• Rubella (measles)

AIRBORNE PRECAUTIONS
In Addition to Standard Precautions

Visitors - Report to Nurses' Station Before Entering Room

BEFORE CARE	DURING CARE	AFTER CARE

BEFORE CARE

1. Private room and closed door with monitored negative air pressure, frequent air exchanges, and high-efficiency filtration.

2. Wash hands.

3. Wear respiratory protection appropriate for disease.

DURING CARE

1. Limit transport of patient/resident to essential purposes only. Patient resident must wear mask appropriate for disease.

2. Limit use of noncritical care equipment to a single patient/resident.

AFTER CARE

1. Bag linen to prevent contamination of self, environment, or outside of bag.

2. Discard infectious trash to prevent contamination of self, environment, or outside of bag.

3. Wash hands.

FIGURE 11-14 Airborne precautions (Courtesy of Briggs Corporation, Des Moines, IA, 800-247-2343)

travel a long distance from the source by natural air currents and through ventilation systems. Tuberculosis is a disease that requires airborne precautions. (See Figure 11-13.) Figure 11-14 shows the required precautions.

- The resident must be in a private room with negative air pressure. This means that air is drawn into the room and leaves the room through a special exhaust system to the outside. Air from the room does not circulate directly into the facility. Portable units that filter the air and create a negative pressure environment are used in facilities that do not have the special ventilation needed for airborne precautions.
- The door to the room is kept closed.
- All care providers who enter the room must wear a high-efficiency particulate air (HEPA) filter mask (Figure 11-15). The special filters in this mask protect the care provider from the very small disease-causing pathogens. A surgical mask does not provide protection. Each care provider must be fitted with a HEPA filter mask. This ensures that air entering the mask comes through the filters only. Follow all facility policies for the use of HEPA filter masks.
- A PFR95 respirator mask or N95 respirator mask are other masks that may be used in air-

borne precautions (Figure 11-16). They are lighter in weight and are preferred by some workers. The same precautions regarding fit and use for HEPA masks apply to these masks as well.

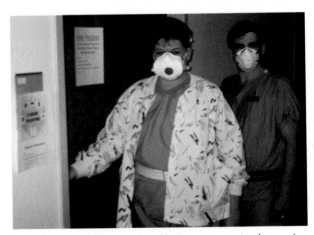

FIGURE 11-15 High-efficiency particulate air (HEPA) filter masks are required for care providers who work with residents placed in airborne precautions. The masks are carefully fitted to each care provider. The mask must seal around the face so that all air being breathed passes through the filters to remove the very small pathogens.

FIGURE 11-16 (A) The PFR95 respirator filter. (B) The N95 respirator filter (Courtesy of 3M Health Care)

• Nursing assistants should be shown the procedure for using the respirator mask and be checked or approved after this training.
• People who are not immune to measles (rubeola) or chickenpox (varicella) should not enter the room of a resident known or suspected to have either of these infections.
• If transport from the room is necessary, the resident must wear a surgical mask.

Droplet Precautions. Droplet precautions are used for diseases that can be spread by means of large droplets in the air. A person can spread droplets containing infectious pathogens by sneezing, coughing, talking, singing, or laughing. The droplets generally do not travel more than 3 feet from the source. Examples of

FIGURE 11-17 Infections requiring droplet precautions
• Rubella
• Diphtheria
• Mumps
• Pertussis
• Influenza

diseases spread by droplets are shown in Figure 11-17.

Figure 11-18 shows the requirements for droplet precautions.

• If a resident cannot be placed in a private room, then residents requiring the same precautions can be placed together.
• The caregivers should wear surgical masks if they expect to be working within 3 feet of the resident. The door can be open if the bed is more than 3 feet from the door.
• If transport from the room is necessary, the resident must wear a surgical mask.

Contact Precautions. Contact precautions are used when the infectious pathogen is spread by direct or indirect contact. Direct contact occurs when the caregiver touches a contaminated area on the resident's skin or blood or body fluids containing the infectious pathogen. Indirect contact occurs when the caregiver touches items contaminated with the infectious material, such as resident's personal belongings, equipment, and supplies used in the care of the resident, contaminated linens, and so on. Examples of infections requiring contact precautions are listed in Figure 11-19.

Figure 11-20 shows the requirements for contact precautions.

• The resident should be in a private room. If this is not possible, then residents requiring

FIGURE 11-18 Droplet precautions (Courtesy of Briggs Corporation, Des Moines, IA (800) 247-2343)

the same type of isolation precautions can be placed in the same room. The door can be open.

- Gloves are put on before the caregiver enters the resident's room. Gloves are changed whenever there is contact with highly contaminated matter in the room. After removing gloves, always wash your hands before putting on a new pair of gloves. After care is completed, remove gloves and wash hands. Use a paper towel to open the door to leave the room and discard the towel in the trash container inside the room.

- Wear a gown when entering the resident's room if your uniform may contact the resident, blood or body fluids, environmental surfaces, or other items in the room. Remove the gown before leaving the room and dispose of it according to facility policy for biohazardous waste. Be careful not to touch environmental surfaces or other items with your uniform as you leave the room.

- Transport the resident from the room only when necessary. Continue precautions to minimize contamination of environmental surfaces, other residents, and health care personnel.

- Disposable equipment and supplies should be used where possible. Noncritical, nondisposable equipment should be used for one resident only. If equipment must be used for more than one resident, it must be cleaned and disinfected between residents.

- Revised infection control guidelines now state that some conditions, such as varicella (chickenpox), can be spread by both airborne

FIGURE 11-19 Infections requiring contact precautions
• Infections with resistant microbes
• Infected pressure ulcers
• *Clostridium difficile*
• Respiratory syncytial virus
• Hepatitis A in incontinent residents
• Impetigo
• Scabies
• Pediculosis (head lice)
• Varicella (chicken pox)
• Herpes Zoster (shingles)

CONTACT PRECAUTIONS
In Addition to Standard Precautions

Visitors - Report to Nurses' Station Before Entering Room

BEFORE CARE

1. Private room.

2. Wash hands.

3. Wear gown if soiling is likely.

4. Wear gloves when entering room. Change after contact with infective material.

DURING CARE

1. Limit transport of patient/resident to essential purposes only. Patient/resident must wear mask appropriate for disease.

2. Limit use of noncritical care equipment to a single patient/resident.

AFTER CARE

1. Bag linen to prevent contamination of self, environment, or outside of bag.

2. Discard infectious trash to prevent contamination of self, environment, or outside of bag.

3. Wash hands.

FIGURE 11-20 Contact precautions (Courtesy of Briggs Corporation, Des Moines, IA (800) 247-2343)

and contact routes. In this case, both precaution signs must be posted on the room.

Preparing for Isolation

To prepare a resident room for isolation, do the following:

1. Place a card indicating the type of isolation precaution on the door to the resident's room.
2. Place an isolation cart outside the room, next to the door. Place in it quantities of personal protective equipment as needed:
   - Gowns
   - Masks
   - Gloves
   - Goggles or face shields
   - Plastic bags marked for biohazardous waste
   - Plastic bags for soiled linen
3. Line the wastepaper basket inside the room with a plastic bag labeled or color-coded for infectious waste.

4. Place a laundry hamper in the room and line it with a yellow biohazard laundry bag.
5. At the sink, check the supply of paper towels and soap. Soap should be in a wall dispenser or foot-operated dispenser.

Refer to Procedure 8–11 for putting on and removing personal protective equipment. Procedures 10–13 cover common tasks performed in the isolation unit. Procedures 14 and 15 cover transporting the resident and equipment from the isolation unit.

Protective Isolation

Protective isolation is sometimes called *reverse isolation* because the resident is segregated for his or her protection from the infectious organisms of others. This technique is used when the resident has a compromised immune system or some other condition that makes him or her more susceptible to infection.

(text continues on page 193

PROCEDURE 8

Putting on a Mask and Gloves

1. Assemble equipment:
   - Mask
   - Disposable gloves in correct size
2. Wash hands.
3. If gown and gloves are needed, the mask goes on first. (If a face shield is used, it is put on next.)
4. Adjust mask over nose and mouth.
5. Tie top strings of mask first, then bottom strings. If ties are elastic, slip around ears and adjust comfortably.
6. Replace mask if it becomes moist during procedures.
7. Do not reuse a mask and do not let the mask hang around your neck.
8. Pick up one glove by the cuff and place it on the other hand.
9. Repeat with glove for other hand.
10. Interlace fingers to adjust gloves on hands.
11. Remember when using gloves:
    - Wash hands before and after using gloves.
    - Remove gloves if they tear or become heavily soiled. Wash hands and put on a new pair.
    - Gloves are used whenever there is the possibility of contacting body fluids, blood, secretions, or excretions with your mucous membranes or nonintact skin.
    - Change gloves between residents and wash hands.
    - Discard gloves immediately after removing in biohazard waste receptacle.

PROCEDURE 9

Removing Contaminated Gloves

1. Grasp cuff of one glove on the outside with the fingers of the other hand (Figure 11-21A).

2. Pull cuff of glove down, drawing it over the glove and turning the glove inside out (Figure 11-21B). Pull glove off hand.

FIGURE 11-21A Removing contaminated gloves. With fingers of one hand, grasp glove of other hand.

FIGURE 11-21B Pull the glove down over the hand and the fingers and remove it. The glove is inside out with the contaminated side inside.

(continues)

PROCEDURE *9* *(continued)*

3. Hold the glove with the still-gloved hand.
4. Insert fingers of the ungloved hand under the cuff of the glove on the other hand (Figure 11-21C).
5. Pull the glove off inside out, drawing it over the first glove.

6. Drop both gloves together into the biohazardous waste receptacle.
7. Wash hands. Dry with a paper towel and discard towel in proper container. Use a dry towel to turn off water faucet. Discard towel.

FIGURE 11-21C Hold the glove just removed in the gloved hand. Insert fingers of the ungloved hand inside the cuff of the other glove.

PROCEDURE 10 Putting on a Gown

To be effective, a gown should have long sleeves, be long enough to cover the uniform, and big enough to overlap in the back. Gowns should be waterproof.

1. Assemble equipment:
   • Clean gown
   • Paper towel

2. Remove wristwatch; place it on paper towel.
3. Wash hands.
4. If a mask and goggles or face shield are required, put them on first.

(continues)

PROCEDURE *10* *(continued)*

5. After tying on the mask, put on the gown outside the resident's room. Put on gown by slipping arms into sleeves (Figure 11-22A).

FIGURE 11-22A Putting on the clean cover gown before entering the resident's room. After tying on the mask, put on the gown.

FIGURE 11-22B Slip fingers inside the neckband and tie gown.

6. Slip fingers of both hands under inside neckband and grasp ties in back. Secure neckband (Figure 11-22B).
7. Reach behind and overlap edges of gown. Secure waist ties (Figure 11-22C).
8. Take your watch into the isolation unit, leaving it on paper towel.
9. Remember when using gowns:
    * A disposable gown is worn once only and is then discarded as infectious waste.
    * A cloth, reusable gown is worn once only and is then handled as contaminated linen.
    * Carry out all procedures in the unit at one time, to avoid unnecessary waste of gowns.

FIGURE 11-22C Reach behind, overlap the edges of the gown so the uniform is completely covered, and tie the waist ties.

PROCEDURE *11* Removing Contaminated Gloves, Mask, and Gown

1. Assemble equipment:
    * Biohazardous waste receptacle for disposable items

* Waste receptacle for gown if the gown is not disposable
* Paper towels

(continues)

PROCEDURE 11 *(continued)*

2. Follow Procedure 9 for removing contaminated gloves.
3. Undo waist ties of gown (Figure 11-23A).

FIGURE 11-23A Remove gloves. Wash hands and then untie waist tie of gown.

4. Turn faucets on with clean paper towel. Discard towel.
5. Wash hands and dry with clean paper towel.
6. Hold clean, dry paper towel to turn off faucet.
7. Remove goggles if used. Dispose of according to facility policy.
8. Remove mask:
   • Undo bottom ties first, then top ties (Figure 11-23B).
   • Holding top ties, dispose of mask in appropriate waste receptacle.
9. Undo neck ties and loosen gown at shoulders (Figure 11-23C).
10. Slip fingers of dominant hand inside cuff of other hand without touching outside of gown (Figure 11-23D).

FIGURE 11-23B Remove mask by untying bottom ties first and then top ties. Holding mask by ties, place it in the receptacle for contaminated trash.

FIGURE 11-23C Untie neck ties of gown.

(continues)

PROCEDURE _11_ *(continued)*

FIGURE 11-23D Slip fingers of one hand inside the cuff of the other hand. Pull gown down over the hand. Do not touch the outside of the gown with either hand.

11. Using gown-covered hand, pull the gown down over the dominant hand (Figure 11-23E) and then off both arms.

FIGURE 11-23E Using the gown-covered hand, pull the gown down over the other hand.

12. As the gown is removed, fold it away from the body with the contaminated side inward and then roll it up (Figure 11-23F). Dispose of contaminated gown in appropriate receptacle.

FIGURE 11-23F Pull the gown down off your arms, being careful that your hands do not touch the outside of the gown. Hold the gown away from your uniform and roll it up with the contaminated side inside. If gown is disposable, place it in the receptacle for contaminated trash. If gown is not disposable, place it in laundry hamper for contaminated linens.

13. Wash hands.
14. Remove watch from paper towel. Hold clean side of paper towel, and dispose of towel in wastepaper receptacle.
15. Use paper towel to grasp handle to door as you leave resident's room. Discard paper towel in appropriate receptacle before you leave the unit.

PROCEDURE 12
Caring for Linens in Isolation Unit

1. Assemble linen required and place on chair or stand outside isolation unit.
2. Wash and dry hands.
3. Outside the isolation unit, put on PPE as required by type of transmission precautions.
4. Once inside the isolation unit, place clean linen on a chair.
5. Identify the resident and explain what you plan to do.
6. Provide privacy.
7. Allow the resident to help as much as possible.
8. Raise bed to comfortable working height.
9. Remove soiled linen from bed by starting at the edges and working toward the center. Roll the linen toward the center with the soiled side inside.
10. Handle soiled linen as little as possible. Pick up the linen from the bed and hold it away from your uniform and gown (if used).
11. Place soiled linen in a meltaway laundry bag (a bag that dissolves in the wash water in the laundry), or follow facility policy.

12. Place meltaway bag in laundry hamper lined with biohazard plastic bag, or follow facility policy. Bag should be labeled as biohazardous material for laundry.
13. Secure bag and route soiled linen to laundry according to facility policy.
14. If gloves are heavily contaminated from the soiled linens, remove gloves and dispose of in appropriate receptacle. Wash hands, dry, and put on a clean pair of gloves. Then remake the resident's bed with the clean linens.
15. Carry out all procedure completion actions.

You may remove your PPE after you have finished all tasks in the resident's room. Follow the instructions in Procedures 9 and 10.

Note: Meltaway bags are rarely used now. They have been replaced with plastic bags. If your facility uses meltaway bags, remember that they begin to disintegrate when wet linen is placed inside.

PROCEDURE 13
Measuring Vital Signs in Isolation Unit

Note: Equipment to measure vital signs in isolation should be dedicated to the resident, meaning that the equipment will remain in the room with the resident. If the equipment must be shared with other residents, it must be cleaned and disinfected before use with another resident.

1. Before entering the isolation unit:
   - Wash hands.
   - Remove wristwatch and place it on a clean paper towel.
   - Put on PPE as required by the type of transmission-based precautions used.

(continues)

PROCEDURE 13 *(continued)*

2. Pick up the paper towel with the watch. Enter the isolation unit.
3. With the watch still on the paper towel, place it where you can see it during the procedures.
4. Identify the resident and explain what you plan to do.
5. Provide privacy.
6. Allow the resident to help as much as possible.
7. Raise bed to comfortable working height.
8. Using the equipment dedicated to the resident, measure vital signs.
9. Note the readings on a paper towel so you do not forget them.

10. Clean and store the equipment used according to facility policy.
11. Carry out all procedure completion actions.
12. Remove and discard PPE according to facility policy.
13. Wash hands, dry, and pick up watch.
14. Handling only the clean side of the paper towel, discard it in the appropriate receptacle.
15. Pick up your notes. Use a paper towel to open the door and leave the isolation unit. Discard paper towel before you leave the unit.

PROCEDURE 14

Serving a Meal Tray in Isolation Unit

1. Before entering the isolation unit:
   - Wash hands.
   - Obtain the meal tray for the resident. Check the meal card on the tray and check that the correct menu is provided.
   - Ask for the assistance of another member of the team.
   - Place the tray on the isolation cart.
   - Put on PPE as required by the type of isolation precautions used.
2. Enter the isolation room and identify the resident.
3. Explain what you plan to do.
4. Provide privacy.
5. Allow the resident to help as much as possible.
6. Raise the bed to comfortable working height.

7. Pick up the meal tray that remains in the room. Make sure the tray is clean.
8. Return to the door and open it. The team member assisting holds the meal tray while you carefully transfer items to the isolation tray.
9. Place isolation meal tray on overbed table. Prepare the resident for the meal.
10. Check the resident's identification band against the meal tray card.
11. Assist the resident with food preparation and feeding as needed.
12. When the resident finishes, note how much food and liquid have been eaten. Uneaten food (except bones) is flushed down the toilet.
13. All disposable items (bones, dishes, eating utensils, covers, plastic wrap, foil,

(continues)

PROCEDURE 14 *(continued)*

napkins, cups, cartons) are placed in the appropriate waste receptacle.

14. Reusable dishes may be handled as follows:
    - Use a paper towel to open the door to the isolation unit.
    - Prop door open with your foot. Transfer dishes to a tray held by another assistant outside the door.
    - Assistant outside the room covers the dishes and returns the tray to the food cart.

Note: CDC no longer *requires* the use of disposable dishes on transmission-based precautions.

15. Clean meal tray and store in the isolation unit.
16. Carry out all procedure completion actions.
17. Remove PPE and discard in the appropriate receptacle.
18. Wash hands.
19. Use paper towel to open door to leave the isolation unit.

Note: CDC does not require this procedure.

PROCEDURE 15 Specimen Collection from Resident in Isolation Unit

1. Outside the isolation unit, assemble equipment:
   - Clean specimen container and cover
   - Paper towel
   - Biohazard bag for specimen container (Figure 11-24)
   - Two completed labels, one for the specimen container and one for the biohazard bag

   Note: The biohazard bag may have a preprinted block on the bag that can be completed with the required information. In this case, a second label is not needed.

2. Place the equipment on the isolation cart while you put on PPE.
3. The biohazard bag for specimen transport remains outside the isolation unit.
4. Carry the specimen equipment into the isolation unit. Place container and cover on a paper towel.

5. Identify the resident and explain what you plan to do.
6. Provide privacy.
7. Allow the resident to help as much as possible.
8. Raise bed to comfortable working height.
9. Place specimen into container without touching the outside of the container.
10. Cover the container and apply label.
11. Clean equipment used to obtain the specimen according to facility policy.
12. Carry out all procedure completion actions.
13. Remove personal protective equipment as described in Procedures 9 and 11.
14. Wash hands.
15. Use a paper towel to pick up specimen container. Use another paper towel to open door to leave isolation unit.

(continues)

PROCEDURE *15* *(continued)*

16. Outside the unit, gather the towel in your hands so the edges do not hang loosely. Place the specimen container in the biohazard transport bag, being careful not to allow the paper towel to touch the outside of the transport bag.

17. Discard the paper towels in the appropriate receptacle.
18. Follow facility policy for transport of the specimen.
19. Wash hands.

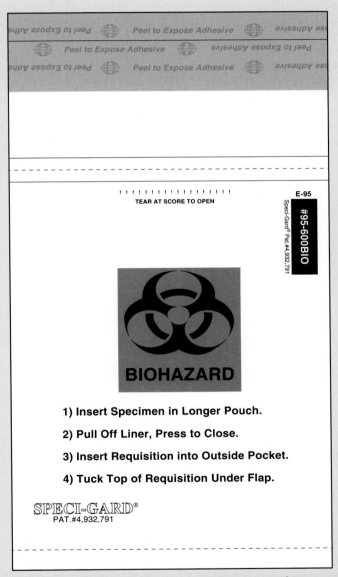

FIGURE 11-24   Specimens taken from residents in isolation can be transported in specimen bags marked with the biohazard symbol.

PROCEDURE 16

Transferring Nondisposable Equipment Outside of Isolation Unit

1. Nondisposable equipment used with a resident in transmission-based precautions may be dedicated to that resident; that is, the equipment remains in the isolation unit and is used only by that resident. Cleaning as required is done in the room by the nursing assistant or the housekeeping staff according to facility policy.
2. If the equipment must be used for other residents, it must be removed from the isolation unit and disinfected or sterilized before use with another resident.
3. Before leaving the isolation unit, clean the equipment with a disinfectant.
4. Place the equipment in a biohazard plastic bag.
5. Follow Procedure 11 for removing contaminated gloves, mask, and gown.
6. Pick up the bag containing the equipment and leave the isolation unit.
7. Once outside the unit, follow facility policy for disinfection or sterilization of the equipment.
8. Some equipment may be terminally (finally and completely) cleaned with disinfectant in the resident's unit when isolation is discontinued.

PROCEDURE 17

Transporting Resident to and from Isolation Unit

1. Wash your hands.
2. Assemble equipment:
   - Transport vehicle (wheelchair or stretcher)
   - Clean sheet
   - Mask for resident, if isolation precautions require it
3. Notify department to which the resident is to be transported that a resident from an isolation unit is being transported.
4. If the resident is to be transported by stretcher, ask for assistance in moving the resident to the stretcher. Two other care providers will be needed.
5. Cover transport vehicle with clean sheet. Do not let the sheet touch the floor.
6. Wash your hands.
7. Put on PPE as required by type of precautions being used. If other care providers are needed to move the resident onto a stretcher, they also must put on PPE.
8. Wheel transport vehicle into isolation unit.
9. Identify the resident. Explain what you plan to do.
10. Provide privacy.
11. Allow the resident to help as much as possible.
12. If the resident is to be transported by wheelchair, the bed must be in the lowest horizontal position. For transport by stretcher, raise the bed to the same height as the stretcher.

(continues)

PROCEDURE *17* (continued)

13. Assist the resident into the wheelchair or onto the stretcher.
14. Put mask on the resident, if required.
15. Wrap the resident in sheet, if required. Make sure sheet does not touch the floor.
16. Remove PPE and wash hands. Open door and take the resident out of isolation unit (Figure 11-25).
17. To return the resident to isolation unit, place wheelchair or stretcher near wall of room as you put on PPE.
18. Enter the isolation unit, unwrap the resident from sheet, and remove mask, if used.
19. Assist the resident from wheelchair or stretcher (with help of other caregivers) and return him or her to bed.
20. Carry out procedure completion actions.
21. Place sheet in laundry hamper for contaminated linens and discard mask in receptacle for biohazardous trash.
22. Remove PPE and wash your hands.
23. Remove transport vehicle from isolation unit. Follow facility procedure for cleaning and storing vehicle used with a resident in isolation.
24. Report completion of procedure: transport of resident in isolation to another department and back to isolation unit.

FIGURE 11-25 This resident is leaving her room, where contact precautions are in effect, and is being transported to another area of the facility.

DISINFECTION AND STERILIZATION

Disinfection is the process of eliminating harmful pathogens from equipment and instruments. A chemical called a *disinfectant* is used for this procedure. You may be required to disinfect personal care items such as wash basins, bedpans, and urinals. You may also use disinfectants to clean wheelchairs and other furniture items. Items are usually washed before they are disinfected. The procedure for disinfecting depends on the chemicals that are used. Follow the directions of the facility for use of disinfec-

tants. Wear disposable gloves and a gown for completing these procedures. You may also need a face shield. Wear PPE that is appropriate to the procedure.

Sterilization removes all microorganisms from an item. This process can be completed in an **autoclave**, which uses steam and pressure to kill organisms. Gas sterilization is also used in some health care facilities. Sterilization procedures are used for all nondisposable equipment that is exposed to potentially infectious materials. Equipment to be sterilized is wrapped in special material. Strips on the packaging material turn a particular color when the package is

FIGURE 11-26 These packages have been sterilized with steam or gas. The strips below each package show how they look before sterilization. The strips shown on the packages have changed color because they have been sterilized.

sterilized (Figure 11-26). Do not use the package if the strip has not turned the appropriate color. Do not use a sterilized package that has been accidentally opened.

STERILE PROCEDURES

Surgical asepsis is the means by which the environment is maintained free of microorganisms, both pathogens and nonpathogens. In procedures where surgical asepsis is used, equipment and supplies must be **sterile**. In other words, items used in the procedure must go through a sterilization process.

In most facilities, nursing assistants are not expected to carry out procedures requiring sterile techniques. If you are responsible for sterile procedures, you should first be given thorough training. Your responsibilities may include opening sterile packages such as gloves.

PROCEDURE
18 Opening a Sterile Package

1. Wash your hands.
2. Assemble equipment:
   * Sterile package
3. If color code has not changed, or seal does not look intact, do not consider article sterile. *If you have any doubt about sterility, consider item unsterile and inform the nurse.*
4. Touch only outside of package. Only sterile surfaces contact other sterile surfaces. Never reach over a sterile field.
5. Commercially prepared products will be sealed. If package is in poor condition or discolored, do not consider item sterile. Discard item.

6. Place package, fold side up, on a flat, clean surface.
7. Remove tape.
8. Unfold flap farthest away from you by grasping outer surface only between thumb and forefinger (Figure 11-27A).
9. Open right flap with right hand using same technique (Figure 11-27B).
10. Open left flap with left hand using same technique (Figure 11-27C).
11. Open final flap (nearest you) (Figure 11-27D). Touch only the outside of flap. Be careful not to stand too close. Do not allow uniform to touch flap as it is lifted free. Be sure the flaps are pulled open completely to prevent them from folding back over sterile items.

(continues)

PROCEDURE *18* *(continued)*

FIGURE 11-27 Opening a sterile package. (A) Open the top flap away from you; handle only the outside. (B) Open the right side. Do not touch the inside of the folded-over portion. (C) Open the left side, drawing the left flap to the side. (D) Without reaching over the sterile field, open the side toward you.

LESSON SYNTHESIS: Putting It All Together

You have just completed this lesson. Now go back and review the Clinical Focus. Try to see how the Clinical Focus relates to the concepts presented in the lesson. Then answer the following questions.

1. What kind of precautions are in use for Mr. Uritz?

2. How is MRSA spread?

3. Why is this resident in a private room?

4. When Mr. Uritz is in his room, is it necessary to keep the door shut?

REVIEW

A. Fill in the blanks by selecting the correct word or phrase from the list.

communicable   sterile
disinfectants   work practice
medical asepsis   controls

1. The process of making an environment pathogen-free is known as _____.

2. An article is _____ when there are no living organisms present.

3. _____ are procedures to prevent the spread of infections in the work area.

4. An easily transmitted disease is called _____.

5. Chemicals that destroy pathogens on articles are called _____.

B. Answer each statement true (T) or false (F).

6. T   F   Items for one resident may be used by another resident.

7. T   F   Food trays should remain covered until they are delivered to the resident.

8. T   F   Laundry dropped on the floor may be used as long as there is no visible dirt.

9. T   F   Soiled linens may be placed on the floor until all the linen is gathered together and put in the laundry hamper.

10. T   F   Hands need not be washed after gloves are removed as long as there are no tears in the gloves.

11. T   F   Gloves are always used when handling bedpans and urinals.

12. T   F   Occupational exposure means coming in contact with potentially infectious material as you work.

13. T   F   Standard precautions require the wearing of gloves for any contact with blood or body fluids.

14. T   F   The biohazard symbol is a green square with a line through it.

15. T   F   A used razor may be disposed of by dropping it in the wastebasket.

C. Select one best answer for each of the following.

16. Housing and caring for a person with an infection is known as
    (A) segregation
    (B) isolation
    (C) sequestration
    (D) separation

17. To remove PPE after caring for a resident on isolation precautions, you should
    (A) remove the gown first
    (B) remove the gloves first
    (C) remove the mask first
    (D) remove PPE in any order

18. If a nursing assistant is sensitive to latex gloves
    (A) gloves need not be worn
    (B) wear the latex gloves anyway
    (C) ask the supervisor for nonlatex gloves
    (D) put powder in the gloves

19. The basic foundation of medical asepsis is
    (A) handwashing
    (B) wearing goggles
    (C) wearing a mask
    (D) wearing a gown

20. If there is an exposure incident, you should
    (A) ignore the situation
    (B) report it at once to the supervisor
    (C) call the doctor
    (D) tell other nursing assistants

SECTION 4

Characteristics of the Long-Term Care Resident

LESSONS

12 The Long-Term Care Resident

13 The Psychosocial Aspects of Aging

14 Alternative Health Practices

LESSON 12

The Long-Term Care Resident

Clinical Focus

Think about how stereotypes and myths about the elderly and those who live in long-term care make it difficult to recognize the uniqueness of each person as you study this lesson and meet:

Sam Jacobzinski, age 84, who was admitted to Riverview Skilled Care Facility in acute cardiac failure 4 years ago. There was little hope for his recovery, but Sam fooled everyone. He recovered and was transferred to your facility, where he has been a resident ever since. He is alert and involved in facility activities, acting as the Resident Council president. He uses a motorized wheelchair and makes a daily round of visits to other residents. Periodically he "overdoes it" and needs bed rest, but even then his spirit is felt throughout the unit.

OBJECTIVES

After studying this lesson, you should be able to:

- Define and spell vocabulary words and terms.
- Identify four physical changes that are expected to occur in normal aging.
- List five common functional changes that occur in the aging process.
- List four reasons why residents are admitted to long-term care facilities.
- List three facts about the over-65 population.
- Describe three considerations required for giving care related to the physical and functional changes of aging.
- Describe five facts to remember when caring for younger adults.
- Identify the unique needs of younger residents in long-term care facilities.
- List five procedures you can do to increase the resident's comfort.

VOCABULARY

chronic disease   (**KRON**-ick dih-**ZEEZ**)

developmental disability   (dee-vel-op-**MEN**-tal dis-ah-**BILL**-ah-tee)

disability   (dis-ah-**BILL**-ah-tee)

functional changes   (**FUNK**-shun-al **CHAYN**-jez)

impairment   (im-**PAIR**-ment)

instrumental activities of daily living (IADL)   (**in**-strew-**MEN**-tal ack-**TIV**-ih-tees of **DAY**-lee **LIV**-ing)

myth   (mith)

self-care (functional) deficit   (self-kair [**FUNK**-shun-al] **DEF**-ih-sit)

senescent changes   (see-**NESS**-ent **CHAYN**-jez)

stereotype   (**STEH**-ree-oh-type)

trauma   (**TRAW**-mah)

value system   (**VAL**-you **SIS**-tum)

ABOUT AGING

Some general thoughts about aging can be stated:

• Aging is progressive and universal.
• No diseases are specific to aging.
• Aging and disease are not the same thing.
• Not all functional changes from age are related to disease. Interest, personal and financial resources, family structure, genetics, attitude, and life-style all play a part. Elements of life-style that contribute to the aging process include smoking, misuse of alcohol and drugs, type of diet, and lack of exercise.
• A wider range of what is considered "normal" function exists among older people than among younger people. A greater variability occurs among older people in physical abilities, sizes, and characteristics compared to younger groups.
• All older adults are not alike. People in their sixties, seventies, eighties, and nineties are all different.

THE PROCESS OF NORMAL AGING

Aging is a natural process and is not a result of disease. The term *gerontology* means the study of aging. It is used to describe a specialty area for health care workers and other professions. The term *geriatrics* refers to the diagnosis and treatment of disorders that occur with aging. Although some changes are expected from aging, no disorders are unique to older people.

Aging is a progressive process that begins at birth and ends at death. It is a normal process experienced by all living things. During the life span, a unique person of value emerges and makes contributions to society. When elderly, this same person of value needs and deserves respect, support, and care. The elderly make many contributions to society.

CHANGES CAUSED BY AGING

Normal aging changes are called **senescent changes**. These changes occur in every body system, but not at any specific time or at any specific rate (Figure 12-1). Some changes are more obvious than others. Aging is both a physical and psychological process. One person may feel and act old at 60, and another may be spry at 80. Both will usually show some physical evidence of their ages. In general, with increasing age:

• The body's systems become less effective.

FIGURE 12-1   Note the many signs of aging.

- This results in **functional changes**; that is, the ability to carry out activities of daily living decreases.
- The risk of acquiring a disease and disability increases.

Most older adults have at least one chronic health condition and many have several. Some of the most common conditions are

- Arthritis
- Hypertension
- Heart disease
- Hearing impairments
- Vision impairment

Normal aging changes are listed in Figure 12-2. Some of these changes are usually seen in all older adults. For example, hair begins to turn gray, the skin becomes dry, wrinkles develop, and posture changes.

Functional Changes

Functional changes may occur as people age. Consider these changes as you care for your residents.

1. Changes in the muscles and joints result in slower movements and decreased flexibility. Residents will take longer to accomplish an activity. Less flexible fingers mean that residents may need help to open and close things, to write, to dial a telephone (Figure 12-3) and to button clothing.
2. Residents have a greater risk of falling because of loss of balance when walking or moving from a sitting to a standing position. Encourage residents to use handrails and to move carefully, without haste. Exercise helps to decrease the loss in flexibility and increase bone density. Be sure that residents have the necessary aids to help them keep their mobility (Figure 12-4).
3. Changes in the urinary system may make it more difficult to empty the bladder completely. This puts the older adult at risk for bladder infections. Providing adequate fluids is important in preventing such infections. Older adults generally have to go to the bathroom more often than younger people. Provide privacy and help the residents assume a comfortable position when you help them to the toilet.
4. Changes in the intestinal tract lead to loss of muscle tone and slower peristalsis, resulting in constipation. Flatulence is more common. Provide the residents with adequate fluids and food. Help them to remain physically active.

FIGURE 12-2 Senescent changes

Body System	Physical Changes of Aging
Integumentary	• Hair loses color and becomes thinner • Skin dries, is less elastic, and wrinkles develop • Skin is fragile and tears easily • Bruises easily (senile purpura common) • Fingernails and toenails thicken • Sweat glands do not excrete perspiration as readily • Oil glands do not secrete as much oil • There is increased sensitivity to cold • Skin discolorations (age spots) become more common
Nervous	• Problems with balance • Temperature regulation is less effective • Sensation of pain decreases • Deep sleep is shortened, more awakenings during the night • Brain cells are lost but intelligence remains intact unless disease is present • Decreased sensitivity of nerve receptors in skin (heat, cold, pain, pressure)
Senses	• More difficult to see close objects • Night vision may decrease

(continues)

FIGURE 12-2 *(continued)*			
Body System	**Physical Changes of Aging**	**Body System**	**Physical Changes of Aging**
Senses *(continued)*	• Cataracts (clouding of the lens of the eye) are more common • Side vision and depth perception diminish • Hearing diminishes in most elderly persons • Smell receptors and tastebuds are less sensitive so foods have less taste	Digestive *(continued)*	• Constipation increases • Flatulence increases • Movement of food through the digestive system slows
Musculoskeletal	• Less muscle strength • Less flexibility • Slower movements • Arthritis and osteoporosis common • Body becomes more stooped	Cardiovascular	• Blood vessels less elastic, more narrowed • Heart may not pump as efficiently leading to decreased cardiac output and circulation
Respiratory	• Breathing capacity lessens	Endocrine	• Decrease in levels of estrogen, proges-terone • Hot flashes, nervous feelings • Higher levels of parathormone and thyroid-stimulating hormone • Weight gain • Insulin production less efficient • Diabetes mellitus
Urinary	• Kidneys decrease in size • Urine production is less efficient • Emptying bladder completely may become more difficult • Stress incontinence may develop	Reproductive	*Females:* • Ovulation and men-strual cycle cease • Vaginal walls are thinner and drier *Males:* • Scrotum less firm • Prostate gland may enlarge
Digestive	• Primary taste sensations of salt, sweet, and sour decrease		

5. Visual changes mean that most older adults need to wear glasses for reading. Make sure glasses are clean and readily available. Evening hours can be hazardous because of poor lighting and shadows. Position lights for maximum illumination. Do not turn corridor lights lower in evening hours. Older adults may also be more sensitive to glare, so lights should not be shining directly into their eyes. Use indirect lighting whenever possible.

FIGURE 12-3 The large numbers on the telephone help the resident remain independent.

6. Hearing loss is common as people age. They may not respond as quickly because they do not hear you. They may act irritated when they hear only part of a conversation or instruction. Be patient and repeat the message using only the essential words.

7. The senses of taste and smell influence one another. Loss of appetite may occur when the ability to taste and smell decreases. Taste buds lose their sensitivity, especially for salt and sugar. As a result, older adults may use more sugar and salt in an attempt to add more flavor to foods.

8. Changes in the cardiovascular system mean the elderly may tire more easily with exertion. As a result, they require more time to complete an activity. More time for resting between activities may be needed. Circulation may be impaired. Residents should be cautioned to sit with the legs uncrossed and to change positions slowly to avoid postural hypotension.

9. The sex drive in men and women may last throughout life. However, decreased estrogen production in women means there is less vaginal moisture. This may make sexual intercourse uncomfortable or painful. Men may need more time to attain an erection during sexual activity. More time may also be needed for ejaculation to occur.

FIGURE 12-4 Older residents may need help to remain physically active. The walker provides support and stability, giving the resident more confidence in walking.

The changes described here occur slowly, over many years. Because they take place so gradually, people compensate for many of these changes; that is, they learn to deal effectively with the changes.

ILLNESS AND DISABILITY

The residents are in the long-term care facility for several reasons. Many have a chronic illness or a **disability**. A disability occurs when there is an impairment that interferes with the individual's ability to perform the activities normal for a person of that age. A disability is present if any adult is unable to perform the activities of daily living. An **impairment** is a loss or abnormality of the body structure and function. The damage to brain cells in Alzheimer's disease, for example, interferes with the person's ability to perform activities of daily living. A disability or impairment could be the result of:

1. Chronic disease

   A **chronic disease** is one that begins slowly and is expected to continue for a long time, perhaps for life. Some chronic diseases are progressive, which means the symptoms will increase in severity as time goes on. Examples of chronic diseases are:

   • Arthritis
   • Neurologic disorders such as multiple sclerosis, Parkinson's disease (Figure 12-5), Huntington's disease, or Alzheimer's disease
   • Heart or lung disease
   • Diabetes
   • Illnesses with acute onset that have chronic aftereffects, such as stroke

2. Trauma

   Trauma refers to injuries received in an accident. These accidents may result in brain injuries, spinal cord injuries, multiorgan damage, or amputation of one or more extremities. The injuries may prevent the individual from being independent.

FIGURE 12-5 Note the typical bent posture in this front view of a resident with Parkinson's disease.

FIGURE 12-6 This woman has had a developmental disability since birth.

3. Developmental disabilities

   A **developmental disability** is a permanent condition that is present at birth or occurs before the age of 21. Developmental disabilities limit the ability to care for oneself in an independent way (Figure 12-6). This topic is discussed further in Lesson 31.

4. Acquired immune deficiency syndrome (AIDS)

   An increasing number of persons with AIDS are being cared for in long-term care facilities. This disease makes the individuals more susceptible to other infections and diseases. Admission generally occurs when the person is in the terminal stages of disease and needs continual care.

5. Many long-term care facilities have residents with cancer. Sometimes they are receiving treatments specific for the cancer (chemotherapy or radiation). Other residents may be in the terminal stage of the illness.

6. A growing number of residents in long-term care are admitted directly from hospitals for additional care after surgery or illness or for rehabilitation after fractures or strokes. These residents generally stay for a short time, with stays ranging from several weeks to several months. The goal is to return these residents to their homes or to another facility

FIGURE 12-7   This resident needs assistance in completing her activities of daily living.

where more independent living is possible. In many facilities these residents are cared for in the subacute care unit (see Lesson 33).

Most residents in long-term care facilities are women because women have a longer life expectancy than men. The older a person gets, the greater the chance that a chronic illness will develop. Most residents have multiple health problems. A resident may be admitted because of a stroke, but also have diabetes and a heart problem. Because of the health problems, residents have **self-care (functional) deficits**. This means they are unable to care for themselves in one or more areas of activities of daily living (ADL) (Figure 12-7). The activities of daily living include:

- Personal grooming and hygiene
- Bathing
- Dressing and undressing
- Eating
- Toileting
- Mobility

There are also **instrumental activities of daily living (IADL)** (Figure 12-8). The IADL include activities such as:

- Managing a household
- Managing money
- Driving a car

FIGURE 12-8   Cooking is an example of an instrumental activity of daily living.

STEREOTYPES AND MYTHS

Stereotypes of people are rigid ideas about people as a group. A stereotype may partly be true, or it may be true for some people, but all members of a group are never totally alike. For example, many elderly people are hearing impaired, but not all of them. Beliefs of this kind that are not even partly true are **myths**.

Imagine someone asking you to describe a cat if you had only seen two small, black, short-haired cats in your life. You would undoubtedly say that cats are small, black, and short-haired. As you know, this does not even begin to describe all the different cats throughout the world. Describing all cats with one narrow set of characteristics establishes a stereotype for cats; it is only partly true. It is easy to form stereotypes, because limited experience tends to make us think that everyone in a certain group has the same characteristics as the few people we know in that group.

The Dangers of Stereotyping

Stereotypes about the elderly are limiting to both the people who believe them and to the elderly themselves. This is true for several reasons.

- *Stereotyping does not consider the uniqueness of the individual.* Although they have certain characteristics in common, the elder members of society have developed from their own special life experiences. This makes each person different, in some ways, from all others.
- *Stereotyping may make people devalue themselves because they see themselves as a reflection of what others think.* If people are treated with respect, they feel respectable and behave in respectable ways. If people are viewed as helpless and unable to make their own decisions, some may lose confidence in their ability to handle their own affairs and become increasingly dependent on others.

It is unwise and unfair to take stereotypes at face value. It is especially important for those who work in long-term care facilities to realize that the people in their care are not representative of all people in the age group.

You can help residents by:

- Resisting the temptation to stereotype
- Accepting them as individuals
- Giving them as much control over their lives as possible
- Supporting their efforts to remain as independent as possible
- Treating all residents with respect and courtesy

Myths

A *myth* is an untruth that some people believe. It is a myth that age alone causes the diseases that are often associated with elderly residents. Although many elderly residents have cancer,

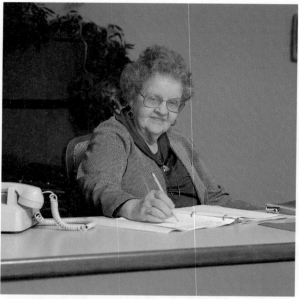

FIGURE 12-9 Age alone does not determine a person's abilities or activities.

heart disease, diabetes, or strokes, younger people also have these conditions.

Another myth is that age alone determines the value of the contributions a person can make to society. Many people make their most valuable contributions to society in their later years. Civic groups and charities could not survive without the involvement of older people (Figure 12-9).

Commonly Held Beliefs

- *As people age, they experience the same characteristic changes in the structure and function of their bodies.* This stereotype is partly true. Aging is usually shown by graying of the hair, diminished eyesight, and slower reaction times. The rate and type of changes due to aging are different for different people. In general, the functioning of the body is slowed but is still adequate to meet the needs of the older life-style.
- *Older people are incompetent and unable to make correct judgments and decisions.* This is a myth. Sensory losses occur with aging, but most older people remain mentally sound until they die. They manage their own affairs, can learn new skills, and process new information (Figure 12-10).
- *Older people are unhappy, without focus in their lives, and have little interest in sex.* In general, the older population is no less and no more content with life than younger people.

Clinical Focus:

Think of Sam, the resident described in the clinical focus. Does Sam meet any stereotyped ideas that you may have had before you took this course? Think about what your ideas about aging were prior to this course and now.

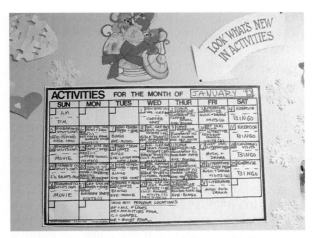

FIGURE 12-10 Activities can provide opportunities for acquiring new skills and information.

They fill their lives with activities suitable to their needs. Their views of life in later years are usually a reflection of the attitudes they had in younger years. They are still sexual beings and can express sexual feelings and fulfill sexual needs (Figure 12-11).

• *Old people are sent to nursing homes because society does not want to be bothered with them.* Compared to the general population, a small number of people over 65 years live in long-term care facilities. The percentage increases with age. For persons aged 64 to 74 years, only 1% live in these facilities. This number increases to 6% for persons 75 to 84 years and to 24% for persons over 85 years. Admission to a long-term care facility is often a difficult decision for the individual and the family. The decision is usually based on the fact that the person needs the type of care available only in the long-term care facility.

• *Being "old" is determined solely by the number of years a person has lived.* This is not necessarily true. The term *old* is subjective and relative and has a great deal to do with a person's outlook on life. To a child 5 years old, someone of 35 years is old.

Myths Versus Facts About the Aged

The first list is made up of myths about the aged. The second is based on facts. Note that the facts in List 2 are true for most elderly people in general, but not all of them.

LIST 1: MYTHS Many people believe that *all* older persons:

• Cannot care for themselves
• Are unable to learn
• Have no interest in life
• Are neglected by family, friends, and society
• Are living in poverty
• No longer contribute to society
• Have no interest in sexuality
• Become "old" at a certain age, such as 65
• Are incompetent to make decisions

LIST 2: FACTS It is true, in general, that the elderly:

• Have sensory losses (changes in vision and hearing)
• Have changes in sleep patterns
• Have slower sexual responses
• Are more prone to certain chronic conditions
• Undergo postural changes
• Have less efficient elimination
• Have less tolerance to glucose
• Experience physical changes such as graying of the hair and drying of the skin

Positive Stereotypes

Many stereotypes are negative, but some may be positive. For example, some positive stereotypes are that older people:

• Are more peaceful
• Are wiser and more self-confident
• Have a well-developed **value system** and know what is important to them
• Have more time to do the things that are important to them

Even these stereotypes do not apply to all the residents in your care.

FIGURE 12-11 Older people have the same emotional needs as younger people.

THE YOUNGER RESIDENT IN THE LONG-TERM CARE FACILITY

You may care for younger people in the long-term care facility. These young people may be there because of injuries from accidents, birth defects, or disease. Common reasons for admission are:

- Traumatic brain injuries
- Spinal cord injuries
- Developmental disabilities
- Chronic diseases (Figure 12-12)
- AIDS

The health care team must recognize that although the needs of all humans are the same, regardless of age, the ways in which individuals meet these needs may vary with age.

Young residents have the same needs as other persons their age. Their natural development has often been interrupted during a critical stage of life. Some of them may have been unable to complete their education, to experience a career, to marry, or to have children. Others may have a spouse and young children at home. It is often difficult for these residents to adapt to and accept the change in their lifestyle.

Adjustment to a long-term care facility may be more difficult for the younger resident. Young people have had fewer years in which to accumulate the resources for dealing with crises. Their lives have been interrupted and they still have more years of living ahead of them.

FIGURE 12-12 Multiple sclerosis is an example of a chronic disease that may affect a younger person.

Because of improved medical technology, young persons with a chronic disease or disability can expect to live almost as long as they would have without the disease or disability.

- Privacy for all residents is essential. For younger people, privacy is necessary to allow them opportunities to think things through and to daydream (which is normal if not used to excess).
- Assist the activities department in providing activities that are appropriate to the resident's age and interests. It is good for them to participate in some activities with older people, but the total program should include activities just for younger residents. If there are not enough younger residents to form a group, then one-to-one activities may be necessary.
- As a caregiver, you may find yourself identifying with younger residents. For example, you may begin to treat a resident your own age as a personal friend. If you are a parent, you may think of a younger resident as your child. It is important that you be aware of this possibility. It is appropriate to have empathy for all residents, but at the same time you need to remember the distinction between caregiver and friend and caregiver and parent.
- Keep in mind that visitors of younger residents may be more boisterous than those of your older residents. Young residents may exhibit unacceptable behavior just as they might if they were home. For example, friends may try to bring in alcoholic beverages to a resident who is not of legal drinking age. You need to report this to your supervisor so that appropriate action can be taken.

Opportunities for continuing education may be provided. Vocational training may be a part of the care plan for some younger residents.

BUILDING CULTURAL AWARENESS

The aging process is thought of differently by different cultural groups. Think of racial and ethnic persons you have known and whether their treatment of the elderly differed from that of this country.

*G*uidelines for

Caring for Younger Residents

Remember when caring for younger residents that:

1. Many younger residents may be your peers. You will need to learn how to have empathy (putting yourself in the other person's place) without becoming emotionally involved to the extent that you cannot remain objective.
2. They may be frustrated and angry because their lives have been interrupted; they may never have the opportunity to marry, have a family, or earn a living.
3. Sexual feelings are at the most intense level during young adulthood. These feelings do not decrease just because the person is in a long-term care facility. Residents may act out these feelings. Discuss these situations with the nurse so that you are prepared to handle them. Like all res-

idents, they need to have privacy and an opportunity for intimacy with a companion, whether a spouse or "significant other."

4. If the young resident has children, try to provide a place where the family can visit together without interruption.
5. Socialization with other people of the same age is essential to the continuing development of the individual. Younger residents may not wish to be constantly with the elderly residents. If there are several younger residents in a facility, they may enjoy age-related activities together.
6. Emotional problems such as depression may be present in residents of any age. These problems must be addressed by the interdisciplinary health care team.

COMFORT, REST, AND SLEEP

Comfort, rest, and sleep are physical needs. If these needs are not met, the resident may suffer complications. *Comfort* refers to the absence of mental and emotional distress and physical pain. Rest and sleep are not usually possible when discomfort is present. Comfort is not possible when rest and sleep are insufficient.

Comfort

A level of comfort is necessary for healing and human survival. A lack of comfort may result from either internal or external factors. Internal factors include:

- Pain
- Nausea
- Hunger and thirst
- Elevated temperature
- Anxiety
- Confusion and disorientation
- Agitation
- Anger

External causes of discomfort include environmental factors:

- Temperature
- Ventilation
- Noise
- Lighting
- Unpleasant odors
- Appropriate furnishings

When all internal and external factors are in balance, comfort is present and rest and sleep are possible. As a nursing assistant, you can do much to increase the comfort of the residents.

Internal Factors

- Observe the resident carefully for signs of discomfort (see Lesson 6). Report these signs to the nurse immediately. Remember that persons of other cultures may express their feelings of pain differently than you might expect.
- Feelings of nausea create distress. Try to avoid these feelings by eliminating unpleasant odors and sights from the environment, especially during meals. Report nausea to the

nurse, as medication may be needed to control the nausea and prevent vomiting.

- Hunger pains are unpleasant and can also cause nausea. For complaints of hunger, provide a small snack that follows the resident's dietary orders.
- Thirst may be due to inadequate fluid intake and is also a symptom of some medical conditions such as diabetes. Make sure the resident always has fresh water at the bedside (unless ordered otherwise) and offer water frequently to those who need assistance.
- An elevated temperature causes restlessness. As the temperature goes up, the resident feels chilly and may have "goose pimples." You may need to provide another blanket for warmth. Feeling "hot" occurs as the temperature reaches its peak and the resident becomes restless. You may need to remove the extra covers. After the temperature begins to fall, the resident perspires. To increase comfort, you may need to give a sponge bath, assist the resident to change clothes, and put clean linens on the bed.
- Anxiety is a reaction to stressful situations. It is noted by excessive activity such as pacing or thrashing about in bed. Persons in long-term care facilities may be worried about families and finances as well as their medical conditions.
- Confusion and disorientation are symptoms of brain disorders and may be temporary or permanent. A resident may be aware that he is confused or disoriented and also know that he is unable to change the situation. The resident then feels very stressed and anxious.

Lessons 13, 20, and 30 provide more information on these topics. It is usually easier to control the external factors that can lead to discomfort and restlessness. Refer to Lesson 16 for environmental factors.

Rest and Sleep

Rest and sleep are essential for good health. As a caregiver, you can do much to help the resident fulfill these needs. Performing these tasks at certain times (such as at bedtime) can increase comfort:

- A bath and backrub can help the resident feel refreshed, relaxed, and comfortable (See Lesson 16.)
- Fresh linens on the bed, free from wrinkles, increase comfort.
- Provide a snack and noncaffeinated beverage if the resident is hungry or thirsty.
- Provide a quiet, well-ventilated, odor-free room with a comfortable temperature.
- Assist the resident to a position of comfort. (See Lesson 22.)
- Assist the resident to empty the bowel and bladder as necessary.
- Inquire as to whether the resident has any habits that help to induce sleep, such as listening to soft music, having a nightlight on, wearing socks to bed, or using two pillows.

You will find that a resident who is physically, mentally, and emotionally comfortable is a satisfied resident.

LESSON SYNTHESIS: Putting It All Together

You have just completed this lesson. Now go back and review the Clinical Focus. Try to see how the Clinical Focus relates to the concepts presented in the lesson. Then answer the following questions.

1. How does Sam indicate his desire to stay an active participant in life?

2. How does Sam compare with the common stereotypes and myths about aging?

3. What situations might lead to a younger person's entering a long-term care facility?

4. What needs do nursing assistants have to meet that are the same for the elderly and for young residents in long-term care? What needs must nursing assistants meet that are different for the elderly and young residents?

REVIEW

A. Select the one best answer for each of the following.

1. Residents are admitted to long-term care facilities because they
   (A) are old
   (B) need health care
   (C) have no loved ones
   (D) have no other place to live

2. A chronic disease
   (A) results from an injury
   (B) comes on suddenly and is usually cured
   (C) is a form of cancer
   (D) begins slowly and is expected to continue for a long time

3. The need to receive long-term health care because of trauma may be due to
   (A) spinal cord injury
   (B) heart attack
   (C) stroke
   (D) dementia

4. The aging process begins
   (A) during middle age
   (B) after age 65 years
   (C) at birth
   (D) at age 21

5. Instrumental activities of daily living include
   (A) bathing
   (B) toileting
   (C) eating
   (D) household management

6. Most older persons
   (A) are unable to learn
   (B) have no interest in sexuality
   (C) have sensory losses
   (D) are incontinent

7. It is generally true that older persons
   (A) become very forgetful
   (B) become incontinent
   (C) usually have sensory losses
   (D) lose all interest in sexual activity

8. The elderly are at greater risk for falls because
   (A) they tend to be constipated
   (B) of decreased flexibility
   (C) of decreased appetite
   (D) of increased sensitivity to cold

9. The elderly are more likely to suffer skin injuries because
   (A) fingernails grow longer
   (B) wrinkles develop
   (C) the skin becomes drier and more fragile
   (D) fluid intake is inadequate

10. Changes in the urinary system mean the elderly need to
    (A) void more often
    (B) empty the bladder less often
    (C) limit liquid intake
    (D) eat more fiber

11. Changes in the cardiovascular system mean that when you care for the older adult, you should remember to
    (A) encourage vigorous exercise
    (B) allow more rest time between activities
    (C) have residents breathe deeply before exercise
    (D) continue exercise even if fatigue develops

12. Older adults may add more sugar and salt to their food than younger people because
    (A) the food served has no flavor
    (B) they are fussy eaters
    (C) tastebuds are less sensitive
    (D) they cannot see as well

13. A resident's comfort may be increased by
    (A) providing adequate room ventilation
    (B) hunger
    (C) pain
    (D) not disturbing the resident to remove wrinkles from bed linens

14. A resident may be assited to sleep by
    (A) watching a science fiction movie
    (B) reading the newspaper
    (C) having a backrub
    (D) having a cup of regular coffee

15. If a resident appears to be having pain, you should first
    (A) tell him to think of something else to distract his mind
    (B) tell him to take deep breaths until the pain subsides

(C) report the pain to the nurse
(D) give him pain medication

B. Match each term with the correct definition.

a. injury received in accident
b. permanent condition present at birth or occurs during childhood
c. one that begins slowly and is expected to last a long time
d. loss or abnormality of the structure or function
e. inability to perform activities normal for one's age
f. an untruth that some people believe
g. rigid ideas about a group of people

16. _____ impairment

17. _____ disability

18. _____ trauma

19. _____ chronic disease

20. _____ developmental disability

21. _____ myth

22. _____ stereotype

C. Answer each statement true (T) or false (F).

23. T   F   A developmental disability is always present at birth.

24. T   F   Parkinson's disease is an example of a chronic illness.

25. T   F   The inability to feed oneself is an example of a self-care deficit.

26. T   F   There are more men over age 65 than women over age 65.

27. T   F   The over-65 population is the fastest growing age group.

28. T   F   Stereotypes are true generalizations about specific types of groups.

D. Indicate which of the following is myth (M) and which is stereotype (S) regarding residents of advanced age.

29. S   M   Age alone causes diseases.

30. S   M   All older people have gray/white hair.

31. S   M   Only people who are young are of value to society.

32. S   M   Elderly people are always more peaceful.

33. S   M   Eyesight diminishes in all elderly people.

34. S   M   All elderly people are unable to manage their own affairs.

35. S   M   All elderly people have little interest in sex.

36. S   M   Reaction time is prolonged in all of the elderly.

37. S   M   Being old is only determined by the number of years lived.

38. S   M   All elderly people have less energy.

39. S   M   All elderly people live in poverty.

40. S   M   All elderly people are self-confident.

The Psychosocial Aspects of Aging

Clinical Focus

Think about how you can assist residents in meeting their psychosocial needs as you study this lesson and meet:

*M*r. Warner, age 87, who has been a resident of your facility for 2 years since his wife of 51 years died. During that time you have come to know him well. He uses a wheelchair but his mind is still very clear. He confides to you one morning that he really misses "having a woman" and wishes that he had a way to relieve his sexual tension. The staff is sensitive to his needs.

OBJECTIVES

After studying this lesson, you should be able to:

- Define and spell vocabulary words and terms.
- Identify the needs common to all human beings.
- Describe the developmental tasks of older adults.
- List the ways in which you can help residents feel safe and secure.
- List the ways in which you can help residents fulfill psychosocial needs.
- Describe how you can assist a resident to maintain sexuality.
- Discuss the challenges to adjustment faced by residents.
- Recognize signs of stress reaction.
- Describe actions to take when residents display unusual behaviors.

VOCABULARY

amulet (*AM-you-let*)

compensation (*kom-pen-SAY-shun*)

defense mechanism (*dee-FENS MECK-ah-niz-em*)

denial (*dih-NIGH-al*)

deteriorate (*dee-TER-ee-or-ayt*)

developmental tasks (*dee-vel-op-MEN-tal tasks*)

VOCABULARY

manipulative behavior (*mah-**NIP**-you-lah-tiv bee-**HAY**-vyour*)

masturbation (***mass**-tur-**BAY**-shun*)

personality (***per**-son-**AL**-ih-tee*)

projection (*proh-**JECK**-shun*)

rapport (*rah-**POHR***)

rationalization (***rash**-un-al-ih-**ZAY**-shun*)

self-esteem (*self-es-**TEEM***)

suppression (*suh-**PRESH**-un*)

talisman (***TAL**-iz-man*)

BASIC HUMAN NEEDS

Basic human needs are the things and activities required by all persons to successfully and satisfactorily live their lives and realize their full potential as human beings. The needs are the same for all people at all ages, although individuals' abilities to meet these needs may vary widely.

Cultural backgrounds influence the way in which individuals fulfill these basic needs. *Culture* refers to those customs and practices that are common to groups of people, including beliefs, habits, health practices, expressions of spirituality, and ways of celebrating. These cultural patterns are part of the uniqueness of each individual and must be considered when providing for the person's care.

Abraham Maslow and Eric Erikson are two leaders in the field of human behavior. They helped us understand basic human needs and how people go about satisfying these needs.

Maslow's Hierarchy of Needs

Maslow originally proposed five steps in the continuum of needs: physical needs, safety and security needs, love and belonging needs, self-esteem needs, and self-actualization (accomplishment) needs. He later expanded the hierarchy to seven levels to include the growth needs of knowing, understanding, exploring, and appreciating symmetry, order, and beauty; and the ability to help others find self-fulfillment

FIGURE 13-1 Maslow's Hierarchy of Needs. People meet needs in order of their importance to survival. Physical needs must be satisfied first.

and realize their potential. This step he called *transcendence*.

The five original steps of the hierarchy help us understand the basic needs that must be met (Figure 13-1). Within the five original steps, Maslow described the basic needs as:

- Physical (physiological) needs
- Security and safety needs
- Psychosocial needs

Maslow believed that the order in which needs are satisfied is based on their importance to survival. Physical or physiological needs must be satisfied first. Safety and security needs are next in importance to survival. Only after these needs are satisfied can the psychosocial needs (emotional) be considered.

Physical Needs (Physiological)

The most basic human needs relate to the physical functioning of our bodies. These needs must be met to maintain life:

- Oxygen
- Water

On the Job

Health care workers often excel at giving physical care but neglect the psychosocial needs of residents.

- Food
- Sleep/rest
- Activity
- Elimination
- Sexuality

Safety and Security Needs

Residents who do not feel safe will experience anxiety and fear. Living in a state of fear prevents an individual from achieving psychosocial well-being. You can help residents feel safe by:

- Being dependable and trustworthy
- Being kind and considerate
- Providing care promptly, gently, and safely
- Helping the residents maintain a life-style structured to their choice
- Protecting their possessions from theft
- Letting residents know that the facility is protected against fire and other disasters

Psychosocial Needs

The psychosocial needs of the elderly are the same as those at any age. There is a need to:

- Love and be loved
- Be treated with respect and dignity
- Feel needed
- Feel important as an individual
- Feel appreciated

When residents first enter a long-term care facility, they often feel depressed and frightened. They are in a strange environment and they fear that they will lose all privacy and control of their own lives.

Their self-esteem is threatened. Each person has in his or her own mind an idea of how they appear and wish to appear to others. This idea of self is referred to as **self-esteem** and must be protected. How residents respond to a threat to their self-esteem depends on how the resident has handled such threats previously and how those who are caring for the resident understand and respond to these feelings.

Some residents react to a threat of self-esteem with an aggressive response and complaints about all levels of care. Others may become quiet, withdrawn, and depressed. The nursing assistant must be aware of the residents' underlying feelings. Remain open and receptive and do not take personal offense at things the resident may say or do in frustration.

You can help residents meet their psychosocial needs if you:

- Treat each resident as an individual with specific characteristics and needs.

FIGURE 13-2 Assist the resident whenever necessary, but encourage her to make her own decisions.

- Give the resident choices whenever possible (Figure 13-2).
- Honor the residents' identities. Call residents by the names they choose. Allow them to reflect their identity by the way they dress, the way they arrange their rooms, and the activities they choose.
- Allow residents to do as much as possible for themselves. Encourage their independence to the level their conditions permit.
- Respect the residents' rights.

Personality

The way each resident satisfies psychosocial needs depends on personality. **Personality** is the sum of the ways we react to the events in our lives. Personality is gradually formed through life experiences.

Erikson suggests that as we mature from infancy to old age, we pass through several developmental stages. During each stage, certain tasks must be accomplished. These are called **developmental tasks** (Figure 13-3).

The developmental tasks specific to older adults are just as important as those for younger people. They include the need to:

- Adjust to decreased abilities such as physical limitations caused by the aging process
- Integrate life experiences through reminiscing
- Accept the onset of chronic illness
- Accept one's place in the community structure
- Adapt to possible changes in social and financial security
- Recognize and accept that life is limited
- Act as a role model for others

FIGURE 13-3 Erikson's tasks of personality development from infancy through old age

Physical Stage	Year of Occurrence	Tasks to Be Mastered
Oral-sensory	Birth–1 year (infant)	To learn to trust (Trust)
Muscular-anal	1–3 years (toddler)	To recognize self as an independent being from mother (Autonomy)
Locomotor	3–5 years (preschool years)	To recognize self as a family member (Initiative)
Latency	6–11 years (school-age years)	To demonstrate physical and mental skills/abilities (Industry)
Adolescence	12–18 years	To develop a sense of individuality as a sexual human being (Identity)
Young Adulthood	19–35 years	To establish intimate personal relationships with a mate (Intimacy)
Adulthood	35–50 years	To live a satisfying and productive life
Maturity	50+ years	To review life's events and examine how they have influenced the development of a unique individual (Ego integrity)

Nursing assistants can play an important role in helping residents accomplish the developmental tasks by:

- Allowing residents to talk about their experiences and feelings
- Creating an atmosphere of acceptance where the residents are not judged

If these stages are interrupted and not completed because of illness, the individual may display behavior that is inappropriate for the age and the culture we live in.

CULTURAL INFLUENCES

The residents you care for may come from different cultures. More complete care is given if nursing assistants are sensitive to the cultural influences on a resident's behavior. People from the same culture usually share similar values, customs, clothing, and food preferences.

Even the cause of illness is influenced by cultural beliefs. Many European-Americans share in the belief that illness is punishment for sins and self-abuse. Many African Americans believe that illness is caused by spirits and demons and is punishment from God. Cultural values and customs are passed from generation to generation and are

the foundation for accepted behavior. Cultural influences play an important role in how a person views and reacts to illness. For example, it is a common cultural practice in Asian American cultures to seek care from traditional healers. The healer reestablishes the balance between the negative (*yin*) energy that is believed to be the cause of illness and the positive (*yang*) energy of health.

Each culture may have its own belief system and religious faith. Belief systems influence choices in various cultures. For example, some Native American peoples create elaborate sand paintings to diagnose and treat illness. Hispanic Americans may treat illness with prayer, wearing of medals, and consumption of special food. An understanding of some of the major belief systems will help you assist your residents to meet their needs. Always remember that you are caring for an individual within a cultural framework. Within the framework of each belief system, there are individual differences in depth of belief and extent of practice.

SPIRITUALITY

Spirituality is the part of a person that gives a sense of wholeness by fulfilling the human need

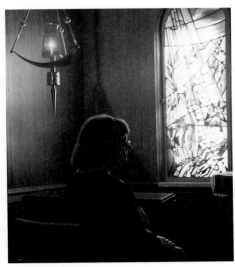

FIGURE 13-4 Spiritual needs must be respected and supported.

to feel connected with the world and to a power greater than self. Spirituality and religion (an organized system of belief) are products of the individual's cultural background and experience. Spiritual values form the guiding principles that people may use to determine right or wrong.

Facing death, coping with loss, and accepting life as it really is are all spiritual tasks for the elderly.

A person's spiritual feelings play an important part in helping him or her through crises and stress periods. Spiritual feelings are personal, are expressed in different ways, and may or may not be associated with a specific religion (Figure 13-4).

RELIGION

Religion is not the same as spirituality, although spiritual people are frequently religious. Religion is a formal system that includes rituals and ceremonial acts that are an outward expression of faith. Many religions have objects of special significance, ranging from **amulets** (protective charms), **talismans** (engraved stones, rings, or other objects to ward off evil), copper or silver bracelets, and religious medals, to holy books such as the Bible, Koran, and Torah. You must be careful to handle all items having religious significance with respect and to protect them from damage or loss.

Residents may wish to talk to you about their beliefs or may need help in carrying out certain practices or rituals. Be open to discussions with the resident even if you do not share the same beliefs. The nursing assistant supports the resident's spirituality and religious practices by:

- Being a willing listener
- Respecting the resident's belief system
- Never trying to convert the resident to your belief system
- Respecting religious symbols
- Not interrupting during religious rituals
- Reading aloud resident's favorite passages from religious books such as the Bible, Talmud, Koran, or Book of Mormon, for example
- Providing privacy during prayers and meditation and when clergy visits
- Being sensitive at all times to information that residents share with you about their cultural beliefs and practices

SEXUALITY AND INTIMACY

Sexuality is a lifelong characteristic that defines the maleness or femaleness of each person. This definition may be different for each person. All individuals are sexual beings.

Being old or disabled does not decrease human sexuality. However, our society tends to define sexuality as youth, beauty, and physical agility. Applying this definition, older people would not be considered sexual beings.

The human person within the aging body does not change. Although the hair is gray, the skin is wrinkled, and the body not so agile, the person inside still has the basic human need to love and to be loved. When this need is not met, self-esteem decreases. (Self-esteem is how one feels about oneself.) With low self-esteem, human beings do not feel good about themselves.

As people age it becomes more difficult to share love. Relationships that provided love, affection, and friendship may be lost through death or geographic distance. In addition, not all people understand that older persons are still interested in and capable of sexual expression and experience. Some caregivers ignore these needs or pretend they do not exist. Others feel that there is something wrong or childish about residents who want to express their sexuality.

Sexual Expression

Sexual expression may take many forms. Sexual intercourse, genital and nongenital caressing, tender communications, **masturbation** (self-stimulation), and mental imaging (fantasizing) are examples of ways that people satisfy their sexual needs.

Sexual Intercourse. Sexual intercourse is desired and can be achieved by many older couples. Before sexual intercourse actually occurs, there is an excitement phase. This phase is brought about by sexual thoughts or physical caressing. Erection occurs as the tissues of the penis fill with blood and the penis becomes firm and enlarged. During this phase, the vagina becomes moist. The excitement reaches a plateau of arousal and is then followed by orgasm (climax) and a release of sexual tension.

- In the woman, the sexual sensations are centered in the vagina, uterus, rectum, and clitoris.
- In the man, they are associated with ejaculation (release of semen).

Orgasm for both men and women is a series of pleasurable muscular contractions that are strong initially and gradually slow and stop.

Men must wait a while before repeating intercourse, but women may experience another orgasm very soon if stimulated adequately.

Sexual intercourse has psychological and physical benefits because it meets sexual needs and is good physical exercise. Even those with severe physical limitations can have successful sexual experiences.

Self-Stimulation. Remember that masturbation is the act of stimulating oneself sexually. Many men and women find this sexual outlet satisfying. It is a common way of gaining comfort when stressed and when other sexual opportunities are not available (Figure 13-5).

FIGURE 13-5 Self-stimulation is one way some elderly people reduce built-up sexual tension.

You may feel uncomfortable when you notice such an activity, but you must remember that the appropriate response is to:

- Treat the situation calmly
- Draw the curtains to provide privacy or move the resident to a more private area
- Not criticize or make fun of the resident

Helping Residents Express Their Sexuality

Health care providers now recognize that the elderly have sexual needs and that satisfying these needs often has beneficial results. Many facilities are revising their procedures to allow couples living in the facility to express their sexuality without fear of interruption by staff or other residents. Some facilities now provide a secure area where a spouse living outside the facility can have a sexual relationship with the spouse living in the facility in privacy and without fear of embarrassment.

Nursing Assistant Actions

Nursing assistants can help residents maintain their sexuality. First, however, you must think honestly about your own sexuality and your attitude regarding the sexuality of the elderly people in your care. These feelings may influence your actions. You can help residents if you:

1. Help them to maintain their appearance and look their best. Give sincere compliments to residents about their appearance. This assures them of their attractiveness (Figure 13-6).
2. Use touch frequently. Touch is the only sense that does not usually diminish with aging and yet it is the sense most likely to be neglected and deprived. Remember, however, to use touch according to the cultural preferences of the resident. Some cultures consider the casual touch of a nonfamily member or member of the opposite sex to be improper. This is especially true in the Islamic culture.
3. Support friendships among residents. Treat all relationships with dignity and respect.
4. Residents who are mentally competent have the right to do in private whatever is pleasing to them both unless there are medical reasons to prevent it.
5. Always knock before entering a room. If you accidentally interrupt sexual activity, leave the room and quietly shut the door.
6. Provide privacy for residents and visiting mates. They have a need to talk and to hold

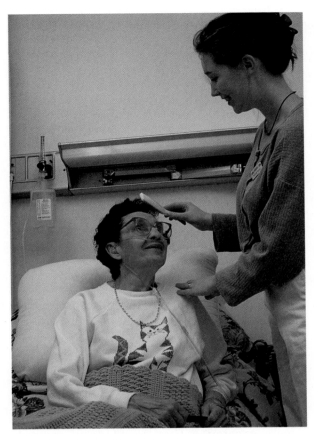

FIGURE 13-6 Sincere compliments assure residents that they are still worthy of respect.

each other (Figure 13-7). Some couples may wish to continue a sexual relationship.

7. Provide privacy for a resident who is masturbating.
8. Protect the rights of residents who do not want to be involved in sexual activity.

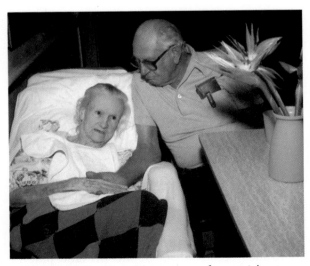

FIGURE 13-7 Provide privacy for residents and spouses when spouses are visiting.

The health care staff is responsible for protecting residents who are mentally incompetent or physically unable to protect themselves from sexual advances. Care providers, visitors, and other residents cannot be allowed to sexually abuse residents. Report any observations of potential sexual abuse to your supervisor immediately.

MAJOR CHALLENGES TO ADJUSTMENTS

Each phase of life brings with it challenges to be met and adjustments to be made. The challenges that develop personality often come as the result of a major life crisis. Three crises older people are likely to experience are:

- Loss of a loved one (spouse or companion)
- Living with illness and disability
- Loss of independence

For many people, these events occur in close succession, and the stress can be overwhelming.

Loss of a Loved One

A person who loses a loved one faces major psychological adjustments. This is a time of great uncertainty at any age. It is particularly difficult when one is old, with failing health and limited resources. Many important decisions about the future must be made at a time when loneliness, confusion, and grief are at a peak.

When a spouse dies, the surviving spouse may sense a loss of identity or place in social situations. If able, he or she will eventually adjust to a new life alone. Although family and friends can help in the process, it is the individual who must face the loss and make the adjustment.

Sometimes a pet is a beloved member of the family to an elderly person. The loss of the pet through death can also require major psychological adjustments similar to those experienced when a human family member dies. Most facilities do not allow personal pets. The person who leaves a pet behind to enter a long-term care facility also feels a great sense of loss as well as guilt about leaving the pet. The separation is painful for the resident.

Having someone to confide in can help the elderly person work through the grief and adjustment period. The nursing assistant who has good **rapport** (sympathetic and understanding relationship) with the resident can help fill this role (Figure 13-8).

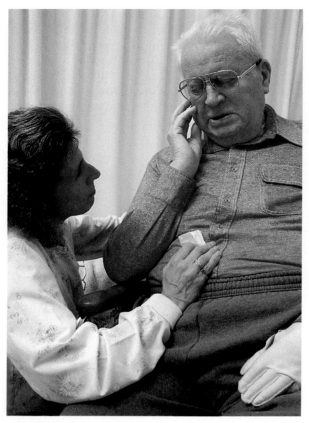

FIGURE 13-8 The nursing assistant can help residents work through a period of grieving.

Giving the resident the opportunity to talk about lost loved ones helps to put feelings and memories into a proper perspective. Working through feelings gives the resident a sense of strength and better understanding of himself.

Chronic Illness

Many older people must adjust to the changes caused by aging and the problems associated with a chronic illness.

Some people try to deny these changes. They become angry when they realize they cannot control the changes going on in their bodies. Over time, most people adjust to and accept their limitations. Eventually they accept that life does not go on forever and that death is inevitable.

Loss of Independence

The third crisis involves the loss of independence that comes with the move to a long-term care facility. Dependency is natural for a child but not for a mature adult. The emotional dis-

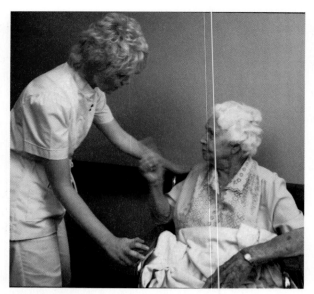

FIGURE 13-9 Residents may become frustrated with the changes occurring in their lives.

tress before admission is high. Making the decision to enter a long-term care facility is never easy for the family or the person involved. It may require separation from loved ones, personal possessions, and pets. A person's sense of independence is threatened just by knowing that this type of care and support is necessary.

The anxiety and stress levels may be even higher once the person is admitted to the facility. New surroundings, new people, a room shared with another resident, and new procedures and rules now define the resident's world. Feelings of fear and frustration grow as the resident comes to know the degree to which independence is sacrificed (Figure 13-9). The calm manner, caring attitude, and patience of the nursing assistant are vital factors in helping the new resident adjust to life in the facility.

USING DEFENSE (COPING) MECHANISMS

Making positive psychological adjustments in later life depends to a large extent on how well the developmental tasks of earlier life periods were mastered and how the personality was formed. The ways of adjusting that a person used successfully through life become part of the person's **defense** (or coping) **mechanisms**.

Residents will react to situations using defense mechanisms that worked for them in the past. Residents may use defense mechanisms to protect their self-esteem. The use of defense mechanisms is harmful only when they become the major way of dealing with stressful situations. If this occurs, a mental health professional may counsel the resident. Here are some definitions for common defense mechanisms:

1. **Suppression:** refusing to recognize a painful thought, memory, feeling, or impulse. A person who has been abused, for example, may refuse to admit the memory of the abuse.
2. **Projection:** attributing one's own unacceptable feelings, thoughts, and actions to others. For example, a resident may tell you the bed is wet because you did not bring the bedpan on time. The resident is blaming you rather than admitting that she is incontinent.
3. **Denial:** pretending that a problem does not exist. For example, a resident is in denial when he or she talks about going home but there is little realistic chance that this will occur. This is different from similar expressions in dementia.
4. **Rationalization:** giving false but believable reasons for a situation. A resident may be rationalizing when he or she tells you that he or she must stay in bed all day because there was too much noise to sleep the night before.
5. **Compensation:** making up for a situation in some other way. A woman who received much satisfaction from caring for a husband and children may compensate for this loss by caring for and protecting other residents (Figure 13-10).

FIGURE 13-10 Treat relationships between residents with respect.

MEETING RESIDENTS' PSYCHOSOCIAL NEEDS

It is important to see each resident as a whole person. The psychological needs of each resident must be recognized and met. Unmet psychological needs have a great effect on physical needs and status. For example, if psychological needs go unmet, the resident may become depressed and refuse to cooperate in therapy. Such a refusal may start a physical and emotional decline that rules out any chance of the resident returning home and could lead to death.

Nursing assistants can do much to help the residents meet their needs. If the residents' rights are respected at all times, you will be helping the residents to fulfill their psychosocial needs.

1. Remember that emotional needs cannot be fulfilled unless the residents' physical and safety needs are first met.
2. New residents must adjust to living in the long-term care facility. Help them to:
   - Develop trust in staff members
   - Meet other residents
   - Adapt to the routine of the facility
   - Adjust to having less personal space. You must respect the space that is theirs
   - Adjust to the loss of a home and many personal belongings
   - Use their own personal possessions, such as clothing or books
   - Display family photos and mementos
   - Find activities that have meaning and contribute to the resident's sense of self-worth
3. Always give residents the opportunity to be as independent as possible. Allow choices whenever possible.
4. Attend to the residents' comfort. Report complaints of pain or signs of anxiety immediately.
5. Explain procedures and routines to residents; notify your supervisor if the resident does not understand procedures and routines.
6. Listen carefully to everything residents say.
7. Recognize that each resident is an individual with likes and dislikes.
8. Answer signal lights promptly.
9. Treat all residents as adults.
10. Help residents feel loved and accepted by:
    - Accepting each resident in a nonjudgmental manner

- Using touch appropriately to indicate your acceptance of the person

11. Help residents feel positive self-esteem and respect from others by:
    - Calling them by the names/titles of their choice
    - Learning about them, their families, and their histories

12. Unless they choose not to, residents should have the opportunity to contribute to facility life. These activities must be voluntary and written into the care plan so no violation of the resident's rights occurs. Activities may include:
    - Visiting other residents who may have no family and few visitors
    - Sharing their knowledge of a hobby with other residents
    - Working on the facility newsletter
    - Creating items for a facility craft sale
    - Delivering mail to other residents
    - Stuffing envelopes for mailings
    - Caring for nursing home pets such as birds or fish
    - Serving on the Residents' Council
    - Playing the piano or leading singing groups
    - Leading current events groups

STRESS REACTIONS

When defense mechanisms are inadequate, stress reactions develop and can take several forms. Examples are:

- Chronic complaining without reason
- Agitation
- Restlessness
- Sleeplessness
- Depression
- Withdrawal

Some residents may just give up and begin to **deteriorate** physically and mentally. This means their condition weakens. Others may become combative in an attempt to assert themselves.

REACTIVE BEHAVIORS

Residents display reactive behaviors when they are not able to meet their psychosocial needs. They are frustrated by their lack of control and use these behaviors in an attempt to satisfy the unfulfilled needs and to ease anxieties. Some reactive behaviors include:

- Demanding behavior—expressing excessive wants or needs
- Manipulative behavior—directing the actions of others for one's own purposes
- Maladaptive behavior—abnormal responses

Demanding Behavior

Demanding behavior occurs when residents make unreasonable requests for service, special meals, or special treatment. For example, a resident may ask to be repositioned every 10 to 15 minutes.

Try to learn and appreciate the factors that are causing the behavior. Demands and complaints are often due to the residents' feelings about their loss of control over their lives. Give the residents as much personal control as possible and offer choices.

Listen to the resident and be sensitive to body language. The resident may feel more secure if caregiving is consistent, with all staff members completing procedures in a consistent manner. Try to talk with the resident at times other than when care is needed. Do not take the resident's behavior personally.

Manipulative Behavior

Residents who develop devious methods to get staff members to do what residents want them to do are using **manipulative behavior**.

Residents may become manipulative in an attempt to control their lives. They may try to develop a special relationship with you. If the resident with manipulative behavior compliments you, accept the compliment graciously and in a matter-of-fact manner. Do not allow the compliments to influence your judgment or cause you to show favoritism to the resident. The resident with manipulative behavior may voice criticisms of other staff members to you. Avoid agreeing with critical comments. If the resident persists in the comments, tactfully tell the resident to talk to the nurse or social worker about the problems.

Do not falsely label a resident as manipulative. Compliments may be sincere and the resident may have real problems with another staff member. Relay concerns to the nurse if the behavior becomes a pattern.

All staff members should treat the resident in a consistent manner. Develop a sense of trust with the resident. Do not make promises you cannot keep; respond to requests promptly.

Maladaptive Behaviors

Maladaptive behaviors are abnormal behaviors. These behaviors may be noted when a resident is unable to function smoothly with staff, other residents, and perhaps family. Depression and disorientation are examples of maladaptive behaviors. These situations require assessment and planning by members of the interdisciplinary team. Interventions by a mental health professional or psychiatrist are often necessary. However, you can also help residents with maladaptive behaviors.

Depression.   Depression is a serious condition that requires professional treatment. If you are caring for any residents who are suffering from depression:

1. Stress the resident's worth and assist him or her in using available support systems.
2. Do not pity the resident. This validates depressed feelings.
3. Make sure the resident has eyeglasses and hearing aids if these are needed. Residents who cannot see or hear well may not interact successfully with others. This often causes the resident to withdraw.
4. Provide the resident with activities that help him think beyond himself.
5. Avoid tiring activities.
6. Use simple language and speak slowly.
7. Encourage and assist the resident to participate in activities involving physical exercise.

8. Monitor intake, elimination, and sleep patterns. Depression may cause major changes in these functions.
9. Monitor skin condition. Depression often results in less movement, increasing the risk for skin breakdown.

Be alert for the potential for suicide. Watch for and report:

1. A change in response or mood
2. Withdrawal or secretiveness
3. Sudden loss of a support system
4. Refusal of medications, food, fluids, or nursing care
5. Sudden interest or disinterest in religion
6. Attempts to obtain scissors, knives, or other dangerous objects
7. Statements about "ending it all," "killing myself," or "nothing to live for"
8. An inability to complete simple tasks without a physical reason
9. Deep preoccupation with something that they cannot explain

Disorientation.   Residents who are disoriented do not know one or all of the following:

- The time of day, day of the week, month, year
- Where they are: facility, city, state
- Who they are

This is discussed in more detail in Lesson 29.

LESSON SYNTHESIS: Putting It All Together

You have just completed this lesson. Now go back and review the Clinical Focus. Try to see how the Clinical Focus relates to the concepts presented in this lesson. Then answer the following questions.

1. What factors make it more difficult for the resident in long-term care to meet sexual and psychological needs?

2. How does the attitude of the staff help or hinder the expression and satisfaction of psychosocial needs of residents?

3. What ways do residents have to indicate that their needs are not being met? Do they always act directly?

4. What losses do you think Mr. Warner has suffered that have contributed to his level of stress? Are these stresses common to many older residents in long-term care?

REVIEW

A. Fill in the blanks by selecting the correct word from the list.

deterioration   self-esteem
personality   sexuality
masturbation

1. The sum of the ways we react to the events in our lives: _____

2. A lifelong characteristic that describes the maleness or femaleness of a person: _____

3. Gradual weakening of physical and mental abilities: _____

4. Feelings about oneself: _____

5. Self-stimulation for sexual pleasure: _____

B. Select the one best answer for each of the following.

6. A resident who uses her call bell repeatedly even though she frequently does not require immediate attention is showing
   (A) loss of independence
   (B) manipulative behavior
   (C) demanding behavior
   (D) depression

7. When caring for a resident who is depressed, the nursing assistant should
   (A) show pity
   (B) engage the resident in many activities to produce fatigue so the resident will sleep
   (C) stress the resident's problems so he understands you care
   (D) use simple language and speak slowly

8. According to Maslow, which human needs must be met first?
   (A) psychological needs
   (B) social needs
   (C) security needs
   (D) physical needs

9. Helping the residents maintain a lifestyle structured to their choices helps meet the residents'
   (A) psychological needs
   (B) social needs
   (C) security needs
   (D) physical needs

10. A nursing assistant helps residents meet psychological needs by
    (A) selecting the residents' clothing
    (B) making sure the door is always open during care
    (C) protecting residents' possessions from theft
    (D) calling residents by the names of their choice

11. Which of the following is a physical need?
    (A) to be treated with kindness
    (B) to be loved
    (C) elimination
    (D) to feel needed

12. People of the same culture tend to
    (A) look alike
    (B) have the same life experiences
    (C) share similar values and customs
    (D) share the same faith

13. Spirituality
    (A) is an organized system of beliefs
    (B) gives an individual a sense of wholeness
    (C) is a type of religion
    (D) is present at birth

14. The nursing assistant can promote self-esteem in a resident by
    (A) being respectful and touching the resident as little as possible
    (B) ignoring what the resident says because the elderly tend to ramble
    (C) giving sincere compliments
    (D) insisting that residents contribute by serving on the Residents' Council

15. A resident is withdrawn and secretive and has suddenly shown an interest in religion. You report this to the nurse because you suspect the resident is
    (A) manipulative
    (B) demanding
    (C) angry
    (D) depressed

C. Answer each statement true (T) or false (F).

16. T F At each stage of human development, the individual has certain tasks to complete.

17. T F Cultural values affect the residents' response to illness.

18. T F People lose interest in sexual activity as they become older.

19. T F When a spouse dies, the surviving spouse may feel a loss of identity.

20. T F If a resident is depressed, it is important to provide him with activities that help him think beyond himself.

D. Match each defense mechanism (items a.–d.) with the correct example.

a. projection c. compensation
b. denial d. rationalization

21. _____ Mr. Brooks spills a glass of water and explains that it happened because the glass was too close to the edge of the overbed table.

22. _____ Miss Alcott wants to stay in her room because, she says, the other residents do not like her.

23. _____ Mrs. Jones spends most of her time out of bed helping other residents, even when they do not want or need the help.

24. _____ When the nursing assistant tries to talk to Miss Anderson about her incontinence (she had wet the bed the night before), Miss Anderson says, in a tone of injured innocence, "Why, I don't know what on earth you are talking about!"

25. _____ Mr. Ramirez tells everyone how much his family loves him and that they would visit him more often if they lived closer. You know that his family lives in the same town as the facility and that they have transportation.

E. Clinical Situation

Mr. Williams is 85 and confined to a wheelchair. He has been a resident in your facility for years. He came to the facility after his wife of 50 years died. He never tires of describing how happy they were. Recently the staff has noticed that he has occasionally been masturbating alone in his room. Answer the following questions by circling yes (Y) or no (N).

26. Y N Are Mr. Williams' actions abnormal for a man his age?

27. Y N Should the staff try to stop his actions?

28. Y N Do you think Mr. Williams is trying to meet a basic human need?

29. Y N If Mr. Williams acted this way in front of others, would you leave him in their presence?

30. Y N Will masturbating cause Mr. Williams harm?

Alternative Health Practices

Clinical Focus

Think about how your knowledge of alternate health practices can be supportive of residents' right to individual choice as you study this lesson and meet:

Millicent Milburn, who is 67 years old and has advancing Alzheimer's disease. She spent many years in India where her husband was stationed. There are times when she states her strong reliance on the alternative health practice of Ayurveda.

OBJECTIVES

After studying this lesson, you should be able to:

- Define and spell vocabulary words and terms.
- Identify the steps of the scientific (western) approach to health care.
- Define alternative therapy.
- Explain, in simple terms, seven common alternative therapies.
- Identify five adjunctive therapies.
- State the value to the nursing assistant of an understanding of alternative practices.

VOCABULARY

acupressure *(ak-you-**PRESH**-ur)*

acupuncture *(**AK**-you-punk-tjer)*

adjunctive (complementary) therapy *(**ADD**-junk-tihv **THER**-ah-pee)*

alternative therapy *(all-**TURN**-uh-tihv **THER**-ah-pee)*

antioxidant *(**ann**-tee-**OKS**-ih-dent)*

aromatherapy *(uh-**roam**-uh-**THER**-ah-pee)*

Ayurveda *(eye-ur-**VEE**-duh)*

biofeedback *(buy-oh-**FEED**-bak)*

body work *(**BAH**-dee wurk)*

Chinese medicine *(chy-**NEEZ MED**-ih-sin)*

chiropractic *(ky-row-**PRAK**-tik)*

VOCABULARY

circadian   (sir-**KAY**-dee-un)

folk medicine   (**fohk MED**-ih-sin)

holistic   (hoh-**LISS**-tik)

homeopathy   (**HOH**-mee-oh-**path**-ee)

hydrotherapy   (**high**-droh-**THER**-ah-pee)

light therapy   (**LITE THER**-ah-pee)

magnetic therapy   (mag-**NET**-ik **THER**-ah-pee)

naturopathic medicine   (**nayt**-jer-oh-**PATH**-ik **MED**-ih-sin)

protocol   (**PROH**-tuh-kahl)

spiritual healing   (**SPIH**-riht-joo-ul **HEE**-ling)

tai chi   (**TIE CHEE**)

touch therapy   (**TUTCH THER**-ah-pee)

SCIENTIFIC (WESTERN) APPROACH TO HEALTH CARE

The prevalent approach to health care practices in the United States is based on biomedical principles (natural science related to physical life processes). A great deal of emphasis and value are placed on the technical aspects of care. The technique follows a specific pattern, including:

- Gathering information through
  - Assessment of body systems
  - Identifying signs and symptoms
  - Carrying out laboratory tests such as cultures, blood tests, and body scans
- Establishing a diagnosis by comparing gathered data against known disease or injury status
- Prescribing treatment following a **protocol** (plan of treatment) designed to correct the underlying disease pathology, including:
  - Medicine
  - Surgery
  - Radiation

ALTERNATIVE AND ADJUNCTIVE THERAPIES

Alternative therapies are nontraditional health practices (compared to the Western approach to health care) used alone or in combination with scientific techniques. The use of alternative therapies is believed to lead a person to a healthier life-style, maintain health, improve a health problem, or increase the effectiveness of a treatment.

Alternative health practices focus on and stress a **holistic** (applying to the whole) approach to treatment and care. Holistic care considers the mental, emotional, and spiritual health of the individual as well as the person's physical health. The holistic approach recognizes that the person is an integrated whole and that the health of each part has an influence on the health of the total individual. For example, emotional stress can have a negative effect on the physical immune system of an individual, making that person more susceptible to disease.

Culture and cultural values often influence a person's belief in and acceptance and use of alternative therapies. The most common alternative therapies (Figure 14-1) include:

- Ayurveda
- Chinese medicine
- Chiropractic
- Folk medicine
- Homeopathy
- Naturopathic medicine

In addition to the major therapies described in this figure, there are many other **adjunctive (complementary) therapies** that people try and in which they have faith. These therapies include:

- Acupressure
- Acupuncture
- Aromatherapy
- Biofeedback
- Body work
- Hydrotherapy
- Light therapy
- Magnetic therapy
- Spiritual healing
- Tai chi
- Touch therapy

Figure 14-2 describes these therapies.

Cultural values greatly influence a person's choice of alternative practices or remedies and

FIGURE 14-1   Common alternative therapies

- **Ayurveda**—Natural system developed in India that focuses on prevention of disease and return to optimum health through exercise, herbal remedies, minerals, massage, and nutritional counseling, according to an individual's specific body type.

- **Chinese medicine** (traditional)—Emphasizes herbal remedies, acupuncture, acupressure, tai chi, cupping, and bleeding

- **Chiropractic**—Treatments related to aligning the neuromuscular segments of the spinal column through manipulation, exercise, and life-style changes.

- **Folk medicine**—Culturally based; emphasizes traditional remedies passed from one generation to the next.

- **Homeopathy**—Employs plant, animal, and mineral substances to encourage the immune system to accelerate healing and strengthen the individual's own body to achieve the healing process.

- **Naturopathic medicine**—Employs fasting, special diets, and supportive approaches to assist the healing process.

his or her willingness to share this information with health care workers. The resident may fear that others may not be open to or understand her beliefs. It is very important to listen carefully to residents, without making value judgments, as they discuss their personal health practices with you.

Ayurveda

Ayurveda is a holistic approach to alternative health maintenance. It is an ancient philosophy that originated in India and has been practiced for more than 5,000 years. This system is based on the physical and health characteristics of the individual. These characteristics are determined by body types known as *prakriti*. There are three body types known as *doshas*. Each person

is a combination of each dosha. One dosha predominates and it is this dosha that determines the individual's personality and physical disposition. This same dosha may be changed or unbalanced by illness. The three doshas are known as:

- *Vata*—characterized as unpredictable, slim, and nervous. Responsible for respiration, blood, circulation, digestion, and nervous system functioning and movement throughout and in and out of the body.
- *Pitta*—characterized as fervent, intelligent, and filled with drive. Responsible for metabolism and utilization of nutrients.
- *Kapha*—characterized as slower moving, muscular, relaxed, and stable. Responsible for body-building processes and mental processes like loyalty, forgiveness, and sympathy.

Balanced health represents harmony of the doshas in conformity with the four biological and spiritual instincts of religion, finances, procreation, and freedom. Using the individual's prakriti as a guide, the Ayurvedic practitioner can prescribe the best plan of foods, exercise, herbal treatment, and living practices that will return the harmony of the doshas. Many of the Ayurvedic herbs are powerful antioxidants. **Antioxidants**, including vitamins C and E, help to neutralize free radicals. Naturally occurring free radicals are molecules that damage body cells. These free radicals are a factor in cancer, heart disease, and aging. Meditation is an important general recommendation of therapy.

Chinese Medicine

Chinese medicine is an ancient holistic-based practice that has been passed down through many generations. The basic concept of Chinese medicine is that there is a universal energy present in every living person. The energy is called *qi* or *chi* (pronounced "chee") and travels along specific pathways called meridians. When qi runs freely there is health; but when qi is blocked, illness and pain result. Yin and yang must be balanced or disharmony occurs. The Chinese medicine practitioner looks for a pattern of disharmony and then attempts to correct it through one or more of the following:

- Acupressure—pressure with fingers, palms, or elbows along specific meridians to stimulate and regulate the flow of energy.

FIGURE 14-2 Common complementary (adjunctive) therapies

- **Acupressure**—Pressure applied with the finger or a ball-pointed instrument to acupuncture points. Similar to acupuncture but noninvasive.

- **Acupuncture**—Insertion of fine needles in specific areas of the skin to influence body functions. Sometimes heat (moxibustion) or electrical stimulation is used in conjunction with the needle placement.

- **Aromatherapy**—Oils from aromatic plants and flowers are blended and inhaled. This is believed by some to have restorative effects on the body, mind, and spirit.

- **Biofeedback**—Uses machines to assist the person to become aware of changes in body functions. The person then exerts his or her own mental will to alter his or her own physiology.

- **Body work**—Includes chiropractic in addition to other hands-on massage techniques such as foot reflexology, lymphatic massage, Rolfing, and Swedish massage.

- **Hydrotherapy**—Uses water in any form, internally or externally, for healing purposes.

- **Light therapy**—Exposure to controlled light is used to influence and regulate the daily biorhythmic (**circadian**) functions of the body. Includes exposure to blue light to cure jaundice in newborns and ultraviolet to treat psoriasis.

- **Magnetic therapy**—May reduce pain and support healing by increasing blood flow, blocking pain impulses through nerves, or altering the acidity of bodily fluids. Conflicting studies regarding effectiveness in treatment.

- **Spiritual healing**—Individual, alone or with help, attempts to reach a unity with a higher power. This may be achieved through prayer. *Shamans* are folk healers who use natural and supernatural forces to help others.

- **Tai chi**—Slow, graceful, and precise body movements combined with breathing techniques which are believed to improve posture, spiritual and mental clarity, and improve the life energy flow (*qi*) within the body.

- **Touch therapy**—Healer's hands move 3–5 inches above the body of an individual to restore the balance of energy flow and promote self-healing.

- Acupuncture—insertion of thin needles on the meridian. Sometimes heat is applied to the needles (moxibustion) as a supplement to stimulate and balance the energy flow.
- Herbal remedies—use of selected roots, stems, seeds, flowers, and leaves. Some eliminate toxins, some redistribute the life force (qi), and some strengthen specific organs or the body as a whole.
- Qigong—a series of slow stretches, breathing exercises, meditation, and visualization designed to balance the flow of qi.
- Tai chi—a noncombative series of gentle exercises and meditation designed to unite body and spirit and to improve muscle tone.
- Tui ma—a traditional therapy combining acupuncture and chiropractic.

Chiropractic

The chiropractic system considers the spine the core of human health. The condition of the spinal column is viewed as a critical factor in a person's well-being. It is also considered a key to maintaining the health of the nervous system. Chiropractic also teaches that a body that is functioning correctly will cure itself.

Poor posture or trauma cause misalignment of the vertebrae, resulting in pressure on the spinal nerves. Diminished function and illness may result from this pressure.

Chiropractic treatment seeks to restore the proper flow of nerve impulses to and from the spinal column. Chiropractors adjust the position of the spinal vertebrae through manipulation and massage.

Folk Medicine

Folk medicine is culturally based, and is usually conducted in the individual's own home under the guidance of a "healer" or family member. The treatment choices, which have been passed down from generation to generation, include remedies that have been found effective. Often these remedies are derived from plants and flowers. There is a strong holistic emphasis and prevention is stressed. Members of some cultures believe there are two kinds of folk illnesses:

• Personalistic—ill will directed by someone else or punishment for wrongdoing. Some cultures (Haitians and Puerto Ricans) believe that witchcraft is the source of illness. Italian, Greek, and Spanish-speaking cultures may place the blame on an "evil eye." In either case, the evil spirit must be driven out by rituals.
• Naturalistic—an imbalance between impersonal internal factors. The most common imbalance is between "hot" and "cold" (see Figure 14-3). These temperatures have no relationship to body temperature or to the temperature of the substances used to treat the condition. This belief of imbalance is culturally true of Hispanics, Mideastern cultures, and Asians. The Chinese share the same concepts but refer to cold as "yin" and hot as "yang."

Homeopathy

Homeopathy, although gaining in popularity, today remains one of the most controversial areas of alternative therapy. Homeopathy is based on three principles:

1. *Similarities*—Substances that can bring on symptoms of illness in a healthy person are able to control the same symptoms in an ill person. Therefore, if an individual is ill because of an infection, a very small amount of that same infectious agent introduced into the ill person will stimulate the ill person's immune system to the extent that the signs and symptoms of the infection are controlled.
2. *Individualism*—An ill individual presenting many signs and symptoms can be healed by a single homeopathic remedy. For example, if someone has both fever and a rash, he or she presents a "symptoms picture" that will respond to a single remedy.
3. *Infinitesimals*—Ultrasmall dilutions of the causative agents can stimulate the immune system of a person to destroy the disease and control the signs and symptoms. The curative agent must be diluted in saline or water and shaken to be effective.

Believers in homeopathy see signs and symptoms as the way the body heals itself. Therefore, symptoms are encouraged to be fully expressed, not suppressed. Restraint of symptoms is believed to force the illness deeper into the body. Plants, roots, and mineral substances are given to promote signs and symptoms rather than suppress them.

Naturopathic Medicine

Naturopathic medicine is a holistic approach based on three major philosophies:

1. The body has the ability to heal itself. The physician identifies the cause of the symptoms and prescribes treatments that are drawn from many disciplines, such as therapeutic massage, hydrotherapy, homeopathy, Chinese medicine, and herbal medicine. All therapy must be complementary to the body's healing process.
2. The cause of illness must be identified. Signs and symptoms are believed to be the attempts of the body to heal itself and to rid itself of toxins and therefore should not be repressed.
3. Treat the individual from a holistic approach, considering not only emotional and mental aspects but also environmental, social, and related genetic factors.

FIGURE 14-3 Examples of hot/cold conditions and hot/cold treatments

Hot Conditions	Cold Treatments
Hypertension	Herbs
Infections	Milk of magnesia
Pregnancy	Sage
Ulcers	Linden

Cold Conditions	Hot Treatments
Cancer	Aspirin
Headache	Garlic
Pneumonia	Penicillin
Depression	Vitamins

Naturopathic medicine emphasizes the healing power of nature. Much emphasis is placed on teaching and helping individuals understand their illnesses and assume responsibility for management of their conditions. The naturopathic physician uses dietetics, with stress on nutrition and nutritional supplements for natural hygiene. There is not a large body of scientific evidence proving that the naturopathic approach is really effective.

Osteopathy

The practice of osteopathy includes diagnosis and treatment of illness as well as the prescription of drugs. Osteopathic practitioners (doctors of osteopathy) provide comprehensive medical care, including preventive medicine, diagnosis, prescription of medications, surgery, ordering of laboratory tests, and manipulations.

Four principles guide osteopathic medicine:

1. The body tends to be self-healing. Treatments should be given to support the body's efforts.
2. The structure and function of the body are integrated through a complex communication network of circulatory and neuromuscular pathways.
3. Most diseases are related to abnormalities of the neuromuscular system and can be corrected through manipulation.
4. Preserving proper health requires constant regulation, including manipulation and other means of diagnosis and treatment.

Doctors of osteopathy today are as likely to be as well prepared as other medical doctors. Osteopathic manipulation techniques have been proven to be of value by many scientific studies.

IMPORTANCE FOR THE NURSING ASSISTANT

Despite changes in living arrangements, people often continue to use health practices they found helpful in the past. Therefore, the nursing assistant must be prepared to understand alternative health practices and be open to residents as they share these practices. Faith in the alternative practices often alters the willingness of the resident to follow the care plan. Remember that many of the alternative practices are accepted and used in conjunction with conventional Western therapy. It is important that you:

• Continue to learn about alternative practices to better understand and support the residents
• Make sure the supervising nurse is aware of any practices that residents are employing
• Accept practices that residents wish to share with you
• Be supportive of practices that are not harmful to current therapy

LESSON SYNTHESIS: Putting It All Together

*Y*ou have just completed this lesson. Now go back and review the Clinical Focus. Try to see how the Clinical Focus relates to the concepts presented in the lesson. Then answer the following questions.

1. Why would Mrs. Milburn naturally become interested in Ayurveda as an alternative therapy?

2. What dosha do you think predominates in Mrs. Milburn?

3. Mrs. Milburn meditates every morning and every evening and practices yoga. Why would she do these things?

REVIEW

A. Select the one best answer for each of the following.

1. Biomedical principles include all but which one of these?
   (A) assessment
   (B) praying to a higher power
   (C) identifying signs and symptoms
   (D) carrying out laboratory tests

2. Culturally based traditional remedies passed from generation to generation best describes:
   (A) folk medicine
   (B) naturopathic medicine
   (C) biofeedback
   (D) hydrotherapy

3. Residents who use oils from plants and flowers for restorative effects practice the adjunctive therapy known as
   (A) hydrotherapy
   (B) aromatherapy
   (C) acupressure
   (D) biofeedback

4. The insertion of fine needles in specific areas of the skin to influence body function is known as
   (A) biofeedback
   (B) acupressure
   (C) tai chi
   (D) acupuncture

B. Answer each statement true (T) or false (F).

5. T   F   Today, homeopathic therapy remains one of the least controversial areas of alternative therapy.

6. T   F   Homeopathy sees signs and symptoms as the way the body heals itself.

7. T   F   Naturopathy emphasizes helping the individual assume responsibility for personal health.

8. T   F   Chiropractors may perform manipulation to properly align the spine.

9. T   F   Cultural values are an important aspect of alternative therapies.

10. T   F   People can learn to become aware when their blood pressure is rising and then to voluntarily lower their blood pressure.

11. T   F   Folk medicine is based on biomedical principles.

12. T   F   Cupping and bleeding are techniques used in traditional Chinese medicine.

13. T   F   Chiropractors believe that light therapy and herbal medicine are the best ways to treat illness.

14. T   F   Ayurveda is an ancient system to prevent disease and help people return to wellness.

C. Match the term for each adjunctive therapy with its description.

a. acupressure   d. biofeedback
b. hydrotherapy   e. light therapy
c. magnetic therapy   f. tai chi

15. _____ Uses machines to assist a person to become aware of changes in body physiology.

16. _____ Uses slow, graceful body movements to improve the flow of qi.

17. _____ Uses water for healing purposes.

18. _____ May relieve pain and speed healing by increasing blood flow.

19. _____ Noninvasive; may apply a ball-pointed instrument to selected places on the body.

20. _____ Used to influence and regulate the daily biorhythm.

SECTION 5

Meeting the Residents' Basic Needs

LESSONS

15 Care of the Residents' Environment

16 Caring for the Residents' Personal Hygiene

17 Meeting the Residents' Nutritional Needs

18 Meeting the Residents' Elimination Needs

LESSON 15

Care of the Residents' Environment

Clinical Focus

Think about how controlling the environment for the resident contributes to the resident's sense of well-being and comfort as you study this lesson and meet:

*E*dith Curry, a resident who is 96 and constantly complains of feeling cold. She has congestive heart failure and non–insulin-dependent diabetes mellitus. She also suffers from chronic respiratory infections. She shares a room with two other residents whose grandchildren visit and the noise bothers her. She reads but requires extra lighting. She becomes disoriented during the early evening hours. When out of bed in a wheelchair, she enjoys watching television. On warm days, she likes to sit on the sheltered and enclosed patio.

OBJECTIVES

After studying this lesson, you should be able to:

- Define and spell vocabulary words and terms.
- State three components of the resident's environment.
- Name four ways in which a safe, comfortable, and pleasant environment can be maintained for the resident.
- Describe two actions to be taken at the beginning and end of each resident care procedure.
- Demonstrate the following:
  Procedure 19 Unoccupied Bed: Changing Linens
  Procedure 20 Occupied Bed: Changing Linens

VOCABULARY

draw sheet   *(draw sheet)*

environment   *(en-**VIRE**-on-ment)*

mitered corner   *(**MY**-terd **KOR**-ner)*

occupied bedmaking   *(**OCK**-you-pyed **BED**-may-king)*

procedure   *(proh-**SEE**-djur)*

square corner   *(skwair **KOR**-ner)*

unoccupied bedmaking   *(un-**OCK**-you-pyed **BED**-may-king)*

RESIDENT ENVIRONMENT

The resident's **environment** is the surroundings in which the resident now lives. Anything that is part of the environment affects the resident's sense of comfort, happiness, and security. The environment includes:

- Physical surroundings
- People who interact with the resident
- Quality of care given
- General atmosphere of the facility and staff

Nursing assistants have a responsibility for maintaining a safe, clean, and pleasant environment for the residents (Figure 15-1).

The resident's sense of well-being is a reflection of how the resident believes he or she is being treated. Residents respond positively when they are treated with respect, are viewed as persons with value, are encouraged to exercise some control over their lives, and experience some personal

On the Job

Residents who are more independent may have many items in their rooms, causing a cluttered environment. It may be difficult to maintain a safe, orderly room for these residents.

independence. Negative feelings result when residents feel neglected, unimportant, unworthy, and powerless. A warm and friendly atmosphere promotes the well-being of both residents and health care providers.

PERSONAL SPACE

Personal space is the area immediately around a person's body. The boundaries of personal space are viewed differently by different cultures and by individuals within a culture. For example, people of some Asian cultures stand very close to each other when speaking. People of other cultures are uncomfortable and feel threatened if someone stands too close. Eye contact is another factor that defines personal space. Some cultures, such as some Native American groups, view eye contact as rude and a personal space violation (Figure 15-2).

For a resident in a long-term care facility, personal space is often extended to include personal articles and the room in which the resident lives. You can show respect for a resident's personal space by:

- Making sure a resident's personal articles are not placed in another resident's area when a room is shared.
- Allowing the resident to arrange personal possessions as desired as long as safety is not an

FIGURE 15-1 The nursing assistant contributes greatly to the friendly and comfortable atmosphere that creates a pleasant environment.

FIGURE 15-2 Personal space is interpreted differently by people of different cultures.

Culture	Definition of Personal Space	Eye Contact
American	About 3 feet	Yes
Asian	Close, no contact	No
African	Close	Yes
European	Distant	Yes
Native American	Distant	No
Hispanic	Close	Yes

issue. Do not rearrange the resident's personal possessions without permission. Residents are encouraged to keep a favorite chair or chest, as space permits. Moving these items can upset the resident. Because the residents become used to the placement of furniture in the room, moving furniture may cause accidental injury.

- Treating personal belongings with respect. Residents are encouraged to keep blankets, spreads, pillows, plants, photos, and mementos of family and their lives before their admission to the facility. These reminders help residents make the transition to living in the facility.
- Being sensitive to the clues the resident gives you about how the resident views personal space
- Knocking before entering the room
- Speaking before drawing back a privacy curtain
- Closing privacy curtains before carrying out procedures
- Explaining procedures and asking permission before starting the procedure
- Being patient with residents and treating each as a person of value

The unit equipment includes:

- Bed
- Privacy curtain
- Bedside table
- Closet space
- Call or signal cord/lights
- Bathroom equipment
- Overbed table
- Chair
- Sink and running water

Note that residents are not usually allowed to keep certain items in their rooms because these items are a safety hazard. Items that are not permitted vary from state to state. Some of these items include:

- Uncovered food
- Perishable food
- Matches and lighters
- Razor
- Knife
- Medications
- Cigarettes
- Alcohol

Check the facility regulations for items residents are not allowed to keep in their rooms.

RESIDENT UNIT

The resident's immediate environment is the unit or room where the resident lives. This room is often shared with another resident. The most important item in the room for the resident's comfort is the bed. Although many residents can be dressed and up for the day, some residents must remain in bed. The comfort and safety of the bed are important considerations for all residents.

Beds

The typical bed is adjustable and can be raised to make giving care easier. At the end of care, the bed is lowered to make it easier and safer for residents to get into and out of the bed. The back and foot of the bed can be raised to different positions for comfort and therapeutic reasons. Beds may be provided with adjustable side rails. Unless needed for safety, most facilities do not use the side rails, because they are restrictive and restraining.

Electric control of the bed positions is used in many facilities, but some manually, crank-operated beds may still be used. If the bed has cranks to change positions, be sure they are returned to the nonuse position so that no one will be injured by hitting them. The wheels of the bed should be locked to prevent the bed from rolling. If the bed has large wheels, they should be turned inward to prevent tripping over them.

Call Signal/Lights

Each bed is equipped with a call signal. This may be a simple cord with a pushbutton or a more elaborate panel that is attached to the side rail. When the resident signals, a light is activated both over the door to the room and at the nurses' station. Make sure that the resident knows how to use the system. A special system is found in the bathing area and bathroom. This signal is an emergency signal, which rings loudly and has a flashing red light. This signal indicates the need for immediate help and must be answered at once. Make sure that residents can always reach their call signals. For example, a resident who is paralyzed on the left side should have the signal readily available on the right side.

EXTENDED RESIDENT ENVIRONMENT

All facility employees are responsible for ensuring that safety, physical comfort, and a spirit of well-being are maintained throughout the extended resident environment, which includes the:

- Dining room
- Bathing area
- Activity area
- Therapy rooms
- Lounges
- Lobby
- Dayroom

To achieve these conditions the following factors must be managed:

- Cleanliness and order
- Adequate air circulation
- Proper temperature
- Adequate lighting
- Noise control
- Odor control

Cleanliness and Order

Dust and dirt, crumbs from food, and dirty dishes and glasses are contaminated by microbes that can contribute to the spread of disease. Food left in the residents' rooms may attract insects such as cockroaches and ants. The food can also cause unpleasant odors. Remove all dishes as soon as the resident finishes a meal or nourishment. Clean up any spills and crumbs immediately. Remember that residents are not usually allowed to store food in their rooms. Some facilities permit candy in the room if it is sealed or in a closed container.

The routine cleaning of the windows, bathroom, and floor is the responsibility of housekeeping, but the nursing department is expected to keep the rest of the environment safe and orderly.

Disposable items such as latex gloves and paper products should be disposed of in the proper receptacle in the dirty utility rooms. Reusable equipment must be cleaned and disinfected or sterilized before being used with another resident. Reusable equipment, such as bed cradles, basins, or commodes, is usually very expensive and should be properly handled in the following manner:

- Wear gloves and follow standard aseptic procedure.
- Rinse article with cold water; never use hot, because heat tends to cause blood and body tissues to harden on the article.
- Wash with warm, soapy water.
- Dry carefully.
- Check carefully for breakage or defects. Report defects if found.
- Disinfect or sterilize according to facility policy.
- Return article to proper storage area.

Clutter is a safety hazard and often is disturbing to the older adult. Return all equipment to its proper place as soon as you finish using it. Move equipment carefully to avoid hitting walls and furniture.

Adequate Air Circulation (Ventilation)

Everyone feels refreshed when fresh, clean air is available. Most facilities have central controls to manage ventilation. Some facilities have controls in each resident room so ventilation can be controlled to meet individual needs.

Circulating air may produce drafts. Blankets, screens, and curtains are used to control the flow of air to meet the residents' comfort needs.

Temperature Control

Older adults often prefer warmer temperatures than do younger people. The facility temperature is usually controlled at 70 to 72 °Fahrenheit. A resident may use a lap robe, sweater, or shawl for comfort and to protect dignity when wearing a dress (Figure 15-3).

Adequate Lighting

Make sure there is adequate lighting for resident and staff safety. This is especially important at dusk and during the night. The light level can be controlled by adjusting the overbed light, any lamps that may be in the room, and the room light

FIGURE 15-3 A lap robe provides comfort and protects the resident's dignity if she is wearing a dress.

(Figure 15-4). The overbed light usually has more than one level of brightness. The cord for controlling the overbed light should be within reach of the resident whenever the resident is in bed or sitting near the bed. A nightlight near the floor will not disturb the resident at night and is an added safety feature. Lights must be left on in the hallways and on stairways at night. Bright sunlight can be controlled using curtains and shades.

Noise Control

Loud noises are disturbing to most people. Older adults are often more sensitive to noise and find a noisy environment upsetting. Noisy equipment, banging trays, loud radios or televisions, ringing telephones, squeaking wheels, and loud or excited voices all add to the noise level in the facility. Health care providers can make the environment more pleasant by controlling noise when they work (Figure 15-5). Many surveyors will write a deficiency for too much noise in the facility.

Odor Control

Odors can be a problem in a long-term care facility unless everyone makes an effort to control them. Odors should be eliminated, not covered up. Residents who are incontinent must be cared for immediately. Soiled pads, garments, and linens must be placed in covered containers and handled according to facility policy.

FIGURE 15-4 The best lighting is indirect lighting.

FIGURE 15-5 Handle equipment carefully to control noise. Position equipment according to facility policy to prevent clutter.

*G*uidelines for

Ensuring a Safe and Comfortable Environment

The nursing assistant makes important contributions to maintaining a safe and comfortable resident environment.

Follow all infection control guidelines and use standard precautions for the care of all residents.

Cleanliness

1. Remove dishes immediately after use and clean up crumbs and spills.
2. Check that the resident is not storing food in the room. If food is permitted, check that it is wrapped or in a closed container.
3. Clean overbed table after use; use disinfectant, if necessary.
4. If the floor is soiled with blood or body fluids, call housekeeping for immediate cleanup, or follow facility policy.
5. Pick up resident clothing and place in laundry hamper if soiled or hang in closet.
6. Each time you enter the room, check it for cleanliness and order.
7. Provide a bag for used tissues and change it often.
8. Empty wastebaskets if full and reline with a plastic bag (this is usually done by housekeeping, but a basket may become full before the scheduled change).
9. Try to keep dresser and table tops uncluttered, but remember that the resident has the right to display personal items and to expect that they will not be disturbed. Ask permission to clean around them when necessary.

Noise

1. Exercise care in using and moving equipment to keep the noise level down.

2. Speak in a conversational tone of voice. Call out to other staff members only if the resident has had an incident, you cannot leave the resident, you cannot reach the call button, and you need assistance; otherwise, walk to another staff member to talk.
3. Keep radio and television volumes at a reasonable level on a station desired by the resident.
4. Close the door to the resident's room, and tell the resident why you are doing so, if cleaning or construction is underway in the hallway or a nearby room.

Odor

1. Control odors by caring for incontinent residents immediately.
2. Follow facility policy for handling of clothing and bed linens soiled by feces, urine, vomitus, respiratory secretions, wound drainage, or food spills.
3. Empty bed pans, urinals, and commodes promptly. Clean and disinfect after each use or according to facility policy.

Other Environmental Concerns

1. Be aware of residents' needs for ventilation and air circulation, temperature control, and adequate lighting; assist the resident as necessary to ensure comfort.
2. Check that all equipment used by the resident is in good repair and safe to use.
3. Be sensitive to residents' wishes relating to cultural preferences and accommodate them as much as possible without violating facility policy.

Bedpans, urinals, commodes, and emesis basins should be emptied, cleaned, and disinfected immediately after use, or as dictated by facility policy. Utility rooms and dining areas must be cleaned regularly.

Nursing assistants have a major responsibility for influencing the environment in which the residents live. Each day you will care for the residents' belongings and ensure that the resident unit and other areas are safe and clean.

CRITICAL PROCEDURE ACTIONS

Caring for residents safely means you must perform tasks in a manner specified by facility policy. Such tasks are called **procedures**. As you continue your study, you will learn the procedures for many nursing assistant tasks. You have already learned several emergency care and infection control procedures, including handwashing. The procedures that follow give you step-by-step directions for performing tasks that involve personal care of residents.

Certain steps must be done before you perform the actual resident care procedure. These steps are called beginning procedure actions. When the resident care procedure is completed, another series of steps, called procedure completion actions, must be done (Figure 15-6).

FIGURE 15-6 Beginning procedure actions and procedure completion actions	
Beginning Procedure Actions	**Rationale**
1. Assemble equipment needed and take to resident's room.	1. Improves the efficiency of the procedure. Means you do not have to leave the resident.
2. Knock on the resident's door and identify yourself by name and title.	2. Respects the resident's right to privacy. Notifies the resident who is giving care.
3. Identify the resident by checking the identification bracelet.	3. Ensures that you are caring for the correct resident.
4. Ask visitors to leave the room and advise where they may wait.	4. Respects the resident's right to privacy. Shows hospitality to visitors by advising them where to wait.
5. Explain what you are going to do and how the resident can assist. Answer questions about the procedure.	5. Informs the resident of what is going to be done and what is expected. Gives the resident an opportunity to get information about the procedure and the extent of resident participation.
6. Provide privacy by closing the door, privacy curtain, and window curtain.	6. Respects the resident's right to privacy. All three should be closed even if the resident is alone in the room.
7. Wash your hands.	7. Applies the principles of standard precautions. Prevents the spread of microorganisms.
8. Apply gloves if contact with blood, moist body fluids, secretions, excretions, or nonintact skin is likely.	8. Applies the principles of standard precautions. Protects the care provider and resident from transmission of pathogens.
9. Apply a gown if your uniform will have substantial contact with linen or other articles contaminated with blood, moist body fluids (except sweat), secretions, or excretions.	9. Applies the principles of standard precautions. Protects your uniform from contamination with bloodborne pathogens.
10. Apply a gown, mask, and eye protection if splashing of blood or moist body fluids is likely.	10. Applies the principles of standard precautions. Protects the care provider's mucous membranes, uniform, and skin from accidental splashing of bloodborne pathogens.
11. Raise the bed to a comfortable working height.	11. Prevents back strain and injury caused by bending at the waist.
12. Lower the side rail on the side where you are working.	12. Provides an obstacle-free area in which to work. *(continues)*

FIGURE 15-6 *(continued)*

Procedure Completion Actions	Rationale
1. Check to make sure the resident is in good alignment.	1. All body systems function better when the body is correctly aligned. The resident is more comfortable when the body is in good alignment.
2. Remove gloves.	2. Prevents contamination of environmental surfaces from the gloves.
3. Raise the side rail.	3. Resident's right to a safe environment. Prevents accidents and injuries.
4. Remove other personal protective equipment, if worn, and discard according to facility policy.	4. Prevents unnecessary environmental contamination from used gloves and protective equipment.
5. Wash your hands.	5. Applies the principles of standard precautions. Prevents the spread of microorganisms.
6. Return the bed to the lowest horizontal position.	6. Resident's right to a safe environment. Prevents accidents and injuries.
7. Open the privacy and window curtains.	7. Privacy is no longer necessary unless preferred by the resident.
8. Leave the resident in a position of comfort and safety with the call signal and needed personal items within reach.	8. Prevents accidents and injuries. Ensures that help is available. Eliminates the need to call or reach for needed personal items.
9. Wash your hands.	9. Although the hands were washed previously, they have contacted the resident and other items in the room. Wash them again before leaving to prevent potential transfer of microorganisms to areas outside the resident's unit.
10. Inform visitors that they may return to the room.	10. Courtesy to visitors and resident.
11. Report completion of the procedure and any abnormalities or other observations.	11. Inform the nurse that your assigned task has been completed so further resident care can be planned and you can be reassigned to other duties. Notifies the nurse of abnormalities and changes in the resident's condition for further assessment.
12. Document the procedure and your observations.	12. Ongoing progress and care given is documented. Provides a legal record. Provides a record of what has been done, for other members of the interdisciplinary team.

BEDMAKING

You will learn two basic methods of making the resident's bed:

- **Unoccupied bedmaking** (when the resident is not in the bed)—see Procedure 19
- **Occupied bedmaking** (when the resident is in the bed)—see Procedure 20

The following linens are used to make the resident's bed:

- Sheets, top and bottom (the bottom sheet may be contoured or have elastic edges to fit over the edges of the mattress)
- Pillowcases, usually two although more may be required if several pillows are used to position and support the resident in bed
- **Draw sheet** or lift sheet, a small sheet or a regular top sheet folded in half and placed sideways across the bed to cover the area between the resident's upper back and thighs
  - The sides of the draw sheet may or may not be tucked under the mattress.
  - The draw sheet can be changed frequently without changing the rest of the bed linen if the bottom sheet is not soiled.
  - The draw sheet can be used to lift the resident to change position in bed (in this case, the edges of the draw sheet would not be tucked under the mattress).
- Underpad (protective pad) may be placed on top of the bottom sheet or draw sheet to provide additional protection. Underpads may be disposable, paper-type pads with a moisture-resistant layer that are placed under the resident and changed when soiled. Other types of reusable moisture-resistant materials can also be used.
- Blanket
- Spread (when the resident is out of bed, the spread is usually placed on the bed and covers the pillows)

Bed linens that are not soiled by blood, body fluids, body secretions or excretions, or spilled food are changed according to a schedule set by the facility. All soiled linens are changed immediately.

*G*uidelines for

Handling Linens and Making the Bed

Handling Linens

1. Wash hands and use gloves as required; other personal protective equipment may be required.
2. Laundry hampers placed in the hallway should be at least two rooms away from clean linen carts.
3. The clean linen cart is always covered; replace covers after removing required linen.
4. Take only the linens you need into the resident's room.
5. Linens that touch the floor are considered dirty and placed in the laundry hamper; they are not used.
6. Avoid contact between the linens and your uniform (for both clean and soiled linens).
7. Unused linen is never returned to the clean linen cart; it is placed in the laundry hamper.
8. As soiled linen is removed from the bed, keep the soiled areas on the inside and fold or roll the linen toward the center.
9. Never shake soiled bed linens, because microbes will be released into the air.
10. Soiled linen is never placed on environmental surfaces in the room, such as overbed table, chair, or floor; soiled linens are placed in the appropriate laundry hamper (follow facility policy).
11. Fill laundry hampers no more than two-thirds full.
12. Many facilities do not permit laundry hampers or barrels to be taken into the resident's room. Soiled linen may be placed in a plastic bag or a pillowcase in the room. Make a cuff at the top of the bag or open end of the pillowcase and place the cuff over the back of the chair. When the bag or case is two-thirds full, secure the top and place it in the hamper in the hallway.
13. Laundry hampers or barrels are returned to utility room after use, or as directed by facility policy.

(continues)

---

*G*uidelines *(continued)*

Making the Bed

1. Use proper body mechanics at all times to prevent back injury.
2. Work on one side of the bed at a time to complete removing soiled linen and placing clean linen (see Procedures 19 and 20).
3. Make sure the bottom sheet and draw sheet (if used) are smooth and unwrinkled (wrinkles in bed linens can lead to skin breakdown, especially for residents who remain in bed).
4. Follow the care plan for the positioning of the head and foot of the bed, the number of pillows to be used, and the need for pillows for positioning.

PROCEDURE 19

Unoccupied Bed: Changing Linens

1. Carry out the beginning procedure actions (Figure 15-7).

FIGURE 15-7 Remember to start and end each procedure by washing your hands.

2. Assemble equipment:
   - Disposable gloves (if linens are soiled with blood or body fluids, secretions, or excretions)
   - Pillowcases
   - Spread
   - Blankets, as needed
   - Two large sheets (90 × 109) (substitute one fitted, if used)

   - Draw sheet, for selected residents
   - Laundry hamper (Figure 15-8)

FIGURE 15-8 If facility policy permits, take a laundry hamper or barrel into the room with you.

3. Lock bed wheels so the bed will not roll and place chair at the side of the bed.
4. Raise bed to comfortable working height.
5. Arrange linens on chair in order in which they are to be used. Make a cuff at the top of a plastic bag or pillowcase. Place the cuff over the back of the chair and use the bag or case for the disposal of soiled linen.

(continues)

PROCEDURE *19* (continued)

6. Remove soiled linen as follows:
   a. Loosen the bedding on one side of the bed by lifting the edge of the mattress with one hand and drawing the linens out with the other.
   b. Remove the pillow from the bed. Grasp pillow with one hand. Using the other hand, gather the pillowcase and pull it back over the pillow so it is inside out. Place pillow on chair and put pillowcase in bag for soiled linen.
   c. If the spread is clean and to be reused, fold it lengthwise by bringing the far edge toward the near edge. Fold it once more from the center lengthwise. Then fold the spread from top to bottom and place it over the back of the chair.
      Note: If the spread is soiled, it must be handled as the sheets are handled.
   d. Gather the top sheet by folding the edges inward so that the dirtiest side is on the inside. Place sheet in bag.
   e. Gather up the draw sheet (if used) by folding the dirtiest side inward. Place draw sheet in bag.
   f. Repeat process with the bottom sheet. Before putting the linen in the hamper or pillowcase, remember to check it for items such as dentures, eyeglasses, hearing aids, equipment, supplies, syringes, and so on. Remove the items and follow facility policy for cleaning, disinfection, storage, or disposal. Mattresses have a plasticized top for protection against soiling. If the top of the mattress is wet from the linens, wipe dry using a disinfectant. Secure top of plastic bag or pillowcase and place in hamper in hallway. Remove gloves and dispose of properly. Wash hands, dry, and put on fresh gloves, if required.
7. Position mattress to head of bed by grasping handles on mattress side.
8. Work from one side of the bed until that side is completed, and then go to the other side of the bed.
9. Place bottom sheet lengthwise on mattress with fold at center of bed. Be sure the smooth side (hemside) is up and

the narrow hem is even with the foot of the mattress (Figure 15-9A). See Figure 15-9B if a fitted bottom sheet is used.

FIGURE 15-9A Place flat bottom sheet even with end of mattress at foot of bed.

FIGURE 15-9B If a fitted bottom sheet is used, fit it properly and smoothly around the corner of the mattress.

10. Tuck 12 to 18 inches of sheet smoothly over the top of the mattress.
11. Make a **mitered** (Figure 15-10) or **square corner**.
12. Tuck in the sheet on one side, keeping it straight. Work from the head to the foot of the bed. If a fitted sheet is used, adjust it over the head and bottom ends of the mattress.
13. Unfold the top sheet and place wrong side up, top hem even with the upper edge of the mattress, and center fold on the center of the bed. Tuck in sheet at

(continues)

PROCEDURE 19 *(continued)*

FIGURE 15-10 Making a mitered corner.
A. The sheet is hanging loose at the side of the bed. B. Pick up the sheet about 12 inches from the head of the bed to form a triangle. Pull back toward the bed to smooth out the sheet and lay triangle on bed.
C. Tuck in sheet at head of bed. D. Pick up triangle and place other hand at edge of bed near head to hold edge of sheet in place. Bring triangle over edge of mattress and tuck smoothly under mattress. Tuck in the rest of the sheet along the side of the mattress. Make sure sheet is smooth.

FIGURE 15-11A Gather about 12 to 18 inches of the top sheet at bottom of bed.

FIGURE 15-11B Face foot of bed and lift mattress with near hand.

FIGURE 15-11C Using other hand, bring sheet smoothly over end of mattress.

the bottom of the bed, as shown in Figures 15-11A–C.

14. Spread blanket over the top sheet and foot of mattress. Keep blanket centered.

15. Tuck top sheet and blanket under mattress at the foot of the bed as far as the center only and make a mitered or square corner (Figure 15-12A–C).
16. Place spread with top hem even with head of mattress.
17. Unfold to foot of bed.
18. Tuck spread under mattress at the foot of one side of bed (Figure 15-13) and make mitered or square corner.
19. Go to other side of bed and fanfold the top sheet, blanket, and spread to the center of the bed to work with lower sheets and pad.
20. Tuck bottom sheet under head of mattress and make mitered or square cor-

(continues)

PROCEDURE 19 *(continued)*

FIGURE 15-12A Make the square (box) corner following the steps of Figure 15-10A–C. Then, holding the corner with one hand, grasp the bottom of the sheet and pull it straight down until fold is even with the edge of the mattress.

FIGURE 15-12B Holding the square corner in place, tuck sheet under mattress.

ner. Working from top to bottom, smooth out all wrinkles and tighten sheet as much as possible, or adjust fitted bottom sheet smoothly and securely around mattress corners.
21. Tuck in top sheet and blanket.
22. Fold top sheet back over blanket, making an 8-inch cuff.

FIGURE 15-12C Finished square corner should look like this.

FIGURE 15-13A Gather top sheet and spread together and smooth evenly over end of mattress.

23. Tuck in spread at foot of bed and make a mitered or square corner.
24. Bring top of spread to head of mattress.
25. Insert pillow in pillowcase properly. Be sure corners of pillows are in corners of pillowcases.
26. Place pillow at head of bed with open end away from the door.
27. Spread is brought up to cover pillow.
28. Lower bed to lowest horizontal position.
29. Replace bedside table parallel to bed. Place chair in assigned location. Place

(continues)

PROCEDURE 19 *(continued)*

FIGURE 15-13B Tuck sheet and spread under mattress together.

FIGURE 15-13C Continue as in the procedure for a mitered corner.

FIGURE 15-13D Slide finger to the end to make a smooth edge.

FIGURE 15-13E The completed top bedding. The procedure is repeated on the other side.

overbed table over the foot of the bed opposite the chair.

30. Wash hands.
31. Perform procedure completion actions.
32. Report completion of task.

PROCEDURE 20 Occupied Bed: Changing Linens

OBRA

1. Carry out each beginning procedure action.
2. Assemble equipment:
  • Disposable gloves (if linens are soiled with blood, body fluids, secretions, or excretions; gown is required if there may be contact between your uniform and soiled linens)
  • Draw sheet, for selected residents
  • Two pillowcases
  • Two large sheets (or one large sheet and one fitted sheet)
  • Laundry hamper
3. Place bedside chair at the foot of the bed.
4. Arrange bed linen on chair in the order in which it is to be used.

(continues)

PROCEDURE *20* *(continued)*

5. The bed should be flat with wheels locked, unless otherwise indicated. Raise to working horizontal height.
6. If bed linens are soiled with blood or body fluids, wash hands and put on disposable gloves.
7. Loosen the linens on one side by lifting the edge of the mattress with one hand and drawing bedclothes out with the other.
8. Adjust mattress to head of bed. If resident's condition permits, have resident bend knees, grasp side rails or headboard of bed with hands, and pull on frame as you draw mattress to the top (Figure 15-14) or have another person help from the opposite side.

FIGURE 15-14 The resident grasps the head of the bed and pushes in with the heels while two nursing assistants pull the mattress to the head of the bed.

9. Remove covers, except for top sheet, one at a time. Fold to bottom and pick up in center. Place over the back of chair.
10. Place a clean sheet over top sheet. Have the resident hold the top edge of the clean sheet, if possible. If not, tuck the sheet beneath the resident's shoulder.
11. Slide out the soiled top sheet, from top to bottom. Place in hamper.
12. Ask the resident to roll toward you and assist if necessary. Move one pillow with the resident. Pull up side rail for safety.

13. Go to the other side of the bed. Fanfold the draw sheet, if used, and the bottom sheet close to the resident (Figure 15-15).
14. Place a clean bottom sheet on the bed so that the narrow hem comes to the edge of the mattress at the foot and the lengthwise center fold of the sheet is at the center of the bed.

FIGURE 15-15 Note that the bottom linen is flat and the resident is positioned on the far side of the bed.

15. Tuck top of clean bottom sheet under the head of the mattress.
16. Make a mitered or square corner. Tuck side of bottom sheet under mattress, working toward the foot of the bed.
17. Position clean draw sheet if used. Tuck it under the mattress. If used, place protective underpad on top of draw sheet.
18. Ask the resident to roll toward you and assist as needed. Move the pillow with the resident.
19. Raise side rail for safety.
20. Go to the other side of the bed. Remove soiled linen by rolling the edges inward.
21. Keep soiled linen away from your uniform, and place in hamper, plastic bag, or pillowcase.
22. Complete the bed as for an unoccupied bed. Some residents prefer not to have the blanket, top sheet, or spread tucked in.

(continues)

PROCEDURE 20 *(continued)*

23. Turn resident on back. Place clean case on pillow. Replace pillow. If other pillows are used for positioning, change pillow-cases each time bed linens are changed, or according to facility policy.
24. Remove and dispose of gloves (if used) according to facility policy. Wash hands.
25. Adjust bed position for the resident's comfort.

26. Be sure side rails are up and secure, if needed. Lower bed to lowest horizontal position.
27. Replace bedside table and chair.
28. Make sure call signal and fresh water are within reach of resident.
29. Carry out each procedure completion action.
30. Report completion of task.

LESSON SYNTHESIS: Putting It All Together

You have just completed this lesson. Now go back and review the Clinical Focus. Try to see how the Clinical Focus relates to the concepts presented in the lesson. Then answer the following questions.

1. What actions could you take to increase Edith Curry's comfort when the grandchildren of her roommates visit?

2. How should the environment be adjusted to increase safety during evening hours?

3. How can you help Mrs. Curry to be comfortable when she is sitting on the patio area and the sun is shining in?

4. How does a well-made bed, properly positioned, contribute to the safety and well-being of the resident?

REVIEW

A. Match each term (items a.–e.) with the proper definition.

a. side rails
b. draw sheet
c. environment
d. mitered corner
e. unoccupied bed

1. _____ half-sheet

2. _____ bed without a resident

3. _____ sheet tucked in at a 45° angle

4. _____ safety feature on beds that can be regarded as a restraint

5. _____ surroundings in which the resident lives

B. Select the one best answer for each of the following.

6. Most facilities regulate the room temperature to approximately
   (A) 60–62 °F
   (B) 64–66 °F
   (C) 70–72 °F
   (D) 78–80 °F

7. A positive atmosphere is created when
   (A) radios play loudly
   (B) residents are treated with respect
   (C) odors are covered up
   (D) equipment is out of place

8. Which of the following is not usually permitted to be stored in the resident's room?
   (A) uncovered food
   (B) books
   (C) radio
   (D) pictures

9. To ensure privacy, you should
   (A) arrange the resident's belongings to please yourself
   (B) enter rooms without knocking
   (C) close curtains around the bed before carrying out procedures
   (D) leave curtains open around a resident receiving care if only her roommate is present

10. Underpads
   (A) are half-sheets
   (B) reduce pressure
   (C) can be easily changed when soiled
   (D) are also called draw sheets

C. Answer each statement true (T) or false (F).

11. T   F   Adjustable beds provide for resident comfort and therapeutic positioning.

12. T   F   Bed linens are completely changed every day even if they are not soiled.

13. T   F   A draw sheet is a half-sheet placed over the bottom sheet.

14. T   F   When making an unoccupied bed, make one side completely before going to the opposite side.

15. T   F   It is important that the bottom sheet be smooth.

16. T   F   When making a bed, linens should be arranged on a chair in the order in which they are to be used.

17. T   F   The mattress should be positioned to the top of the bed before clean linen is applied.

18. T   F   If the linen is soiled with blood, the nursing assistant should wear gloves when making the bed.

19. T   F   The occupied bed should be left in a high horizontal position with the side rails down.

20. T   F   Side rails should be checked for security when up in place.

21. T   F   If a crank is left protruding, it can cause an injury.

22. T   F   Beds should be raised to a comfortable working height before linens are changed.

23. T   F   The nursing assistant is responsible for maintaining a safe and comfortable environment for the resident.

24. T   F   Side rails must be up and secured for all residents, regardless of condition.

25. T   F   When stripping soiled linen from a bed, the linens should always be gathered so the dirtiest part is inside.

LESSON 16

Caring for the Residents' Personal Hygiene

Clinical Focus

Think about ways you can assist residents in meeting their personal hygiene needs as you study this lesson and meet:

Mary Mandell, one of your residents, who is a charming lady, full of stories about growing up on an Oklahoma cattle ranch. She is right-handed. A stroke 2 years ago left her paralyzed on the right side. She is up in a wheelchair most of the day, and a small reddened area has developed over her sacrum.

OBJECTIVES

After studying this lesson, you should be able to:

- Define and spell vocabulary words and terms.
- Name the parts and functions of the integumentary system.
- Review changes in the integument due to aging.
- Describe common skin conditions affecting the long-term care resident.
- Identify factors that contribute to skin breakdown.
- List actions that prevent skin breakdown.
- Explain the use of comfort and positioning devices.
- Demonstrate the following:

  Procedure 21 Backrub
  Procedure 22 Bed Bath Using Basin and Water
  Procedure 23 Bed Bath Using a Rinse-Free Cleanser and Moisturizer
  Procedure 24 Tub Bath or Shower
  Procedure 25 Partial Bath
  Procedure 26 Female Perineal Care
  Procedure 27 Male Perineal Care
  Procedure 28 Daily Hair Care
  Procedure 29 Shaving Male Resident

  Procedure 30 Hand and Fingernail Care
  Procedure 31 Foot and Toenail Care
  Procedure 32 Assisting Resident to Brush Teeth
  Procedure 33 Cleaning and Flossing Resident's Teeth
  Procedure 34 Caring for Dentures
  Procedure 35 Assisting with Oral Hygiene for the Unconscious Resident
  Procedure 36 Dressing and Undressing Resident

VOCABULARY

axilla   (ack-**SILL**-ah)

bridging   (**BRIJ**-ing)

caries   (**KAIR**-eez)

constricting   (kon-**STRICK**-ting)

cuticle   (**KYOU**-tih-kul)

decubiti   (dee-**KYOU**-bih-tie)

dentures   (**DEN**-churz)

dermis   (**DER**-mis)

dilating   (**DIE**-lay-ting)

dry sterile dressing (DSD)   (dri **STER**-ill **DRESS**-ing)

epidermis   (ep-ih-**DER**-mis)

friction   (**FRICK**-shun)

genitalia   (jen-ih-**TAIL**-ee-ah)

halitosis   (hal-ih-**TOH**-sis)

integumentary system   (in-**teg**-you-**MEN**-tair-ee **SIS**-tem)

lesion   (**LEE**-zhun)

oil gland   (oil gland)

oral hygiene   (**OR**-al **HIGH**-jeen)

perineal care   (**pair**-ih-**NEE**-al kair)

pore   (por)

pressure ulcer   (**PRESH**-zhur **UL**-sir)

pubic   (**PYOU**-bick)

receptor   (ree-**SEP**-tor)

senile lentigines   (**SEE**-nile len-**TIJ**-ih-nees)

shearing   (**SHEER**-ing)

skin tear   (skin tair)

subcutaneous tissue   (sub-kyou-**TAY**-nee-us **TISH**-you)

sweat gland   (swet gland)

The **integumentary system** consists of the skin, oil and sweat glands of the skin, hair, nails, teeth, and the environmental sense organs. The teeth are formed from the tissues of the integument (body shell) but also make a major contribution to the digestive system.

The outermost layers of the skin make up the **epidermis** (Figure 16-1). Under the epidermis is the **dermis**, and under the dermis is the **subcutaneous tissue** that attaches the skin to the muscles.

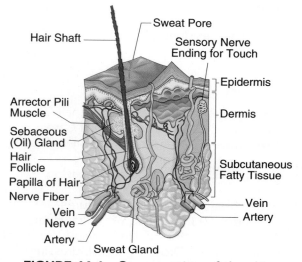

FIGURE 16-1 Cross-section of the skin

Labels:
Hair Shaft
Sweat Pore
Sensory Nerve Ending for Touch
Epidermis
Dermis
Arrector Pili Muscle
Sebaceous (Oil) Gland
Hair Follicle
Papilla of Hair
Nerve Fiber
Subcutaneous Fatty Tissue
Vein
Nerve
Artery
Sweat Gland
Vein
Artery

EPIDERMIS

The epidermis consists of dead outer cells that are constantly shed as new cells move upward from the dermis. There are no blood vessels in the epidermis, so injury to this level does not produce bleeding. Nerve endings reach into this outer covering. The nerves form sense organs that keep us in contact with changes in the environment. Nerve endings called **receptors** receive information about temperature, pressure, and pain.

DERMIS

The dermis contains blood vessels, nerve fibers, and two kinds of glands:

- **Sweat glands**
- **Oil glands**

Sweat Glands

The sweat glands produce perspiration that reaches the skin surface through tubes or ducts that end in openings called **pores**. Heat from deep in the body is brought to the skin by blood vessels. This heat is transferred to the perspiration. At the skin surface, the perspiration and the heat are lost through the pores to the air. The heat of the body is controlled by changes in the size of the blood vessels in the skin.

- **Dilating** (enlarging) blood vessels bring more heat to the body surface.
- **Constricting** (narrowing) blood vessels bring less heat to the body surface.

Oil Glands

Oil glands lubricate and keep flexible the hairs found in the skin. Hair covers almost all the body surfaces except for the palms of the hands and the soles of the feet.

SKIN FUNCTIONS

The skin has many functions that are critical to the well-being of the body:

- Protection—forms a continuous membranous covering and regulates body temperature
- Storage—stores fat and vitamins
- Elimination—loses water, salts, and heat through perspiration
- Sensory perceptions—contains nerve endings that keep us aware of environmental changes

FIGURE 16-2   Look carefully at the skin of the hands of the nursing assistant and the resident. Note the aging changes in the skin of the resident.

SKIN CHANGES CAUSED BY AGING

Common Changes in the Aging Skin

As people age, changes occur in the integumentary system (Figure 16-2). These changes include:

1. Sweat glands decrease in activity and number.
2. Loss of elasticity and fatty tissue causes wrinkling. The eyelids tend to droop.
3. The skin becomes drier as oil gland secretions decrease, and it becomes thin like tissue paper.
4. Areas of pigmentation seem more pronounced. In light-skinned people, the skin becomes more sallow or yellow and less pink. Skin tags and moles are more common.
5. The hair loses its color, becoming first gray and then white. Less oil causes the hair to become drier and duller. The amount of hair, especially in men, diminishes.
6. Nails on both fingers and toes thicken, becoming more brittle and likely to split.
7. Peripheral blood vessels weaken. These are more easily seen under the thinned epidermis. Small hemorrhages occur due to the weakness of the blood vessels. Peripheral circulation to the skin decreases so that general skin nutrition is less satisfactory.
8. Loss of teeth may result in the need for **dentures** (artificial teeth).

Injury and Healing

The skin is exposed to the environment and is constantly in danger of trauma and infection. The skin of the older adult is fragile because of aging changes. Injuries to the skin of older adults are slower to heal. Compared to younger people, the skin receives less blood flow and, as a result, fewer nutrients to help the healing process.

Caution is always required when caring for the elderly to prevent injury to the skin. Bathing, dressing, positioning, and bedmaking (occupied bed) are all situations in which the elderly may experience skin injuries if the nursing assistant is not careful.

SKIN LESIONS

Changes in the structure of the skin are called **lesions**. The lesions may be caused by the aging process, disease, trauma, or wear. It is the nursing assistant's responsibility to observe the residents carefully. Observations about the condition of the skin and changes in the skin are important. Any changes noted should be reported immediately and described accurately. The following types of lesions are discussed: skin cancer, senile lentigines, skin breakdown, and pressure ulcers.

Skin Cancer

Cancers of the skin are fairly common in the older individual. Be sure to report any changes you note in the size or shape of a wart or mole or indications of inflammation (redness) around the area of a wart or mole. Skin cancer can also appear as an area of darkened pigmentation in the skin. Skin that has been exposed to the sun for long periods of time over the years is susceptible to skin cancer. The earlier any changes noted are reported, the earlier treatment can begin.

Senile Lentigines

Areas of skin pigmentation seem to become more pronounced with advancing years. **Senile lentigines** (Figure 16-3) are sometimes called liver spots although they are not related to liver function. They are thought to be a response to environmental exposure. They appear as yellowish or brownish spots on exposed skin surfaces.

A professional evaluation may be needed to determine if a lesion is a relatively harmless senile lentigine or an early indication of skin cancer.

Skin Breakdown

Friction, shearing, pressure, poor nutrition, and moisture are common causes of skin break-

FIGURE 16-4 The rubbing of nasal catheters, nasogastric tubes, or urinary catheters can cause skin breakdown.

down. **Friction** occurs when the skin moves against a firm or rough surface, including bed linens, wheelchair parts, a crutch or brace, or tubing, such as a nasogastric tube or urinary catheter (Figure 16-4). Friction also occurs when parts of the body rub together, for example, ankles or knees rubbing against each other. The rubbing action may cause skin abrasions that can lead to deeper tissue injury.

Shearing occurs when the skin moves in one direction while the structures under the skin, such as the bones, remain fixed or move in the opposite direction. This can happen when residents are dragged rather than lifted up in bed, when positions are changed, or when residents slide down in bed or in a wheelchair (Figure 16-5). Blood vessels become twisted and stretched, causing the tissues being served to lose essential oxygen and nutrients, leading to breakdown. In addition, shearing may cause actual tears in fragile skin. These **skin tears** are painful, a portal of entry for infectious pathogens, and commonly lead to further breakdown.

When pressure is put on tissues for a long time, skin breakdown can occur. The tissues are

FIGURE 16-3 Senile lentigines

On the Job

Residents often slip from proper alignment after you have positioned them properly. Check frequently to make sure correct position is maintained.

FIGURE 16-5 Shearing can occur when the resident's position is poorly supported. As the resident slides down in bed or in a chair, the skeleton remains stationary but the skin slips, causing tension both on the skin and on the underlying blood vessels, leading to tissue damage.

usually trapped between a bony prominence such as the heel, hip bone, or sacrum and the source of the pressure. The pressure causes the collapse of tiny blood vessels. Skin surfaces receiving less nourishment through the damaged vessels quickly break down.

Pressure Ulcers

Skin breakdown may progress to the formation of deep, painful lesions called **pressure ulcers** (also known as **decubiti**). They are a serious problem, especially for older adults. Residents are assessed by the interdisciplinary team for the probability of developing pressure ulcers. A care plan is developed with specific actions to prevent the formation of pressure ulcers. In some facilities, this activity is performed by a nurse who is specially trained in skin and wound care.

Factors Leading to Breakdown. Pressure ulcers can frequently be prevented by conscientious care and attention. Nursing assistants must be alert to the factors that contribute to their formation, including:

- Impaired circulation due to pressure
- Prolonged contact with moisture
- Prolonged contact with excretions/secretions
- Poor nutrition and debilitation
- Dehydration
- Shearing forces and friction
- Immobility
- Incontinence

Signs of Tissue Breakdown. Tissue breakdown is described and classified in four stages. Unless action is taken, the damage is progressive.

1. Stage one: The intact skin surface shows redness or blue-gray discoloration over a pressure point, which does not disappear when the pressure is removed (Figure 16-6). In darker-skinned people, the area may seem drier, and under pressure, become darker or purplish in color, and feel warm to the touch.
2. Stage two: The reddened skin is accompanied by an abrasion, blisters, or a shallow crater (Figure 16-7). The epidermis alone or the epidermis and dermis may be involved. The area around the site is reddened.
3. Stage three: The deeper subcutaneous tissues break down and a deep crater is formed (Figure 16-8).
4. Stage four: The deeper tissues of muscles and bones are involved. At this stage, residents

FIGURE 16-6 First indication of tissue damage (stage one) is redness and heat over a pressure point, such as this heel. (Courtesy of Emory University Hospital, Atlanta, GA)

FIGURE 16-7 Stage two is marked by destruction of the epidermis and partial destruction of the dermis. *Note:* The area shown is the sacrum. (Courtesy of Emory University Hospital, Atlanta, GA)

FIGURE 16-9 This pressure ulcer developed over the hip of a resident. It involves deep tissues (stage four). (Courtesy of Emory University Hospital, Atlanta, GA)

experience fluid loss and pain and are at great risk for infection (Figure 16-9).

Actions to Take When Breakdown Occurs. It is easier to prevent skin breakdown than to treat the results. It is also more cost-effective. Residents with existing skin breakdown may be admitted to the long-term care facility from home or another health care facility. At other times, despite careful preventive care, skin breakdown occurs. In these situations, the nursing assistant actions include:

- Performing the actions listed in the guidelines to prevent further breakdown
- Following the care plan exactly
- Reporting indications of infection, such as fever, odor, drainage, bleeding, and changes in size

FIGURE 16-8 In stage three, all layers of skin have been destroyed. A deep crater has been formed. *Note:* Photo shows right hip. (Courtesy of Emory University Hospital, Atlanta, GA)

- Keeping the area around the breakdown clean and dry
- Assisting with whirlpool baths, if ordered, to keep the area clean

The nurse or physician may perform other procedures to care for areas of skin breakdown. For example:

- The area may be covered with a **dry sterile dressing (DSD)**. Holding a DSD in place without causing additional injury is not easy. The skin of older adults may be sensitive to regular tape. In this case, silk tape, paper tape, cellophane tape or other hypoallergenic tape may be used. To prevent injury when removing the tape before a dressing change, a saline solution is applied to loosen the tape.
- Residents may be placed on alternating-pressure mattresses or pressure-reducing mattresses or beds.
- In some facilities, the open lesions are packed loosely with gauze soaked in a wound gel. The gel keeps the lesions moist, breaks down dead cells, and promotes healing.
- The area may be protected and kept moist by using special dressings. They have a clear plastic covering that permits air to reach the tissues as well as keeping them moist to promote healing. The dressing must extend beyond the wound edge. It is held in place with a frame of either paper or silk tape. The dressing must be changed every 3 to 5 days unless there is leakage, or according to facility policy.
- The wounds may be cleaned by the nurse or physician with saline solution and debrided (dead tissue removed) using instruments and proteolytic enzymes.

*G*uidelines for

Preventing Skin Breakdown

Nursing assistant actions are vital in identifying potential causes of breakdown and taking steps to eliminate or minimize them.

1. Carefully inspect the resident's skin during care and report findings to the nurse.
2. Bathe resident regularly. Handle the skin gently and use a mild cleansing agent. Avoid hot water and do not scrub the skin. Dry thoroughly by patting the skin with the towel. Closely inspect potential pressure or friction areas.
3. Immediately remove feces, urine, or moisture of any kind, including perspiration, from the resident's skin. Prolonged contact is irritating to the skin. Keep the skin clean and dry.
4. Use underpads or briefs that absorb moisture, to help keep the resident dry.
5. Use lotion on dry skin areas but do not use on broken skin. Pat lotion on skin gently; do not rub vigorously.
6. Encourage good nutrition and adequate fluid intake.
7. Change the position of an in-bed resident at least every 2 hours to reduce pressure in any one area. Some residents may need repositioning more often than others. The care plan for each resident must be followed carefully. The turning schedule will be posted in the care plan and in the room. Figure 16-10 shows an example of the sequence of turns.
8. Keep bed linens wrinkle-free.

9. Encourage residents sitting in geri-chairs or wheelchairs to raise themselves or change position to relieve pressure every 15 minutes. If the resident is not able to do so, assist the resident in repositioning at least every hour.
10. Check for improperly fitted or worn braces, shoes, and restraints that may rub the skin.
11. Check nasogastric tubes and urinary catheters to be sure they are positioned so they do not irritate the skin. Keep nasal and urinary openings clean and free of drainage. These areas must be checked frequently and carefully.
12. Do passive range of motion exercises twice daily.
13. Use a turning sheet to help move dependent residents in bed. Some residents may be able to help reposition themselves in bed by using a trapeze. Do not drag the resident over the bed linens.
14. Do not elevate the head of the bed too high. This may cause shearing of tissues as the resident slides down in bed. An elevation of no more than 30° is recommended for residents who are at risk for pressure ulcers.
15. Separate body areas likely to rub together, especially over bony prominences, by using pillows or foam wedges, according to the care plan.
16. For residents sitting in geri-chairs or wheelchairs, use foam, gel, or air cushions to reduce pressure on buttocks and sacrum.
17. For residents in bed, relieve pressure on heels by supporting feet off the bed.
18. Use special pressure-reducing mattresses or alternating-pressure mattresses for residents in bed.
19. Report signs of infection, such as fever, odor, drainage, inflammation, or bleeding to the nurse.
20. OBRA and the Joint Commission on Accreditation of Healthcare Organizations (JCAHO) require that the health care team develop an individualized care plan to prevent pressure ulcers in residents at risk.

FIGURE 16-10 Example of a turning schedule with a position change every 2 hours

- Antiseptic sprays, antibiotic ointments, and dressings are used to control infection.
- Surgery may be needed to close the ulcerated area in severe cases.

Residents are encouraged to participate to whatever extent is possible in their own care. Attentive nursing care is essential in preventing skin breakdown. Remember that it is far easier to prevent pressure ulcers than to heal them.

Blood Circulation to Tissues. Ensuring adequate circulation to tissues is a major factor in preventing skin breakdown. This can be accomplished by:

- Positioning the resident properly
- Using mechanical aids
- Providing backrubs
- Performing active or passive range of motion exercises

The most common sites for skin breakdown are shown in Figure 16-11.

Positioning. Five basic in-bed positions are used to relieve pressure as the resident's condition permits. Each position must be supported for comfort. The nursing assistant must remember that not all residents can assume the full range of positions, because of disabilities such as arthritis, contractures, or breathing limitations. Residents who sit in geri-chairs or wheelchairs for long periods of time must also change position to relieve pressure.

Residents with special problems require extra care when they are positioned in bed. For example:

- Be sure the resident can breathe properly.
- Remember that a fractured hip is never rotated over the unaffected leg.
- If the resident had a stroke, elevate the weak arm to reduce edema.
- Always maintain proper body alignment.
- The resident with a recent stroke is turned on the unaffected side.

The five basic positions residents assume in bed are:

- Supine position
- Semisupine position
- Lateral position
- Semiprone position
- Fowler's position

These positions are described fully and illustrated in Lesson 22 on restorative care.

Mechanical Aids

Mechanical aids are used to reduce pressure. Examples are

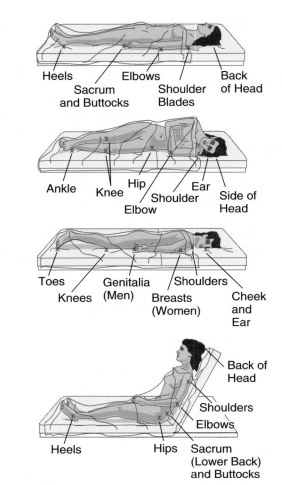

FIGURE 16-11 Most common sites for skin breakdown

- Sheepskin pads (or artificial sheepskin)
- Foam pads and pillows
- Protectors for areas such as heels and elbows (Figure 16-12) that are subject to friction as the resident moves in bed
- Bed cradles (foot cradles)
- Alternating pressure mattresses
- Flotation mattresses
- Pillows
- Gel-filled mattresses

Sheepskin Pads (or Artificial Sheepskin). These absorb moisture and reduce friction when placed under the resident (Figure 16-13).

Foam Pads and Pillows. These are used to bridge areas to reduce pressure. Watch residents for signs of disorientation that might be caused by the feeling of weightlessness. Adequate fluid intake to prevent urinary stasis must be provided and conscientious range of motion exercises must be carried out. Rubber or hard doughnut-shaped pads may not be effective. Although they

FIGURE 16-12   A. Heel protector B. Elbow protector (Courtesy of J. T. Posey Company, Arcadia, CA)

FIGURE 16-13   A soft, synthetic fleece pad takes pressure off the back. (Courtesy of J. T. Posey Company, Arcadia, CA)

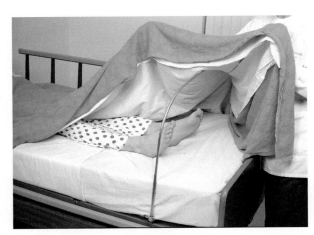

FIGURE 16-14   A bed cradle keeps the sheet and blanket from putting pressure on the feet.

shield the affected areas, they create pressure by their own shape.

Bed (Foot) Cradles. These devices can lift the weight of bedding but must be carefully positioned and may be padded, because injury can occur if the resident strikes them (Figure 16-14).

Alternating-Pressure Mattress (Air Mattress). This type of mattress (Figure 16-15) is used in some facilities. Air pressure is reduced in a different area of the mattress on an alternating basis. The pressure alteration reduces pressure

FIGURE 16-15   Alternating air pressure mattress overlay. Alternating air pressure in the mattress cells changes pressure points against the resident's skin and gently massages the skin. (Courtesy of Hill-Rom, Charlestown, SC)

FIGURE 16-16 Mattress filled with water helps to minimize pressure points on the body.

FIGURE 16-17 Clinitron® air-fluidized mattress (Courtesy of Support Systems International, Inc., Charleston, SC)

against the body so that no skin area is continuously subjected to pressure.

Flotation Mattress. This mattress (Figure 16-16) is a water bed with controlled temperature. The weight of the resident's body displaces water to the extent that pressure is consistently equalized against the skin. Sheets should not be tucked tightly over the flotation mattress because this will restrict the function of the mattress.

Special Equipment. Specialized beds or overlays are available for residents who need continuous pressure relief. One type of bed is the Clinitron® bed (Figure 16-17). It is filled with a sandlike material. Warm, dry air circulates through the material to maintain an even temperature and support the body evenly.

Gel-Filled Mattress. The gel in this type of mattress has a consistency similar to body fat. It allows for a more equal distribution of body weight by conforming to the body contours.

Pillows. Pillows are used in a technique called **bridging**. In bridging, body parts are supported by pillows in such a way that spaces are left to relieve pressure on specific areas.

Each of these aids reduces pressure, but nothing can take the place of nursing observation and care.

BACKRUB

Regular back care is given after the bath. It may also be given after use of the bedpan or after changing a resident's position. When performed

properly, with long, smooth strokes, it stimulates the resident's circulation and aids in preventing skin breakdown. It is also soothing and refreshing. (See Procedure 21.)

BATHING RESIDENTS

A complete bath two or three times a week will maintain cleanliness. Too frequent bathing can lead to skin dryness and itching. Many facilities require a daily partial bath. Incontinent residents are bathed as often as necessary.

Bathing may be performed as:

- Complete bed bath
- Partial bed bath
- Perineal care
- Tub bath

On the Job

The odor of a facility reveals much about how carefully personal care is being provided for the residents.

1. Carry out each beginning procedure action.
2. Assemble equipment:
   - Disposable gloves
   - Basin of water (105°F)
   - Bath towel
   - Soap and lotion
3. Put up far side rail.
4. Place lotion in basin of water to warm (Figure 16-18).

FIGURE 16-18 Before the backrub, the bottle of lotion can be placed in a basin of warm water for several minutes so the lotion will not be cold when applied to the resident's back.

5. Put on disposable gloves if resident has open lesions.
6. Turn the resident on his or her side with back toward you.
7. Expose and wash back, dry carefully. This step is not necessary if backrub is given after a bath.
8. Pour a small amount of lotion into one hand.
9. Apply to skin and rub with gentle but firm strokes. Give special attention to all bony prominences (Figure 16-19).
10. Begin at base of spine:
    - With long, soothing strokes rub up the center of back, around the shoulders, and down sides of back and buttocks (Figure 16-20, left).
    - Repeat previous step four times, using long, soothing upward strokes and circular motion on downstroke (Figure 16-20, middle).
    - Repeat, but on downward stroke rub in small circular motions with palm of

FIGURE 16-19 Use long, smooth strokes as you apply the lotion.

   hand. Include areas over coccyx (over base of spine) (Figure 16-20, right).
    - Repeat long, soothing strokes on muscles for 3 to 5 minutes (Figure 16-20, left).
    - Dry area well.
    - If redness on pressure areas is noted, report to nurse. Straighten and tighten bottom sheet and draw sheet.
11. Change resident's gown if needed.
12. Replace equipment.
13. Carry out each procedure completion action.

FIGURE 16-20 Strokes to be used during the backrub

- Shower bath
- Whirlpool bath
- Therapeutic

During bathing, special attention should be given to skin areas that touch, including:

- Between the legs
- Under the arms
- Under the breasts
- Under the scrotum
- Between the buttocks
- Around the anus
- For obese people, under folds of skin or fat

Gently sponge and pat these areas dry. Follow facility policy for the use of talcum or cornstarch.

A partial bath, bed bath, and tub and shower bath are all ways to meet resident needs for cleanliness. The most stimulating form of bathing for residents is a therapeutic bath that is given in a whirlpool tub (Figure 16-21). The whirlpool bath is beneficial for the resident because:

1. The temperature of the water can be regulated to an optimum 97°F.
2. The movement of the water stimulates circulation.
3. Being surrounded by warm circulating water is relaxing and invigorating.

Safety Issues

General safety issues must be considered when giving a tub or shower bath:

- The tub or shower must be clean before and after use (Figure 16-22).

FIGURE 16-21 This tub is a whirlpool tub in which the water circulates around the resident's body to give a mild therapeutic massage that helps tone muscles and relieve tension. (Courtesy of Arjo-Century, Inc.)

FIGURE 16-22 The shower is cleaned with a disinfectant before and after each use.

- Be sure that there is adequate help.
- Check that all safety aids such as hand rails, shower seats, and hydraulic lifts are in good repair and proper working order.
- Wipe up all water spilled on the floor immediately to prevent falls.
- Keep the temperature of the room comfortable and the area free of drafts.
- Wear gloves if there may be contact with open lesions, body fluids, mucous membranes, or the perineum.
- Observe the skin for any changes or irregularities. Do not disturb or injure any warts or moles. Report anything unusual.
- Protect the resident from fatigue by transporting the resident to and from the tub room and carrying out the bathing procedure as efficiently as possible.
- Use good body mechanics to protect yourself and the resident.
- Use a bath thermometer to be sure the temperature of the water is correct. If a bath thermometer is not available, test the water with your wrist. (See Procedures 22–24.)

PROCEDURE 22

Bed Bath Using Basin and Water

1. Carry out each beginning procedure action.
2. Assemble equipment (Figure 16-23).
   - Disposable gloves (for perineal care)
   - Bed linen
   - Bath blanket
   - Laundry bag or hamper
   - Bath basin
   - Bath thermometer
   - Soap and soap dish
   - Washcloth
   - Face towel
   - Two bath towels
   - Facility gown or the resident's clothes
   - Lotion
   - Equipment for oral hygiene
   - Nail brush, emery board, and orange-wood stick (if available)
   - Brush and comb
   - Bedpan and cover or urinal

FIGURE 16-23 Assemble equipment. Place bed linens on chair next to bed and remaining items (except bedpan) on overbed table. If used, the bedpan or urinal will be removed from bedside stand, used, cleaned immediately, and returned to stand.

3. Close the door and windows to prevent chilling the resident.
4. Close privacy curtain.
5. Put towels and linen on chair in order of use.
6. Place laundry hamper so that it is convenient.
7. Offer bedpan or urinal. Put on gloves if resident wants to use bedpan or urinal. Empty and clean before proceeding with bath. Return to storage. Remove gloves and discard according to facility policy. Wash hands.
8. Put on disposable gloves (if facility requires or resident has open lesions).
9. Lower the back of bed and side rails on side you are working. Be sure opposite side is up.
10. Loosen top bedclothes. If blanket is to be reused, remove it from bed, fold it, and place it over the back of the chair. Otherwise, place bath blanket over top bedclothes and remove top bedclothes by sliding them out from under the bath blanket. Place in laundry hamper.
11. Leave one pillow under resident's head. Place other pillow on chair.
12. Remove resident's nightwear and place in laundry hamper.
13. Fill bath basin two-thirds full with water at 105°F.
14. Assist resident to move to the side of the bed nearest you.
15. Fold face towel over upper edge of bath blanket to keep blanket dry.
16. Form a mitten by holding washcloth around hand (Figure 16-24). Wet washcloth; wash eyes, using separate corners of cloth for each eye. Do not use soap near eyes.
17. Rinse washcloth and apply soap if resident desires. Squeeze out excess water.
18. Wash and rinse resident's face, ears, and neck (Figure 16-25). Use towel to dry.

(continues)

PROCEDURE *22* *(continued)*

FIGURE 16-24 To make a bath mitt, wrap the washcloth around one hand. Then bring the free end back over palm and tuck in the end. Thumb is free to hold washcloth in place. *Note:* If gloves are used in the procedure, make the bath mitt over the glove.

FIGURE 16-25 Wash face carefully, doing eyes separately. Do not use soap on washcloth when cleaning around eyes.

19. Expose resident's far arm. Protect bed with bath towel placed under arm. Wash, rinse, and dry arm and hand. Be sure **axilla** (armpit) is clean and dry. Apply deodorant if resident agrees. Repeat for other arm.
20. If necessary, care for hands and nails as follows:
    a. Wash each hand carefully. Rinse and dry. Push back cuticle (base of fingernails) gently with towel while wiping the fingers. Be sure to dry the areas between the fingers.
    b. Clean under nails with orangewood stick and shape with emery board. Be careful not to file nails too close. If resident is diabetic, inform the nurse if nail care is needed.
21. Discard used bath water and refill basin two-thirds full with water at 105°F.
22. Put bath towel over resident's chest, and then fold blanket to waist. Under towel, wash with soap, rinse, and dry chest. Rinse and dry under breasts of female resident. Wash carefully to avoid irritating skin.
23. Fold bath blanket down to **pubic** area. Wash with soap, rinse, and dry abdomen. Replace bath blanket over abdomen and chest. Slide towel out from under bath blanket.
24. Ask resident to flex far knee if possible. Fold bath blanket up to expose thigh, leg, and foot. Protect bed with bath towel, and put bath basin on towel. Place resident's foot in basin (Figure 16-26). Wash and rinse leg and foot. When moving leg, support leg properly.

(continues)

PROCEDURE 22 *(continued)*

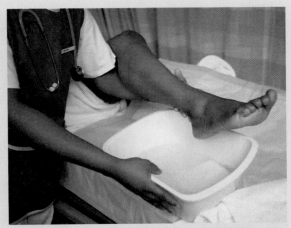

FIGURE 16-26 Support leg and place the foot in the basin.

25. Lift leg and move basin to other side of bed. Dry leg and foot. Dry well between toes.
26. Repeat for other leg and foot. Take basin from bed before drying leg and foot.
27. Care for toenails as necessary. File nails straight across. Do not round edges. Do not push back the cuticle because it is easily injured and infected. Apply lotion to feet of resident with dry skin, except between toes. Observe toenails carefully so that you can report condition of nails to nurse. If resident is diabetic, inform nurse if toenail care is needed.
28. Discard used bath water and refill basin two-thirds full with water at 105°F. Several water changes are suggested in this procedure, but you may need to change water more often.
29. Help resident to turn on side away from you and to move toward center of bed. Place towel lengthwise next to resident's back. Wash, rinse, and dry neck, back, and buttocks. Use long, firm strokes when washing back.

30. A backrub is usually given at this time. (See Procedure 21.)
31. Help resident turn on back.
32. Place towel under buttocks and upper legs. Place washcloth, soap, basin, and bath towel within convenient reach of resident. Instruct resident to wash **genitalia**, assisting if necessary. (You must assume responsibility for this procedure if resident has difficulty. Residents often are reluctant to acknowledge the need for help. Wear gloves when assisting.) When assisting female resident, always wash from front to back, drying carefully. When assisting male resident, carefully wash and dry penis, scrotum, and groin area. If male is uncircumcised, gently push foreskin back and carefully wash and dry penis. Then gently pull foreskin down when you are finished. Ask the resident to turn to the side so that you can wash, rinse, and dry the buttocks and anal area. Remove gloves (if used) and discard according to facility policy. Wash your hands.
33. Carry out range of motion exercises as ordered.
34. Cover pillow with towel and comb or brush hair. Oral hygiene is usually given at this time. (See procedures later in this lesson.)
35. Place used towels and washcloth in hamper.
36. Provide clean gown.
37. Clean and replace equipment, according to facility policy.
38. Change bed linen, following occupied bed procedure. Put soiled linen in laundry hamper.
39. Remove and discard disposable gloves according to facility policy. Wash your hands.
40. Raise side rails if required.
41. Carry out each procedure completion action.

Waterless Bed Bathing

Some facilities use a bathing system that uses a rinse-free cleanser and moisturizer rather than the usual basin of water and soap and a rinsing procedure (Figure 16-27). The solution-saturated cloths are heated in the microwave oven. After use, the skin does not require drying. The procedure is similar to that of the bed bath, with cleansing performed in the same order:

- Face and neck
- Far arm and hand
- Near arm and hand
- Far leg and foot
- Near leg and foot
- Back and buttocks
- Perineum

Advantages of the system include:

- Less fatigue for the resident
- Refreshing and cleansing without soap
- Less friction, because the drying step is eliminated

The following precautions are taken to prevent injury to the resident:

- Monitor temperature of the cleansing cloths carefully
- Do not heat in the microwave for more than one minute
- Discard cleansing cloths 72 hours after opening the package or immediately if they are dry

- Label should be peeled open without completely removing it before heating the package
- Cloths are for individual use only

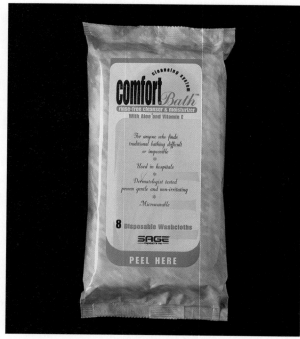

FIGURE 16-27 Package containing eight cleansing washcloths. Washcloths may be warmed in microwave or in warmer. One cloth is used for each of the following body areas: (1) face, neck, and chest; (2) right arm; (3) left arm; (4) perineum; (5) right leg; (6) left leg; (7) back; and (8) buttocks. (Courtesy of Sage Products, Inc.)

PROCEDURE 23

Bed Bath Using a Rinse-Free Cleanser and Moisturizer

1. Carry out each beginning procedure action.
2. Assemble equipment:
   - Same as bed bath using basin and water (see Procedure 22), but omit:
     - Bath basin
     - Soap
     - Wash cloth
     - Bath thermometer
     - Soap dish
3. Follow steps 3–12 of the regular bed bath procedure (Procedure 22).
4. Open pack of cloths. Extract one, make a mitt, and cleanse resident's face and neck (solution can safely be used around the eyes)
5. Place towel over resident's chest. Fold blanket down to waist and cleanse chest. Be sure area under breasts is carefully cleaned.

(continues)

PROCEDURE *23*   *(continued)*

6. Fold bath blanket down to pubic area and wash abdomen. Replace bath blanket over abdomen and chest. Remove towel by sliding it out from under the bath blanket. Dispose of washing cloth per facility policy.

7. Uncover resident's far arm. Protect bed with bath towel placed under arm. Use a new cloth and wash arm and hand (Figure 16-28). Be sure axilla is clean. Apply deodorant if resident desires. Dispose of used cloth. Using another new cloth, repeat for near arm and hand.

8. Care for hands and nails as needed.

9. Ask resident to flex far knee, if possible. Fold bath blanket up to expose thigh, leg, and foot. Protect bed with bath towel. Use a new cloth and cleanse thigh, leg, and foot. Be sure area between toes is left dry. Care for toenails as needed. Remove bath towel. Cover with bath blanket.

10. Repeat with near thigh, leg, and foot.

11. Be sure opposite side rail is up. Help resident move to the center of the bed and turn on side away from you. Place a bath towel lengthwise next to resident's back.

FIGURE 16-28   Washing resident using the cleansing washcloth. (Courtesy of Sage Products, Inc.)

Use a new cloth to cleanse neck, back, and buttocks. A backrub is usually given at this time. Remove towel.

12. Assist resident to turn on back. Place towel under buttocks and upper legs. Hand resident a new cloth to cleanse the perineum. Assist as necessary.

13. Complete nursing care following steps 33–41 of the regular bed bath (Procedure 22).

PROCEDURE
24   Tub Bath or Shower

1. Carry out each beginning procedure action.

2. Assemble equipment:
   - Disposable gloves
   - Soap
   - Washcloth
   - Two to three bath towels
   - Bath blanket
   - Resident's gown, robe, and slippers
   - Bath thermometer
   - Chair or stool
   - Bath mat

3. Take the supplies to the bathroom and prepare it for resident. Make sure tub is clean.

4. Fill tub one-third full with water at 105°F or adjust shower flow. Use your elbow to test the water temperature if a shower is being given. The water should feel comfortably warm.

(continues)

PROCEDURE *24* *(continued)*

5. Assist resident to bathroom and help him or her with robe and slippers.
6. Help resident undress. Give resident a towel to wrap around midriff. Cover resident with bath blanket when going to and from bath or shower.
7. Assist resident into tub or shower. For resident's safety, the bottom of the tub and the shower floor are covered with a nonskid surface. In addition, a tub chair or a shower chair can be provided so the resident can sit safely while bathing.
8. Put on disposable gloves if there are open lesions.
9. Wash resident's back. Observe skin for signs of redness or breaks. If resident's condition permits, allow resident to assist as much as possible in the procedure. Give resident the choice of washing genitalia. If you assist with this part of the procedure, put on gloves. On completion, remove gloves and discard according to facility policy. Wash your hands.
10. If resident shows any signs of weakness, remove plug and let water drain out, or turn off shower. Allow resident to rest until feeling better before making any attempt to assist him or her out of tub or shower. Keep resident covered with bath towel to avoid chilling.
11. If resident wants a shampoo and you have permission to do so:
    - Ask resident to hold washcloth over eyes.
    - Pour small amount of water on hair (enough to wet hair thoroughly).
    - Use a small amount of shampoo to lather hair.
    - Massage scalp gently.
    - Rinse hair with warm water.
    - Repeat lathering, massaging, and rinsing, if necessary.
    - Towel hair dry.
12. Hold bath blanket around resident when he or she is stepping out of tub or shower. A resident may choose to remove wet towel under bath blanket.
13. Assist resident to dry, apply deodorant, dress, and return to unit.
14. Put on gloves and clean bathtub. Remove gloves and discard according to facility policy. Wash your hands. Put supplies away.
15. Carry out each procedure completion action.

Partial Bath

A partial bath is cleaning of the hands, face, axilla, buttocks, and genitals. It is very refreshing. Many residents will be able to help with the bath process and, whenever possible, should be encouraged to do so. (See Procedure 25.)

**PROCEDURE
25 Partial Bath**

1. Carry out each beginning procedure action.
2. Assemble equipment:
   - Disposable gloves
   - Bed linen
   - Bath blanket
   - Bath thermometer
   - Soap and soap dish
   - Washcloth
   - Face towel

(continues)

PROCEDURE 25 *(continued)*

- Bath towel
- Gown or robe
- Laundry bag or hamper
- Bath basin
- Lotion
- Equipment for oral hygiene
- Nail brush, orangewood stick, and emery board
- Brush, comb, and deodorant
- Bedpan or urinal and cover
- Paper towels or bed protector

3. Close the door and any windows to prevent chilling resident.
4. Put towels and linen on chair, in order of use. Place laundry hamper so that it is convenient.
5. Put on disposable gloves.
6. Offer bedpan or urinal. Empty and clean before proceeding with bath. Remove gloves and discard according to facility policy. Wash hands and put on pair of new gloves.
7. Elevate head rest, if permitted, to comfortable position.
8. Loosen top bedclothes. Remove and fold blanket and spread and place over back of chair. Place bath blanket over top sheet and remove sheet by sliding it out from under bath blanket.
9. Leave one pillow under resident's head. Place other pillow on chair.
10. Assist resident to remove gown. Place gown in laundry hamper. Wrap bath blanket around resident.
11. Place paper towels or bed protector on overbed table.

12. Fill bath basin two-thirds full with water at 105°F and place on overbed table.
13. Push overbed table comfortably close to resident.
14. Place towels, washcloth, and soap on overbed table within easy reach.
15. Instruct resident to wash as much as he or she is able and that you will return to complete the bath.
16. Place call bell within easy reach. Ask resident to signal when ready.
17. Remove gloves and discard according to facility policy. Wash hands and leave unit.
18. Wash hands and return to unit when resident signals. Put on a new pair of gloves.
19. Change bath water. Bathe those areas the resident could not reach. Make sure the face, hands, axilla, buttocks, anal area, back, and genitalia are washed and dried.
20. Give a backrub with lotion.
21. Assist the resident in applying deodorant and fresh gown.
22. Cover pillow with towel and comb or brush hair. Assist with oral hygiene if needed.
23. Clean and replace equipment according to facility policy.
24. Change bed linen, following occupied bed procedure. Discard soiled linen in laundry hamper.
25. Remove and dispose of gloves according to facility policy.
26. Carry out each procedure completion action.

Therapeutic Bath

A therapeutic bath is one in which a specific substance is added to the water to treat a problem such as a rash. Follow the care plan's directions for the type of therapeutic bath you are giving.

Perineal Care

Perineal care is the cleaning of the area between the resident's legs. Keeping this area clean is especially important when residents are unable to control bladder and bowels. Excreta left on the skin is unpleasant and uncomfortable. If left unattended, it can lead to skin breakdown.

Perineal care may be performed as part of general bathing or as a separate procedure as needed. (See Procedures 26 and 27.)

PROCEDURE

26

Female Perineal Care

1. Carry out each beginning procedure action.
2. Assemble equipment:
   - Disposable gloves
   - Bath blanket or topsheet
   - Bedpan and cover
   - Liquid soap
   - Basin with warm water (105°F)
   - Bath thermometer
   - Bed protector
   - Washcloth and towel
3. Lower side rail on side where you will be working. Be sure opposite side rail is up and secure.
4. Remove bedspread and blanket. Fold and place on back of chair.
5. Resident is to be on back. Cover resident with bath blanket and fanfold sheet to foot of bed.
6. Put on disposable gloves.
7. Ask resident to raise hips while you place bed protector underneath resident.
8. Offer bedpan to resident. If used and resident is on intake and output, record amount. Then empty and clean the bedpan before continuing with the procedure. Remove gloves and discard according to facility policy. Wash hands and put on a new pair of gloves.
9. Position bath blanket so only the area between the legs is exposed.
10. Ask resident to separate her legs and flex knees. *Note:* If resident is unable to spread legs and flex knees, turn the resident on her side with legs flexed. This position provides easy access to the perineal area.
11. Wet washcloth, make mitt, and apply a small amount of liquid soap. *Note:* Heavy soap application may be difficult to rinse off completely. Soap residue is irritating.
12. Use one gloved hand to stabilize and separate the vulva (Figure 16-29). With the other gloved hand, proceed as follows.
    a. Bring soaped washcloth in one downward stroke over urethra. Rinse

washcloth, remake mitt, and rinse off urethra.
    b. Bring soaped washcloth in one downward stroke along the far side of outer labia to perineum.
    c. Rinse washcloth, remake mitt, and rinse area just cleaned.
    d. Repeat steps b and c, washing and rinsing inner far labia.
    e. Repeat steps b and c, washing and rinsing inner near labia.
    f. With gloved hands, separate labia. Clean and rinse inner part of vulva to perineum.
    g. Dry washed area with towel.

FIGURE 16-29 Spread the vulva with one hand. With the washcloth in the other hand, start at the front and stroke downward along the outer labia.

13. Turn resident away from you. Flex upper leg slightly if permitted.
14. Make a mitt, wet, and apply soap lightly.
15. Expose anal area. Wash area, stroking from perineum to coccyx (front to back) (Figure 16-30).
16. Rinse well in the same manner.
17. Dry carefully.
18. Return resident to back.

(continues)

PROCEDURE *26* *(continued)*

19. Remove and dispose of bed protector according to facility policy.
20. Cover resident with sheet.
21. Remove and dispose of gloves according to facility policy. Wash hands.
22. Remove, fold, and store bath blanket according to facility policy.
23. Replace top covers, tuck under mattress, and make mitered corners. (Resident may prefer that the top covers not be tucked in.)
24. Put up side rail.
25. Put on gloves. Empty water, clean equipment, and dispose of or store, according to facility policy.
26. Remove gloves and discard according to facility policy. Wash hands.
27. Carry out each procedure completion action.

FIGURE 16-30   With one hand, lift up on the buttocks to expose the rectal area. Wipe from the perineum back toward the anus.

PROCEDURE
27
Male Perineal Care

1. Carry out each beginning procedure action.
2. Assemble equipment:
   - Disposable gloves
   - Bath blanket
   - Bath thermometer
   - Urinal and cover
   - Soap, washcloth, and towel
   - Plastic bag
   - Bed protector or bath towel
   - Ordered solution (if other than water)
3. Fill basin with warm water at approximately 105°F.
4. Lower side rail and position bed protector (or towel) under resident's buttocks.
5. Fanfold blanket and spread to foot of bed.
6. Cover resident with bath blanket and fanfold sheet to foot of bed.

7. Put on disposable gloves.
8. Offer bedpan or urinal. If used and resident is on intake and output, record amount. Then empty and clean the bedpan or urinal before continuing with the procedure. Remove gloves and discard according to facility policy. Wash hands and put on a new pair of gloves.
9. Have resident flex and separate knees. *Note:* If the resident is unable to spread legs and flex knees, the perineal area can be washed with the resident on the side with legs flexed. This position provides easy access to the perineal area.
10. Draw bath blanket upward to expose perineal area only.
11. Make a mitt with washcloth and apply a small amount of soap. *Note:* Heavy soap application may be difficult to rinse off completely. Soap residue is irritating.

(continues)

PROCEDURE 27 *(continued)*

12. Grasp penis gently with one hand and wash. Begin at the meatus and wash in a circular motion toward the base of the penis (Figure 16-31).

FIGURE 16-31 Grasp penis gently with one hand. With the other hand, wipe in a circular motion from the glans (head) down to the base of the penis.

13. If resident is not circumcised, draw foreskin back (Figure 16-32). Be sure entire penis is washed. Rinse thoroughly.
14. Wash scrotum. Lift scrotum and wash perineum.
15. Rinse washcloth, remake mitt, and rinse area just washed.
16. Dry washed area with towel. Reposition foreskin if necessary.
17. Turn resident away from you. Flex upper leg slightly if permitted.
18. Make a mitt, wet, and apply soap lightly.
19. Expose anal area. Wash area, stroking from perineum to coccyx.

FIGURE 16-32 If the resident is not circumcised, gently push the foreskin back so the glans can be washed. Once the penis is washed and dried, the foreskin is returned to its normal position.

20. Rinse well in the same manner.
21. Dry carefully.
22. Return resident to back.
23. Remove and dispose of bed protector according to facility policy.
24. Cover resident with sheet.
25. Remove and dispose of gloves according to facility policy. Wash hands.
26. Remove, fold, and store bath blanket, according to facility policy.
27. Replace top covers, tuck under mattress and make mitered corners. (Resident may prefer that the top covers not be tucked in.)
28. Put up side rail.
29. Put on gloves. Empty water, clean equipment, and dispose of or store, according to facility policy.
30. Remove gloves and discard according to facility policy. Wash hands.
31. Carry out each procedure completion action.

DAILY HAIR CARE

Neat, attractively arranged hair contributes to a feeling of being well groomed. Daily hair care is part of the morning care but should be done whenever it is needed to keep the resident groomed. Residents should be encouraged to take care of their hair and choose the style they prefer.

In many facilities, barbers and beauticians visit once a week to cut, wash, and style the hair of residents who desire the service. Often there is a charge for the service. Normally the residents are prescheduled for their hair care. Some residents may have standing appointments every week or every 2 weeks. The nursing assistant should know which residents have hair appointments. The hair would not be washed just before the appointment.

The hair should be combed and brushed each morning. Tangles can be loosened by sectioning the hair with a comb or brush, working with one section at a time. Grasp the hair near the scalp to reduce pulling (Figure 16-33). Start combing or brushing tangles out starting at the ends and working toward the scalp. Braiding long hair after brushing can help reduce tangles. Tangles can be reduced in wiry, dry hair by using conditioner and keeping the hair short or in braids.

Some residents prefer to have their hair washed in the tub or shower. Be sure you have specific instructions. When assisting with a shampoo in the tub or shower, you must:

- Protect the resident's eyes
- Towel dry the hair thoroughly

When a resident must remain in bed and a shampoo is ordered, it can be given using a shampoo tray and pitchers of water to wet and rinse the hair. The water is collected in a pail or bucket placed on the floor next to the bed. The water is collected in the shampoo tray and drains into the pail (Figure 16-34).

FIGURE 16-34   The shampoo tray collects the water used to wet and rinse the hair and directs it into a bucket or pail on the floor next to the bed.

FACIAL HAIR

Men feel better groomed when they are shaved regularly (Figure 16-35). This procedure is usually done during the morning care. For safety, use an electric razor or rotary razor.

FIGURE 16-33   To remove tangles from long hair, divide the hair into sections. Work with one section at a time. Hold hair near the scalp to reduce pulling and start combing at the ends of the hair, working toward the scalp.

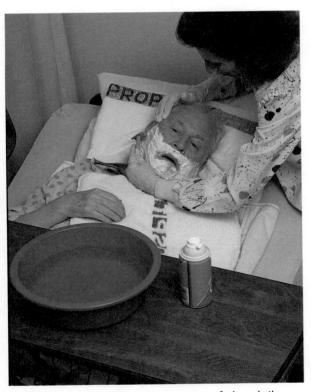

FIGURE 16-35   Shaving is part of the daily routine for most men.

PROCEDURE
28

Daily Hair Care

1. Carry out each beginning procedure action.
2. Assemble equipment:
   - Towel
   - Comb and brush
3. Ask resident to move to the side of bed nearest you, or resident may sit in chair if permitted. If a resident is sitting up, put a towel around her shoulders.
4. Cover pillow with towel.
5. Remove eyeglasses and store safely.
6. Part or section hair and comb with one hand between scalp and end of hair.
7. Brush carefully and thoroughly.
8. Have resident turn so hair on back of head may be combed and brushed. If hair is snarled, work section by section to unsnarl hair, beginning near ends and working toward scalp. Check scalp carefully for breaks in the skin or any abnormalities.
9. Complete brushing and arrange attractively. Braid long hair to prevent repeated snarling, or style hair according to resident's preference.
10. Clean and replace equipment according to facility policy.
11. Carry out each procedure completion action.

Refer to Figure 16-36 for safety considerations for shaving.

Older women have an increase in the growth and coarseness of hairs on the chin and upper lip. Many women find this distressing. Tweezers can be used to remove some of the hairs, but a more permanent method is to have the hairs removed professionally with an electric needle. Some women may require a shave. In some facilities nursing assistants are not permitted to shave women residents. Be sure to check the policy of your facility.

FIGURE 16-36 Special shaving precautions		
• Wear disposable gloves.		
• Use the resident's own shaving equipment if possible. Otherwise, use disposable, one-use safety razors.		
• If the resident is receiving anticoagulants, a special procedure may be required. For example, an electric razor provides the greatest safety. Check with your supervisor for the proper procedure.		
• If oxygen is being given, it may be possible to discontinue it during this procedure. Consult your supervisor and follow facility policy.		

PROCEDURE
29   Shaving Male Resident

1. Carry out each beginning procedure action.
2. Assemble equipment:
   - Disposable gloves
   - Electric shaver or safety razor
   - Shaving lather or preshave lotion for electric razor
   - Basin of water (105°F)
   - Face towels
   - Mirror
   - Washcloth
   - Aftershave lotion
3. Put on gloves.
4. Raise the head of the bed. Place equipment on overbed table.
5. Place one face towel across resident's chest and one under head.
6. Moisten face and apply lather (or preshave lotion).
7. Starting in front of ear:
   a. Hold skin taut and bring razor down over cheek toward chin (Figure 16-37).
   b. Repeat until lather on cheek is removed and area has been shaved. Rinse frequently.
   c. Repeat on other cheek.
   d. Use firm short strokes. Shave in direction of hair growth.
   e. Rinse razor frequently.
8. Lather neck area and stroke up toward the chin. Rinse and repeat until all lather is removed.
9. Wash face and neck and dry thoroughly.
10. Apply aftershave lotion if desired.

FIGURE 16-37 Hold the skin taut with one hand. Using short strokes, bring razor down over cheek toward chin. Start near the ear. Rinse the razor often in basin.

11. If the skin is nicked, apply pressure directly over the area and then apply an antiseptic and Bandaid. Report incident to nurse.
12. Clean and replace equipment. Dispose of razor according to facility policy. Remove head of electric razor. Use razor brush to remove clippings. Store according to facility policy. Remove and dispose of gloves according to facility policy.
13. Carry out each procedure completion action.

HAND AND FINGERNAIL CARE

Fingernails are routinely cleaned during the morning care. Use a soft brush and orangewood stick to gently clean under the nails. Fingernail care can also be carried out as a separate procedure. Soak the hands in warm soapy water. Creams can be used to soften the **cuticles**, which can then be gently pushed back with a towel. When cutting the fingernails, follow the curve of the finger and then file any rough edges. Be careful not to injure the corners of the fingers when cutting the nails.

Some facilities do not permit nursing assistants to perform nail care on diabetic residents.

PROCEDURE 30

Hand and Fingernail Care

Note: Check with nurse and nursing care plan to learn if this procedure is permitted for the resident or if it is to be modified because of the resident's condition.

This procedure can be carried out independently or can be modified and added to the bath procedure.

1. Carry out each beginning procedure action.
2. Assemble equipment:
   - Basin with water at 105°F
   - Bath thermometer
   - Soap
   - Bath towel and washcloth
   - Lotion
   - Plastic protector
   - Nail clippers
   - Nail file
   - Orangewood stick
   - Nail polish (optional)
3. Elevate head of bed, if permitted, and adjust the overbed table in front of resident. If resident is allowed out of bed, assist to transfer to a chair and position overbed table waist-high across lap.
4. Place plastic protector on overbed table.
5. Fill basin with warm water at approximately 105°F using bath thermometer to test temperature. Place basin on overbed table.
6. Use a soft brush or orangewood stick to clean under nails.
7. Instruct resident to put hands in basin and soak for approximately 5 minutes. Place towel over basin to help retain heat. Add warm water if necessary. Remember to remove resident's hands before adding water.
8. Wash hands. Push cuticles back gently with washcloth. (A cream may be used to soften the cuticles first.)
9. Dry hands with towel.
10. Use nail clippers to cut fingernails straight across. Do not cut below tips of fingers. Keep nail cuts on protector to be discarded.
11. Shape and smooth fingernails with nail file. Apply polish to nails if resident desires.
12. Pour small amount of lotion in your palms and gently smooth on resident's hands.
13. Empty basin of water. Gather equipment, clean, and store according to facility policy.
14. Return overbed table to foot of bed. If resident has been sitting up for the procedure, assist into bed.
15. Carry out each procedure completion action.

FOOT AND TOENAIL CARE

Residents should be given routine foot care, including bathing, massage of the feet, and attention to the toenails. Proceed carefully:

- Dry feet carefully after soaking in warm water.
- Give special attention to drying between the toes.
- Carefully inspect the feet and apply lotion to dry areas. Pat, rather than rub, lotion on skin. Do not apply lotion between toes. Use towel to wipe off excess lotion.
- Check the resident's toenails. If the nails are thick or curved and need trimming, inform the nurse.

In some facilities only the RN is allowed to cut toenails. A podiatrist provides this service for residents with poor circulation or diabetes. The podiatrist may do toenail care for all residents in some facilities.

Part of good foot care includes being sure that the resident's shoes fit well and are securely laced so that they offer optimum support.

Note: Be sure to check with the nurse and the nursing care plan to learn if this procedure is permitted for the resident. In some cases, this procedure may be modified according to the resident's condition.

PROCEDURE
31 Foot and Toenail Care

1. Carry out each beginning procedure action.
2. Assemble equipment:
   - Basin
   - Soap
   - Bath mat
   - Bath thermometer
   - Lotion
   - Nail brush
   - Disposable bed protector
   - Bath towel and washcloth
   - Orangewood stick
3. If permitted, assist resident out of bed and into chair.
4. Place bath mat on floor in front of resident. Fill basin with warm water (105°F). Put basin on bath mat.
5. Remove slippers and allow resident to place feet in water. Cover with bath towel to help retain heat.
6. Soak feet approximately 20 minutes. Add warm water as necessary. Lift feet from water while warm water is being added.
7. At end of soak period, wash feet with soap.
8. Rinse and dry. Note any abnormalities such as corns or calluses.
9. Remove basin, covering feet with towel.
10. Use orangewood stick to gently clean toenails. If nails are long and need to be cut, report this fact to the nurse. Follow facility policy.
11. Pour lotion into palms of hands. Hold hands together to warm lotion and apply gently to feet. Do not apply lotion between toes. Wipe off excess lotion using a towel.
12. Assist resident with socks or stockings and shoes if ambulatory. Otherwise, return resident to bed.
13. Make resident comfortable.
14. Gather equipment, clean, and store according to facility policy. Leave unit neat.
15. Carry out each procedure completion action.

ORAL HYGIENE

The elderly need good **oral hygiene** just as much as younger people. Regular cleansing by brushing (Figure 16-38A) and flossing should be carried out routinely three times daily when the resident has any teeth of his or her own. Visits by a dentist can help maintain existing dental function. Older people can develop dental **caries** (cavities) just as readily as younger people. Regular cleaning helps make the breath fresh and eliminates **halitosis** (bad breath). Improved appetite can also result. (See Procedures 32 and 33.)

FIGURE 16-38A Place the head of the toothbrush beside the teeth, with the bristle tips at a 45° angle against the gumline. Move the brush back and forth in short (half-a-tooth-wide) strokes several times, using a gentle scrubbing motion. Brush the outer surfaces of each tooth, upper and lower, keeping the bristles angled against the gumline. (Toothbrushing photos and descriptions compliments of American Dental Association)

Dentures

Many residents wear dentures. Care of dentures includes:

- Cleaning dentures daily under cool running water
- Storing dentures in a safe place when out of the resident's mouth

  In addition, you will care for the resident by:
- Cleaning and checking the resident's mouth daily for signs of irritation
- Checking resident's lips for cracking and dryness
- Applying creams, petroleum jelly, or glycerin to lips for excessive dryness

Many residents have partial plates, which are removable but attached by small metal clips.

Partial plates should be given the same care as full dentures.

Dentures should be stored in a denture cup inside the bedside stand when not in use. Some residents prefer storing dentures dry, but most prefer to store dentures in a special solution. If in doubt, store dentures in water when out of the mouth to keep them moist and prevent cracking. (See Procedure 34.)

Residents who are unconscious still require oral hygiene. Premoistened swabs may be used, followed by glycerine and lemon. Because the resident cannot participate, the staff must carry out this procedure for the resident. (See Procedure 35.)

FIGURE 16-38B Use the same method on the inside surfaces of all teeth, still using short back-and-forth strokes.

FIGURE 16-38D To clean the inside surfaces of the front teeth, tilt the brush vertically and make several gentle up-and-down strokes with the "toe" (the front part) of the brush.

FIGURE 16-38C Scrub the chewing surfaces of the teeth.

FIGURE 16-38E Brushing the resident's tongue will help freshen breath and clean the mouth by removing bacteria.

PROCEDURE
32   Assisting Resident
to Brush Teeth

OBRA

1. Carry out each beginning procedure action.
2. Assemble equipment:
   - Disposable gloves
   - Emesis basin
   - Toothbrush
   - Toothpaste
   - Glass of cool water
   - Mouthwash (if permitted)
   - Hand towel
   - Bed protector
   - Dental floss
3. Elevate head of bed. Help resident into comfortable position.
4. Lower side rails and position overbed table across resident's lap.
5. Cover table with protector and place equipment on table.
6. Place towel across resident's chest.
7. Be prepared to help as resident brushes and flosses teeth. Use gloves if you do assist (Figure 16-39).
8. After resident has brushed teeth, push overbed table to foot of bed.
9. Gather equipment, clean, and store according to facility policy. Place soiled linen in proper receptacle.
10. Remove disposable gloves, if used, and discard gloves according to facility policy.
11. Lower head of bed. Help resident to assume comfortable position and adjust bedding.

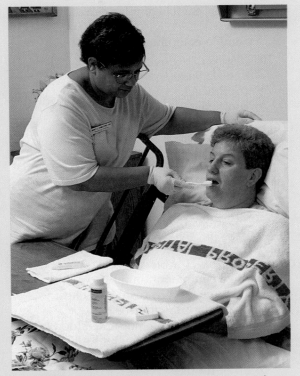

FIGURE 16-39   If necessary, assist resident to brush teeth.

12. Raise side rails.
13. Carry out each procedure completion action.

PROCEDURE
33

Cleaning and Flossing Resident's Teeth

1. Carry out each beginning procedure action.
2. Assemble equipment:
   - Disposable gloves
   - Emesis basin
   - Toothbrush
   - Toothpaste
   - Glass of cool water
   - Mouthwash (if permitted)
   - Hand towel
   - Bed protector
   - Dental floss
3. Elevate head of bed. Help resident into a comfortable position.
4. Lower side rails and position overbed table across resident's lap.
5. Place protector on overbed table and arrange equipment on table.
6. Place towel across resident's chest.
7. Put on disposable gloves.
8. Place toothpaste on moistened toothbrush.
9. Clean all surfaces of each tooth. Use a sweeping motion working from gumline to tip of tooth.

10. Have resident rinse mouth into emesis basin.
11. Select a piece of dental floss about 12 inches long. Wrap ends of dental floss around middle fingers, leaving center area free (Figure 16-40).
12. Ask resident to open his or her mouth. Gently insert floss between each tooth down to, but *not into*, gumline.
13. Ask resident to rinse mouth using emesis basin.
14. Wipe resident's face dry with towel.
15. Push overbed table to the foot of bed.
16. Gather equipment, clean, and store according to facility policy. Place soiled linen in proper receptacle.
17. Remove and discard gloves according to facility policy.
18. Position resident comfortably. Be sure that water and call bell are close at hand.
19. Raise and secure side rails.
20. Carry out each procedure completion action.

FIGURE 16-40 Floss is wrapped around the middle fingers (left). The proper method of using the floss is to clean between the teeth (right).

PROCEDURE
34   Caring for Dentures

1. Carry out each beginning procedure action.
2. Assemble equipment:
   - Disposable gloves
   - Tissues
   - Emesis basin
   - Tongue depressor
   - Brush
   - Toothpaste or tooth powder
   - Mouthwash, if permitted
   - Gauze squares
   - Applicators
   - Denture cup
3. Apply disposable gloves.
4. Allow resident to clean dentures if he or she is able to do so. If resident cannot, give tissue to resident and ask him or her to remove dentures. Assist if necessary.
   To remove upper dentures: Grasp dentures firmly, ease downward and then forward, and remove from the mouth.
   To remove lower dentures: Grasp dentures firmly, ease upward and then backward, and remove from the mouth.
5. Place dentures in denture cup padded with gauze squares. Take to bathroom or utility room.
6. Place a paper towel or washcloth in the bottom of the basin to protect the dentures. Add a small amount of cool water.
7. Dentures may be soaked in a solution with a cleansing tablet before brushing, if necessary.
8. Put toothpaste or tooth powder on brush. Hold dentures and brush until all surfaces are clean (Figure 16-41).
9. Rinse dentures thoroughly under cool or warm running water. Never use hot water. Rinse denture cup.

FIGURE 16-41   Place a paper towel or washcloth on the bottom of the sink and partially fill the sink with water. Place toothpaste or denture cleaning paste on the brush and hold the dentures over the sink while you brush them clean. Rinse with warm water. Never use hot water on dentures.

10. Place fresh gauze squares in denture cup with clean cool water unless instructed otherwise.
11. Place dentures in cup and take them to bedside.
12. Assist resident to rinse mouth with mouthwash, if permitted. Otherwise use water. Hold mouth open gently with wooden tongue depressor. Clean gums and tongue with applicators moistened with mouthwash or use foam "toothettes."
13. Use tissue or gauze to hand wet dentures to resident. Insert if necessary.
14. Clean and replace equipment according to facility policy.
15. Remove and dispose of gloves according to facility policy.
16. Carry out each procedure completion action.

Assisting with Oral Hygiene for the Unconscious Resident

1. Carry out each beginning procedure action.
2. Assemble equipment:
   - Disposable gloves
   - Emesis basin
   - Bath towel
   - Plastic bag
   - Premoistened applicators
   - Tissues
   - Padded tongue depressor
   - Water-based lubricant for lips
3. Put on disposable gloves.
4. Cover pillow with towel and turn resident's head to one side. Place emesis basin under resident's chin.
5. Gently pull down on chin to open mouth and gently separate teeth with padded tongue depressor.
6. Using premoistened applicators, wipe gums, teeth, tongue, and inside of mouth (Figure 16-42).
7. Repeat procedure with premoistened swab.
8. Discard used applicators in plastic bag.
9. Using clean applicators, apply lubricant to lips. Place used applicators in plastic bag.

FIGURE 16-42 Using premoistened applicators, wipe gums, teeth, and tongue.

10. Clean and replace equipment.
11. Remove and discard gloves according to facility policy.
12. Carry out each procedure completion action.

DRESSING RESIDENT

Residents are encouraged to wear their own clothes because it contributes to their sense of identity. If residents are not confined to bed, they dress after morning care every day.

Some residents will be able to dress themselves with assistance; those who are totally dependent will have to be dressed by the staff. It is part of your responsibility to see that the clothing is clean and neat and in good repair. You should remember to:

- Whenever possible, allow the resident to choose the clothing to be put on. The clothing should be lightweight but provide adequate warmth. Do not offer too many choices because that may confuse the resident.

- Encourage resident to participate in the dressing or undressing procedure, to the extent of the resident's ability.

The resident who requires complete help is easiest to dress in bed. Residents who can help themselves may wish to sit in a chair with clothing placed nearby. You can help by:

- Arranging the clothing in the order that it will be put on.
- Being prepared to assist with shoes and stockings, even for residents who can do much themselves. Bending over to adjust shoes and stockings can result in dizziness and loss of balance.
- Removing clothing from unaffected or strongest side first if the resident has difficulty moving one side or is paralyzed.

PROCEDURE 36 Dressing and Undressing Resident

1. Carry out each beginning procedure action.
2. Select appropriate clothing and arrange in order of application. Encourage resident to participate in selection.
3. Cover resident with bath blanket and fanfold top bedclothes to foot of bed.
4. Elevate head of bed to sitting position.
5. Assist resident to comfortable sitting position.
6. Remove night clothing, keeping resident covered with bath blanket. Remove from strong side first and then from weaker side. Place in laundry hamper.
7. If the resident wears a bra, slip straps over resident's hands (weak side first), move straps up arms, and position on shoulders. Adjust breasts in cups of bra. Then hook bra in back (assist resident to lean forward so bra can be fastened).
8. For an undershirt, or any garment that slips on over the head:
   a. Gather undershirt and place it over the resident's head.
   b. Grasp resident's hand and guide it through the arm hole by reaching into the arm hole from the outside.
   c. Repeat procedure with opposite arm.
   d. Assist resident to lean forward, and adjust undershirt so it is smooth over upper body.
9. Alternate procedure for slipover garments:
   Note: Garment must be large enough or made of stretchy fabric for this procedure.
   a. Place garment front side down on resident's lap with bottom opening facing the resident.
   b. Put resident's hands into bottom of garment and, one at a time, into the sleeve holes.
   c. Pull the sleeves up as far as possible on the resident's arms and pull hands through at wrist if it is a long-sleeved garment. The garment should now be high on the resident's chest.
   d. Gather up the back of the garment with your hand and slip the garment over the resident's head.
   e. Smooth the garment down and position it comfortably about the resident's body. Adjust sleeves and shoulders as needed.
10. Shirts or dresses that fasten in the front:
    a. Insert your hand through sleeve of garment and grasp hand of resident, drawing sleeve over your hand and resident's.
    b. Adjust sleeve at shoulder.
    c. Assist resident to sit forward. Arrange clothing across back.
    d. Gather sleeve on opposite side by slipping your hand in from the outside.
    e. Grasp resident's wrist and pull sleeve of garment over your hand and resident's hand. Draw upward and adjust at shoulder.
    f. Button, zip, or snap garment.
11. Underwear or slacks:
    a. Facing foot of bed, gather resident's underwear from waist to leg hole.
    b. Slip underwear over one foot at a time. Pull underwear up legs as high as possible.
    c. Assist resident to raise buttocks and draw garment over buttocks and up to waist. If resident cannot raise buttocks, assist resident to roll first to one side as you pull up the garment and then the other side. Adjust garment until it is comfortable.
    d. Fasten garment if required.
12. Socks or knee-high (or thigh-high) stockings:
    a. Roll sock or stocking with heel in back and place over toes.
    b. Draw sock up over foot and adjust until smooth. Pull stockings smoothly up to knee or thigh.
    c. Repeat for other foot.

(continues)

PROCEDURE *36* (continued)

13. Pantyhose:
    a. Gather pantyhose and adjust over toes and feet. Draw up legs as high as possible.
    b. Draw over hips as described in step 11c. Adjust until comfortable at waist.
14. Shoes:
    a. Slip shoe on, using shoe horn if necessary.
    b. Be sure shoe is fastened securely (Velcro tabs or ties). If the shoes tie, be sure that ends of shoelaces do not drag on the floor. The shoes should be fastened tight enough to prevent them from slipping off the resident's feet but not so tight that circulation is impaired.
    c. Shoes should have rubber soles for better traction. Leather soles slide easily on tile and linoleum floors.
15. To undress, reverse order of steps.
16. Carry out each procedure completion action.

LESSON SYNTHESIS: Putting It All Together

You have just completed this lesson. Now go back and review the Clinical Focus. Try to see how the Clinical Focus relates to the concepts presented in the lesson. Then answer the following questions.

1. Do older persons really care about how they look? What relationship does appearance have to self-esteem?

2. What danger does Mary Mandell face because of sitting in a wheelchair for so many hours?

3. What evidence is there to concern the staff and what steps must be taken?

4. How can the nursing assistant help Mary Mandell feel that she still has some control over her personal hygiene?

REVIEW

A. **Match each term (items a.–e.) with the proper definition.**

   a. caries
   b. pressure ulcer
   c. lesions
   d. dentures
   e. skin tears

   1. _____ skin breakdown due to prolonged pressure over bony prominences

   2. _____ artificial teeth

   3. _____ changes in skin structure

   4. _____ small breaks in the skin

   5. _____ dental cavities

B. **Brief answers**

   6. Name five factors that contribute to skin breakdown.

   7. List three ways you can encourage adequate circulation to tissues.

   8. Briefly describe each of the four stages of pressure ulcer development.

9. Name five basic positions that are routinely used to ensure that pressure is not prolonged on any body part.

10. List five ways to relieve pressure on body parts.

C. Fill in the blanks by selecting the correct word or phrase from the list.

dentures   senile lentigines
diabetes   skin tears
friction   strong
oral hygiene   turning schedule
pressure ulcers   weak
sacrum

11. Liver spots are more properly called _____.

12. Small breaks that occur in fragile skin are called _____.

13. When body parts rub together, _____ results, which may cause tissue damage.

14. Skin breakdown may progress to the formation of deep, painful lesions called _____.

15. For residents who are confined to bed, a _____ is followed to relieve pressure on body parts.

16. One of the most common sites for skin breakdown is the _____.

17. Generally, nursing assistants are not allowed to perform nail care, especially toenail care, on residents with _____.

18. The process of cleaning teeth, the tongue, and the inside of the mouth is called _____.

19. Artificial teeth are known as _____.

20. When dressing a resident with a weakness on one side due to a stroke or other condition, clothing is applied to the _____ side first. Clothing is removed from the _____ side first.

D. Select the one best answer for each of the following.

21. Which of the following is not a function of the skin?
    (A) perception of sensations
    (B) regulation of body temperature
    (C) protection of structures under the skin
    (D) production of insulin

22. Which of the following is a characteristic of the aging skin?
    (A) skin glands produce more oil
    (B) fingernails and toenails thin
    (C) sweat glands increase activity
    (D) circulation to the skin decreases

23. Shearing of tissues is most likely to occur when the resident
    (A) is resting on her abdomen
    (B) is positioned with the head of the bed elevated
    (C) is walking around
    (D) is resting flat on her back in bed

24. Select the best position for the resident considering the condition given.
    (A) Position the resident with respiratory problems flat in bed.
    (B) Position the resident who has had a recent stroke by turning her on the affected side.
    (C) Position the resident who has had a recent stroke by turning her on the unaffected side.
    (D) Position the resident who has a fractured hip by rotating her over the unaffected leg.

E. Clinical Experience

25. Janine was assisting Mrs. Docker with her tub bath when Mrs. Docker said she felt dizzy. What action should Janine take?

26. Carl is giving foot care to Mr. Dobrinski. The toenails are long and thick. What action should Carl take?

27. Chris is shaving Mr. Gates, who moves suddenly. The razor makes a small nick in the skin. How should Chris handle this situation?

28. Mrs. Marks has long curly hair that frequently tangles. How can Holly, her nursing assistant, care for Mrs. Marks's hair during morning care to reduce the amount of tangles?

29. Mrs. Gonzales has very thin, fragile skin. How can Jean, her nursing assistant, try to prevent skin tears?

LESSON 17

Meeting the Residents' Nutritional Needs

Clinical Focus

Think about how food is processed by the body and how you can help residents meet their nutritional needs as you study this lesson and meet:

Mrs. Hartley, a Christian Scientist, who is 92 and almost blind. Although she can make out light and dark, everything is blurred and shadowy. She has a cold and wants to rest in bed instead of going to the dining room to eat. Nursing assistants are serving trays and assisting residents to eat. Mrs. Hartley has dentures and an order for a soft diet. The nursing assistant serving trays notes that Mrs. Hartley seems listless and her skin is dry.

OBJECTIVES

After studying this lesson, you should be able to:

- Define and spell vocabulary words and terms.
- Identify the parts and function of the gastrointestinal system.
- Review changes in the digestive system as they relate to the aging process.
- Name the six classes of nutrients.
- List the functions of each class of nutrients.
- Name the six food groups.
- Provide the resident with fresh water.
- List four diets commonly provided in long-term care facilities.
- Name six therapeutic diets ordered in long-term care facilities.
- Measure intake correctly using the metric system.
- State ways the nursing assistant can promote adequate nutrition.
- Assist the resident who can feed herself or himself.
- Feed the dependent resident.
- Provide between-meal feedings.
- List alternate ways of delivering nutrition.

OBJECTIVES

- Briefly describe seven gastrointestinal disorders.
- Demonstrate the following:
  Procedure 37 Measuring and Recording Fluid Intake
  Procedure 38 Assisting the Resident Who Can Feed Self
  Procedure 39 Feeding the Dependent Resident

VOCABULARY

anus *(AY-nus)*

carbohydrate *(kar-boh-HIGH-drayt)*

colon *(KOH-lon)*

constipation *(kon-stih-PAY-shun)*

cubic centimeter (cc) *(KYOU-bick SEN-tih-mee-ter)*

defecation *(def-eh-KAY-shun)*

dehydration *(dee-high-DRAY-shun)·*

digestion *(die-JEST-shun)*

diverticuli *(die-ver-TICK-you-lie)*

diverticulitis *(die-ver-tick-you-LIE-tis)*

duodenum *(dew-oh-DEE-num)*

dyspepsia *(dis-PEP-see-ah)*

dysphagia *(dis-FAY-jee-ah)*

edema *(ee-DEE-mah)*

electrolytes *(ee-LECK-troh-lights)*

enzymes *(EN-zighms)*

esophagus *(eh-SOF-ah-gus)*

fats *(fats)*

feces *(FEE-cees)*

fiber *(FYE-ber)*

flatulence *(FLAT-you-lens)*

gastritis *(gas-TRY-tis)*

gastrointestinal tract *(gas-troh-in-TES-tih-nal trackt)*

gastrostomy (G) tube *(gas-TROS-toh-mee toob)*

hemorrhoids *(HEM-oh-royds)*

hernia *(HER-nee-ah)*

hiatal hernia *(high-AY-tal HER-nee-ah)*

high density *(high DEN-sih-tee)*

homeostasis *(hoh-mee-oh-STAY-sis)*

hyperalimentation *(high-per-al-ih-men-TAY-shun)*

ileum *(ILL-ee-um)*

inguinal hernia *(ING-gwih-nal HER-nee-ah)*

intake and output (I&O) *(IN-tayk and OUT-put)*

jejunum *(jeh-JOO-num)*

metric system *(MET-rick SIS-tum)*

milliliter (mL) *(MILL-ih-lee-ter)*

mineral *(MIN-er-al)*

nasogastric (NG) tube *(nay-zoh-GAS-trick toob)*

obesity *(oh-BEES-ih-tee)*

pharynx *(FAR-inks)*

protein *(PROH-tee-in)*

regularity *(reg-you-LAIR-ih-tee)*

rupture *(RUP-chur)*

therapeutic *(ther-ah-PYOU-tick)*

total parenteral nutrition (TPN) *(TOH-tal pah-REN-ter-al new-TRISH-un)*

USDA

vitamin *(VYE-tah-min)*

water *(WOT-er)*

THE DIGESTIVE SYSTEM ———

The digestive system processes the foods eaten, releasing simple nutrients that are needed by the body. There are six nutrients: vitamins, minerals, water, fats, proteins, and carbohydrates. The nutrients pass through the wall of the intestine into the bloodstream; they are carried in the blood to where they are used by the body cells.

Chemicals **(enzymes)** help break down or digest the food, and the nondigestible portion of what is eaten is eliminated from the body as solid waste called **feces**. This process is called a bowel movement (BM) or **defecation**.

The digestive system (Figure 17-1) is also called the **gastrointestinal tract**. It is a tube about 30 feet long, stretching from the mouth to the end opening called the **anus**. The walls of

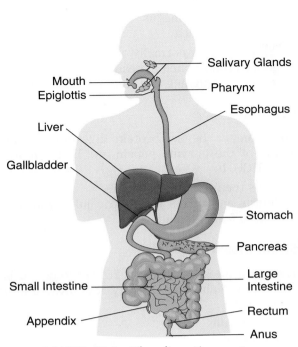

FIGURE 17-1   The digestive system

the tube are made of smooth muscle and the entire tract is lined with mucous membrane. The digestive system consists of the true digestive organs:

- Mouth (Figure 17-2)
- **Pharynx**

- **Esophagus**
- Stomach
- Small intestine
- Large intestine

The true digestive organs receive the help of other organs in breaking food into simpler substances. These organs are called accessory organs and include the:

- Tongue
- Salivary glands
- Teeth
- Liver
- Pancreas
- Gallbladder

The liver produces bile, which is stored in the gallbladder. The pancreas produces digestive enzymes as well as the hormones insulin and glucagon. The tongue and teeth mechanically break down the food and direct it toward the rest of the tract.

THE DIGESTIVE PROCESS

The process of **digestion** is both mechanical and chemical. Foods are broken up and moved along the tract by rhythmic muscular contractions. At the same time, digestive enzymes and bile are mixed with the food. The digestive enzymes from the stomach, pancreas, and small intestine (Figure 17-3), together with

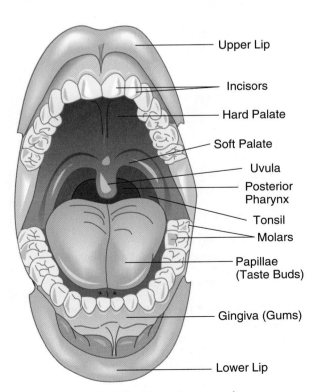

FIGURE 17-2   The mouth

FIGURE 17-3   Enzymes and digestion

Organ	Important Enzymes	Food Acted On
Salivary glands	Salivary amylase	Starches
Stomach	Pepsin Lipase Renin (infants)	Proteins Fats Milk protein
Pancreas	Lipase Amylase Trypsin	Fats Starches Proteins
Small intestine	Lactase Sucrase Maltase Peptidase	Lactose (sugar) Sucrose (sugar) Maltose (sugar) Protein

bile, chemically break the foods into simple nutrients:

- Proteins are changed to amino acids.
- Carbohydrates are changed to simple sugars like glucose.
- Fats are changed to fatty acids and glycerol.

The undigestible portion of food is moved along in the intestines and finally excreted from the body as feces.

Mouth

Digestion begins in the mouth. The teeth and tongue break the food into smaller pieces, mix it with saliva, and form a rounded mass of food. The food is swallowed into the pharynx and moves down the esophagus into the stomach.

The tongue is a skeletal muscle covered with taste buds. It:

- Pushes the food between the teeth
- Propels the food backward to aid swallowing
- Assists in speech

Salivary glands secrete saliva. It contains an enzyme, salivary amylase, to start carbohydrate digestion. Saliva:

- Moistens food for easier swallowing
- Amounts to about 1½ quarts daily in the average adult. The amount of fluid varies with the person and may be altered by specific health problems.

Teeth mechanically break up the food. They:

- Number 32 in the adult
- May be replaced by dentures when lost

The pharynx is a common passageway for:

- Food to the esophagus
- Air to the trachea

The gag reflex normally occurs if food begins to go into the trachea instead of the esophagus. This causes coughing and clearing of the airway.

Stomach

The stomach begins protein digestion by the action of the enzyme pepsin and hydrochloric acid (HCl). It:

- Holds the food about 4 hours
- Churns and mixes the gastric juice with the food to form a liquid

Small Intestine

The small intestine is about 20 feet long and is coiled in the abdominal cavity. It is divided into three parts:

- **Duodenum**
- **Jejunum**
- **Ileum**

The small intestine is attached by the duodenum to the stomach and by the ileum to the large intestine.

The small intestine produces a fluid containing digestive enzymes and receives:

- Food from the stomach
- Bile from the liver and gallbladder to begin fat breakdown
- Pancreatic fluid from the pancreas, which completes the breakdown of:
  - Proteins to amino acids
  - Carbohydrates to simple sugar (glucose)
  - Fats to fatty acids and glycerol

FIGURE 17-4 Basic nutrients and their functions

Nutrient	Form Used	Function
Complex carbohydrates	Glucose	Supply blood sugar—primary energy for body
Proteins	Amino acids	Build and repair tissues
Fats	Fatty acids Glycerol	Supply stored energy Needed to benefit from fat-soluble vitamins
Water	Water	Needed to carry on body chemistry
Vitamins	Fat-soluble—A,D,K,E Water-soluble—B,C	Act as co-enzymes in promoting body activities
Minerals	Calcium, phosphorus, potassium, sodium, and traces of others	Important in formation of body tissues and body chemistry

Most of the digestion and absorption of nutrients occur in the small intestine. Figure 17-4 shows the functions of the basic nutrients and the forms in which they are used in the body.

As food moves slowly through the small intestine, the simple nutrients pass through the wall of the intestine and into the bloodstream, where they are carried to the liver for more action before being used by the body cells.

Once released from foods, the following nutrients can be absorbed directly:

- Water
- Vitamins
- Minerals

Large Intestine

The large intestine is called the **colon**. It extends from the end of the small intestine to the rectum, which ends in the anus. It is not as long as the small intestine. Its main purpose is to carry the unused food out of the body, but some vitamins and water are absorbed through the colon walls. A muscle holds the anus closed and can be voluntarily relaxed to permit defecation.

AGING CHANGES

As the body ages, some changes take place in the digestive process.

- The flow of enzymes is somewhat decreased.
- The muscular walls of the tract lose some tone and strength so that movement along the tract is slower.
- The gag reflex that prevents food from slipping into the trachea is not as active, so choking is possible.
- Absorption of nutrients is slower.

Figure 17-5 is a summary of the changes in the digestive process that are the result of aging. Some older persons find they may not tolerate foods they previously enjoyed.

NUTRIENTS

Nutrients provide us with essential materials to:

- Build and repair tissues
- Perform body functions
- Provide energy for the work the body does

It takes energy to perform activities such as walking or getting in and out of bed. Even when a person is quiet and inactive, energy is needed

FIGURE 17-5 Changes in the digestive system caused by aging
• Decreased number and function of taste buds
• Reduced digestive enzymes
• Thicker saliva
• Tongue more sensitive
• Movement of food not as efficient
• More **flatulence** (gas production)
• Less effective gag reflex
• Poorer tolerance of some foods
• Slower absorption of nutrients
• Decreased chewing/poor dentures
• Weaker muscular walls
• **Constipation** (difficult defecation) more common

for the heart to beat and for the kidneys to produce urine. These are examples of vital body activities that sustain life.

Energy is supplied by the nutrients in the foods we eat. The amount of energy from nutrients is measured in units of heat called calories. When not enough nutrients are eaten, the body gradually uses up its stored supply and becomes depleted; loss of weight and illness follow.

Classes of Nutrients

There are six classes of nutrients. Many foods contain more than one nutrient. The basic nutrients are:

- Carbohydrates
- Fats
- Proteins
- Vitamins
- Minerals
- Water

Carbohydrates are the primary source of immediate body energy. One gram of carbohydrates provides 4 calories of energy. Many foods contain this nutrient. Fruits, vegetables, breads, cereal, and pasta products are good sources. Carbohydrate foods supply the body with **fiber**. Fiber helps maintain **regularity** (bowel activity).

Fats provide energy and are found in both plant and animal foods. One gram of fat provides 9 calories of energy. Sources of fats include butter, meat, nuts, egg yolks, and vegetable oils.

Proteins are essential for tissue building and repair. One gram of protein provides 4 calories. Foods rich in protein include meats, fish, poultry, eggs, beans, nuts, and lentils.

Vitamins and **minerals** regulate body processes. The different kinds of vitamins are represented by letters. Vitamins A, D, K, and E are fat soluble and are found in fatty foods as well as in fruits and vegetables. Vitamins B and C are water soluble and are found in fruits, vegetables, and whole grain products. The minerals include sodium, potassium, calcium, and iron.

Water is essential to life. Each person needs to take in about 2½ quarts (2½ liters or 2,500 milliliters [mL]) of water in some form daily. (In certain circumstances, under a doctor's order, water intake may be limited.) Water is consumed in drinks such as plain water, tea, coffee, and other beverages. Water is also taken in with foods such as fruits and vegetables that have high water content.

ELECTROLYTE BALANCE

Electrolytes are minerals that are essential to the chemical functioning of the body. The electrolytes in the body fluids must be balanced for proper functioning. You may be familiar with electrolytes as solid substances, such as sodium chloride (table salt) and sodium bicarbonate, an antacid used to relieve indigestion.

In the body fluids, the electrolytes break apart to form ions that take part in the body's chemical reaction. Two important electrolytes are:

- Sodium
- Potassium

The **homeostasis** (balance) of body functions depends on many body activities. The endocrine system plays an important part in this process.

When there is an electrolyte imbalance in the body, many problems—sometimes serious—can occur.

Two common problems are:

- Increased levels of sodium in the blood. The sodium causes body tissues to hold fluid, resulting in swelling or edema. This is often seen in the feet and legs of elderly residents

FIGURE 17-6 Edema of the feet and legs as a result of electrolyte imbalance

(Figure 17-6). Fluid may also accumulate in the lungs, causing respiratory distress.

- Decreased levels of potassium in the blood. This leads to a slower heart rate, feelings of weakness, and a lack of interest in surroundings.

Figure 17-7 lists observations to report for residents with electrolyte imbalance.

FIGURE 17-7 Observations to be reported for the resident with electrolyte imbalance

- Swelling of feet and legs
- Respiratory distress
- Slower than normal pulse rate
- Lack of interest in surroundings
- Feelings of weakness
- Intake and output (if ordered)

FOOD GROUPS

Food can be classified into six food groups. Adequate selections from each group ensure proper nutrition. The six food groups are the:

- Bread, cereal, rice, and pasta group
- Fruit group
- Vegetable group
- Milk, yogurt, and cheese group
- Meat, poultry, fish, dry beans, eggs, and nuts group
- Fats, oils, and sweets group

In 1990, the United States Department of Agriculture (**USDA**) revised the guidelines for healthy nutrition. The guidelines explained the food groups from which selections could be made. They also named the number of servings that should be taken from each group. The report emphasized that for most adult Americans:

- The overall calories should be decreased.
- Sugars and salts should be used in moderation.
- Fats, oils, and cholesterol (animal fat) should be limited.
- Alcohol, if consumed at all, should be used in moderation.

Food Guide Pyramid

In 1992, the USDA first presented the Food Guide Pyramid. This is the official visual guide to help people understand the written guidelines (Figure 17-8).

Look carefully at the pyramid. You will see that the bread, cereal, rice, and pasta group is at the base of the pyramid. Selections from this group should make up the biggest part of the diet. Fats, oils, and sweets are at the very small top of the pyramid, meaning that these foods should be only a very small part of the total diet.

Selections must be made from each group in the amounts indicated because important nutrients for the body's well-being are found in each group.

Food Guide Pyramid for People Aged 70 Years and Over

Recently a food guide pyramid for the elderly was developed by researchers at Tufts University, the USDA, and the Human Nutrition Research Center for Aging. This pyramid differs from the original pyramid (shown in Figure 17-8) by recommending the following:

- At the base of the pyramid, eight glasses of water daily to prevent dehydration, kidney dysfunction, and constipation
- Revised servings of the food groups:
  - 6 or more servings of bread, fortified cereal, rice, and pasta
  - 2–3 servings of vegetables
  - 2 or more servings of fruits

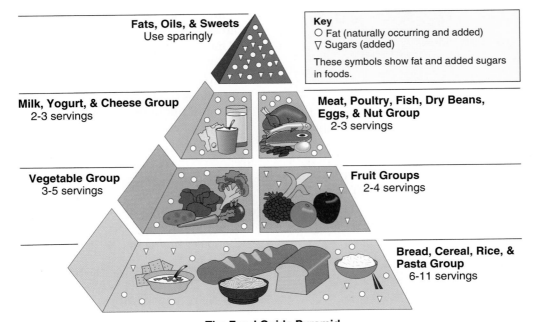

Key
○ Fat (naturally occurring and added)
▽ Sugars (added)

These symbols show fat and added sugars in foods.

Fats, Oils, & Sweets
Use sparingly

Milk, Yogurt, & Cheese Group
2-3 servings

Meat, Poultry, Fish, Dry Beans, Eggs, & Nut Group
2-3 servings

Vegetable Group
3-5 servings

Fruit Groups
2-4 servings

Bread, Cereal, Rice, & Pasta Group
6-11 servings

The Food Guide Pyramid
A guide to daily food choices

FIGURE 17-8 The Food Guide Pyramid illustrates the fundamentals of healthy nutrition for the average individual through mid-life. (Courtesy of USDA)

- 3 servings of milk, yogurt, and cheese group
- 2 or more servings of meat, poultry, fish, dry beans, eggs and nut group
- sparing use of fats, oils, and sweets

Note that upper limits are not set for some foods.

- Supplements of calcium, vitamin D, and vitamin B12.

The Bread, Cereal, Rice, and Pasta Group (6–11 Servings Daily)

This food group provides:

- Carbohydrates for energy
- Vitamins such as vitamin B
- Minerals such as iron
- Roughage or fiber

Members of this group generally have little fat and provide fiber. The fiber adds bulk, which helps to satisfy appetite and promotes bowel activity and elimination. Whole grains and enriched products provide the richest source of fibers and nutrients. Making varied selections ensures that different types of fibers will be included in the diet.

Examples of single servings from this group are:

- 1 slice of bread
- ½ bun, or bagel, or English muffin
- 1 ounce of ready-to-eat cereal
- ½ cup of cooked cereal, rice, or pasta

The Fruit Group (2–4 Servings Daily)

This food group provides:

- Vitamins
- Minerals
- Fiber
- Carbohydrates

Include melons, berries, and citrus fruits regularly. Citrus fruits are a good source of vitamin C, which must be replaced daily. Fruits may be served as juices and make good desserts.

Examples of single servings from this group are:

- 1 medium apple, orange, or banana
- ½ cup small or diced fruit
- ¾ cup fruit juice

The Vegetable Group (3–5 Servings Daily)

This food group provides:

- Vitamins such as A and C and folic acid
- Minerals
- Carbohydrates
- Fiber

Include dark green leafy and deep yellow vegetables often. Dried beans and peas may be counted as either a vegetable serving or may be substituted for 1 ounce of meat. Dried beans and peas provide the nutrients of the vegetables and contain some of the important proteins found in meat.

Starchy vegetables, such as potatoes, provide complex carbohydrates as well as other nutrients and should be considered as part of the vegetable selections.

Fruits and vegetables can be made easier to chew by:

- Cooking
- Chopping
- Dicing
- Pureeing

Examples of single servings from this group are:

- 1 cup raw, leafy vegetables
- ½ cup dry beans or peas
- ½ cup other vegetables

The Milk, Yogurt, and Cheese Group (2–3 Servings Daily)

This food group provides:

- Protein for tissue building and repair
- Minerals such as calcium and phosphorus
- Vitamins such as A, B, and D

Low-fat milk and yogurt provide the same essential nutrients without as many calories from fat.

One serving of milk has about the same amount of calcium as:

- 1 cup of yogurt
- 2½ slices of cheese
- 1 cup of pudding
- 2 cups of cottage cheese

Examples of single servings from this group are:

- 1 cup milk
- 1 cup yogurt
- 1½ ounces cheese
- 1 cup pudding
- 2 cups cottage cheese

The Meat, Poultry, Fish, Dry Beans, Eggs, and Nuts Group (2–3 Servings Daily)

This food group provides:

- High-quality protein
- Vitamins such as D and B
- Minerals such as iron and zinc
- Fats

The amount of fat in this food group can be reduced by:

- Preparing properly, for example, baking rather than frying
- Choosing lean cuts of beef and poultry
- Removing poultry skin because the fat immediately under it adds to the total calories if eaten

An example of a single serving from this group is:

(Total intake = 6 ounces)

- ½ cup dry beans or peas = 1 ounce meat serving

The Fats, Oils, and Sweets Group

This food group provides:

- Energy
- Vitamins such as A and D

These nutrients can be obtained from other food sources that will not raise the calorie level as high. It is recommended that less than 30% of the daily calories come from fat sources. Eating less fat from animal sources will help lower the cholesterol and the total fat in the diet. High levels of cholesterol and other fats in the blood can cause serious health problems. Therefore, use fats and oils sparingly.

Sugars and Salt

Added sugar and salt may make food pleasing to the taste but often mask the natural flavors of the foods. Sugar and salt should be used in moderation.

Sugars left in the mouth favor bacterial growth, contributing to dental cavities. Many so-called sweets, such as desserts and candy, provide calories but little nourishment.

Salt (sodium chloride) is widely found in food. Therefore, a varied diet will provide adequate amounts of salt for health. It should not be necessary to add it to the cooking process or at the table. Salt does increase the pleasure of eating for many people, but it should be used in moderation.

Alcoholic Beverages

Alcoholic beverages add nothing to the diet but calories and are not essential to a healthy diet. Because of the potential for addiction, injuries due to impaired behavior, and birth defects, it is wise to avoid routine consumption of alcoholic beverages.

If alcohol is consumed, it should be done moderately. At present, moderate drinking is considered to be:

- No more than 2 drinks per day for men
- No more than 1 drink per day for women

Count as one drink:

- 12 ounces of regular beer
- 5 ounces of wine
- 1½ ounces of distilled spirits (80 proof)

NUTRITIONAL STATUS

Eating to meet nutritional needs is one of the major activities of daily living. Eating also meets important social and emotional needs when dining is carried out in the proper environment and with the proper support. Elderly people who live independently may prepare foods that satisfy their appetites, yet do not meet basic nutritional needs.

Easy-to-chew, high-calorie foods may provide energy in excess of body needs; the extra energy is stored as fat. Although the person's appetite is satisfied by these foods, they do not necessarily provide the nutrients needed. Essential vitamins, minerals, and proteins may be lacking.

Elderly people are at risk for becoming malnourished. An important part of the job of a nursing assistant is to monitor and report the food and fluid intake of the residents. Malnutrition can result in unintended weight loss and pressure ulcers. A guide called "Nutrition Care Alerts" has been developed by experts in nutrition and long-term care. The guide is to be used not only by nursing assistants but also by other members of the interdisciplinary health care team. Nutrition Care Alerts list the warning signs for unintended weight loss and dehydration and provides a list of actions that caregivers should take to avoid resident malnutrition.

Warning signs for unintended weight loss:

- Needs help to eat or drink
- Eats less than half of the meals/snacks that are served
- Has mouth pain
- Has dentures that do not fit
- Has a hard time chewing or swallowing
- Has sadness, crying spells, or withdraws from others
- Is confused, wanders, or paces
- Has diabetes, chronic obstructive lung disease, cancer, HIV, or other chronic disease

If any of these signs are present. the nursing assistant should follow these steps:

- Report observations and warning signs to nurse and dietician
- Encourage resident to eat
- Honor food preferences
- Offer many kinds of foods and beverages
- Help residents who have trouble feeding themselves
- Allow adequate time to finish eating
- Notify nurse if resident has trouble using utensils
- Record meal/snack intake
- Provide oral hygiene before meals
- Position resident correctly for feeding

Facilities shoud have a protocol for standards of care for residents who experience weight loss of 5% or more in 30 days or 10% or more in the last 6 months. All residents should be weighed at least monthly and those at risk more often. It is important always to use the same scale, at about the same time of the day, and to take into account the weight of wheelchairs, leg rests, and lapboards.

DEHYDRATION

Water in adequate amounts is essential to normal body functioning. Most older adults need to consume about 2,000 to 3,000 mL or 2 to 3 quarts of liquid each day. If the body is functioning properly, the amount of fluids taken in will be balanced by the amount lost.

Dehydration (inadequate fluid level in the body) develops when fluid intake is not adequate. In addition, some drugs cause excessive amounts of fluids to be lost from the body. It is important to recognize the signs of dehydration. All signs of dehydration must be reported immediately so corrective actions can be taken.

Warning Signs of Dehydration. The Nutrition Care Alerts have identified the warning signs of dehydration:

- Drinks less than 6 cups of liquids daily
- Has one or more of the following:
  - dry mouth
  - cracked lips
  - sunken eyes
  - dark urine
- Needs help drinking from a cup or glass
- Has trouble swallowing liquids
- Frequent vomiting, diarrhea, or fever
- Is easily confused or tired

Many residents do not take in enough fluids. This is especially true when they feel ill, have a fever, or have a decreased appetite. An essential task of nursing assistants is to remind and encourage residents to drink water or other fluids frequently.

- Always follow the care plan for each resident for fluid intake. Some residents may be on limited intake because of their medical conditions and should not be offered fluids.
- For other residents, be sure fresh water is within reach. Keep pitchers full. Some residents may request that ice be added to the water.
- Remind the resident to drink whenever you have contact with the resident.
- A resident who has a fever requires careful monitoring of fluid intake.
- Increase attention to fluid intake during hot weather.
- If residents cannot drink unaided, offer fluids frequently and assist as needed.
- If a resident is on intake, record the amount of fluid consumed each time the resident drinks. If this is not possible, the amount of water left in a pitcher can be measured before the pitcher is refilled. The amount left is subtracted from the total amount of water in the pitcher originally.
- Fluid intake over 24 hours is usually consumed during the day and evening shifts (0700 to 2300). It is important for nursing assistants on these shifts to encourage residents to drink adequate fluid.
- Provide alternatives for residents who do not like water. Check dietary card for beverage preferences. Check if resident prefers and is allowed ice in beverages
- Serve water as well as other beverages at mealtime

The procedure for changing water is outlined in the facility procedure manual. Be sure you know the requirements for changing water, especially the steps to prevent the spread of infection. For example, if pitchers are taken to a central area to be refilled, be sure each resi-

On the Job

Residents may still become dehydrated even if they eat well-prepared, balanced meals.

dent receives her own pitcher and not one belonging to another resident. Pitchers must be covered before being taken back to the residents' rooms and should remain covered in the room.

INTAKE AND OUTPUT (I&O)

The amount of fluid taken into the body and the amount of fluid lost should be just about equal. The **intake and output (I&O)** is frequently measured and recorded. Imbalances in intake and output can result in fluid imbalances such as **edema** (water retention) and dehydration.

Intake

Intake includes everything taken in that is liquid at room temperature. For example, included in the intake fluids are:

- Water or tea
- Gelatin, junket, pudding, ice cream
- Fluids given directly into a vein (IV)
- Fluids given by nasogastric tube or gastric tube

Output

The output includes all fluids lost. This includes:

- Urine
- Perspiration
- Blood
- Diarrhea
- Vomiting
- Wound drainage

Calculating Fluid (Liquid) Intake (Output is covered in Lesson 18)

Calculating oral fluid intake is the responsibility of the nursing assistant. To do this correctly, you must know:

- The amount of fluid the container holds when full
- How to calculate the amount of fluid the resident drank from the container

The containers used include cups, glasses, soup bowls, water pitchers, milk cartons, ice cream cups, and gelatin and pudding cups. There are many types of containers and facilities do not all use the same kinds. Your facility will have a chart listing the sizes (amount of fluid the container can hold when full) of the containers used in the facility.

Fluids can be measured using either a standard system (ounce, pint, quart) or the **metric system** (milliliter or cubic centimeter). A comparison of these measurements follows. Note that the abbreviation for milliliter is mL.

drop (gtt)	= .06 mL	
teaspoon (tsp)	= 5 mL	
tablespoon (tbsp)	= 15 mL	
ounce (oz)	= 30 mL	
pint (pt) = 16 oz	= 480 mL	
quart (qt) = 32 oz	= 2 pt	= 960 mL
gallon (gal) = 128 oz	= 4 qt = 8 pt	= 3,840 mL

You cannot actually measure what is gone from the container. Therefore, your calculation will be an estimate. It is important that the estimate be as accurate as possible. In facilities, fluid is recorded in **cubic centimeters (cc)** or **milliliters (mL)**. These measurements are the same amount. The preferred measurement is mL, but many facilities still use cc. All liquids and all foods that become liquid at room temperature (ice cream, sherbet, gelatin) are recorded as fluid intake. All fluids taken with meals and between meals are recorded.

To simplify the calculation, some facilities consider a pint to be 500 mL, a quart 1,000 mL, and a gallon 4,000 mL. Some containers may be marked in ounces. The amount measured in ounces must be converted into mL. For example, a can of soda may be marked as 12 ounces. This equals 360 mL (12 × 30 mL where 30 mL is the same as 1 ounce).

To calculate intake when the resident has finished drinking:

- Pick up the container and hold it at eye level.
- Determine whether ¼, ⅓, ½, ⅔, or ¾ of the container of liquid has been consumed. Remember that containers are not filled to the top when full.
- Look at the facility's chart to see how much that type of container holds when it is full (Figure 17-9).
- Calculate the intake by multiplying the amount consumed times the amount the container holds when it is full.

Examples:

1. A juice glass holds 120 mL when full. The resident has consumed half of the juice. The intake is calculated: ½ × 120 (2 into 120) = 60 mL intake.
2. A water glass holds 180 mL when full. The resident has consumed ¾ of the water. The

FIGURE 17-9 Average container amounts
Water glass = 6 oz = 180 mL
Styrofoam cup = 6 oz = 180 mL
Juice glass (small) = 4 oz = 120 mL
Juice glass (large) = 8 oz = 240 mL
Full water pitcher (1 qt) = 32 oz = 960 mL
Coffee or tea pot = 10 oz = 300 mL
Coffee cup = 5 oz = 150 mL
Milk carton = 8 oz = 240 mL
Soup bowl (small) = 6 oz = 180 mL
Soup bowl (large) = 10 oz = 300 mL
Gelatin = 4 oz = 120 mL
Ice cream cup = 5 oz = 150 mL
Creamer = 1 oz = 30 mL

intake is calculated: $\frac{3}{4} \times 180$ (take 4 into $180 = 45$) and multiply 45 times 3 which equals 135 mL intake.

3. An ice cream cup holds 150 mL when full. The resident has consumed all of the ice cream. Intake is recorded as 150 mL.
4. A soup bowl holds 180 mL when full. The resident has consumed $\frac{2}{3}$ of the soup. The intake is calculated: $\frac{2}{3} \times 180$ (take 3 into $180 = 60$) and multiply 60 times 2. The intake is 120 mL.

When calculating fluids for a meal you may need to calculate the separate quantities, add them, and record the total intake for the meal. For example:

$\frac{2}{3}$ carton of milk	= 160 mL
1 small orange juice	= 120 mL
$\frac{1}{2}$ cup coffee	= 75 mL
$\frac{1}{3}$ glass water	= 60 mL

Total breakfast intake: 415 mL

A special form for recording I&O may be kept at the bedside to be used each day. Fluids taken in and lost are listed on the I&O sheet in the resident's health record.

PROCEDURE 37 Measuring and Recording Fluid Intake

1. Carry out each beginning procedure action.
2. Assemble the following:
   - Intake and output record at bedside
   - Pen for recording
3. Record intake on the I&O record at the bedside (Figure 17-10) by listing all fluids taken in. Total intake includes:
   - The amount of liquid the resident takes with meals
   - The amount of water and other liquids taken between meals
   - All other fluids given by mouth, intravenously, or by tube feeding. How these fluids are taken should also be recorded.
4. Copy information on the resident's chart from the bedside I&O record, according to facility policy. Report low intake to the nurse. The average person should take in between 2,000 and 3,000 mL (cc) daily.
5. Carry out each procedure completion action.

(continues)

PROCEDURE *37* (continued)

INTAKE AND OUTPUT

Room: 103 B   Name: Simon, Grace   Date:

Instructions: Record all I and O

2300-0700		0700-1500		1500-2300	
Intake	Output	Intake	Output	Intake	Output
Total		Total		Total	

Drinking Glass.........200 mL   Full Water Pitcher....950 mL   Milk Carton..............236 mL   Jello...........................90 mL
Styrofoam Cup........200 mL   Coffee or Teapot.....300 mL   Soup Bowl...............250 mL   Ice Cream Cup..........90 mL
Juice Glass (small)..100 mL   Coffee Cup.............150 mL   Soup Bowl (small)...100 mL   Creamer....................50 mL
Juice Glass (large)..250 mL

FOLEY CATHETER DRAINAGE: (Circle the following when applicable)

Color: Yellow   Amber   Brown   Red

Appearance: Cloudy   Clear   Sediment   Mucous   Bloody   24 hour INTAKE_____

Abdomen Distended   Catheter Irrigated   Catheter Changed   24 hour OUTPUT_____

FIGURE 17-10   An intake and output chart becomes part of the resident's record.

DIETS

Some residents may need to have their diets modified because of health problems. Special diets are based on the food groups described previously, but consistency and method of preparation may be altered.

Standard Diets

Four standard diets are offered in long-term care facilities. They are the:

1. Regular diet
2. Mechanical soft diet
3. Pureed diet
4. Clear liquid diet

Regular Diet.   The regular diet is prepared for most residents. It includes varied selections from the food groups. It is rich in vitamins and minerals and provides adequate bulk and balanced calories (Figure 17-11).

FIGURE 17-11   Well-balanced, smaller servings are more appealing to the elderly appetite.

Mechanical Soft Diet.   The mechanical soft diet is based on the regular diet but includes liquids and semisolid foods that are more easily chewed and digested (Figure 17-12).

Pureed Diet.   The pureed diet meets nutritional needs with foods that can be put into

FIGURE 17-13 The pureed diet includes foods from each of the food groups. The foods were pureed in a blender.

semiliquid or liquid form at room temperature (Figure 17-13). It may be given to residents with diseases of the intestinal tract or those who are unable to chew because of infection, stroke, or lack of teeth.

Clear Liquid Diet. The clear liquid diet is usually prescribed when a resident is ill and needs to have fluids replaced. This diet is not

FIGURE 17-12 The mechanical soft diet is easy to chew and digest.

given for prolonged periods because it does not provide adequate nutrition. Milk is not included in the clear liquid diet because the liquids must be clear (that is, you can see through them), but broths and filtered fruit juices are permitted.

Therapeutic Diets

Therapeutic diets, also called special diets, are prepared for residents with specific needs (Figure 17-14). They include the:

1. Diabetic diet
2. Low-sodium diet
3. Low-fat diet
4. Calorie-restricted diet
5. High-protein diet
6. Low-residue diet

The diabetic diet is usually a carefully balanced diet for residents who have diabetes mellitus and who must restrict concentrated sugar (for example, candy or pastry) in their diet. They may eat only foods on their diet, but they must eat everything that is ordered for them. It is important that you report the exact amounts of foods eaten by the diabetic resident because their medication is calculated based on food intake.

The low-sodium diet is prescribed for the resident with a heart condition or one who retains fluids. The low-fat diet limits the amounts of fats in the diet and is served to residents who have gallbladder, cardiovascular, or liver disease. The calorie-restricted diet is given to residents in need of weight control (to avoid or correct **obesity**). The high-protein diet is provided for residents who are underweight and poorly nourished and when diseases such as cancer make unusual nutritional demands.

FIGURE 17-14	Summary of therapeutic diets
Diabetic	Amounts of carbohydrates, fats, and proteins are balanced and prescribed. Concentrated sweets are restricted.
Low-Sodium (Sodium-Restricted)	Amounts of sodium specifically prescribed, such as 500 mg sodium. Sodium-rich foods, such as milk, bacon, and salted nuts, are excluded.
Low-Fat	Foods with high fat content are restricted, such as whole milk and eggs. Eliminates use of fats in preparation of food.
Calorie-Restricted	Limits the number of calories while ensuring an adequate intake of nutrients.
High-Protein	High in protein, iron, and vitamins, served in six small meals per day. Hot, spicy foods excluded.
Low-Residue	Roughage, fresh fruits, and vegetables (except bananas and potatoes), nuts, and whole grains are limited.

The low-residue diet is served to residents who need to limit roughage intake. It is given when residents have lower bowel problems such as colitis and diarrhea.

Remember, special diets are *therapeutic*, which means they are used as *treatments*. Always check to be sure that the resident receives the right tray.

A progressive diet is ordered for many residents after digestive upset, as their conditions permit. The usual progression is:

- Ice chips/sips of water
- Clear liquids
- Full liquids
- Soft or light diet
- Regular diet

NURSING ASSISTANT RESPONSIBILITIES

Nursing assistants have a personal responsibility to provide good nutrition for themselves so they will stay healthy and have the energy to do their work. They also play an important role in helping residents to meet their nutritional needs.

It is important that each nursing assistant know and understand:

- The nutrients and amounts needed for health
- The importance of adequate water to prevent dehydration
- Ways diets can be modified to meet individual health needs

Mealtime is a busy time in the long-term care facility. The nursing assistant has a major responsibility to see that it goes smoothly and pleasantly. You will:

- Make sure the area is pleasant and odor-free.
- Assist residents to reach the dining room.
- Serve trays.
- Help residents who need assistance in eating.
- Always be sure the resident receives the proper diet (standard or therapeutic) by checking the tray card.
- Be sure foods are served at the proper temperature.
- Make sure that used trays are not returned to the serving cart until all clean trays have been served.
- Keep food trays covered until served.
- Housekeeping carts and laundry hampers must be out of the corridor when food is served or kept at least two room widths away from the food cart when it is placed in the corridor.
- Place the food cart against the wall when it is brought into the dining room.
- Doors to the food cart should be closed until the trays are served.

Eating may be one of the few generally enjoyable activities left to the elderly. In addition to meeting nutritional needs, meals should also be sensually and socially satisfying. Large dining areas permit residents to eat together and promote a social atmosphere. The meals are prepared by the dietary staff in large kitchens

FIGURE 17-15 Residents' diets are prepared in the dietary department. The dietary aide takes the marked tray from the tray cart to serve to the resident. If a dietary aide is not available, the nursing assistant delivers the tray to the resident.

and brought to the dining area on tray carts (Figure 17-15).

In many facilities, special evening meals are organized so that residents who are able will dress up and eat in a restaurant-like atmosphere. Dining tables are set up home style and dinner is not served on trays.

This activity meets both social and nutritional needs and is greatly appreciated by residents.

Assisting with Feeding

If residents can go to the dining room:

- Assist them to the toilet before mealtimes.
- Help them wash their hands.
- Help them into the dining room.

Wheelchairs and geri-chairs can be rolled into the dining room if residents cannot walk. Some residents may remain in their wheelchairs. Other residents will transfer to dining room chairs. After washing your own hands, help serve the trays and assist as necessary (Figure 17-16).

- Cut meat into small bite-size pieces. Allow resident time to chew thoroughly.

FIGURE 17-16 If residents need assistance, nursing assistants help them eat.

- Pour liquids. Do not fill containers too full. Cool hot drinks with milk or water to prevent burns.
- Butter bread and cut into small pieces.
- Unfold and position napkin or towel over clothing.

Feeding the Resident

Even when a resident is confined to bed or must be fed, you can make the experience more pleasant if you:

- Position the resident comfortably upright
- Remove all unpleasant things from sight
- Never hurry the resident
- Allow the resident to help as much as possible
- Identify the food offered
- Always identify hot liquids
- Season food as resident desires
- Use a different straw with each liquid
- Place food on unaffected side if resident is paralyzed
- Feed food from tip of spoon
- Provide a clothing protector

PROCEDURE 38   Assisting the Resident Who Can Feed Self

1. Carry out each beginning procedure action.
2. Assemble equipment:
   - Bedpan/urinal
   - Wash water
   - Oral hygiene items
   - Tray of food
3. Offer bedpan/urinal. (If used, follow steps in Procedure 40 in Lesson 18.)
4. If permitted, elevate head of bed or assist resident out of bed.
   Note: The nursing assistant in the photos for this procedure is wearing gloves while preparing the resident to eat. Some facilities require the wearing of gloves; others do not. Follow your facility policy.
5. Clear overbed table and position in front of resident (Figure 17-17A). Remove

unpleasant equipment from sight. Remove sources of odors.
6. Provide water, soap, and towel to wash resident's hands and face (Figure 17-17B).

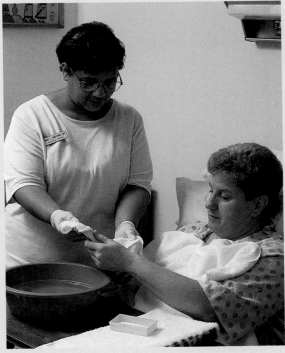

FIGURE 17-17B   Give resident water to wash hands.

7. Assist with oral hygiene if desired.
8. Wash your hands. Obtain tray from dietary cart.
9. Check the diet with the dietary card and with the resident's identification band (Figure 17-17C).
10. Place tray on overbed table and arrange food in a convenient manner.
11. Assist in food preparation as needed (Figure 17-17D). Encourage resident to do as much as possible.
12. Remove tray as soon as resident is finished. Be sure to note what the resident has and has not eaten.

(continues)

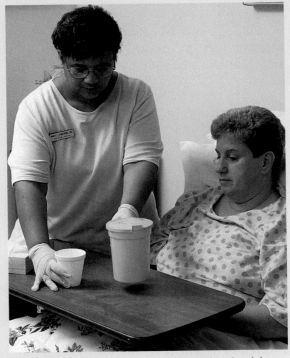

FIGURE 17-17A   Clear off overbed table to make room for food tray.

PROCEDURE 38 *(continued)*

FIGURE 17-17C Check resident's arm band against the tray card to ensure that the resident is getting the right diet.

13. Record fluids on intake record, if necessary.
14. Push overbed table out of the way.

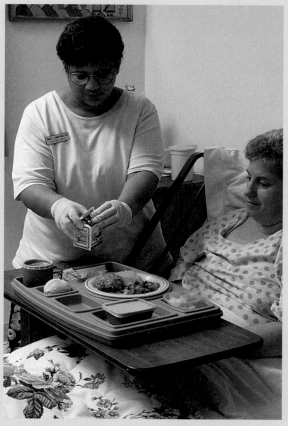

FIGURE 17-17D Assist resident in food preparation as needed.

15. Help to perform oral hygiene to clean teeth or dentures and mouth.
16. Carry out each procedure completion action.

Use of Food Thickeners

If the resident has difficulty swallowing, commercial food thickeners may be added to the diet. The type and amount of thickener is usually ordered by the speech therapist. The nursing staff, including nursing assistants, usually add the thickener at the time of feeding. When adding thickener, the nursing assistant must be sure that the:

• Correct thickener is added
• Correct amount of thickener is added

• Thickener is added according to the manufacturer's instructions

When using food thickeners, follow the procedure for feeding the dependent resident. (See Procedure 39.) Be sure to allow enough time so the resident is not rushed. Direct the food and liquids toward the unaffected side of the mouth. Feed with the tip of a spoon that is not more than one-half full.

PROCEDURE 39 Feeding the Dependent Resident

1. Carry out each beginning procedure action.
2. Assemble equipment:
   - Bedpan/urinal
   - Wash water
   - Oral hygiene items
   - Tray of food
3. Offer bedpan or urinal. (If used, follow steps in Procedure 40 in Lesson 18.)
4. Provide oral hygiene if desired.
5. Remove unnecessary articles from the overbed table.
6. Elevate head of bed. Assist resident into a sitting or upright position with head slightly bent forward. If resident is out of bed, position resident in chair in an upright position with feet flat on the floor.
7. Place napkin, bib, or towel under resident's chin (Figure 17-18A).
8. Obtain tray and check diet with the dietary card and resident's identification band.

9. Place tray on overbed table (Figure 17-18B). Sit down facing resident so you are at eye level. The environment should be quiet and calm.

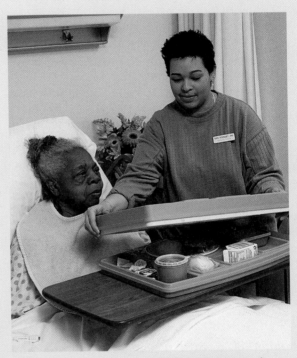

FIGURE 17-18B Uncover the food and place it on the overbed table.

10. Butter bread and cut meat. Do not pour hot beverage until resident is ready for it. Be sure, however, that the beverage is cool enough to drink before offering it to the resident.
11. Use different drinking straws for each fluid or use a cup. Thick fluids are more easily controlled by using a straw.
12. Holding spoon at a right angle:
    - Give solid foods from point of spoon (Figure 17-18C).
    - Alternate solids and liquids.
    - Rotate the offerings of food to give variety.

(continues)

FIGURE 17-18A Place a towel or clothing protector under the resident's chin

PROCEDURE 39 *(continued)*

- Describe or show resident what kind of food you are giving.
- If resident has had a stroke, direct food to unaffected side of mouth and check for food stored in affected side.
- Test hot foods by dropping a small amount on the inside of your wrist before feeding them to the resident.
- Never blow on the resident's food to cool it.
- Never taste the resident's food.
- Do not hurry the meal.

13. Allow resident to hold bread or assist to the extent possible.
14. Use napkin to wipe resident's mouth as often as necessary.
15. Remove tray as soon as resident is finished. Make sure you note what the resident has or has not eaten.
16. Provide oral hygiene.
17. Carry out each procedure completion action.

FIGURE 17-18C Give solid foods from the tip of the spoon.

Choking

Choking is always a danger when feeding dependent or elderly residents because their swallowing ability is not always effective. Be sure to check the resident care plan for any precautions and suggestions before feeding. Watch carefully for signs of aspiration during intake. All health care providers working with the elderly should know how to do abdominal thrusts for choking victims (Heimlich maneuver). Be especially careful with dry, grainy foods such as bran or corn bread, because these are more difficult to swallow. Put such foods in milk or give in small amounts followed by liquid. Visually check the resident's mouth after eating for food that may have been pocketed in the cheeks. Provide mouth care. Keep seated residents upright for 30 minutes following a meal and residents who are fed in bed at a 45° to 60° angle. Care of the choking resident is covered in Lesson 8.

NOURISHMENTS AND SUPPLEMENTS

Nourishments are tasty refreshments, such as crackers, milk, juice, custards and gelatins, which residents enjoy between meals. Supplements are liquids or foods ordered by the physician to improve the nutritional status of the resident. Supplements are often given to increase weight. It is important that all ordered supplements are served in a timely manner and not be allowed to sit on the table for long periods of time.

Nursing assistants may be asked to serve nourishments or supplements, encourage residents to eat or drink them, and assist as necessary. If this is your assignment, be sure that you:

- Wash your hands before serving nourishments or supplements.
- Check the care plan and follow the dietary instructions carefully.

- Check that the right nourishment or supplement is given to the right resident.
- Allow a choice of nourishments if possible.
- Assist the resident if help is needed.
- Serve supplements at scheduled times. If they are served too close to meal time, the resident may feel too full to eat.
- Do not offer nourishments or supplements to residents who are not scheduled to receive them.
- If a resident asks for a supplement or a different supplement, check with your supervisor.
- Do not allow partially eaten nourishments or supplements to remain in the residents' rooms. Most nourishments or supplements are served in disposable containers.
- Record the nourishment or supplement served and the amount consumed according to facility policy. Record fluids on the intake form if required.

ALTERNATE METHODS OF FEEDING

There are several alternate ways to provide nutrition to a resident. They include:

- Enteral feedings
    - Nasogastric tube (NG tube) feedings (Figure 17-19A)
    - Gastrostomy tube (G tube) feedings (Figure 17-19B)
    - Jejunostomy tube (Figure 17-19C)
- Total parenteral nutrition (TPN)

Enteral Feeding

A **nasogastric (NG) tube** is a small tube introduced into the nose and through the pharynx and esophagus and into the stomach by the physician or nurse. A **gastrostomy (G) tube** is a small tube surgically placed directly into the resident's stomach (Figure 17-20A). Feedings may be introduced through the gastrostomy or nasogastric tube using a syringe or feeding pump.

Tube feedings require special training and are performed by the nurse. Commercially prepared formula or liquid food is introduced directly into the tube (Figure 17-20B). The head of the bed must be elevated at 45°, or according to facility policy, during the feeding and for 30 minutes after. Great care must be taken to ensure that the tubes are properly positioned and are not pulled out or moved even slightly. You must inform the nurse if:

A. Nasogastric Route   B. Gastrostomy Route

C. Jejunostomy Route

FIGURE 17-19 Enteral feeding methods. A. Nasogastric route. B. Gastrostomy route. C. Jejunostomy route

- You find the tube in the bed
- The resident complains of discomfort
- The resident is coughing or choking
- The resident feels nauseated or vomits or retches
- The resident has diarrhea, constipation, a swollen stomach, or cramping
- There is redness, pain, heat, swelling, or oozing of fluid from the site where the tube is inserted into the body

Other actions the nursing assistant can take include:

- Maintain the head of the bed at least 30° or more while the feedng is being given.
- Maintain the head of the bed at least 30° for at least 30 minutes after a feeding.
- Check taping of the tube. If taping is loose, inform the nurse.
- Report any retching (straining to, but not vomiting), nausea, or vomiting immediately.
- Ensure that the end of the tube is closed between feedings.
- Provide frequent mouth hygiene.

FIGURE 17-20 A. Feeding a resident through a gastrostomy tube B. Using a feeding pump and prepared liquid nutrients

- Do not permit tension on the tubes.
- Be alert for kinks in the tubing.
- Report signs of irritation near the tube entrance.
- If food is given by pump, inform the nurse if:
  - The alarm goes off
  - The bag holding the solution is empty
  - The resident is coughing or choking.

Total Parenteral Nutrition (TPN)

Total parenteral nutrition (TPN) or **hyperalimentation** is a technique in which **high density** (concentrated) nutrients are introduced into a large vein such as the subclavian vein or the superior vena cava. The nurse manages TPN.

DISORDERS OF THE DIGESTIVE SYSTEM

Constipation

Constipation is a common problem for the elderly. Hard feces that are difficult to expel are a sign of constipation. This can be very uncomfortable for the resident and can cause bleeding if hemorrhoids are present. Regular bowel movements are aided by:

- Enough fluid intake to lubricate the colon and soften the feces
- Adequate fiber in the diet to act as bulk to promote intestinal activity
- Regular exercise to promote muscle tone
- Regular toileting opportunities

Dysphagia

Dysphagia (difficult swallowing) may be caused by decreased saliva production, paralysis due to a stroke, or obstructions such as malignancy of the esophagus. The resident with dysphagia can more easily consume thick liquids and pureed foods than solid foods. If the difficulty is prolonged, it may be necessary to provide nourishment directly into the stomach or through hyperalimentation.

Hernias

A **hernia** occurs when a structure such as the intestine pushes out of its normal body position. Hernias are also known as **ruptures**. These may develop as the intestines push through a weakened area in the abdominal wall.

There are different kinds of hernias, depending on location. Two types of hernias are common in elderly persons:

- Inguinal hernias
- Hiatal hernias

Inguinal Hernia.   This is a protrusion of the intestines through the wall in the groin area. It is felt as a small lump, especially when the resident strains.

Hiatal Hernia.   In a hiatal hernia, the stomach pushes upward into the thoracic cavity, through the normal opening that allows the esophagus to pass through the diaphragm to the stomach. Signs and symptoms of hiatal hernia are:

- Dysphagia
- Pain and pressure in the chest as food and gastric fluid become trapped in the esophagus

The hydrochloric acid in the trapped gastric fluid can be very irritating, causing inflammation and ulceration of the esophagus.

Hiatal hernias tend to be a chronic problem. Residents feel better when they:

- Eat smaller meals
- Eat sitting up

They also feel more comfortable sleeping when the head of the bed is slightly raised. Antacids are sometimes ordered to overcome the acidity and reduce discomfort. Residents should avoid lying flat after meals.

Inflammation

Inflammation anywhere along the gastrointestinal tract can cause distress and the possibility of tissue breakdown and the formation of ulcers. Inflammation of the stomach (**gastritis**) can lead to **dyspepsia** (indigestion). A combination of overeating, foods that are too spicy, and natural aging changes can cause gastric distress.

Also, ulcerations in the colon can cause blood in the stool and painful defecation.

Diverticulosis

Diverticuli are small, weakened areas in the wall of the colon. These areas form small pockets. Seeds and other hard food particles sometimes become trapped, causing inflammation (**diverticulitis**). When the diverticuli become inflamed, the resident complains of constipation and pain and is more susceptible to infection.

Usually diverticuli are multiple and the condition is then called diverticulosis. Residents who have diverticulosis feel best when:

- A bland diet is eaten
- Weight is controlled
- Constipation is avoided

Sometimes part of the bowel must be removed to correct the problem.

Malignancy

Malignancies, or cancers, of the digestive system occur frequently in older people. Cancers may occur anywhere along the tract, but commonly occur in the lower colon. Because the lumen of the large intestine is fairly big, cancer can grow inside the colon for a relatively long time before it becomes large enough to cause an obstruction or change the character of the feces.

Hemorrhoids

Hemorrhoids are varicose veins of the rectum. Their presence can make defecation painful, and they sometimes bleed. Regularity and keeping feces soft to avoid straining are important in preventing complications.

LESSON SYNTHESIS: Putting It All Together

*Y*ou have just completed this lesson. Now go back and review the Clinical Focus. Try to see how the Clinical Focus relates to the concepts presented in the lesson. Then answer the following questions.

1. Why is it especially important for Mrs. Hartley to receive proper nutrition and hydration at this time?

2. What kind of supplemental nourishments might be beneficial for her and when might you offer them?

3. From your observations, what might you suspect about Mrs. Hartley's level of hydration?

4. What beverage would you not serve to this resident?

REVIEW

A. Match each term with the proper definition

a. digestive system   f. flatulence
b. defecation   g. gastritis
c. digestion   h. nasogastric tube
d. dehydration   i. hyperalimentation
e. enzymes   j. obesity

1. _____ chemicals that help digest foods

2. _____ inflammation of the stomach

3. _____ bowel movement

4. _____ the condition of being overweight

5. _____ feeding tube

6. _____ total parenteral nutrition

7. _____ gastrointestinal tract

8. _____ gas

9. _____ excessive water loss

10. _____ mechanical and chemical process that breaks down food

B. Identify the parts of the digestive system by inserting the correct number of each part.

_____ appendix   _____ mouth
_____ colon   _____ pharynx
_____ esophagus   _____ rectum
_____ gallbladder   _____ small intestine
_____ liver   _____ stomach

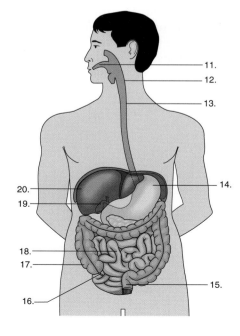

C. Indicate which of the following changes are associated with aging by circling yes (Y) or no (N).

21. Y N More sensitive taste

22. Y N Thinner saliva

23. Y N Reduced digestive enzymes

24. Y N More rapid absorption of nutrients

25. Y N Poorer tolerance to some foods

D. Select the one best answer for each of the following.

26. The primary source of energy for the body is
    (A) fat
    (B) minerals
    (C) carbohydrates
    (D) proteins

27. Which basic nutrient is essential for tissue building and repair?
    (A) fats
    (B) carbohydrates
    (C) minerals
    (D) proteins

28. Vitamins B and C are found in
    (A) beef
    (B) fruits and vegetables
    (C) eggs
    (D) vegetable oils

29. How much water should be taken in daily?
    (A) 1 pint
    (B) 3 glasses
    (C) 2 cups
    (D) 2 to 3 quarts

30. Cottage cheese belongs in which food group?
    (A) vegetable group
    (B) fruit group
    (C) milk, yogurt, and cheese group
    (D) meat, poultry, fish, dry beans, eggs, and nut group

31. Which of the four common diets prepared for long-term care residents includes liquids and semisolid foods that are more easily chewed and digested?
    (A) pureed
    (B) clear liquid
    (C) regular
    (D) mechanical soft

32. Which food is likely to be restricted on a low-fat diet?
    (A) apples
    (B) whole milk
    (C) bananas
    (D) white fish

33. Which food is excluded from a low-sodium diet?
    (A) potato
    (B) bacon
    (C) whole-grain cereal
    (D) carrot

34. Which food may be included on a low-residue diet?
    (A) celery
    (B) orange
    (C) banana
    (D) bran flakes

E. Match the therapeutic diet (items a.–e.) with the specific requirements.

a. diabetic   d. calorie-restricted
b. low-sodium   e. high-protein
c. low-fat

35. _____ prescribed for resident with heart condition or one who retains fluid

36. _____ served to residents who are underweight or poorly nourished

37. _____ served to residents with cardiovascular, gallbladder, or liver disease

38. _____ carefully balanced, concentrated carbohydrates restricted

39. _____ given to residents who need weight control

F. Determine the resident's intake using the chart in Figure 17-10. The resident has consumed: mL

40. ⅔ of a drinking glass of water   _____

41. ¾ of a small glass of orange juice   _____

42. ⅔ of a small glass of apple juice   _____

43. ½ of a water pitcher   _____

44. ¾ of a water pitcher _____

45. ⅓ of a cup of coffee _____

46. ¼ of a carton of milk _____

47. ¾ of a dish of gelatin _____

Total intake _____

G. On the chart provided below, make a record of the resident's intake and output for an 8-hour period.

48.

Time	Item	Amount
0730	urine	300 mL
0800	orange juice	90 mL
	coffee	120 mL
0930	water	60 mL
1130	tea	120 mL
	soup	120 mL
1300	urine	400 mL
1315	water	80 mL
1500	cranberry juice	100 mL
1515	vomitus	120 mL
1620	tea	120 mL
	sherbet	120 mL
1730	urine	300 mL
1800	water	150 mL
2100	ginger ale	100 mL
2130	urine	300 mL
2200	water	90 mL

H. Match the metric amounts with their approximate equivalents.

a. 500 mL   d. 3,840 mL
b. 0.06 mL   e. 1,000 mL
c. 30 mL

49. _____ 1 minim

50. _____ 1 quart

51. _____ 1 gallon

52. _____ 1 pint

53. _____ 1 ounce

I. Show your understanding of fractions by completing the following problems.

54. ½ + ½ = _____

55. ⅔ + ⅓ = _____

56. ¼ + ¼ = _____

57. ¾ + ¼ = _____

58. Your resident drinks ⅔ of her juice. The glass held 120 mL. How much juice did she drink? Show how you determined your answer.

INTAKE AND OUTPUT

Room: _____ Name: _____ Date: _____

Instructions: _____

Intake	Output	Intake	Output	Intake	Output
Total		Total		Total	

Drinking Glass.........200 mL   Full Water Pitcher....950 mL   Milk Carton..............236 mL   Jello...........................90 mL
Styrofoam Cup........200 mL   Coffee or Teapot.....300 mL   Soup Bowl...............250 mL   Ice Cream Cup..........90 mL
Juice Glass (small)..100 mL   Coffee Cup.............150 mL   Soup Bowl (small)...100 mL   Creamer...................50 mL
Juice Glass (large)..250 mL

FOLEY CATHETER DRAINAGE: (Circle the following when applicable)

Color: Yellow   Amber   Brown   Red

Appearance: Cloudy   Clear   Sediment   Mucous   Bloody

Abdomen Distended   Catheter Irrigated   Catheter Changed

24 hour INTAKE_____
24 hour OUTPUT_____

59. You picked up an empty coffee cup when your resident finished eating. How much did he drink if the cup held 150 mL and you filled it twice? Show how you determined your answer.

60. Your resident consumed a bowl of soup that contained 300 mL. How many ounces of soup did your resident consume? Show how you determined your answer.

J. Clinical Experiences

Read the clinical experiences and answer the questions about each long-term care resident.

Amelia Drage, age 92, spent her life as a homemaker. She contributed many hours to civic organizations. Her current frail condition means that she requires assistance in feeding. She is on a soft diet and receives nourishments.

61. The best combination of foods for her soft diet is
    (A) coleslaw and milk
    (B) toast and fresh fruit salad
    (C) chicken and cottage cheese
    (D) garden salad and eggs

62. When feeding her, remember
    (A) do not remove equipment such as the emesis basin
    (B) allow her to help herself as much as possible
    (C) taste foods first to be sure they are not too hot
    (D) offer the bedpan following the meal

63. When serving her nourishments,
    (A) offer a full meal, since she is so frail
    (B) leave the used dishes and glasses at the bedside because someone else can pick them up
    (C) do not record the nourishments
    (D) follow the dietary instructions carefully, using the nourishment list as a guide

Russell Barnes, age 82, has a large obstructing tumor of the esophagus. He is unable to take nourishment by mouth and transfer it to his stomach because of the tumor. A commercial nutritional formula is provided for him through a feeding tube. He has a gastrostomy tube in place.

64. The gastrostomy tube is in Mr. Barnes's
    (A) esophagus
    (B) pharynx
    (C) stomach
    (D) colon

65. While taking care of Mr. Barnes, you note the tube is out of place and lying in the bed. You should
    (A) throw the tube away as it probably is not needed
    (B) notify the nurse immediately
    (C) reinsert the tube so you will be ready for the next feeding
    (D) leave the tube alone because the nurse can take care of it when she checks the resident

66. Your care of Mr. Barnes following a feeding includes
    (A) elevating the head of the bed at 40° for one-half hour
    (B) allowing him to lie on the tube
    (C) keeping the bed flat for one-half hour
    (D) keeping the end of the tube open between feedings

Joe Spando is 78 years old and has chronic obstructive pulmonary disease, a hiatal hernia, and diverticulosis. He was a jockey as a young adult and smoking was a way of life. Even now he insists on his smoking time, which he enjoys under supervision.

67. Mr. Spando's hiatal hernia means that his
    (A) intestines protrude through the wall in the groin area
    (B) colon is inflamed
    (C) rectum has varicose veins
    (D) stomach protrudes up into the thoracic cavity

68. This resident probably suffers from
    (A) painful defecation
    (B) dysphagia
    (C) blood in his stool
    (D) pain in his rectum

69. He will probably be most comfortable if he
    (A) eats while lying down
    (B) eats three big meals a day
    (C) sits up after meals
    (D) sleeps with the head of the bed flat

LESSON 18

Meeting the Residents' Elimination Needs

Clinical Focus

Think about how you may help a resident meet elimination needs as you study this lesson and meet:

*J*essica Beebe, age 79, who has been assigned to your care. She seems listless, complaining of an upset stomach and cramps. She refused breakfast and you note some fecal soiling on the bedding. When you ask her about her last bowel movement, she cannot remember. You report the situation to the charge nurse, who examines Ms. Beebe for fecal impaction. It is decided that Ms. Beebe will benefit from a soapsuds enema.

OBJECTIVES

After studying this lesson, you should be able to:

- Define and spell vocabulary words and terms.
- Identify ways people eliminate wastes.
- Identify the parts and functions of the digestive system.
- Identify the parts and function of the urinary tract.
- Review changes in the urinary system as they relate to the aging process.
- Collect and care for urine and stool specimens.
- Measure and record fluid output.
- Describe common urinary system conditions affecting long-term residents.
- Demonstrate the following:
  Procedure 40 Giving and Receiving the Bedpan
  Procedure 41 Giving and Receiving the Urinal
  Procedure 42 Assisting with Use of the Bedside Commode
  Procedure 43 Assisting Resident to Use the Bathroom

OBJECTIVES

Procedure 44 Giving an Oil-Retention or Commercially Prepared Enema
Procedure 45 Giving a Soapsuds Enema
Procedure 46 Inserting a Rectal Tube and Flatus Bag
Procedure 47 Giving Routine Stoma Care (Colostomy)
Procedure 48 Collecting a Stool Specimen
Procedure 49 Giving Indwelling Catheter Care
Procedure 50 Emptying a Urinary Drainage Unit and Disconnecting the Catheter
Procedure 51 Measuring and Recording Fluid Output
Procedure 52 Connecting the Catheter to Leg Bag and Emptying the Leg Bag
Procedure 53 Collecting a Routine or Clean-Catch Urine Specimen
Procedure 54 Applying a Condom for Urinary Drainage

VOCABULARY

anuria   (ah-**NEW**-ree-ah)

bladder   (**BLAD**-er)

Bowman's capsule   (**BOH**-manz **KAP**-syoul)

catheter   (**KATH**-eh-ter)

colon   (**KOHL**-on)

colostomy   (koh-**LAHS**-toh-mee)

condom   (**KON**-dum)

constipation   (kon-stih-**PAY**-shun)

continent   (**KON**-tih-nent)

cystocele   (**SIS**-toh-seel)

diarrhea   (die-ah-**REE**-ah)

distended   (dis-**TEN**-ded)

dysuria   (dis-**YOU**-ree-ah)

emesis   (**EM**-eh-sis)

enema   (**EN**-eh-mah)

excreta   (ecks-**KREE**-tah)

fecal impaction   (**FEE**-kal im-**PACK**-shun)

glomerulus   (gloh-**MER**-you-lus)

hematuria   (**hem**-ah-**TOO**-ree-ah)

ileostomy   (**ill**-ee-**OS**-toh-me)

incontinence   (in-**KON**-tih-nens)

indwelling catheter   (**IN**-dwell-ing **KATH**-eh-ter)

meatus   (mee-**AY**-tus)

micturition   (**mick**-too-**RISH**-un)

nephron   (**NEF**-ron)

nocturia   (nock-**TUR**-ee-ah)

oliguria   (**ol**-ih-**GYOU**-ree-ah)

ostomy   (**OS**-toh-mee)

prostate gland   (**PROS**-tayt gland)

rectocele   (**REC**-toh-seel)

renal calculi   (**REE**-nal **KAL**-kyou-lee)

retention   (ree-**TEN**-shun)

sepsis   (**SEP**-sis)

septicemia   (**sept**-tih-**SEE**-mee-ah)

specimen   (**SPES**-ih-men)

sphincter   (**SFINK**-ter)

stoma   (**STOH**-mah)

stool   (stool)

suppository   (sup-**POZ**-ih-**toh**-ree)

uremia   (you-**REE**-mee-ah)

uremic frost   (you-**REE**-mick frost)

ureter   (you-**REE**-ter)

urethra   (you-**REE**-thrah)

urinalysis   (**you**-rih-**NAL**-ih-sis)

urination   (**you**-rih-**NAY**-shun)

voiding   (**VOYD**-ing)

INTRODUCTION

The human body produces waste products continuously. Eliminating waste products regularly is one of the basic human needs.

Waste products (**excreta**) that must be eliminated (excreted) include:

• Solid wastes
  • Feces from the digestive tract

- Liquid wastes
  - Urine from the urinary system
  - Perspiration (water and salts) from the skin
  - Water in the feces
  - Water from the lungs
- Gaseous wastes
  - Carbon dioxide (CO_2) from the lungs

In Lesson 17 you learned how nutrients are processed from foods. The undigested portion of the food (roughage or bulk) continues to move through the colon to the anus, where it leaves the body as feces.

In this lesson you will learn ways to:

- Help residents maintain regular elimination
- Assist residents who need special help in eliminating wastes
- Care for residents as they eliminate solid wastes from the digestive system and liquid wastes from the urinary system

A resident who is **continent** is able to control the elimination of waste products. **Incontinence** is the inability to predict and control elimination. Therefore, an incontinent resident has no control over elimination. Incontinence leads to emotional and physical problems that hinder social interaction.

THE CONTINENT RESIDENT

Nursing assistant responsibilities in helping continent residents to meet their elimination needs (Figure 18-1) include:

- Being aware of the resident's need to reach the proper facilities in time
- Being observant so that you can be available to help the resident reach the toilet or commode. Answer call bells promptly for residents who use a bedpan. Be ready to assist them when they are finished.
- Always noting and reporting the frequency and character of the excreta

EQUIPMENT TO ASSIST ELIMINATION

Residents are encouraged to use regular bathroom facilities if their conditions permit. They may need help to reach the toilet in time and assistance with their clothing.

FIGURE 18-1 Nursing assistant actions when assisting with elimination procedures
When assisting with elimination procedures:
• Wear disposable gloves.
• Wash hands immediately before and after procedure.
• Provide privacy.
• Make resident as comfortable as possible during elimination procedures.
• Ensure safety.
• Immediately answer call light, as resident may be finished.

Several devices can make it easier and safer for residents to achieve more independence in elimination. An elevated toilet seat (Figure 18-2) means the resident does not have to bend as much compared to a regular toilet seat. Grab bars on the wall next to the toilet help stabilize the resident when sitting down and getting up.

FIGURE 18-2 An elevated toilet seat promotes independent toileting.

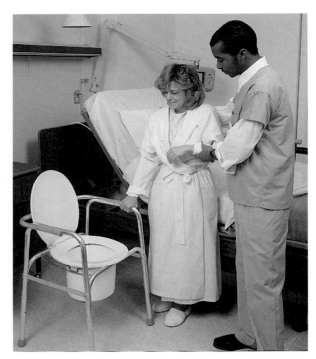

FIGURE 18-3   A bedside commode allows the resident to assume the best position for elimination.

FIGURE 18-4   (Left) Orthopedic (fracture) bedpan; (Right) regular bedpan

They also help stabilize the resident in the proper position for toileting. Proper positioning makes it easier for the resident to void. The preferred position for women is to sit upright with the feet flat on the floor. Men may prefer to stand.

A commode or portable toilet (Figure 18-3) may be left in the room for convenience, but the container must be emptied and cleaned after each use and the cover closed. A commode with a rolling base and support arms may be placed over the toilet for security. The wheels of this type of commode must be locked once it is in place. Residents in bed who can be placed on a commode probably will be more comfortable and have a more natural elimination than when using a bedpan.

Often, a bedpan must be used (Figure 18-4). The resident may be more comfortable if the bedpan is placed on the edge of the bed and the resident sits with the feet resting on a chair. For comfort, the bedpan can be padded and the resident supported by pillows. Always make sure the resident is safely and comfortably supported.

Bedpans are not comfortable in any position when left in place for any length of time. An orthopedic bedpan (fracture pan) is used when it is difficult for the resident to move. This type of bedpan is preferred for the resident who does not get out of bed.

As you provide care, remember to perform all beginning procedure and ending actions. Always follow the principles of medical asepsis.

- Apply principles of standard precautions when handling, emptying, and cleaning bedpans, urinals, and commodes.
- Wash hands before and after applying disposable gloves.
- Cover bedpans and urinals and close the covers of commodes after use until emptied.
- Avoid contamination of environmental surfaces with gloves.
- Encourage residents to perform perineal care after toileting, or assist as necessary.
- Restrict use of bedpan or urinal to specific resident; each resident has a personal bedpan or urinal that is stored in the bedside stand.

Safety Precautions

Following certain precautions can help prevent incidents during toileting.

- Be sure that resident knows how to use the emergency signal in the bathroom and can reach it when using the toilet.
- Encourage resident to use grab bars for support.
- Lock wheels of commode after positioning it over toilet.
- Be sure resident is positioned comfortably on toilet before leaving. Do not leave a resident who is confused or disoriented.
- Do not restrain resident on the toilet or commode.
- Provide as much privacy as possible.
- Answer call bell promptly (resident may have completed toileting).

PROCEDURE
40 Giving and Receiving the Bedpan

1. Carry out each beginning procedure action.
2. Assemble equipment:
   - Disposable gloves
   - Bedpan and cover
   - Basin
   - Washcloth
   - Toilet tissue
   - Soap
   - Towel
3. Lower the head of the bed if necessary.
4. Put on gloves.
5. Take the bedpan and tissue from the bedside stand.
   - Place the bedpan on the bedside chair. Never place it on the bedside stand or overbed table, or on the floor.
   - Put the remainder of the equipment on the bedside table.
6. Place bedpan cover at the foot of the bed. *Note:* Never carry or allow a used bedpan to sit uncovered. If a bedpan cover is not available, cover the bedpan with a towel, pillowcase, or paper towels.
7. Fold top bed covers back at a right angle. Raise the resident's gown. If the resident is thin or has a pressure sore, consult the nurse for the appropriate action. The nursing care plan may have specific instructions for such cases. For example, it may be necessary to pad the bedpan with a folded towel or take some other action.
8. Ask resident to flex knees and rest weight on heels, if able.
9. Help the resident to raise buttocks by:
   - Putting one hand under the small of the resident's back and lifting gently and slowly with one hand.
   - With the other hand, place the bedpan under the resident's hips.
   - If the resident is unable to raise the buttocks, two assistants may be needed to lift the resident.

- The bedpan may also be placed by rolling the resident to one side, positioning the bedpan against the buttocks and rolling the resident back on it (Figure 18-5).
- Alternatively, if a trapeze is in place over the bed, place the bedpan under the resident as the resident lifts self using the trapeze.
- The resident's buttocks should rest on the rounded shelf of the regular bedpan. The narrow end should face the foot of the bed.

FIGURE 18-5   Roll resident away from you while supporting resident with one hand on resident's hip. Place bedpan against resident's buttocks with other hand. Then roll resident back onto bedpan.

10. Remove gloves and dispose of properly. Wash hands. Replace top bedcovers. Raise the head of the bed to a comfortable height.
11. Make sure the toilet paper and signal cord are within easy reach of the resident. Leave the resident alone unless

(continues)

PROCEDURE *40* *(continued)*

contraindicated in the nursing care plan.

Note: If a specimen is to be taken, instruct the resident that toilet tissue is not to be placed in the bedpan. In this case, the nursing assistant will clean the resident and provide perineal care.

12. Watch for resident's signal.

13. Answer resident's call signal immediately. Wash hands and put on disposable gloves. Use a paper towel to turn faucet on and another one to turn faucet off.

14. Fill the basin with warm water (105°F) and place next to soap, washcloth, and towel on overbed table.

15. Remove bedpan from under resident.

- Ask the resident to flex knees and rest weight on heels. Place one hand under the small of the back and lift gently to help raise the buttocks off bedpan. Take the bedpan with the other hand. Cover it and place it on the chair.

16. Assist the resident to a clean area of the bed, if necessary. Provide perineal care.

- If the resident is unable to raise the buttocks, two assistants may be needed to lift. Otherwise, roll the resident off the pan to the side and remove the pan. Lift and move carefully. Hold the pan firmly with one hand.

17. Change linen or protective pads as necessary. Replace bedclothes.

18. Assist the resident to wash hands after the procedure.

19. Take the bedpan to the bathroom or utility room and observe contents. Measure, if required.

20. Empty bedpan.

21. Turn faucet on holding a paper towel in the hand. Rinse with cold water and disinfectant. Rinse, dry, and return bedpan to storage in resident's bedside stand.

22. Remove gloves and discard according to facility policy. Wash hands.

23. Carry out each procedure completion action.

PROCEDURE 41 Giving and Receiving the Urinal

1. Carry out each beginning procedure action.

2. Assemble equipment:
   - Disposable gloves
   - Urinal and cover (Figure 18-6)
   - Basin
   - Soap
   - Washcloth
   - Towel

3. Put on gloves, Lift the top bedcovers and place the urinal under the covers so the resident may grasp the handle. Instruct resident to place his penis in the urinal

FIGURE 18-6 Male urinal with cover

(continues)

PROCEDURE 41 *(continued)*

opening. If he cannot do this, you must place the urinal in position and ensure that the penis is placed in the opening.

4. Remove gloves and dispose of them properly. Wash hands. Make sure the signal cord is within easy reach of the resident. Leave resident alone if possible. Watch for his signal.

5. Answer resident's signal immediately. Wash hands. Use a paper towel to turn on faucet. Fill a basin with warm water (105°F), and place next to the soap, washcloth, and towel, so resident can wash and dry hands.

6. Put on gloves. Ask resident to hand the urinal to you. Cover it. Rearrange bedclothes if necessary.

7. Take the urinal to the bathroom or utility room and observe the contents. Measure, if required. Do not empty urinal if anything unusual (such as blood) is observed. Rather, save the contents of the urinal for your supervisor's inspection.

8. Empty the urinal. Use a paper towel to turn on the faucet and another paper towel to turn the faucet off. Rinse with cold water and clean with warm soapy water. Rinse, dry, and cover urinal. Remove gloves and dispose of them properly. Wash hands.

9. Place urinal inside resident's bedside table. Clean and replace other articles.

10. Carry out each procedure completion action.

PROCEDURE 42 Assisting with Use of the Bedside Commode

1. Carry out each beginning procedure action.
2. Assemble equipment:
   - Disposable gloves
   - Portable commode
   - Toilet tissue
   - Basin
   - Washcloth
   - Soap
   - Towel
3. Position commode beside bed, facing head. Lock wheels and open lid. Be sure receptacle is in place under seat.
4. If bed and side rails are elevated, lower side rail nearest you and place bed in lowest horizontal position. Make sure bed wheels are locked.
5. Put on gloves.
6. Assist resident to sitting position. Swing resident's legs over edge of bed.
7. Assist resident to put on robe. Put shoes on resident. Assist resident to stand. If needed, use a transfer belt.
8. Support resident with hands on either side of the belt. Remember to use proper

body mechanics. Pivot resident to the right and lower to commode. Do not restrain resident on the commode.

9. Leave call bell and tissue within reach.
10. Remove gloves and discard according to facility policy. Wash hands.
11. When resident signals, return promptly. Wash hands and put on gloves. Use a paper towel to turn on the faucet and another paper towel to turn the faucet off. Fill the basin with warm water (105°F). Bring basin to bedside along with soap, towel, and washcloth.
12. Assist resident to stand. Wipe anal area or perineum if required.
13. Allow resident to wash and dry hands. Remove gloves and dispose of according to facility policy. Wash hands.
14. Assist resident to return to bed. Adjust bedding and pillows for comfort.
15. Leave signal cord within easy reach.
16. Put on gloves. Remove receptacle from commode and cover. Close lid of commode.

(continues)

PROCEDURE 42 *(continued)*

17. Take receptacle to bathroom. Note contents and measure if required.
18. Empty and clean receptacle per facility policy. Replace in commode. Remove and dispose of gloves properly.

19. Put commode in proper place. If it remains in the room, place it out of the way.
20. Carry out each procedure completion action.

PROCEDURE 43 Assisting Resident to Use the Bathroom

1. Answer call bell promptly.
2. Carry out each beginning procedure action.
3. Assist resident to toilet. Shut door for privacy.
4. Help resident position himself with the back of his legs against the toilet and facing you.
5. Assist as needed to:
   • Lift skirt or gown
   • Undo belt and lower trousers
   • Lower underwear
6. Assist resident to sit comfortably on toilet with feet flat on floor.
7. Place call bell within reach of resident.
8. Adjust clothing to cover resident as much as possible or place towel over lap.
9. Leave toilet tissue close at hand. Indicate your willingness to return and assist

resident to clean genital/anal area after toileting.
10. Leave resident alone if safe. Do not leave a resident who is confused, disoriented, or weak.
11. Return immediately when resident signals.
12. Wash hands. Put on disposable gloves. Assist resident to stand. (Gather up skirt with one hand to keep clean.)
13. Clean genital/anal area as needed.
14. Remove gloves and discard according to facility policy. Wash hands.
15. Help resident redress.
16. Note contents of toilet and flush.
17. Help resident wash and dry hands.
18. Wash your hands.
19. Assist resident to a comfortable area with call bell and water close at hand.
20. Carry out each procedure completion action.

ELIMINATION FROM THE LOWER DIGESTIVE TRACT

Solid wastes are eliminated through the lower digestive tract or large intestine (**colon**) (Figure 18-7). The colon is divided into the:

• Ascending colon—located up the right side of the abdomen
• Transverse colon—wastes are moved through it to the opposite side

• Descending colon—located down the left side of the body
• Rectum in the pelvis and the anal opening to the outside of the body

Digested food leaves the stomach in liquid form and enters the small intestine. Here water and some vitamins are absorbed. As the wastes move into the large intestine, they have changed to the more solid form known as feces. The more water the body needs, the more is absorbed from the wastes and

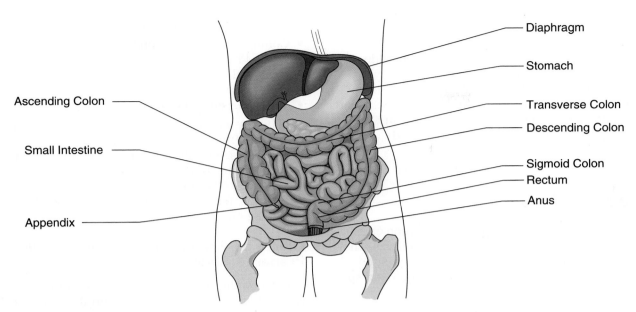

FIGURE 18-7 Elimination of solid wastes involves the organs of the lower digestive tract.

the harder the feces become. Normal feces should be brown in color and formed but soft.

Bowel movements are recorded in the resident's record. Observe the bowel movement and report anything unusual about the feces (also known as **stool**).

- Infections and some medications, such as antibiotics, can cause loose, watery stools (**diarrhea**).
- Iron can make the stool black; in some residents iron can cause loose stools, whereas others experience **constipation** (difficult bowel movements).
- Dark stool may also indicate the presence of blood from the intestines; bright red blood in the stool may be from distended and bleeding blood vessels in the rectum (hemorrhoids).

Conditions resulting from lower digestive tract dysfunction include:

- Constipation
- Flatus (gas)
- Diarrhea
- Anal incontinence

THE RESIDENT WITH CONSTIPATION

Constipation (difficulty in emptying the bowels) is a problem for many residents in long-term care. This is due to food passing more slowly through the digestive tract. In addition, the residents do not:

- Take in adequate fluids
- Exercise sufficiently
- Take in enough bulk to stimulate peristalsis

Other causes include depression, disease, and certain drugs.

The resident with constipation may not have an appetite and may complain of abdominal discomfort. The abdomen may be **distended** (stretched). If **fecal impaction**—the most serious form of constipation—is present, there may be frequent instances of diarrhea.

Fecal impaction results when the fecal mass loses so much water that it becomes dehydrated (dry and hard) and impossible to eliminate. The dried waste acts as an irritant to the bowel. Mucus tends to dissolve the outer part of the mass, which then drains from the bowel as diarrhea. Whenever there are frequent, small amounts of diarrhea, report this to the nurse who will check the resident for fecal impaction.

Checking for Fecal Impaction

In some facilities, nursing assistants are permitted to check for fecal impaction. If it is determined that a resident has a fecal impaction, an order is placed for a **suppository** or **enema** to provide relief. To check for fecal impaction, the resident must be in bed on the left side with the right leg flexed. *Be sure your facility permits nursing assistants to perform this procedure.*

Nursing assistant actions to help residents who are constipated include:

- Encouraging as much activity as possible
- Encouraging a high roughage diet
- Offering fluids frequently
- Assisting the resident to the bathroom and allowing adequate time for defecation
- Administering bowel aids as ordered

BOWEL AIDS

Nursing assistants may give oil-retention enemas and soapsuds enemas. In some facilities, they may be permitted to insert lubricating suppositories. Each of these procedures requires a specific order.

Enemas

An enema is the introduction of fluid into the rectum, through the anal sphincter, to remove feces (stool) or flatus (gas). The fluid is expelled a short time after introduction, along with the waste products. The need to empty the bowel is signaled by a feeling of urgency. Sometimes a small amount of warm oil is given to soften the stool (oil-retention enema). This is followed by a cleansing soapsuds enema.

Prepackaged commercial enema solutions may be used. A specific order is required for an enema before it is given. Some facilities do not permit nursing assistants to give enemas of any kind. You are responsible for knowing the regulations of your facility.

General Considerations. Some general considerations to keep in mind when giving an enema are:

- If the resident is to use the bathroom after the enema, make sure the bathroom is not in use before giving the enema.
- When possible, the enema should be given before breakfast or morning care.
- Do not give an enema within an hour after a meal.
- Remember that you must have a physician's order for any enema and that you can give an enema only if it is a nursing assistant responsibility in your facility.

Enemas commonly ordered are:

- Commercial preparations
  - Phosphosoda
  - Oil
- Soapsuds enema (SSE)
- Tap water enema (TWE)

The procedure for administering an oil-retention enema and a commercially prepared enema is essentially the same. The only difference is in the solution that is administered.

The oil-retention enema is administered to soften the feces and is usually followed by a cleansing enema.

Giving an Enema with a Commercially Prepared Chemical Enema Solution

Commercially prepared enemas are convenient to administer and more comfortable for the resident.

- The chemical solution is already measured and ready to use.
- A small amount of fluid will remain in the container after administration.
- The solution in a prepared enema draws fluid from the body to stimulate peristalsis.
- The amount of solution administered is about 4 ounces.
- The tip of the container is prelubricated.
- The enema solution is in an easy-to-handle plastic container.
- The solution is sometimes used at room temperature.
- You may be asked to warm the solution by placing the container in warm water before administration. Check with the nurse regarding your facility's policy.

Rectal Suppositories

Rectal suppositories are used to stimulate bowel evacuation or administer medication. Medicinal suppositories must be inserted by the nurse. You may be asked to insert the type of suppository that softens stool and promotes elimination. Check your facility policy to be sure this is a nursing assistant function. The suppository must be placed beyond the rectal **sphincter** (circular muscle that controls the anal opening) and against the bowel wall so it can melt and lubricate the rectum.

PROCEDURE 44

Giving an Oil-Retention or Commercially Prepared Enema

1. Carry out each beginning procedure action.
2. Assemble equipment:
   - Disposable gloves
   - Bedpan and cover
   - Toilet tissue
   - Towel, soap, basin
   - Prepackaged oil for retention enema or disposable prepackaged enema
   - Bed protector
   - Bath blanket
3. If this is an oil-retention enema, instruct resident that it will be necessary to hold the solution at least 20 minutes.
4. Place chair at foot of bed and cover with towel. Place bedpan on it.
5. Cover resident with bath blanket and fan-fold linen to foot of bed.
6. Place bed protector under buttocks.
7. Help resident turn to the left side and flex the right leg.
8. Open the prepackaged oil-retention or commercially prepared enema.
9. Wash hands and put on gloves.
10. Expose resident's anus. Remove cap from enema (Figure 18-8) and insert the prelubricated tip into anus as resident takes a deep breath.
11. Squeeze container until all the solution has entered the rectum (Figure 18-9).
12. Remove container and place in package box to be discarded.

FIGURE 18-8   Remove cover from prelubricated tip of container.

FIGURE 18-9   Squeeze bottle from bottom until all the liquid has gone into the rectum.

13. Encourage resident to remain on the side.
14. Discard enema box. Remove and dispose of gloves according to facility policy. Wash hands.
15. Check resident every 5 minutes until fluid has been retained for as long as possible.
16. Wash your hands and put on gloves.
17. Position resident on bedpan or assist to bathroom.
18. If resident is on the bedpan, raise head of bed to comfortable height.
19. Place toilet tissue and signal cord within easy reach of resident. If resident is in bathroom, stay nearby. Caution resident not to flush toilet.
20. Discard disposable materials in biohazardous waste according to facility policy.
21. Remove bedpan and cover or assist resident to return to bed.
    - Observe contents of bedpan or toilet.
    - Dispose of contents of bedpan or flush toilet.
22. Cleanse resident's anal area, if required.
23. Remove gloves and dispose of properly. Wash hands.
24. Give resident soap, water, and towel to wash and dry hands.
25. Replace top bedding and remove bath blanket and bed protector. Dispose of according to facility policy.
26. Carry out each procedure completion action.

PROCEDURE
45
Giving a Soapsuds Enema

1. Carry out each beginning procedure action.
2. Assemble equipment:
   - Disposable gloves
   - Disposable enema equipment, consisting of a plastic container, tubing with rectal tube, clamp, and lubricant (equipment is commercially available as a kit)
   - Bedpan and cover
   - Bed protector
   - Toilet tissue
   - Bath blanket
   - Castile soap packet
   - Towel, soap, basin
3. In the utility room:
   a. Connect tubing to solution container (Figure 18-10A).
   b. Adjust clamp on tubing and snap shut (Figure 18-10B).
   c. Fill container with warm water (105°F) to the 1,000-mL line (500 mL for children) (Figures 18-10C and D).
   d. Open packet of liquid soap and put the soap in the water (Figure 18-10E).
   e. Using the tip of the tubing, mix the solution (mix gently so that no suds form) or rotate the bag to mix. Do not shake.
   f. Run small amount of solution through tube to eliminate air and warm the

FIGURE 18-10B Slip clamp over tubing.

FIGURE 18-10C Fill container with warm water.

tube (Figure 18-10F). Clamp the tubing (Figure 18-10G).
4. Place chair at foot of bed and cover with bed protector. Place the bedpan on it.
5. Elevate bed to comfortable working height. Be sure opposite side rail is up and secure for safety.
6. Cover resident with a bath blanket and fanfold linen to foot of bed.
7. Wash hands and put on gloves.
8. Place bed protector under buttocks.
9. Help resident turn to left side and flex knees.

FIGURE 18-10A Attach tubing to container.

(continues)

PROCEDURE 45 *(continued)*

FIGURE 18-10D Use a bath thermometer to be sure water temperature is about 105°F.

FIGURE 18-10E Add liquid soap from packet.

FIGURE 18-10F Let a small amount of water flow through the tube to expel air.

FIGURE 18-10G Clamp tubing.

10. Place container of solution on chair so tubing will reach resident.
11. Adjust bath blanket to expose anal area.
12. Expose anus by raising upper buttock.
13. Lubricate tip of tube. Resident should breathe deeply and bear down as tube is inserted, to relax the anal sphincter. Insert tube 2 to 4 inches into the anus.
14. Never force the tube. If tube cannot be inserted easily, get help. There may be a tumor or a mass of feces blocking the bowel.
15. Open the clamp and raise the container 12 inches above the level of the anus so that the fluid flows in slowly (Figure 18-10H).

FIGURE 18-10H Raise container above level of anus so fluid flow is unobstructed.

(continues)

PROCEDURE 45 *(continued)*

- Ask resident to take deep breaths to relax the abdomen.
- If resident complains of cramping, clamp tube and wait until cramping stops. Then open the tubing to continue fluid flow.

16. Clamp the tubing before the container is completely empty.

17. Tell resident to hold breath while upper buttock is raised and tube is gently withdrawn.

18. Wrap tubing in paper towel. Put it in the disposable container.

19. Place resident on bedpan or assist to bathroom.

20. Holding a paper towel in the hand so glove does not contaminate control or crank, raise head of bed to comfortable height if resident is on bedpan. Raise side rail for safety if bed is left in the higher horizontal position.

21. Place toilet tissue and signal cord within reach of resident. If resident is in bathroom, stay nearby. Caution resident not to flush toilet.

22. Discard disposable materials in biohazardous waste according to facility policy.

23. Remove gloves and discard according to facility policy. Wash hands.

24. Return to bedside. Wash hands and put on gloves.

25. Remove bedpan. Place it on a bed protector on chair and cover.

26. Cleanse the anal area.

27. Remove the bed protector and discard according to facility policy.

28. Remove gloves and wash hands.

29. Give resident soap, water, and towel to wash and dry hands.

30. Replace top bedding and remove bath blanket.

31. Put on gloves. Take bedpan to bathroom. Dispose of contents according to facility policy or, using a paper towel, flush toilet.

32. Remove gloves and dispose of according to facility policy.

33. Wash hands.

34. Air the room and leave room in order.

35. Unscreen unit.

36. Clean and replace all other equipment used according to facility policy.

37. Carry out each procedure completion action.

RECTAL TUBE AND FLATUS BAG

The rectal tube is used to reduce flatus (gas) in the bowel. Placing a rectal tube into the rectum provides a passageway for the gas to escape.

Flatus distends the intestines, causing pain and stress on incisions. Flatus is a problem for many residents in long-term care. If unexpelled, it can cause the resident to feel very uncomfortable.

You can assist the resident as follows:

- Encourage activity.
- Promote regularity.
- Accept the expulsion of gas as a natural body function. Do not contribute to the resident's embarrassment.

- Use flatus-reducing procedures when ordered.
- Insert a rectal tube with flatus bag if ordered. (Remember that your facility policies must state that nursing assistants can perform this procedure.)

The disposable tube is used once in a 24-hour period for no more than 20 minutes.

- Relief may occur as soon as the tube is inserted.
- Check the amount of abdominal distention (stretching).
- Question resident about amount of relief.

PROCEDURE 46

Inserting a Rectal Tube and Flatus Bag

1. Carry out each beginning procedure action.
2. Assemble equipment:
   - Disposable gloves
   - Disposable rectal tube and flatus bag
   - Bed protector
   - Lubricant
   - Tissue
   - Tape
   - Paper towel
3. Identify resident and screen unit. Explain what you plan to do.
4. Lower the head of the bed to horizontal position.
5. Wash hands and put gloves on.
6. Assist resident to turn to the left side and flex the right leg. Place bed protector under hips.
7. Adjust bed linen to expose only the resident's buttocks.
8. Lubricate tip of rectal tube.
9. Separate buttocks, exposing anus, and ask resident to breathe deeply and bear down gently.
10. Insert lubricated tip of rectal tube 2 to 4 inches.
11. Secure rectal tube in place with small piece of hypoallergenic adhesive (Figure 18-11).
12. Remove gloves and dispose of properly. Wash hands.
13. Adjust bedding and make resident comfortable. Leave unit neat and tidy. Place signal cord within reach of resident.

FIGURE 18-11   Secure rectal tube with flatus bag in place using a small amount of hypoallergenic tape.

14. Return to unit in 20 minutes. Wash your hands.
15. Put on gloves.
16. Gently remove rectal tube and place on paper towel.
17. Clean area around anus as needed.
18. Dispose of wrapped rectal tube and bag according to facility policy.
19. Remove and dispose of gloves according to facility policy. Wash hands.
20. Carry out each procedure completion action.

OSTOMIES

The surgical removal of a section of diseased bowel requires the creation of an artificial opening (**ostomy**) in the abdominal wall for solid waste elimination. When the colon is brought through the abdominal wall, the opening is called a **colostomy**. The mouth of the opening is called a **stoma** (Figure 18-12). The ostomy may be temporary or permanent. The location of the ostomy (Figure 18-13) determines if the feces are formed, soft and mushy, semiliquid, or liquid.

The resident with a colostomy does not have normal sphincter control. This means the resident cannot voluntarily control emptying of the bowel in the same manner as emptying through the anus. If the colostomy is located in the bowel where stool is formed, regularity of elimination may be established. As elimination is controlled, the stoma may be covered with a simple dressing between evacuations. Liquid to mushy fecal drainage from a stoma is collected in a disposable drainage pouch, called an appliance, that is attached over the stoma.

FIGURE 18-12 Typical colostomy stoma

Stoma Care

Proper care is needed to keep the tissue around the stoma healthy. The waste eliminated from the stoma may be irritating to the tissue, espe-cially the liquid or semiliquid feces. Other prob-lems may include leakage and odor.

You can assist the resident with a colostomy by:

- Encouraging the resident to eat food helpful in controlling elimination. Restricting foods determined to cause flatus or loose feces (depending on location of ostomy) can make management of the ostomy easier.
- Performing routine stoma care
- Keeping the area around the opening clean and dry
- Protecting the skin around the stoma according to facility policy. Follow the care plan exactly.
- Adding deodorizer to ostomy bag, if instructed, to reduce odor
- Attaching the appliance securely over the stoma
- Reporting the nature of the colostomy output
- Reporting to the nurse if area around the stoma is red, irritated, or nonintact

If the colostomy appliance is reusable, it should be washed with soap and water and dried while a clean alternate is applied. If the pouch is not reusable, dispose of it according to facility policy.

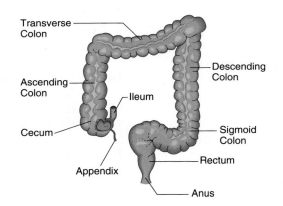

Transverse Colon

Descending Colon

Ascending Colon

Ileum

Cecum

Sigmoid Colon

Rectum

Appendix

Anus

Fluid to Semifluid Feces

Mushy Feces

Semimushy to Solid Feces

Solid (Formed) Feces

Ascending Colostomy

Transverse Colostomy

Descending Colostomy

Sigmoid Colostomy

FIGURE 18-13 The site of the colostomy determines the character of the feces.

PROCEDURE 47 Giving Routine Stoma Care (Colostomy)

1. Carry out each beginning procedure action.
2. Assemble equipment:
   - Disposable gloves
   - Washcloth and towel
   - Basin of warm water
   - Bed protector
   - Bath blanket
   - Disposable colostomy bag and belt
   - Bedpan
   - Skin lotion as directed
   - Prescribed solvent/dropper
   - Cleansing agent
   - Adhesive wafer
   - 4 × 4 gauze square
   - Toilet tissue
3. Place bath blanket over resident. Fanfold top bedding to foot of bed.
4. Wash hands and put on disposable gloves.
5. Place bed protector under the resident's hips.
6. Place bedpan and cover on bed protector on chair.
7. Remove the soiled disposable stoma bag (appliance) and place in bedpan—note amount and type of drainage.
8. Remove belt that holds stoma bag and save if clean.

FIGURE 18-14A The area around the stoma is cleaned well but gently and dried before a new appliance is applied.

9. Gently clean area around stoma with toilet tissue to remove feces and drainage (Figure 18-14A). Dispose of tissue in bedpan.
10. Wash area around stoma with soap and water. Rinse thoroughly and dry.
11. If ordered, apply barrier cream lightly around the stoma—too much lotion may interfere with proper seal of fresh ostomy bag.
12. Position clean belt around resident— inspect skin under belt for irritation or breakdown.
13. It may be necessary to remove the adhesive wafer. To select the proper size of wafer, a commercial guide can be used to size the stoma (Figure 18-14B).

FIGURE 18-14B Check the size of the stoma to be sure the proper size of barrier is used.

14. Replace adhesive wafer (Figure 18-14C). Place clean ostomy bag over stoma and secure belt.
15. Remove bed protector. Check to be sure bottom bedding is not wet. Change if necessary.
16. Remove gloves and discard according to facility policy. Wash hands.
17. Replace bath blanket with top bedding, making resident comfortable.
18. Using a paper towel to protect hands, gather and cover soiled materials and bedpan. Take to utility room. Dispose of materials according to facility policy.

(continues)

PROCEDURE 47 *(continued)*

19. Empty, wash, and dry bedpan. Store according to facility policy.

20. Carry out each procedure completion action.

FIGURE 18-14C A new barrier adhesive wafer is applied around the stoma.

Care of the Resident with an Ileostomy

An **ileostomy** is a permanent artificial opening in the ileum (Figure 18-15) that drains through a stoma on the surface of the abdomen. The drainage from the ileum is in liquid form and contains digestive enzymes that are irritating to the skin.

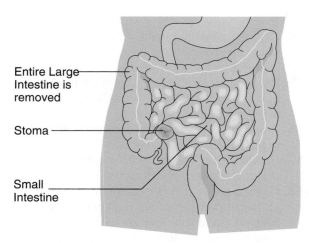

Entire Large Intestine is removed

Stoma

Small Intestine

FIGURE 18-15 An ileostomy brings a section of the ileum through the abdominal wall.

Considerations for caring for a resident with an ileostomy include:

- The professional nurse cares for the resident with a fresh ileostomy.
- Routine care may be given by nursing assistants.
- The drainage from an ileostomy is very irritating to the skin, so care of the skin surrounding the stoma is crucial.
- The fit of the ileostomy ring is critical to prevent leakage. This is true for both the disposable and reusable types of appliances.

FECAL INCONTINENCE

Feces are highly irritating and contain many microbes that can be sources of infection. Fecal incontinence is distressing to residents. Residents must be cleaned immediately after involuntary defecation and every attempt must be made to establish continence through retraining and dietary management.

When there are frequent liquid stools, a drainable fecal incontinence collector may be needed (Figure 18-16).

1. Position patient on side.

2. Clean and dry skin.

3. Trim barrier, if needed.

4. Remove release paper.

5. Fold barrier.

6. Separate buttocks.

7. Position collector.

8. Press and seal barrier.

9. Connect to bedside collector.

10. Remove.

DRAINABLE FECAL INCONTINENCE COLLECTOR WITH FLEXTEND SKIN BARRIER

Preparation and Application

1. Turn patient on one side, bending the upper knee up towards the chest.
2. Clean and dry the perineal area thoroughly.
3. If necessary, trim the skin barrier to fit perineal area.
   - For females with a narrow perineal bridge, the skin barrier should be cut to fit.
   - Follow the cutting guide, leaving as much of the skin barrier as possible. The barrier should not cover the labia or the vaginal opening.
4. Remove the release paper.
5. Fold the skin barrier in half.
6. Separate the buttocks.
7. Position the pre-cut hole over the anus. Do not enlarge pre-cut hole.
8. Apply and press firmly.
   - Apply barrier to perineal area first, pressing firmly after positioning correctly. Using your other hand, press the barrier firmly, holding for thirty seconds to allow it to adhere properly.
9. To empty, open drain cap and direct the stool into an appropriate receptacle. For best results, connect to a bedside drainage collector.
10. To remove, gently ease the barrier from the patient's skin, using fabric tab.

Preparation and Application

- Remove oily substances or powders from the skin which interferes with skin barrier adhesion.
- Skin gel wipes on skin may decrease wear time.
- DO NOT cut the barrier opening.
- Trim excess hair with scissors. DO NOT use a razor.

FIGURE 18-16 Fecal incontinence collection system (Permission to reproduce this copyrighted material has been granted by the owner, Hollister Incorporated, Libertyville, IL)

COLLECTING A STOOL SPECIMEN

A stool specimen is usually required when infection, bleeding, or parasites in the colon are suspected. You may be asked to collect a stool specimen. When carrying out this task:

- Wear gloves.
- Collect the specimen in a bedpan, commode receptacle, toilet insert, or from a fecal collection bag or bed linens.
- Do not place toilet paper in the collection container.
- Do not allow the specimen to touch the outside of the ollection container.
- Use tongue depressors to handle the specimen.
- Make sure that the specimen is properly labeled and promptly transported.

PROCEDURE

48

Collecting a Stool Specimen

1. Carry out each beginning procedure action.
2. Assemble equipment:
   - Disposable gloves
   - Bedpan and cover or collection container
   - Specimen container and cover
   - Biohazard specimen transport bag
   - Label including:
     - Resident's full name
     - Room number
     - Date and time of collection
     - Physician's name
     - Examination to be performed
     - Other information required
   - Toilet tissue
   - Tongue depressors
   - Basin
3. Wash hands and put on disposable gloves.
4. Uncover container used to collect bowel movement (bedpan or commode receptacle). (If toilet insert is used, specimen will be collected from insert.) If resident is incontinent of feces, use tongue depressors to obtain specimen from bed linens, diaper, or protective padding. A specimen may also be obtained from a fecal incontinence collection bag when it is changed.
5. Following defecation, resident is to wash hands. Fill basin with water at 105°F. Assist resident if needed. If resident is incontinent, carefully clean and dry area around anus. Change bed linens as needed.
6. Take container with bowel movement to the bathroom. Use tongue blades to remove specimen and place in specimen container (Figure 18-17). Do not contaminate the outside of the specimen container or the cover. If possible, take a sample (about 1 teaspoon) from each part of the specimen.
7. Empty collection container into toilet. Clean or dispose of collection container according to facility policy. If resident was incontinent, dispose of soiled brief or padding as biohazardous waste. Place soiled linen in proper hamper.
8. Remove and dispose of gloves according to facility policy.

FIGURE 18-17 Use tongue blades to transfer the stool specimen from the collection container (left) to the specimen container (right).

(continues)

PROCEDURE **48** *(continued)*

9. Wash your hands.

10. Cover container and attach completed label. Make sure cover is on container tightly. Place container in biohazard transport bag.

11. Take or send specimen to laboratory promptly. (Stool specimens are never refrigerated.)

12. Carry out each procedure completion action.

URINARY SYSTEM

Most liquid wastes are eliminated from the body through the urinary system in the form of urine.

The urinary system consists of the kidneys (filter blood and form urine) and the ureters and urethra (tubes that carry the urine to the outside of the body) (Figure 18-18). The urinary system:

- Forms urine
- Stores urine
- Excretes urine
- Manages blood chemistry
- Manages fluid balance

Kidneys

The kidneys are two bean-shaped organs about 6 inches long. They are located on either side of the spinal column in the lumbar area. They are made up of the:

- Cortex—the dark reddish-brown outer part that contains the urine-producing unit called the **nephron** (Figure 18-19).
- Medulla—the lighter-colored middle part contains collecting tubules that receive the formed urine.
- Renal pelvis—the central basin-like area into which the urine passes. The renal pelvis directs the urine out of each kidney and into the ureters.

Ureters

The **ureters** are tubes about 12 inches long that lead from each kidney to the urinary bladder.

FIGURE 18-18 Structures of the urinary system

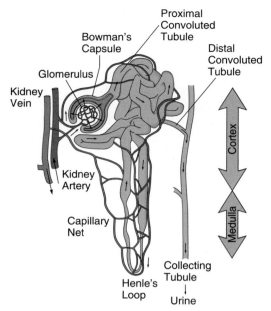

FIGURE 18-19 Nephron and related structures. Small arrows indicate the flow of blood through the nephron. The urine produced by the nephron flows through the collecting tubule.

Urinary Bladder

The **bladder**, a hollow muscular organ in the pelvis, has the following functions:

- Receives the urine from the ureters
- Stores urine until it can be eliminated from the body (holds about 1 cup or 250 mL of urine before urge to void is felt)
- The exit from the bladder is guarded by a small, circular (sphincter) muscle that prevents urine from escaping involuntarily.

Urethra

The **urethra** is a small tube that carries the urine from the bladder out of the body. The opening to the outside is called the **meatus**. The male and female urethra differ as follows.

The female urethra:

- Is about 1½ inches long
- Transports urine only

The male urethra:

- Is 8 to 10 inches long.
- Is surrounded by a gland called the **prostate gland**, which is part of the reproductive system
- Transports urine
- Transports reproductive fluids to the outside. (Urine and reproductive fluids may not pass at the same time.)

Enlargement of the prostate gland can press on the urethra, making the passage of urine diffi-

cult. This often happens in men as they reach later middle age.

Urine Formation

The nephron is a filtering system of tubules and blood vessels that produces urine. It is estimated that each kidney contains one million nephrons.

Blood arriving at the kidneys carries waste products such as acids and salts. These waste products must be eliminated from the body. Urine is a liquid waste solution containing water and dissolved substances. Urine is produced as follows:

- Waste products, helpful products, and large quantities of water are passed (filtered) through the capillary walls of the **glomerulus** (capillary bed) into **Bowman's capsule**, forming a liquid called filtrate. (See Figure 18-19.)
- The filtrate moves slowly along the convoluted tubules where some water and helpful substances like sugar are reabsorbed into the blood.
- The liquid remaining in the convoluted tubules is urine and contains wastes.
- The urine passes into the collecting tubules of the medulla, then out of the kidney to the ureter and into the urinary bladder.
- *Normal* urine is acid in reaction and pale to deep yellow in color.
- *Dilute* urine has more water and fewer dissolved substances, so it is white to pale yellow.
- *Concentrated* urine has less water and more dissolved substances, so it is darker in color and has a stronger odor.
- The amount of urine produced depends on the amount of intake and various physical conditions. Inadequate water intake leading to dehydration results in a small amount of concentrated urine.

The substances in the urine provide good information about the chemistry of the body and how well it is functioning. Tests are frequently performed on the urine (**urinalysis**).

During your care of the resident, note the amount, color, and odor of the urine, and the presence of any sediment.

CHANGES IN THE URINARY SYSTEM CAUSED BY AGING

As a person ages, the kidneys decrease somewhat in size and some renal cells are lost and replaced by scar tissue. This means the kidneys are less efficient filters. The blood vessels carrying the blood to the kidneys for filtration undergo changes that reduce the amount of blood delivered. The lower blood flow decreases urine production.

Loss of pelvic muscle tone and strength makes bladder emptying less efficient. Urine may be retained in the bladder (**retention**). Urine production influences the acid-base and fluid balances of the body.

Urine is produced continuously. In younger persons, it is more concentrated during the night. An older person loses some concentrating ability and experiences more need to empty the bladder at night. This problem is called **nocturia**. Make sure the call bell is available and that lighting is adequate for safe ambulation at night. Figure 18-20 summarizes the urinary system changes caused by aging.

URINE ELIMINATION

The act of eliminating urine from the bladder is known by various terms:

- **Micturition**
- **Urination**
- **Voiding**

A common phrase is "passing water." Voiding or urinating are the terms most frequently used to describe emptying the bladder.

Voiding can occur involuntarily when the bladder fills to about 250 mL. Urine is released as the sphincter muscle relaxes and the bladder walls contract. With training, the signal that the bladder is filling is brought to the level of conscious thought so that voiding can be voluntarily controlled.

URINARY RETENTION AND INCONTINENCE

Elderly residents face two major problems related to the urinary system. The problems are retention and incontinence.

Urinary retention is due to poor bladder tone or incomplete emptying because of an obstruction. Poor tone may be related to the aging process or prolonged catheter drainage. Obstruction may be due to tumor growth. In, men, obstruction is often due to the enlargement of the prostate gland. Urinary retention due to a tumor may require surgery to relieve the obstruction.

Urinary retention is due to one or more factors, including:

- Inability to reach toileting facilities in time
- Emotional withdrawal
- Lack of awareness of need
- Physical changes
- Infection of the urinary tract
- Fecal impaction
- Neurologic damage such as in a stroke
- Inability to communicate the need to use the toilet
- Mental confusion
- Ineffective muscle control

Urinary incontinence may be temporary or established. If attention is given to the underlying causes, the temporary use of incontinence pads may be all that is needed. When the incontinence is prolonged, tests to determine the cause may be ordered. If needed, a urinary retraining program will be started.

Nursing Assistant Actions

Urinary incontinence is uncomfortable and embarrassing to the resident. In addition, prolonged exposure of the skin to urine is a major cause of skin breakdown. The warm, moist conditions also encourage bacterial growth. Pathogens on the skin grow quickly and move upward through the urinary tract to cause serious urinary infections. These can lead to life-threatening **septicemia (sepsis)**. Wet linen that is not changed promptly has a disagreeable odor. Residents who are incontinent fear having "accidents" and tend to limit social interactions with others.

Every effort must be made to help the resident become continent. Little reference should

FIGURE 18-20 Changes in the urinary system as the result of aging
• Kidneys decrease in size
• Scar tissue replaces some renal cells
• Reduced blood flow through the kidneys means lower urine production
• Reduced renal concentration, leading to nocturia
• Less efficient bladder emptying
• Reduced filtration ability

be made to the temporary incontinence. Nursing assistants can do much to give emotional support and reassurance to residents who are incontinent. Nursing assistant responsibilities include:

- Assisting residents to toilet regularly
- Answering call lights promptly
- Always being courteous and patient when assisting residents with toileting
- Maintaining a positive attitude when changing soiled garments and bed linen and never being critical
- Performing good perineal care and being sure resident is clean and dry
- Checking the skin for signs of irritation whenever you toilet or bathe resident or perform perineal care
- Giving special attention to residents who are confused or forgetful because they may be unable to clearly state their need for assistance

INTERNAL URINARY CATHETER DRAINAGE

At times, it may be necessary to assist urinary elimination by the use of an **indwelling catheter**. The **catheter** is a slender rubber or plastic tube that is inserted into the bladder using sterile technique. The urine drains out of the bladder through the catheter. A balloon around the neck of the catheter is inflated once the catheter is in place. The inflated balloon keeps the catheter in place so that it will not easily slip out. The other end of the catheter is connected to a drainage tube and collection bag (Figure 18-21). This is a closed system and is sterile as long as it is not opened. Opening the system greatly increases the risk of infection. The insertion of a sterile catheter is the responsibility of the nurse.

Catheter Care

The nursing assistant provides daily care of the catheter when the resident has an indwelling catheter for urinary drainage. This care consists of the following actions:

- Applying the principles of standard precautions
- Keeping the urinary meatus clean
- Washing the area around the meatus daily with a solution approved by your facility
- Checking regularly for signs of irritation or urinary discomfort and reporting to the nurse

- Securing the tubing in such a way that there is no strain on the catheter or tubing. (A catheter strap should be applied to the leg to secure the tubing.)
- Maintaining the drainage bag below the level of the bladder
- Clamping and unclamping the catheter tubing at specific times. The clamping allows the bladder to fill, stimulating muscle tone.
- Not opening the closed system
- Making sure the tubing is not kinked or obstructed
- Ensuring that the collection bag does not touch the floor
- Measuring the amount of drainage in the collection bag at the end of each shift, noting the character of the urine, and reporting and recording the information
- Checking the entire drainage setup each time care is given and at the beginning and end of your shift
- Reporting changes in the character or quantity of urine

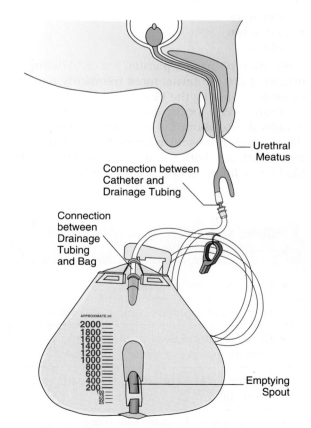

FIGURE 18-21 Indwelling catheter connected to a urine drainage bag

PROCEDURE 49 Giving Indwelling Catheter Care

1. Carry out each beginning procedure action.
2. Assemble equipment:

   - Disposable gloves
   - Bed protector
   - Bath blanket
   - Plastic bag for disposables
   - Daily catheter care kit (if available)
   - Washcloth, towel, basin, and soap if kit is unavailable
   - Antiseptic solution
   - Sterile applicators
   - Tape

3. Elevate bed to comfortable working height. Be sure opposite side rail is up and secure. Position resident on back, with legs separated and knees bent, if permitted.
4. Cover resident with bath blanket and fan-fold bedding to foot of bed.
5. Ask resident to raise hips. Place bed protector underneath resident.
6. Position bath blanket so that only genitals will be exposed.
7. Arrange catheter care kit and plastic bag on overbed table. Open kit.
8. Wash hands and put on gloves and draw drape back.
9. For the male resident:

   - Gently grasp penis and draw foreskin back, if not circumcised (Figure 18-22).
   - Using a new applicator dipped in antiseptic solution for each stroke, cleanse the glans from meatus toward shaft for approximately 4 inches.
   - After one stroke, dispose of each used applicator in plastic bag.
     Alternate Action: Going around the catheter first and then around meatus and glans. Wash with soap and water and rinse using a circular motion. Dry in the same manner. Make sure to return the foreskin (if not circumcised) to its proper position.

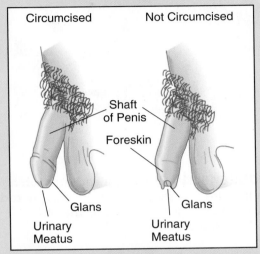

FIGURE 18-22 Comparison of circumcised and uncircumcised penis

For the female resident:

- Separate the labia.
- Using a new applicator dipped in antiseptic for each stroke, cleanse from front to back.
- After one stroke, dispose of each used applicator in plastic bag.
  Alternate Action: Using a clean cloth, soap and water, seperate labia, cleanse, rinse, and dry the labia majora from front to back. Repeat, cleaning labia minora and then wash meatus. Clean catheter down about 4 inches. Rinse and dry carefully.

10. Remove gloves and discard in plastic bag. Wash hands.
11. Check catheter to be sure it is secured properly to the leg. (See Figure 18-23.) Readjust Velcro® strap for slack, if needed. If a Velcro® strap is not available, use tape (Figure 18-24).
12. Check to be sure tubing is coiled on bed (see Figure 18-23) and hangs straight down into drainage container. Empty bag and measure if necessary. Do not raise bag above level of resident's hips.

(continues)

PROCEDURE 47 *(continued)*

FIGURE 18-23 Check the catheter tubing to be sure it is secured but not obstructed by the Velcro® leg band and that it is coiled on the bed.

13. Replace bedding and remove bath blanket.
14. Fold bath blanket and store or put in linen hamper.

FIGURE 18-24 The catheter tubing can also be taped to the thigh using hypoallergenic tape (preferably).

15. Lower bed. Adjust side rails for safety.
16. Carry out each procedure completion action.

Ambulating with a Catheter

When residents are ambulatory or using a geri-chair or wheelchair, you must be careful about placement of the urinary drainage bag. Remember that the drainage bag must always be lower than the bladder so the urine cannot flow back into the bladder. The bag may be secured to the resident's leg or clothing when the resident ambulates.

When the resident is seated in a wheelchair, the tubing should run below and under the wheelchair so the drainage bag can be secured to the wheelchair back. The drainage bag or tubing must never touch the floor.

At times, the catheter may be disconnected to make ambulation easier. However, there is always the danger of contamination.

Infection Risk

You must follow the procedure for disconnecting the catheter carefully. The resident who has an indwelling catheter is at risk for infection. There are several sites where infection can enter the drainage system:

- Urinary meatus, where the catheter is inserted
- Connection between the catheter and drainage tube
- Connection between the drainage bag and drainage tubing
- Opening used to empty the drainage bag

Disconnecting the Catheter

It is preferable never to disconnect the drainage setup, but at times, it is necessary. If sterile caps and plugs are available, they should be used. If not, the disconnected ends must be protected with sterile gauze sponges.

PROCEDURE
50

Emptying a Urinary Drainage Unit and Disconnecting the Catheter

1. Carry out each beginning procedure action.
2. Assemble equipment:
   - Disposable gloves
   - Graduated container
   - Sterile cap or sterile 4 x 4 (needed if container has no bottom drain tube)
   - Antiseptic wipes
   - Clamps
3. Wash hands and put on gloves.
4. Place paper towel on the floor under the drainage bag. Place a graduated container (graduate) on paper towel under drain of collection bag.
5. Remove drain from holder (Figure 18-25) and open. Using aseptic technique, allow the urine to drain into the graduate. Do not allow the tip of the tubing to touch the sides of the graduate.

FIGURE 18-25 Remove drain from holder and wipe with an antiseptic wipe.

6. Close the drain and replace it in the holder (Figure 18-26). If accidental contamination occurs, wipe the drain tip with an antiseptic wipe before returning it to the holder. Dispose of antiseptic wipe in plastic bag.
7. Pick up paper towel, touching top surface only, and discard.
8. Check position of drainage tube.

FIGURE 18-26 Wipe the drain with an antiseptic wipe and return the drain to the holder.

9. Take graduate to bathroom and empty it.
10. Wash and dry graduate and store it according to facility policy.
11. Carry out each procedure completion action.
12. Copy information on resident's record from intake and output sheet according to facility policy.
    - Perspiration and blood loss may be described as little, moderate, or excessive.
    - Also record the number of times linens or dressings have been changed or reinforced because of such fluid losses.
    - Blood loss is determined by the size of the wet area on dressings and by measuring amounts in Hemovac containers.

To disconnect the catheter:
13. Wash hands and put on gloves.
14. Clamp the catheter.
15. Disconnect the catheter and drainage tubing. Do not put the ends down or

(continues)

PROCEDURE 50 *(continued)*

allow them to touch anything. If accidental contamination occurs, wipe the ends with antiseptic wipes before inserting plug or placing tip. Dispose of antiseptic wipes in plastic bag.

16. Insert a sterile plug in the end of the catheter. Place a sterile cap over the catheter. Place a sterile cap over the exposed end of the drainage tube (Figure 18-27).

17. Secure the drainage tube to the bed frame in such a way that the tube will not touch the floor.

18. Remove and dispose of gloves according to facility policy. Wash hands.

19. Carry out each procedure completion action.
Note: Reverse the procedure to reconnect the catheter. If you find an unprotected, disconnected tube in the bed or on the floor, do not reconnect it. Report it at once.

FIGURE 18-27 Sterile catheter plug and protective cap (left). Plug and protective cap in place (right).

INTAKE AND OUTPUT (I&O)

Intake

Intake includes everything taken in that is liquid at room temperature, such as:

- Water or tea
- Gelatin, junket, or pudding
- Fluids given directly into a vein (IV)

Output

Normal fluid output includes all fluids that leave the body, including:

- Urine
- Perspiration
- Moisture from the lungs
- Moisture from the bowels

Excessive fluid loss results in dehydration (inadequate water content in body tissue). This loss can occur through:

- Diarrhea
- Vomiting
- Excessive urine output (diuresis)
- Excessive perspiration (diaphoresis)

Retention of fluids results in edema (swelling of body tissues). This may be caused by:

- Kidney dysfunction
- Cardiovascular disease

Recording Output

An accurate recording of intake and output is basic to the care of many residents. Intake and output totals are usually kept on the same form. Records are kept when ordered by the physician and when residents:

- Are dehydrated
- Receive intravenous infusions
- Have a urinary catheter
- Are perspiring profusely or vomiting

• Have specific diagnoses such as congestive heart failure or renal disease that require accurate monitoring of I&O

If the resident is incontinent, indicate the number of times on the output record. Do not forget to check the resident often and to change the bed linen each time it is wet. After each incident, clean resident and give perineal care. Change soiled clothing.

PROCEDURE 51 Measuring and Recording Fluid Output

 OBRA

1. Carry out each beginning procedure action.
2. Assemble equipment:
   • Disposable gloves
   • Graduate pitcher
   • Pen for recording
3. Wash hands and put on disposable gloves.
4. Save urine **specimen** (amount collected) and take to utility room or resident's bathroom.
   • Instruct a resident who is able to ambulate to the bathroom to use the hat-shaped specimen collection container (Figure 18-28).

Specimen Collector

Lower Toilet Seat Over Collector Before Resident Uses

FIGURE 18-28 Specimen collection container is placed on toilet under seat. Seat is lowered to hold container in place during use.

5. Pour urine from bedpan or urinal into graduate pitcher and measure (Figures 18-29A and B).
6. Empty urine.
   • If specimen is accidentally lost, estimate amount and make notation that it is an estimate.

FIGURE 18-29A Pour urine into graduate pitcher. Make sure there is no toilet paper in the bedpan.

FIGURE 18-29B Read the amount of urine in the graduate pitcher at eye level. The measuring scale is marked in cc or mL.

   • In some cases, the physician will request that the incontinent resident's protective pads or briefs be weighed to determine output.

(continues)

PROCEDURE *51* *(continued)*

Note: Some health care facilities have guidelines for estimating the amount of urine or blood on pads or linen by the diameter of the wet area.

7. Rinse graduate pitcher with cold water. Clean according to facility policy.
8. Clean bedpan or urinal or specimen container and store properly, according to facility policy.
9. Remove and dispose of gloves according to facility policy. Wash hands.
10. Record amounts immediately under output column on bedside intake and output record (Figure 18-30). All liquid

output should be recorded. Output includes:

- Urine
- Vomitus—also called **emesis**
- Drainage from a wound or the stomach
- Liquid stool—record an estimated amount
- Blood loss—record an estimated amount if on sheets or dressings, otherwise measure with a graduate
- Perspiration—record an estimated amount

Note: Fluids used to irrigate the bladder or for an enema are not included in calculating the output.

(continues)

FIGURE 18-30 Bedside intake and output sheet. In this example, the output amounts are highlighted.

Date	Time	Method of Adm.	Solution	Intake Amounts Rec'd	Time	Output Urine Amount	Others Kind	Amount
7/16	0700	PO	water	120 mL		500 mL		
	0830	PO	coffee	240 mL				
			or. ju.	120 mL				
	1030	PO	cran. ju.	120 mL				
	1100					300 mL		
	1230	PO	tea	240 mL				
	1400	PO	water	150 mL				
Shift Totals	1500			990 mL		800 mL		
	1530	PO	gelatin	120 mL				
	1700	PO	tea	120 mL				
			soup	180 mL				
	2000					512 mL		
	2045						vomitus	500 mL
	2205						vomitus	90 mL
Shift Totals	2300			420 mL		512 mL		590 mL
	2345						vomitus	80 mL
	0130	IV	D/W	500 mL				
	0315					400 mL		
Shift Totals	0700			500 mL		400 mL		80 mL
24 Hour Totals				1910 mL		1712 mL		670 mL vomitus

PROCEDURE *51*   *(continued)*

11. Carry out each procedure completion action.
12. Copy information on resident's record from intake and output sheet according to facility policy.
    - Perspiration and blood loss may be described as *little, moderate,* or *excessive.*

- Also record the number of times linens or dressings have been changed or reinforced because of such fluid losses.
- Blood loss is determined by the size of the wet area on dressings and by measuring amounts in Hemovac containers.

LEG BAG DRAINAGE

Some residents find it easier to ambulate when urine drainage is collected in a leg bag instead of the larger urinary drainage bag. The leg bag is held to the resident's leg by Velcro® straps around either the thigh or the lower leg (Figure 18-31). Points to keep in mind when residents use a leg bag are:

- The leg bag is smaller and must be emptied more often.
- The bag must be placed so there is a straight drop down from the catheter.
- Tension on the catheter tubing must be minimal.
- Care must be taken not to introduce germs when connecting and disconnecting the bag and catheter.

FIGURE 18-31   The leg bag is held in place by adjustable straps. Because it is smaller than the standard drainage bag, it must be emptied more often.

PROCEDURE *52*   Connecting Catheter to Leg Bag and Emptying the Leg Bag

Note: Always check with the nurse before using a leg bag.

1. Carry out each beginning procedure action.
2. Assemble equipment:
   - Disposable gloves
   - Antiseptic wipes
   - Leg bag and tubing
   - Emesis basin
   - Bed protector
   - Graduate pitcher
   - Paper towels
   - Sterile cap/plug
   - Clamp
3. Wash hands and put on gloves.
4. Place bed protector under the connection between catheter and drainage tube.
5. Clamp the catheter.

(continues)

PROCEDURE *52* *(continued)*

6. Disconnect the catheter and drainage tubing. Do not put them down or allow them to touch anything.

7. Insert a sterile plug in the end of the catheter. Place a sterile cap over the exposed end of the drainage tube.
   Note: If accidental contamination occurs, wipe the area with antiseptic wipes before inserting the sterile plug or replacing the sterile cap over the exposed end of the drainage tubing. Dispose of antiseptic wipes in plastic bag.

8. Secure the drainage tube to the bed frame. The drainage tube must not touch the floor.

9. Remove catheter plug.

10. Insert the end of the leg bag tubing into the catheter (Figure 18-32).

11. Release the catheter clamp.

12. Secure the leg bag with Velcro® straps to the resident's leg so there is no tension

FIGURE 18-32 Connecting leg bag to catheter tubing. Do not let the catheter tubing touch anything that could contaminate it. Note that the tubing to the drainage bag is covered with a sterile cap to protect it until it is reconnected to the catheter.

on the tubing. Be sure there is a straight drop down of tubing from the catheter to the bag for urine flow. Check for leakage.

13. Remove bed protector and discard.

14. Remove gloves and discard according to facility policy. Wash hands.

15. Assist resident to get out of bed. The single-use leg bag should be discarded in a biohazardous waste container.

16. Carry out each procedure completion action.
    Note: To reconnect the regular drainage bag, reverse the procedure.

To Empty the Leg Bag:

17. Position resident safely.

18. Wash hands and put on gloves.

19. Release Velcro® straps holding leg bag so it can be moved away from leg.

20. Place paper towel on floor under drainage outlet of leg bag.

21. Place graduate on paper towel under drainage outlet.

22. Remove cap, being careful not to touch tip. Drain urine into the graduate. Do not put cap down and do not touch inside of cap. If accidental contamination occurs, wipe the area with antiseptic wipes before replacing cap. Dispose of antiseptic wipes in a plastic bag.

23. Wipe drainage outlet with an antiseptic wipe and replace cap.

24. Refasten Velcro® straps to secure drainage bag to leg.

25. Make sure resident is comfortable and safe.

26. Discard paper towel.

27. Measure urine and note amount if required.

28. Discard urine. Clean graduate and store.

29. Remove gloves and discard according to facility policy.

30. Carry out each procedure completion action.

PROCEDURE 53 Collecting a Routine or Clean-Catch Urine Specimen

1. Carry out each beginning procedure action.
2. Assemble equipment:
   - Disposable gloves
   - Bedpan/urinal
   - Sterile specimen container and cover
   - Label including:
     - Resident's full name
     - Room number
     - Facility identification
     - Date and time of collection
     - Physician's name
     - Examination to be done
     - Other information requested
   - Graduate pitcher
   - Laboratory requisition slip, properly filled out
   - Biohazard specimen transport bag
   - Gauze squares or cotton
   - Antiseptic solution
3. Completely fill out the label of the specimen container.
4. Wash hands and put on disposable gloves.
5. Offer bedpan or urinal.
6. Instruct resident not to discard toilet tissue in the pan with the urine. Provide a small plastic bag in which to place the soiled tissue.
7. After resident has voided, cover pan and place on bed protector on chair. Offer wash water to resident.
8. If resident can ambulate to bathroom, place specimen collector in toilet.
9. Assist resident to bathroom. Ask resident to void into specimen collector. Instruct resident to discard soiled toilet tissue in plastic bag provided. Tissue must not be placed in collector.
10. Provide privacy.
11. Put on gloves. Remove specimen collector from toilet. If resident is on I&O, note amount of urine (Figure 18-33). If resident used bedpan, pour urine into graduate to measure. Note amount. Remove

FIGURE 18-33 Remove specimen collector from toilet. Note amount of urine if resident is on I&O.

gloves and discard according to facility policy. Wash hands.
12. Remove cap from specimen container. Place cap (inside up) on shelf or other flat surface in bathroom or utility room. Do not touch inside of cap or container.
13. Put on gloves. Carefully pour about 120 mL urine into specimen container from collector (Figure 18-34).
14. Remove and discard gloves according to facility policy.
15. Wash your hands.
16. Place cap on specimen container. Do not contaminate outside of container. Attach completed label to container (Figure 18-35). Place specimen container in biohazard specimen transport bag and attach laboratory requisition slip (Figure 18-36).
17. Carry out each procedure completion action.
18. Follow facility policy for transporting specimen to laboratory.

(continues)

PROCEDURE 53 *(continued)*

FIGURE 18-34 Carefully pour about 120 mL of urine from specimen collector into specimen container.

FIGURE 18-35 After specimen is placed in container and cap is put on, place label on container.

To Collect a Clean-Catch Specimen:
Complete steps 1 and 2 noted at the begining of this procedure.

3. Wash hands and put on disposable gloves.
4. Wash resident's genital area properly or instruct resident to do so. If soiled due to incontinence, perform perineal care.

FIGURE 18-36 Properly labeled specimen container is placed in biohazard specimen transport bag and laboratory requisition is attached.

5. For female residents:
   a. Using the gauze or cotton and the antiseptic solution, cleanse the outer folds of the vulva (folds are also called labia or lips) from front to back. Use separate gauze/cotton for each side. Discard the gauze/cotton in plastic bag.
   b. Cleanse the inner folds of the vulva with two pieces of gauze cotton and antiseptic solution, again from front to back. Discard gauze/cotton in plastic bag.
   c. Cleanse the middle, innermost area (meatus or urinary opening) in the same manner. Discard the gauze/cotton in plastic bag.
   d. Keep the labia separated so that the folds do not fall back and cover the meatus.
6. For male residents:
   a. Using the gauze/cotton and the antiseptic solution, cleanse the tip of the penis from the urinary meatus down, using a circular motion.
   b. Discard gauze/cotton in plastic bag.
7. Instruct resident to void, allowing the first part of the urine to escape. Then:
   a. Catch the urine stream that follows in the sterile specimen container.

(continues)

PROCEDURE *53* (continued)

b. Allow the last portion of the urine stream to escape.

Note: If resident's I&O is being monitored, or if the amount of urine passed must be measured, catch the first and last part of the urine in a bedpan, urinal, or specimen collection container.

8. Place the sterile cap on the urine container immediately to prevent contamination of the urine specimen.

9. Allow resident to wash hands. Assist as necessary.

10. With the cap securely tightened, wash the outside of the specimen container. Dry the container.

11. Remove and dispose of gloves according to facility policy.

12. Wash your hands.

13. Attach completed label to the container and place specimen in the transport bag.

14. Carry out procedure completion actions.

15. Follow facility policy for transporting specimen to laboratory.

EXTERNAL URINARY DRAINAGE (MALE)

External urinary drainage is preferred for male residents who require drainage for long periods of time. In this form of drainage, an internal catheter is not inserted in the urethra. Thus, there is less danger of infection.

A **condom** (sheath) or some other type of appliance is placed on the penis. The condom is attached to drainage tubing and a collection bag. The condom is removed every 24 hours and the penis is washed and dried.

PROCEDURE *54* Applying a Condom for Urinary Drainage

1. Carry out each beginning procedure action.

2. Assemble equipment:
   - Disposable gloves
   - Basin of warm water
   - Condom with drainage tip
   - Bed protector
   - Bath blanket
   - Towel

3. Arrange equipment on overbed table.

4. Raise bed to comfortable working height. Be sure opposite side rail is up and secure for safety.

5. Lower side rail on the side where you will be working.

6. Cover resident with bath blanket and fanfold bedding to foot of bed.

7. Wash hands and put on gloves.

8. Place bed protector under resident's hips.

9. Adjust bath blanket to expose genitals only.

10. Carefully wash and dry penis. Observe for signs of irritation. Check to be sure condom has "ready stick" surface.

11. Apply condom and drainage tip to penis by placing condom at top of penis and

(continues)

PROCEDURE 54 *(continued)*

rolling toward base of penis. Leave space between drainage tip and glans of penis to prevent irritation (Figure 18-37). If resident is not circumcised, be sure that foreskin is in normal position.

12. Apply tape provided with condom to secure it to the penis (Figure 18-38).

13. Condom is now ready to be connected to drainage tubing leading to collection bag.

14. Remove gloves and discard according to facility policy.

15. Wash hands.

16. Adjust bedding and remove bath blanket. Fold bath blanket and store in room or place in laundry hamper.

17. Lower bed. Adjust side rails for safety.

18. Carry out procedure completion actions.

FIGURE 18-37   When condom is placed on penis, leave room between the drainage tip and the glans of the penis to prevent irritation. Roll condom to base of penis.

Tape to Hold Catheter in Place

Condom Catheter

Attach Tip to Tubing Leading to Collection Bag

FIGURE 18-38   Correctly applied and secured condom ready to be attached to tubing leading to drainage bag.

COMMON CONDITIONS

Rectocele and Cystocele

The urinary bladder, ureters, and the urethra are found in the pelvic cavity. Some of the female reproductive organs are also in the pelvis. Each group of organs can be affected by disease or stress in the other group.

Frequent pregnancies and general loss of muscle tone due to the aging process may cause the bladder to protrude into the vagina (**cystocele**) and the rectum into the vagina (**rectocele**).

The weakness of the bladder wall can cause urinary incontinence, especially with extra stress such as laughing or coughing. The weakened rectal wall can lead to constipation and

hemorrhoids. Surgery can be helpful in repairing the cystocele and rectocele.

Renal Calculi

Renal calculi, or kidney stones, form as various salts and compounds settle out of the forming urine. Starting as tiny grains of sediment, they become larger and larger until they block part of the drainage system, often a ureter. When blockage occurs the resident experiences extreme pain. Pain associated with urine elimination is known as **dysuria**. Most kidney stones are passed when fluids are forced, but surgery may be required to relieve the obstruction.

The urine may be strained through gauze or filter paper before being measured and discarded to determine when the stone is passed. Blood may cause the urine to become pink to deep red in color. Blood in the urine is called **hematuria**.

Renal Failure

Renal failure (**uremia**) may occur suddenly but it is usually a chronic situation that develops gradually over a period of years. Causes include changes in the blood vessels that serve the kidneys, hypertension, and the aging process.

The resident in chronic renal failure does not eliminate effectively, so water and wastes build up in the body. Urine output is reduced (**oliguria**). In the terminal stage of renal failure, urine output ceases altogether (**anuria**). Blood pressure increases and edema and chemical imbalance develop throughout the body. The resident may complain of headache, nausea, and a bad taste in the mouth. Uric acid is eliminated in the perspiration. The uric acid accumulates as white crystals on the skin and is called **uremic frost**. The perspiration has an unpleasant odor. Careful attention is needed to keep the skin clean and free from breakdown.

Renal failure is treated by:

- Surgery to implant a healthy kidney
- Hemodialysis, a procedure that uses a machine to filter wastes and impurities from the blood (Figure 18-39).

Residents receiving hemodialysis may leave the facility for the treatment, which normally requires several hours. When residents return to the facility after hemodialysis, they are observed closely for dizziness and fainting. They are often placed on fluid restriction, I&O, and a special-

FIGURE 18-39   Hemodialysis filters wastes from the resident's blood. Blood leaves the body from an artery, is filtered by the machine, and is returned to the body through a vein.

ized diet. Hemodialysis is often performed more than once a week. Two connectors (cannulas) are implanted in the resident's body, usually in an arm. One cannula is placed in an artery and the other is placed in a vein.

When caring for the resident with implanted hemodialysis cannulas:

- Be careful not to dislodge the cannulas.
- Notify the nurse if there is pain, swelling, redness, or drainage in the arm.
- Do not use the arm for blood pressure measurements.
- Do not apply tight clothing to the arm.
- Encourage resident to follow any special exercises that may have been ordered.

LESSON SYNTHESIS: Putting It All Together

*Y*ou have just completed this lesson. Now go back and review the *Clinical Focus. Try to see how the Clinical Focus relates to the concepts presented in the lesson. Then answer the following questions.*

1. What do you think Ms. Beebe's problem is?

2. What made the nursing assistant think to ask Ms. Beebe when she had her last bowel movement?

3. What actions could the nursing staff take that might help the resident avoid a similar situation in the future?

4. Why is the attitude of the staff an important factor in the success or failure of managing elimination problems?

REVIEW

A. Match each term (items a.–e.) with the proper definition.

a. constipation   d. micturition
b. diarrhea   e. retention
c. feces

1. _____ loose, liquid stools

2. _____ inability to urinate

3. _____ hard stool that is difficult to evacuate

4. _____ solid waste

5. _____ another term for urination

B. Complete the sentence by providing the proper term.

6. Elimination of feces is called _____.

7. Blood in the urine is called _____.

8. Painful urination is _____.

9. Inability to control elimination is _____.

10. An artificial opening in the wall of the abdomen for the elimination of feces is called a(an) _____.

C. Fill in the blanks by selecting the correct word or phrase from the list.

liquid	sit upright
left side	I&O sheet
floor	incontinent
coiled	dehydration
oil-retention enema	tongue depressors
voiding	stoma

11. The best position for the resident receiving an enema is on the _____ with the knees flexed.

12. One type of enema that should be retained for 20 minutes is the _____.

13. When collecting a stool specimen, use _____ to transfer the sample from the bedpan to the specimen container.

14. The best position to encourage voiding in a female resident is to have her _____.

15. A person who is unable to control urine output voluntarily is said to be _____.

16. Intake includes everything taken in that is _____ at room temperature.

17. Intake and output are recorded on the _____.

18. When a resident has a colostomy, the opening is called the _____.

19. During a routine urinary drainage check, the tubing should be _____ on the bed.

20. A urine collection bag must never touch the _____.

21. A common term for eliminating urine from the bladder is _____.

22. Excessive fluid loss from the body results in _____.

D. Select the one best answer for each of the following.

23. The proper temperature for a soapsuds enema is
(A) 80°F
(B) 95°F
(C) 105°F
(D) 120°F

24. A rectal tube should be inserted into the rectum
(A) ½ inch
(B) 1 to 1½ inches
(C) 2 to 4 inches
(D) 6 inches

25. Gloves should be worn in each instance except when
(A) inserting a flatus tube
(B) giving perineal care
(C) applying a leg drainage bag
(D) filling out the label for a specimen container

26. A resident with a colostomy evacuates feces through the
(A) anus
(B) ileum
(C) jejunum
(D) colon

27. Normal urine color is
    (A) red
    (B) yellow
    (C) colorless
    (D) brown

E. Clinical Experience

Mrs. Duff has an indwelling catheter and is in a wheelchair. You are assigned to her care. Answer the following questions.

28. May the collection bag touch the floor at any time?

29. Should the collection bag or tubing be higher or lower than the resident's bladder?

30. Is perineal care necessary?

31. How often should the drainage be emptied?

32. When Mrs. Duff is in her wheelchair, how should the urinary drainage tubing be positioned?

SECTION 6

Special Nursing Assistant Activities

LESSONS

19 Measuring and Recording Residents' Data

20 Admission, Transfer, and Discharge

21 Warm and Cold Applications

Measuring and Recording Residents' Data

Clinical Focus

Think about situations in which the measuring and recording of data are an important part of your duties as you study this lesson and meet:

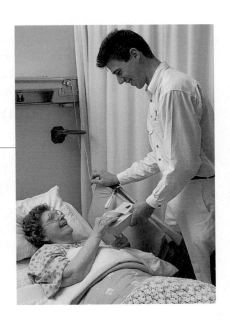

*G*eraldine Hoden, 72 years old, who is a resident in your facility. Mrs. Hoden has heart problems that cause her to retain fluid (edema). She becomes short of breath with any physical exertion. Mrs. Hoden is taking medication to strengthen and regulate her heart activity. She also has a history of hypertension. Mrs. Hoden is alert and cooperative.

OBJECTIVES

After studying this lesson, you should be able to:

- Define and spell vocabulary words and terms.
- Properly select and use equipment to measure vital signs.
- Identify the range of normal values.
- State the reasons for measuring weight and height.
- Demonstrate the following:
  Procedure 55 Measuring an Oral Temperature (Glass Thermometer)
  Procedure 56 Measuring a Rectal Temperature (Glass Thermometer)
  Procedure 57 Measuring an Axillary Temperature (Glass Thermometer)
  Procedure 58 Measuring an Oral Temperature (Electronic Thermometer)
  Procedure 59 Measuring a Rectal Temperature (Electronic Thermometer)
  Procedure 60 Measuring an Axillary Temperature (Electronic Thermometer)
  Procedure 61 Measuring a Tympanic Temperature
  Procedure 62 Counting the Radial Pulse Rate
  Procedure 63 Counting the Apical-Radial Pulse
  Procedure 64 Counting Respirations
  Procedure 65 Taking Blood Pressure

OBJECTIVES

Procedure 66 Weighing and Measuring the Resident Using an Upright Scale
Procedure 67 Measuring Weight with an Electronic Wheelchair Scale
Procedure 68 Weighing the Resident in a Chair Scale
Procedure 69 Measuring and Weighing the Resident in Bed

VOCABULARY

accelerated (*ack-SELL-er-ay-ted*)

antihypertensive (*an-tee-high-per-TEN-siv*)

apex (*AY-pecks*)

apical pulse (*AP-ih-kal puls*)

bradycardia (*brad-ee-KAR-dee-ah*)

Celsius (*SELL-see-us*)

centimeter (*SEN-tih-mee-ter*)

cyanotic (*sigh-ah-NOT-ick*)

depressant (*dee-PRESS-ant*)

diastolic (*die-ah-STOL-ick*)

expiration (*ecks-pih-RAY-shun*)

Fahrenheit (*FAIR-en-hight*)

fasting (*FAST-ing*)

hypertension (*high-per-TEN-shun*)

hypotension (*high-poh-TEN-shun*)

inspiration (*in-spih-RAY-shun*)

kilogram (*KILL-oh-gram*)

mercury (*MER-kyou-ree*)

oral (*OR-al*)

pulse (*puls*)

pulse deficit (*puls DEF-ih-sit*)

pulse rate (*puls rayt*)

radial artery (*RAY-dee-al ARE-ter-ee*)

rales (*rahls*)

respiration (*res-pih-RAY-shun*)

rhythm (*RITH-um*)

sheath (*sheeth*)

sphygmomanometer (*sfig-moh-mah-NOM-eh-ter*)

stethoscope (*STETH-oh-skohp*)

systolic (*sis-TOL-ick*)

tachycardia (*tack-ee-KAR-dee-ah*)

thermometer (*ther-MOM-eh-ter*)

tympanic (*tim-PAN-ick*)

vital signs (*VIGH-tal signs*)

volume (*VOL-youm*)

MEASURING VITAL SIGNS

Each resident must have **vital signs** (*vital* means living) measured and recorded on admission. Vital signs are also frequently measured throughout the resident's stay. The vital signs are:

- Temperature
- Pulse rate
- Respiratory rate
- Blood pressure

The vital signs give information about the general health of the individual and changes in the health status. It is essential that these measurements be accurate and that you record them properly.

To do this accurately you must know how to:

- Read a clinical thermometer using the **Celsius** and **Fahrenheit** scales

- Read a **sphygmomanometer** (blood pressure cuff)

In addition to vital signs, you will also measure residents' weight and height on a regular basis. To do this accurately you must know how to:

- Read a scale for weight in pounds and **kilograms**.
- Read a scale for height in feet and inches and in **centimeters**.

Procedures for measuring weight and height are described later in this lesson.

Celsius, kilograms, and centimeters are metric measurements. Facilities that use the metric system for these temperature, weight, and height measurements will have thermometers and scales with the metric values. You do not have to convert measurements from one system to the other.

Clinical Focus:

Think about Geraldine Hoden and her diagnosis. Why is it important to monitor her weight? Make a correlation between her weight (loss/gain) and her medical condition.

Equipment Needed

Clinical **thermometers** are used to determine temperature. A watch with a second hand is needed to count the pulse and respiratory rate. A **stethoscope** and sphygmomanometer are needed to measure the blood pressure. Each vital sign is discussed separately, although actual measurements are usually done as a combined activity.

TEMPERATURE

Temperature is the measurement of body heat. One of two temperature scales may be used: Fahrenheit or Celsius. Normal body temperature is about 98.6° Fahrenheit (37° Celsius).

Temperatures are usually measured orally. The temperature can also be taken with a thermometer placed and held in the rectum (rectal temperature). Alternatively, the thermometer can be placed in the armpit (axillary temperature) if the resident:

- Is unable to keep the mouth closed
- Has respiratory difficulty
- Is receiving oxygen
- Is receiving oral tube feeding

The rectal temperature registers 1° higher and the axillary temperature registers 1° lower than an **oral** temperature in the same person (Figure 19-1).

The temperature of the blood in the vessels of the eardrum may also be measured. This is known as **tympanic** temperature. It is the most accurate temperature reading. The temperature taken in the axilla is the least accurate reading.

Temperature can be increased by:

- Infection
- Dehydration
- Physical exercise
- Hot water
- Brain damage

It can be decreased by:

- Shock
- Cold weather
- Sponge bath
- Medications
- Approaching death

Clinical Thermometers

Note: The following material describes the use of mercury-filled glass thermometers. Because of the hazards of mercury in the event the thermometer breaks, many facilities no longer use this type of thermometer. Facility policy will dictate the type of thermometer to be used.

Three types of glass clinical thermometers are shown in Figure 19-2:

- Oral
- Security
- Rectal

These thermometers differ mainly in the size and shape of the bulb (the end that is inserted into the resident). When only security or stubby-type thermometers are in use, the rectal thermometers are marked with a red dot at the end of the stem. Figure 19-3 shows rectal thermometers: A has a Fahrenheit scale and B has a Celsius scale.

Reading the Glass Thermometer. **Mercury** is a heat-sensitive liquid metal that appears as a solid color line in the bulb of the thermometer. The mercury rises in the hollow center of the stem. To read the thermometer:

- Hold it at eye level.
- Find the solid column of mercury (Figure 19-4).

	Oral	Axillary	Rectal
FIGURE 19-1 Temperature variations related to method of measurement			
Average Temperature	98.6°F	97.6°F	99.6°F
Acceptable Range	97.6–99.6°F (36.5–37.5°C)	96.6–98.6°F (36–37°C)	98.6–100.6°F (37–38.1°C)

FIGURE 19-2 Clinical thermometers: from left to right—oral, security, rectal

- Look along the sharper edge between the numbers and lines.
- Determine the point where the mercury ends.

Starting with 94°F (34°C), each long line indicates a 1° elevation in temperature. Only every other degree is marked with a number. In between each long line are four shorter lines. Each shorter line equals two tenths ($\frac{2}{10}$ or 0.2) of a degree. The thermometer is "read" at the point at which the mercury ends (stops rising). If it stops between two lines, read it to the closer line.

Note: On a Celsius thermometer, the lines have different values. Each degree is marked (34, 35, 36, etc.). There are 10 small lines in between each number. Each of these small lines equals one tenth ($\frac{1}{10}$ or 0.1) of a degree.

General Thermometer Safety Precautions

- Check glass thermometers for chips.
- Shake mercury down before use, *away* from resident or hard objects.
- Do not leave resident alone with thermometer in place.

A

B

FIGURE 19-3 A. Fahrenheit and B. Celsius thermometers

FIGURE 19-4 Reading a thermometer. This thermometer reads 98.6°F.

- Allow glass thermometer to register for at least 3 minutes orally, 2 minutes rectally, or 10 minutes axillary.
- Hold rectal and axillary thermometers in place.
- When measuring a rectal temperature, lubricate bulb end of thermometer before inserting in rectum.
- Use an alcohol wipe or cotton ball to wipe thermometer from end to bulb before reading.

Contraindications—Oral Temperatures:
An oral temperature is not taken if resident is

- Confused, disoriented
- Restless
- Unconscious
- Chilled
- Coughing
- Unable to breathe through the nose
- Very weak
- On seizure precautions

Contraindications—Rectal Temperatures:
A rectal temperature is not taken if resident has

- Diarrhea
- Fecal impaction
- Combative behavior
- Rectal bleeding
- Hemorrhoids
- Colostomy

Some facilities use other types of thermometers to take temperatures, including

- Electronic thermometer
- Tympanic thermometer

The Electronic Thermometer

The electronic thermometer is battery-operated. The temperature is registered in large numbers on the screen. The *probe* is the portion that is placed into the resident. The probes or probe stems are colored blue for oral or axillary use and red for rectal use. The probe is covered with

FIGURE 19-5 An electronic thermometer. The temperature is registered in large, easy-to-read numerals. The disposable plastic sheath is placed over the probe tip. (The blue probe is for oral temperatures and the red probe is for rectal temperatures.) The blue probe is then inserted into the resident's mouth in the usual manner.

FIGURE 19-6 The cordless, hand-held tympanic thermometer. The lens on the handset indicates the digital temperature reading. (Courtesy of Thermoscan® Inc., San Diego, CA)

a disposable **sheath** that stays on during use and is then discarded (Figure 19-5).

The tympanic (ear) thermometer (Figure 19-6) measures the temperature from blood vessels in the tympanic membrane in the ear. This provides a reading close to the core body temperature. The instrument has a built-in converter that provides the equivalent temperature in rectal or oral values (in both Fahrenheit or Celsius systems). The type of thermometer reading (mode) is selected by the user.

PROCEDURE 55

Measuring an Oral Temperature (Glass Thermometer)

1. Carry out each beginning procedure action.
2. Assemble equipment:
   - Disposable gloves
   - Container with clean thermometer
   - Container for used thermometers
   - Cotton balls
   - Container for soiled tissues
   - Container with tissues
   - Pad and pencil
   - Watch with second hand
   - Disposable sheath for thermometer (if used in facility)

3. Put on gloves.
4. Have resident rest in a comfortable position in bed or chair.
5. Ask resident if he or she has had hot or cold liquids to drink or has smoked within the last 15 minutes. If the answer is "yes," wait 15 minutes before taking oral temperature. Holding stem end, remove thermometer from container. Wipe with tissue. Check to be sure the thermometer is intact with no chips or cracks. Read the mercury column. It should register below 96°F. If necessary,

(continues)

PROCEDURE 55 *(continued)*

FIGURE 19-7 Shake mercury down in column by holding the thermometer by the stem and snapping the wrist. Check the reading. Repeat until the reading is below 96°F.

shake down. To shake down (Figure 19-7), move away from table or other hard objects. Grasp the stem tightly between your thumb and fingers. Shake down with downward motion.

6. Insert thermometer in sheath, if used. Insert bulb end of thermometer under resident's tongue, toward base of tongue (Figure 19-8). Tell resident to hold thermometer gently with lips closed for 3 minutes.

7. Remove thermometer, holding by stem. Remove sheath, if used, and place in proper container. Wipe from stem end toward bulb end.

8. Discard tissue in proper container.

9. Read thermometer (Figure 19-9) and record on pad.

10. Place thermometer in container for used thermometers. If thermometer is to be reused for this resident:

  • Wash it twice in cold water and soap with two separate cotton balls, wiping from stem to bulb.
  • Rinse and dry it.
  • Return it to the individual disinfectant-filled holder.

11. Remove gloves and discard according to facility policy.

12. Carry out each procedure completion action.

13. Report any unusual variations to the nurse at once.

FIGURE 19-8 The bulb end of the thermometer is inserted under the tongue, left 3 minutes, then removed.

FIGURE 19-9 Hold thermometer at eye level, locate the column of mercury, and read to the closest line.

Measuring a Rectal Temperature (Glass Thermometer)

1. Carry out each beginning procedure action.
2. Assemble equipment:

   - Disposable gloves
   - Container with clean rectal thermometer
   - Container for used thermometers
   - Container for soiled tissues
   - Lubricant
   - Container with tissues
   - Sheath for thermometer, if used
   - Pad and pencil
   - Watch with second hand

3. Put up opposite side rail if not already up. Lower back rest of bed. Ask resident to turn on her side. Assist resident, if necessary.
4. Place small amount of lubricant on tissue.
5. Put gloves on. Remove thermometer from container by holding stem end. Read mercury column. Be sure it registers below 96°F. Check thermometer for cracks and chips. Insert thermometer in sheath if used.
6. Using tissue, apply small amount of lubricant to bulb.
7. Fold the top bedclothes back to expose anal area.
8. Refer to Figure 19-10. Separate buttocks with one hand. Insert the thermometer gently into rectum 1½ inches. Hold in place. Replace bedclothes as soon as thermometer is inserted.
9. Thermometer should remain inserted for 3 minutes.
10. Remove thermometer, holding by stem. Remove sheath, if used, and dispose of in proper container. Wipe from stem toward bulb end.
11. Discard tissue in proper container.

FIGURE 19-10 The rectal thermometer is lubricated and then inserted 1½ inches into the rectum and held in place.

12. Read thermometer. Record reading on pad.
13. Wipe lubricant from resident. Discard tissue.
14. Place thermometer in container for used thermometers. If thermometer is to be reused for this resident:

    - Wash it in cold water and soap.
    - Rinse and dry it.
    - Return it to the individual disinfectant-filled holder.

15. Remove gloves and discard according to facility policy.
16. Lower opposite side rail if indicated.
17. Carry out each procedure completion action.
    Note: Remember that when a rectal temperature is recorded, add (R) after the reading.

PROCEDURE 57

Measuring an Axillary Temperature (Glass Thermometer)

1. Carry out each beginning procedure action.
   Note: Use disposable gloves if there may be contact with open lesions, wet linens, or body fluids.

2. Assemble equipment:
   - Container with clean oral thermometers
   - Container for used thermometers
   - Container for soiled tissues
   - Container with tissues
   - Pad and pencil
   - Watch with a second hand
   - Sheath for thermometer, if used

3. Wipe the area dry and place sheath on the thermometer, if used. Place thermometer in armpit.

   a. The resident's arm is kept close to his body if axillary site is used (Figure 19-11).
   b. Leave the thermometer in place 10 minutes.
   c. Remove sheath, if used, and dispose of in proper container. Wipe and read thermometer. Note reading on pad.
   d. Clean and replace as with oral thermometer if it is to be reused.

4. Carry out each procedure completion action.
   Note: Remember that when an axillary temperature is recorded, add (AX) after the reading.

FIGURE 19-11 When the thermometer is placed in the axilla, it must be held in place.

PROCEDURE 58 — Measuring an Oral Temperature (Electronic Thermometer)

1. Carry out each beginning procedure action.
2. Obtain electronic thermometer, disposable sheaths, and gloves (if this is your facility policy). (Gloves are not necessary with an oral temperature using this type of thermometer. Know and follow your facility policy.)
3. Ask resident if he or she has had hot or cold liquids to drink or has smoked within the last 15 minutes. If the answer is "yes," wait 15 minutes before taking oral temperature.
4. Cover probe (blue) with protective sheath.
5. Insert covered probe under resident's tongue, toward side of mouth (Figure 19-12).
6. Hold probe in position.
7. When buzzer signals that temperature has been determined, take reading and record on pad.
8. Discard sheath in wastebasket. Do not touch sheath. Remove gloves and discard according to facility policy.

9. Return probe to proper position and entire unit to charging.
10. Carry out each procedure completion action.

FIGURE 19-12 Inserting the blue probe of the electronic thermometer in the resident's mouth

PROCEDURE 59 — Measuring a Rectal Temperature (Electronic Thermometer)

1. Carry out each beginning procedure action.
2. Assemble equipment:
   - Disposable gloves
   - Electronic thermometer with red probe
   - Sheaths
   - Lubricant
3. Lower back rest of bed. Ask resident to turn on his side. Assist resident, if necessary.

4. Put on disposable gloves.
5. Place a small amount of lubricant on the tip of the sheath (Figure 19-13).
6. Fold the top bedclothes back to expose anal area.
7. Separate buttocks with one hand. Insert sheath-covered probe about 1½ inches into rectum or as recommended by manufacturer. Hold in place. Replace bedclothes as soon as thermometer is inserted.

(continues)

PROCEDURE *59* *(continued)*

FIGURE 19-13 Lubricating the tip of the sheath-covered probe

8. Read temperature when registered on digital display. Note reading on pad.
9. Remove probe and discard sheath. Wipe lubricant from resident. Discard tissue.
10. Remove gloves and discard according to facility policy.
11. Carry out each procedure completion action.

PROCEDURE 60 Measuring an Axillary Temperature (Electronic Thermometer)

1. Carry out each beginning procedure action.
   Note: Use disposable gloves if there may be contact with open lesions, wet linens, or body fluids.
2. Equipment needed: same as for oral temperature measurement using an electronic thermometer (See Procedure 58).

3. Wipe axillary area dry and place covered probe in place. Keep resident's arm close to the body. Hold probe in place until temperature records on digital display and buzzer signals.
4. Remove thermometer probe. Dispose of sheath.
5. Carry out each procedure completion action.

Many facilities use tympanic (aural) thermometers. The temperature is taken by measuring the heat given off by the tympanic membrane (in the ear). This method has several advantages:

• Tympanic thermometers are accurate and easy to use.
• The temperature registers in a few seconds. Because of this, taking the temperature of an agitated resident is safer and faster.
• Temperatures that cannot be taken orally can be taken by the tympanic method, elim-

inating the need to take rectal or axillary temperatures.
• The tympanic thermometer allows you to select a core, oral, or rectal mode. This means the reading will correlate with the mode selected. Choose the mode according to your facility's policy.
• Wait for 15 minutes to take the temperature if the resident has been outdoors or if the resident has been lying on the ear you will use.

PROCEDURE
61

Measuring a Tympanic Temperature

1. Carry out each beginning procedure action.
2. Assemble equipment:
   - Disposable gloves if there may be contact with blood or body fluids, open lesions, or wet linens
   - Tympanic thermometer
   - Probe covers
3. Place a clean probe cover on the probe.
4. Select the appropriate mode on the thermometer.
5. Check the lens to make sure it is clean and intact (Figure 19-14).
6. Put on disposable gloves if you may have contact with blood or body fluids, open lesions, or wet linens.
7. Position the resident so you have access to the ear you will be using.

8. Gently pull the ear pinna back and up (Figure 19-15). This straightens the ear canal so the thermometer can be placed for an accurate reading.
9. Place the probe in the resident's ear, aiming it toward the tympanic membrane. Insert the probe until it seals the ear canal (Figure 19-16). Do not apply pressure.
10. Press the activation button (Figure 19-17). Leave the thermometer in the ear for the time recommended by the manufacturer.
11. When you have a reading, remove the probe from the resident's ear and dispose of the cover.
12. Carry out each procedure completion action.

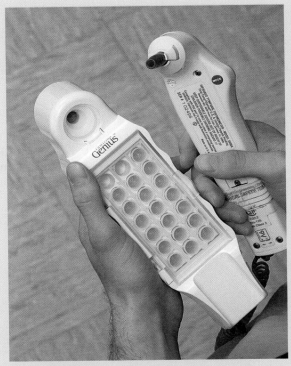

FIGURE 19-14 Check the lens of the tympanic thermometer to make sure it is clean and intact.

FIGURE 19-15 Gently pull the ear pinna back and up.

(continues)

PROCEDURE 61 *(continued)*

FIGURE 19-16   Place the probe in the resident's ear, aiming it toward the tympanic membrane. Insert probe until it seals the ear canal.

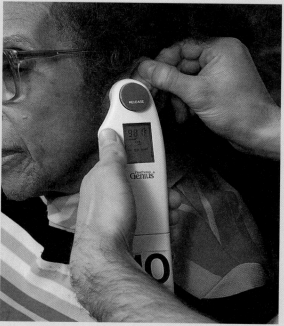

FIGURE 19-17   Press the activation button and leave the thermometer in the ear for the time recommended by the manufacturer.

Clinical Focus:

If Mrs. Hoden was confused and disoriented, what method would you use to take her temperature? Explain your choice.

PULSE AND RESPIRATION

The **pulse** and **respiration** of the resident are usually counted during the same procedure.

Pulse is the pressure of the blood felt against the wall of an artery as the heart alternately beats (contracts) and rests (relaxes). The pulse is more easily felt in arteries that are fairly close to the skin surface and can be gently pressed against a bone by the fingers. The pulse rate and its character provide a good indication of how the cardiovascular system is able to meet the body's needs.

Radial Pulse

The pulse is usually measured over the **radial artery** (at the base of the wrist on the thumb side) (Figure 19-18). The age, sex, size, and con-

FIGURE 19-18   Locate the pulse on the thumb side of the wrist with tips of your fingers.

dition of the resident affect the character of the pulse. Pulse character means:

- Rate (speed)
- **Volume** (fullness)
- **Rhythm** (regularity)

Pulse character should always be noted when counting the pulse.

Apical Pulse

The heart rate is usually the same as the **pulse rate**. At times, however, some of the heartbeats are not strong enough to be transmitted and felt along the radial artery. This results in a difference between the heart rate and the pulse rate. This difference is called a **pulse deficit**. Pulse

---

PROCEDURE
62
Counting the Radial Pulse Rate

1. Carry out each beginning procedure action.
   Note: Use disposable gloves if there may be contact with open lesions, wet linens, or body fluids.
2. Place resident in a comfortable position. The palm of the hand should be down

and the arm should rest across the resident's chest.

3. Locate the pulse on the thumb side of the wrist with the tips of your first three fingers. Do not use your thumb because it contains a pulse that may be confused with the resident's pulse. Refer to Figure 19-19 for the location of other sites on the body where the pulse rate can be counted.
4. When the pulse is felt, exert slight pressure. Use second hand of watch and count for 1 minute. It is the practice in some facilities to count for 30 seconds, multiply the value by two, and then record the rate for 1 minute. For accuracy, a 1-minute count is preferred and must be done if the pulse is irregular. Figure 19-20 lists average pulse rates.
5. Carry out each procedure completion action.

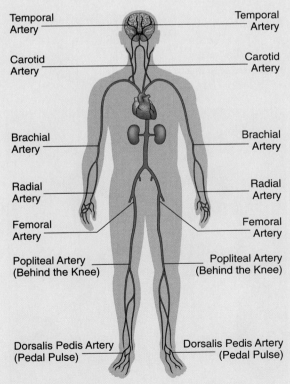

FIGURE 19-19 Pulses may be felt in areas other than the wrist. These are called pulse sites.

FIGURE 19-20 Average pulse rates		
Adult men	60–70	beats per minute
Adult women	65–80	beats per minute
Children over 7 years	75–100	beats per minute
Preschoolers	80–110	beats per minute
Infants	120–160	beats per minute

deficits are found in some forms of heart disease. If a pulse deficit is suspected, it may be necessary to count the heart rate and the pulse rate at the same time. One person determines the heart rate by placing a stethoscope on the chest over the **apex** or point of the heart. The apex is the lowest point of the heart and can easily be located near the left nipple or under a woman's left breast. The second person counts the radial pulse at the same time and the rates are compared. This is called taking an **apical pulse**. The average pulse rate is about 72 beats per minute (bpm). Pulse rates under 60 or over 90 should be reported.

- **Tachycardia**—unusually fast pulse rate (over 90 bpm)

- **Bradycardia**—unusually slow pulse rate (under 60 bpm)

Any irregularities in the rate, rhythm, or volume of the resident's pulse should be reported immediately.

Respiration

Respiration supplies the cells in the body with oxygen and rids the body of excess carbon dioxide. When respirations are inefficient, carbon dioxide gas builds up in the bloodstream, making the skin dusky, bluish, or **cyanotic**.

There are two parts to each respiration:

- One **inspiration** (inhalation)
- One **expiration** (exhalation)

PROCEDURE 63 Counting the Apical-Radial Pulse

1. Carry out each beginning procedure action.
   Note: Use disposable gloves if there may be contact with open lesions, wet linens, or body fluids.
2. Clean stethoscope ear pieces and bell with disinfectant.
3. Two people measure the heart rate and the radial pulse at the same time. The nurse places the stethoscope ear pieces in the ears and the stethoscope diaphragm over the apex of the resident's heart. (The diaphragm may be warmed in the hands before placing it on the resident's chest.) The heartbeats are counted for 1 minute.
4. At the same time, the nursing assistant counts the radial pulse for 1 minute (Figure 19-21).
5. Compare the results and note them on the pad.
6. Clean ear pieces and bell of stethoscope with disinfectant.
7. Carry out each procedure completion action. Record date, time, pulse values as in example, and character, such as weak and irregular.

Example:

Apical pulse	A 108
Radial pulse	R 82

Pulse deficit is 26
(108 − 82 = 26)

FIGURE 19-21 The nurse takes the apical pulse while the nursing assistant takes the radial pulse.

The character (rhythm and volume) and the rate of respirations must be noted. Respirations are described as:

- Normal
- Shallow
- Deep
- Labored
- Difficult

The normal respiration rate for adults is 16 to 20 per minute. If the rate is more than 25 per minute, it is **accelerated** and is reported. If the rate is less than 12 per minute, it is too low and is reported. Special terms are used to describe different types of breathing (Figure 19-22).

The rate is determined by counting the rise and fall of the chest for 1 minute while using a watch equipped with a second hand.

Breathing is partially under voluntary control; that is, a person is able to stop breathing for a short period of time. This frequently happens when a resident realizes that breathing is being watched and counted. The breathing pattern is altered unintentionally. To avoid this, the respirations are counted immediately following the pulse count. The resident's hand is kept in the same position on the chest and your fingers remain on the pulse.

Factors affecting respiratory rates are listed in Figure 19-23.

FIGURE 19-22 Special terms describe different breathing patterns.

- Tachypnea—rapid, shallow breathing
- Dyspnea—difficult or labored breathing
- Shallow—breaths that partially fill the lungs
- Apnea—a period of no respirations
- Cheyne-Stokes respirations—a period of dyspnea followed by periods of apnea
- Stertorous—Snoring-like respirations
- **Rales** (gurgles)—moist respirations. At times, fluid (mucus) will collect in the air passages. This causes a bubbling type of respiration. Rales are common in the dying resident.
- Wheezing—difficult breathing accompanied by a whistling or sighing sound due to narrowing of bronchioles (as in asthma) or an increase of mucus in bronchi

---

FIGURE 19-23 Factors affecting respiratory rates

• Illness	• Exercise
• Emotions	• Position
• Elevated temperature	• Drugs
• Age	

Clinical Focus:

If you take Mrs. Hoden's pulse and respirations right after she has been up to the bathroom, what results would you expect and why?

PROCEDURE

64 Counting Respirations

1. After counting the pulse rate, leave your fingers on the radial pulse.
2. Start counting the number of times the chest rises and falls during a period of 1 minute.
3. Note depth and regularity of respirations.
4. Record the time, rate, depth, and regularity of respirations.

BLOOD PRESSURE

The factors that influence blood pressure are listed in Figure 19-24.

There is greater resistance to blood flow in arteries that have lost their elasticity or ability to stretch due to disease. This causes higher blood pressure. Blood pressure is also increased by:

* Exercise
* Eating
* Stimulants
* Emotional anxiety
* Some drugs

Blood pressure is decreased by:

* **Fasting** (not eating)
* Rest

FIGURE 19-24 Factors influencing blood pressure readings
• Amount of blood in circulatory system
• Force of the heartbeat
• Age
• Sleep
• Weight
• Emotion
• Heredity
• Viscosity of blood
• Condition of blood vessels

On the Job

In some long-term facilities and other health care agencies, blood pressures are taken only by licensed or registered nurses. If this is true where you become employed, it would be wise to occasionally practice this procedure on a coworker or to ask the nurse if you could take the blood pressure of a resident under her supervision. You do not want to lose this skill in case you later seek employment elsewhere.

* **Depressants** (drugs that slow down body functions)
* Excessive loss of blood
* **Antihypertensives** (drugs that lower blood pressure in persons who have hypertension)

If the resident is resting, any reading between 60 and 90 diastolic (lower reading) is considered normal. Blood pressure rises slightly with age.

Hypertension is high blood pressure (greater than 140/90). Uncontrolled hypertension can lead to stroke, kidney disease, or heart damage.

Hypotension is low blood pressure (below 100/70). Excessive hypotension can lead to shock.

In either case, unusual or changed findings must be recorded and reported.

Blood Pressure Equipment

Blood pressure equipment includes the sphygmomanometer (Figure 19-25) and the stethoscope (Figure 19-26). The commonly used sphygmomanometer consists of a cuff with a rubber bladder inside with two tubes—one connected to the pressure control bulb and the other to the pressure gauge (see Figure 19-25). The gauge may be a round dial or a column of mercury. Both are marked in numbers. Be sure to use a cuff of the proper size. Cuffs that are too wide or too narrow for the arm will give inaccurate readings. The length of the bladder portion of the cuff should be about 80% of the circumference of the resident's arm.

How to Read the Gauge. The gauges are marked with a series of large lines at 10-mm (millimeter) intervals (Figure 19-27). In between the large lines are shorter lines, each of which indicates 2 mm. For example, the small line above 80 mm is 82 mm, and the small line below 80 mm is 78 mm. For accuracy, the gauge should be at eye level when reading. The mercury column gauge must not be tilted. The level of the top of the column of mercury or the pointer of the dial is taken for the reading. Two readings are recorded:

* **Systolic**—first sound heard. It represents the highest pressure in the arteries.
* **Diastolic**—the level at which sound stops. The smaller number indicates when this change in sound is heard.

The blood pressure is recorded as a fraction with the larger number on top. For example, 112/68 means:

* 112 is the systolic pressure
* 68 is the diastolic pressure

FIGURE 19-25 Types of sphygmomanometers: (Left) Mercury gravity sphygmomanometer; (Top, right) Dial (aneroid) sphygmomanometer; (Bottom, right) Electronic sphygmomanometer.

FIGURE 19-26 Stethoscope

FIGURE 19-27 The gauges are marked with a series of large lines at 10-mm (millimeter) intervals.

*G*uidelines for

Preparing to Measure Blood Pressure

Before using the stethoscope:

1. Clean the ear pieces with an alcohol wipe and clean the bell with a different alcohol wipe.
2. Point the ear pieces forward when inserting them in your ears.
3. Use the bell portion of the stethoscope (Figure 19-28).
4. Be sure the bell portion is open so you will hear the beats.

Before using a sphygmomanometer:

1. If using a mercury manometer—if the mercury moves up the column very slowly (Figure 19-29), it may have oxidized. Report this to the nurse and use another sphygmomanometer.
2. If using an aneroid manometer—make sure the needle is on zero before inflating the cuff (Figure 19-30). If it is not, report this to the nurse and use another sphygmomanometer.

   Turn off radio and television when taking blood pressure. Ask the resident not to talk. Do not take blood pressure on an arm that:

   • Has an intravenous feeding or other device inserted

   • Is being treated for burns, fractures, or other injuries

FIGURE 19-29 Do not use the sphygmomanometer if the mercury moves up the column very slowly.

FIGURE 19-28 Use the bell portion of the stethoscope when taking a blood pressure.

FIGURE 19-30 Make sure the needle is on zero before inflating the cuff of the aneroid manometer.

PROCEDURE

65   Taking Blood Pressure

1. Carry out each beginning procedure action.
2. Assemble equipment:
   - Sphygmomanometer with appropriate size cuff
   - Stethoscope
   - Alcohol wipes
3. Remove resident's arm from sleeve or roll sleeve 5 inches above elbow; it should not be tight or binding.
4. Locate the brachial artery with your fingers (Figure 19-31).
5. Place resident's arm palm upward, supported on bed or table. Resident should be comfortable.
6. Wrap the cuff smoothly and snugly around resident's arm. Center the bladder over the brachial artery. The bottom of the cuff should be 1 inch above the antecubital space (inner elbow) (Figure 19-32) and should cover about two-thirds of the upper arm.
7. Place the bulb in your dominant hand. In your other hand, place the bell portion of

FIGURE 19-32 The bottom of the cuff should be 1 inch above the antecubital space (inner elbow).

the stethoscope over the brachial artery where you previously located the pulse with your fingers (Figure 19-33).

- Inflate the cuff quickly to about 30 mm Hg above the level where pulse sounds disappear (Figure 19-34).
- Release the air slowly—about 2 to 3 mm Hg per second.
- Listen closely while keeping your eyes on the gauge. The *first* sound you hear is the *systolic pressure*. You will then hear a series of loud beats followed by a series of tapping sounds.
- The sounds then become muffled. After a few of these muffled beats, the sounds disappear. Note the number the needle on the gauge is pointing to between the muffling and the absence of sounds. This number is the *diastolic pressure*. Document both sounds: the point at which the sound becomes muffled and the point at which the sound ceases. The B/P might read 126/82/66

FIGURE 19-31 Locate the brachial artery with your fingers.

(continues)

PROCEDURE 65 *(continued)*

FIGURE 19-33 Place the stethoscope over the brachial artery.

8. Quickly deflate the cuff. If it is necessary to recheck the blood pressure, wait at least 15 to 30 seconds before reinflating the cuff.

FIGURE 19-34 Reinflate the cuff quickly and steadily to about 30 mm Hg above the level where pulse sounds disappear.

9. Clean the ear pieces of the stethoscope with alcohol wipes. Return equipment to appropriate area.
10. Carry out each procedure completion action.

On the Job

Some facilities require only a two-digit reading, for example: 136/88. Ask about your facility's procedure.

WEIGHING AND MEASURING THE RESIDENT

Maintaining a record of the height and weight of all residents is important for several reasons:

- Medication dosages may be calculated based on height and weight.
- Weight is monitored to determine if the resident is retaining fluid (edema).
- Weight indicates if the resident's nutritional intake is adequate.

Baseline (original) measurements are obtained on admission. Residents are weighed at least monthly thereafter. Some residents may need to be weighed more often.

Methods of Measurement

Height and weight may be measured using the metric system: centimeters for height and kilograms for weight. If your facility uses this method, the scales will be calibrated for the metric system. There is no need to convert from the inch and pound system to the metric system. There are several types of scales:

FIGURE 19-35 An upright scale is used only for residents who can stand unattended on the platform.

FIGURE 19-36 Electronic chair scales are used for residents in wheelchairs who cannot stand on an upright scale.

- An upright scale is used only for residents who can stand unattended on the platform (Figure 19-35).
- Chair scales are used for residents in wheelchairs who cannot stand on an upright scale (Figure 19-36).
- A mechanical lift with scale is used to weigh residents in bed who cannot stand on an upright scale and who cannot sit in a wheelchair (Figure 19-37).

Height is measured with the ruler attached to an upright scale or with a tape measure when the resident is in bed.

Obtaining Accurate Weights

To obtain an accurate measurement of weight, you must:

- Weigh the resident at the same time of day each time.
- Have the resident wear the same type of clothing each time.
- Use the same method and the same scale each time, if possible.

You must learn to read the scale correctly. There are two bars on the upright scale shown in Figure 19-35. The balance bar should hang free to start.

- The lower bar indicates weights in large 50-pound increments.
- The upper bar indicates smaller pound weights (Figure 19-38). The even-numbered pounds are marked with numbers.
- The long line between each number indicates the odd-numbered pounds.
- Each small line indicates one quarter of a pound, or 4 ounces.

The two figures are added and recorded as the person's total weight. The sum is recorded according to facility policy in either pounds or kilograms.

Large weight = 100 pounds
Small weight = +22 pounds
　　　Total = 122 pounds

Measuring the resident may be done during the weighing procedure with an upright scale. The information is recorded in feet and inches or in centimeters, according to facility policy.

Example:

A height measurement of 62 inches may be recorded as 62 inches, or 5 feet 2 inches or 155 cm.

FIGURE 19-37 A mechanical lift with scale is used to weigh residents in bed who cannot stand on the upright scale and cannot sit up in a wheelchair.

FIGURE 19-38 The upper bar indicates smaller pound weights. The weight shown on the lower bar is added to the weight shown on the upper bar.

PROCEDURE 66

Weighing and Measuring the Resident Using an Upright Scale

1. Carry out each beginning procedure action.
   Note: Use disposable gloves if there may be contact with open lesions, wet linens, or body fluids.
2. Check previous weight as documented. Then escort the resident to the scales.
3. Place a paper towel on the platform of the scale.
4. Be sure the weights are to the extreme left and the balance bar (bar with weight markings) hangs free.
   - The lower bar (large indicator) is calibrated (marked) in increments (amounts) of 50 pounds.
   - The upper bar (small indicator) is calibrated in increments of single pounds.
   - The even-numbered pounds are marked with numbers.
   - The long line between even numbers indicates the odd-numbered pounds.
   - Each small line indicates one quarter of a pound.
5. Assist the resident to remove shoes and step up onto the scale platform, facing the balance bar. The balance bar will rise to the top of the bar guide. The resident should not hold the bar or other parts of the scale.
6. Move the large weight to the right to the closest estimated resident weight.
7. Move the small weight to the right until the balance bar hangs freely halfway between the upper and lower bar guides.
8. Add the two figures and record the total as the resident's weight in pounds or kilograms, according to the type of scale used.

9. Assist the resident to turn on the platform until facing away from the balance bar. Raise the height bar until it is level with the top of the resident's head.
10. The reading is made at the movable point of the ruler (Figure 19-39).
11. Note the number of inches indicated. Record this information in inches ("), feet (') and inches ("), or centimeters (cm) according to the type of scale. The height shown in Figure 19-39 is 62 inches. This may be recorded as 62 inches or 5 feet 2 inches ($62 \div 12 = 5$ feet 2 inches). Record value on your note pad.
12. Assist the resident off the platform. Help resident to put on shoes, if necessary, and return to the room.
13. Carry out each procedure completion action.

FIGURE 19-39 The resident's height is read at the movable point of the ruler.

PROCEDURE 67

Measuring Weight with an Electronic Wheelchair Scale

1. Carry out each beginning procedure action.
2. Assemble equipment:
   - Wheelchair scale (Figure 19-40A)
3. Determine empty weight of wheelchair by weighing it on the scale.
4. Take wheelchair to resident's room. Help the resident into the wheelchair and take the resident to the electronic wheelchair scale.

5. Open metal ramp sides on scale to rest on floor. This allows wheelchair access to scale.
6. Press "on" button; scale zeros automatically (Figure 19-40B).
7. Roll wheelchair with resident onto platform of scale. Lock wheels of wheelchair.
8. Digital readout will show weight.
9. Record weight of resident and wheelchair. Subtract wheelchair weight to obtain resident weight.
10. Unlock wheels of wheelchair. Roll wheelchair with resident off scale.
11. Fold scale ramps back in place.
12. Carry out each procedure completion action.

FIGURE 19-40A Wheelchair scale

FIGURE 19-40B Press "on" button to zero scale automatically. (Courtesy of Scale-Tronix, White Plains, NY)

PROCEDURE 68 Weighing the Resident in a Chair Scale

1. Carry out each beginning procedure action.
2. Assemble equipment:
   - Chair scale
3. Take resident in wheelchair to chair scale.
4. Apply transfer belt to resident and assist in a pivot transfer to chair on scale. Instruct resident to sit down when the chair is felt against the back of the legs. Be sure resident's feet are on footrest of scale.
5. Walk behind the scale to obtain the reading.
6. Transfer resident back to wheelchair.
7. Carry out each procedure completion action.

PROCEDURE 69 Measuring and Weighing the Resident in Bed

1. Carry out each beginning procedure action.
2. Obtain assistance from coworker.
3. Assemble equipment:
   - Overbed scale
   - Tape measure
   - Pencil
4. Check scale sling and straps for frayed areas or poorly closing straps.
5. Lower side rail on your side. Make sure side rail is up on other side.
6. Fanfold top linen to foot of bed.
7. Position resident flat on back with arms and legs straight and body in good alignment.
8. Make a small pencil mark at the top of the resident's head on the sheet.
9. Make a second pencil mark even with the feet.
10. Using the tape measure, measure the distance between the two pencil marks.
11. Note this on a pad with resident's height in feet and inches.
12. Remove the scale sling from suspension straps and position half under the resident.
    - Turn the resident away from you.
    - Place the sling folded lengthwise under the resident.
    - Return resident to recumbent position and place sling so that the resident rests securely within it.
    - Attach sling to suspension straps. Check to be sure attachments are secure.
13. Position lift frame over bed with base legs in maximum open position and lock.
14. Elevate head of bed and bring resident to sitting position.
15. Attach suspension straps to frame. Position resident's arms inside straps.
16. Slowly raise sling so resident's body is free from bed. Be reassuring.
17. Guide the lift away from the bed so that no part of the resident touches the bed.
18. Balance scale according to manufacturer's instructions.
19. Take and note reading.
20. Reposition sling over center of bed.
21. Release knob slowly, lowering resident to bed.
22. Remove sling by reversing the process in step 12.
23. Assist resident to comfortable position.
24. Move overbed scale out of the way.
25. Replace top bed linen over resident. Raise side rail and lower bed to lowest horizontal height.
26. Carry out each procedure completion action.

RECORDING VITAL SIGNS

Temperature, pulse, and respiration (TPR), and height and weight values are recorded in a notebook and then transferred to the resident's chart (Figure 19-41) by a secretary or a nurse.

Bay Shore Convalescent Home
4782 Bay Shore Drive
Watertown, Mich.

Vital signs are to be checked on all residents once each day unless ordered otherwise.

Date 4/10/XX

Resident	Room	Temp.	Pulse	Resp.	B/P	Comments
Estrada, Luisa	101A					
Hartong, Mary	101B					
Diette, Marie	102A					
Aquino, Lucy	102B					
Ihli, Fred	103A					
Dyment, Frank	103B					
Lightfoot, Wm.	104A					
Lee, Sayo	104B					
Salcido, Rose	105A					
Tham, Peou	105B					
Wilde, Rose Marie	106A					
Hubbard, Marta	106B					
Lam, Lotruc	107A					
Uy, Aime	107B					
Valasco, Mary	108A					
Lobliner, Esther	108B					
	109A					
Moak, Loreta	109B					
Ocha, Vario	110A					
	110B					

FIGURE 19-41 Vital signs may be taken and recorded on the unit sheet and later transferred to the resident's record.

LESSON SYNTHESIS: Putting It All Together

You have just completed this lesson. Now go back and review the Clinical Focus. Try to see how the Clinical Focus relates to the concepts presented in the lesson. Then answer the following questions.

1. The physician has ordered that Mrs. Hoden be weighed daily. Why do you think this is important?

2. Which method would be the most appropriate for weighing Mrs. Hoden?

3. An apical/radial pulse is taken on Mrs. Hoden because she has a pulse deficit. What does this mean?

4. What type of respirations would you expect to note on Mrs. Hoden?

REVIEW

A. Select the one best answer for each of the following.

1. The term vital signs includes
   (A) height and weight
   (B) temperature, pulse, respirations, and blood pressure
   (C) temperature, pulse, and respirations
   (D) blood pressure

2. Temperature can be increased by
   (A) medications
   (B) shock
   (C) dehydration
   (D) cold weather

3. Oral temperatures should be taken on residents who are
   (A) confused and disoriented
   (B) on seizure precautions
   (C) unconscious
   (D) conscious

4. A temperature taken in the ear is called
   (A) oral
   (B) axillary
   (C) rectal
   (D) tympanic

5. The most accurate method of taking temperature is
   (A) oral
   (B) axillary
   (C) rectal
   (D) tympanic

6. The pulse is usually taken at which artery?
   (A) brachial
   (B) radial
   (C) femoral
   (D) carotid

7. The average pulse rate per minute for adult women is
   (A) 80–110
   (B) 60–70
   (C) 65–80
   (D) 75–100

8. Blood pressure can be decreased by
   (A) exercise
   (B) eating
   (C) emotional anxiety
   (D) resting

9. Medications prescribed to lower blood pressure are called
   (A) antihypertensives
   (B) stimulants
   (C) depressants
   (D) antibiotics

10. The first sound heard when taking blood pressure is called
    (A) diastolic
    (B) systolic
    (C) pulse pressure
    (D) apical

B. Match each term (items a.–j.) with the proper definition.

a. sphygmomano-
   meter
b. tachycardia
c. thermometer
d. volume
e. fasting

f. hypotension
g. bradycardia
h. hypertension
i. pulse deficit
j. rales

11. _____ low blood pressure

12. _____ fullness (amount)

13. _____ moist respirations

14. _____ not eating

15. _____ rapid heart rate

16. _____ slow heart rate

17. _____ used to determine blood pressure

18. _____ used to determine temperature

19. _____ high blood pressure

20. _____ difference between radial and apical pulse rates

C. Fill in the blanks by selecting the correct word or phrase from the list.

axillary
bradycardia
centimeters
cyanotic
dyspnea
expiration

rate
rectal
rhythm
sphygmomanometer
stethoscope
tachycardia

inspiration
kilograms
rales

vital signs
volume

21. Temperature, pulse, respiration, and blood pressure are: _____.

22. The instrument used to listen to the heart is a (an): _____.

23. The instrument used to measure blood pressure is a (an): _____.

24. A _____ temperature is usually 1° higher than an oral temperature.

25. An _____ temperature is usually 1° lower than an oral temperature.

26. In the metric system, height is measured in _____.

27. In the metric system, weight is measured in _____.

28. When taking a pulse, you should note _____, _____, _____.

29. A rapid pulse rate is called _____.

30. A slow pulse rate is called _____.

31. The two parts to each respiration are called _____ and _____.

32. The term _____ means a dusky, bluish color to the skin.

33. Moist respirations are called _____.

34. Labored breathing is called _____.

Admission, Transfer, and Discharge

Clinical Focus

Think about situations that require admission to, or transfer and discharge from, the long-term care facility as you study this lesson and meet:

Jack Tyler, 28 years old, who has multiple sclerosis. He is no longer able to care for himself and has made the decision to enter a long-term care facility.

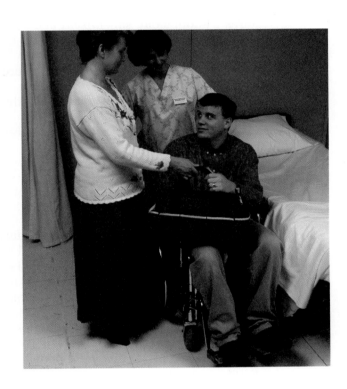

OBJECTIVES

After studying this lesson, you should be able to:

- Define and spell vocabulary words and terms.
- List reasons why residents are admitted to long-term care facilities.
- Describe the emotional reactions of the resident and the family to admission.
- Identify reasons why admission to a long-term care facility may be more difficult for a teenager or young adult.
- Identify the responsibilities of the nursing assistant related to admission procedures.
- List reasons why residents may be transferred out of the facility.
- Identify the responsibilities of the nursing assistant related to transfer procedures.
- List reasons why residents are discharged from long-term care facilities.
- Describe the actions involved in the discharge of a resident.
- Identify the responsibilities of the nursing assistant related to discharge procedures.
- Demonstrate the following:
  Procedure 70 Admitting the Resident
  Procedure 71 Transferring the Resident
  Procedure 72 Discharging the Resident

VOCABULARY

community services *(kom-MYOUN-ih-tee SIR-vih-sez)*

diagnosis-related group (DRG) *(die-ag-NOS-is ree-LAY-ted groop)*

discharge planner *(DIS-charj PLAN-er)*

discharge planning *(DIS-charj PLAN-ing)*

kidney dialysis *(KID-nee die-AL-ih-sis)*

personal inventory *(PER-son-al IN-ven-tor-ee)*

ADMITTING THE RESIDENT

Reasons for Admission

A resident may be admitted to a long-term care facility because the individual:

- Requires 24-hour-a-day supervision and nursing care
- Requires specialized treatments
- Requires rehabilitation services before returning home
- Has a progressive, chronic disease that requires more care
- Has Alzheimer's disease or another dementia and can no longer be cared for at home

The resident may be admitted from

- An acute care hospital
- Home
- Another extended care facility

There may be varying circumstances surrounding the admission. Some residents are admitted to the hospital for emergencies requiring immediate care. An example of this would be a person who fell and broke a hip or the person who had a stroke. The individual can stay in the hospital for a limited number of days according to the **diagnosis-related group (DRG)** that covers the person's diagnosis. At the end of this time most people are not yet ready to care for themselves. The **discharge planner** (the person who arranges care after discharge from the hospital) may arrange for home care or for the person to be admitted to a long-term care facility until the person is more independent. In these situations the family and resident may need to make a quick decision about placement (Figure 20-1).

Some residents are admitted because they have Alzheimer's disease or another dementia. These diseases are progressive and eventually require 24-hour-a-day supervision. Most families do not have the energy or resources to cope with the situation at home. Other chronic diseases such as Parkinson's disease or multiple sclerosis may progress to the point that the individual is unable to perform the activities of daily living without maximal assistance.

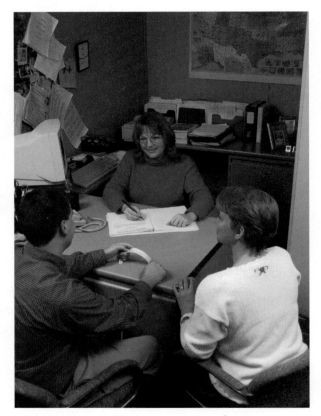

FIGURE 20-1 In some cases, a decision about a long-term care facility may have to be made in a hurry.

In some situations, residents require specialized care because they need:

- Artificial ventilation to breathe
- **Kidney dialysis** (treatment when kidneys fail)
- Complicated wound care
- Rehabilitation services

Anxiety About Admission

Some admissions are considered permanent, which means the resident will live in the facility for the rest of his life. Other admissions are temporary and the resident will eventually be discharged.

The new resident who is considered a permanent admission probably has experienced many losses. Admission means a further loss of independence. He or she may have lost a spouse and now, along with failing strength and health, the comfort and security of familiar surroundings is about to be lost. Families often feel guilty because the family member cannot be provided for at home. They may also be physically and emotionally exhausted from giving care for several years before this admission. Burdens also may be intensified by the financial costs of admission. Residents who need to apply for Medicaid usually feel embarrassed because they cannot pay their own way.

Both the family and the new resident will feel uncertain about and somewhat fearful of the new environment. They will need support and encouragement. Their anxiety may make it difficult for them to remember things that you explain to them. Be prepared to repeat statements. Reassure them that their feelings are natural and help them express these feelings. Make their first impression of you and the facility a positive one.

The admission of a teenager or young adult to the long-term care facility is very difficult, especially if it is considered a permanent admission. The illness of a family member affects every person in the family. The young person as well as the parents may be devastated to learn that the child will not be able to experience the privileges of adulthood. The individual will not be a part of the peer community that is so vital to teenage development. As you complete your admission responsibilities, remember how difficult this process is for both the resident and the family.

Preadmission Activities

Arranging for admission to a long-term care facility involves many activities that occur before the resident arrives. The family is often responsible for participating in these procedures, especially if the resident is in the hospital. The family will need to:

- Choose (with the resident's input if possible) a facility
- Meet with someone from the Social Services Department to arrange for the admission
- Apply for Medicaid, if necessary, to pay for the cost of services

If the resident is coming from a hospital, the discharge planner at the hospital will need to:

- Confirm admission with the Social Services Department of the facility to be sure a bed is available and that the facility can provide the care and treatment the person needs

- Complete transfer forms to ensure continuity of care
- Arrange for the resident's transfer (usually by ambulance) from the hospital to the facility

The Social Services Department staff of the receiving facility will need to:

- Meet with the discharge planner to determine what services are needed. The social worker may visit the resident to make an initial assessment.
- Meet with the nursing staff of the receiving facility to determine if special equipment, such as traction, will be needed
- Meet with the family (and resident if possible) to explain the facility's services and the responsibilities of the family and resident
- Explain and provide a copy of the Residents' Rights to family and resident
- Determine the method of payment for services
- Inform appropriate departments of the resident's pending admission and the services that will be needed
- Inform any residents who may be sharing the room of the new resident's arrival

In-service meetings or training for the staff may be needed if the resident has an unusual diagnosis, requires special treatment, or needs special equipment.

Day of Admission

On the day of admission, you may be expected to check the room to be sure it is ready for the new resident's arrival.

- Check the room lights to be sure they are working.
- Check the call light to be sure it is working. Attach it to the bed.
- Check bed controls and attach them to the bed.
- Check the bed for clean sheets, a pillow, and a spread. Lock the wheels of the bed. Place the bed in lowest position.
- Check the telephone for a dial tone.
- Move the overbed table, if necessary, so it is not in the way.
- Place a pitcher and glass on the bedside table. Wait to fill the pitcher with fresh water until the resident arrives.
- Place personal care items in the bedside table. In the top drawer place:
  - Emesis basin
  - Toothbrush and toothpaste
  - Mouthwash
  - Lotion
  In the middle drawer place:
  - Wash basin
  - Soap in soap dish

In the bottom drawer place:
- Bedpan
- Toilet tissue
- Urinal if resident is male

Note: The arrangement of items may be different for each facility. Remember that "dirty" items such as bedpans and urinals should not be placed with clean items like the wash basin and toothbrush.

- Check the resident's bathroom for:
  - Cleanliness
  - Soap in soap dispenser
  - Paper towels in dispenser
  - Towels and washcloths for the resident
  - Toilet tissue
- Check dresser drawers for cleanliness.
- Check the closet for hangers.

The bed may be opened (top covers folded to end of bed) or left closed depending on the condition of the resident. The nurse or the unit secretary will set up a chart, care plan, and other forms to be used on admission.

Admission Assessments

The members of the interdisciplinary health care team will each make an assessment of the new resident (Figure 20-2). This includes the Minimum Data Set (MDS) 2.0 form required by OBRA and other assessments required by the facility. This information will be used to start the plan of care.

Meeting the New Resident

First impressions are important. Remember that this is a new and strange experience for the resident and family. Someone from the facility is designated to meet the resident and family and

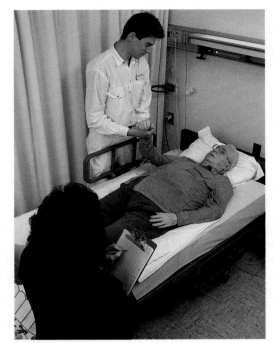

FIGURE 20-2 Each member of the interdisciplinary team will make an assessment of the new resident.

to accompany them to the assigned room. The social worker or nurse may be responsible for this procedure.

The resident's first impression is a lasting one. Your appearance and your attitude will set the tone for the resident's opinion of the facility.

Responsibilities of the Nursing Assistant

The nurse and social worker need to complete a number of procedures once the resident is in the room. At the appropriate time you will need to complete the nursing assistant's part of the admission procedure.

In most facilities the social worker or nurse will inform the resident and family about:

- Facility rules such as limitations on smoking
- Visiting periods
- Availability of services and activities

The resident (if possible) and the family will be taken on a tour of the building so they know the location of:

- Stairs and elevators
- Dining room
- Activity areas
- Visiting areas outside the resident's room
- Offices of administrative staff
- Public telephones

BUILDING CULTURAL AWARENESS

Remember that persons from different cultural groups may respond differently to admission and health care procedures. Consider issues of personal space, touching, and eye contact. Members of some cultures may have beliefs about nature and the cause of illness and types of health care practices that differ from yours.

PROCEDURE
70 Admitting the Resident

1. Wash hands and assemble equipment:
   - Urine specimen container
   - Equipment for taking temperature
   - Worksheet for recording information
   - Stethoscope
   - Sphygmomanometer
   - Watch with second hand
   - Appropriate scales
2. Prepare unit as described earlier in this chapter, if that has not yet been done.
3. Identify the resident both by asking the name and checking the identification bracelet.
4. Introduce yourself.
5. Help the resident undress if instructed by the nurse to do so. If resident will remain dressed, have the resident sit in a chair.
6. Show the resident how to use the call light.
7. Help the resident unpack. Hang up clothing or place it in the dresser drawers.
8. Set up personal items such as photographs, plants, religious articles (Figure 20-3).
9. Fill the pitcher with fresh water and ice (if appropriate).
10. Take the resident's vital signs.
11. Obtain the resident's height and weight.
12. Collect a urine specimen if instructed to do so.

FIGURE 20-3   The nursing assistant can help the new resident set up personal items.

13. Show the resident and family how to operate equipment such as electric bed, telephone, and television.
14. Carry out each procedure completion action.

- Public restrooms
- Rehabilitation services areas

You should be familiar with this information so you can accurately answer any questions the resident may have later.

Completing a Personal Inventory

A **personal inventory** is completed for every resident who is admitted. This is a special form that lists and describes all items the resident brings to the facility (Figure 20-4). All items must be labeled with the resident's name. Follow the facility policy for this procedure. This task may be completed by the nurse, the unit secretary, the nursing assistant, or housekeeping staff.

The personal inventory includes:

- All items of clothing
- Jewelry, including wedding rings and watches
- Personal equipment such as razors, combs, brushes
- Religious items such as bibles, rosaries
- Books, magazines, plants, photographs, afghan, quilt
- Furniture such as a chair, dresser, television
- Assistive devices: glasses, dentures, hearing aid(s), cane, walker

Form 883/2   BRIGGS, Des Moines, Iowa 50306
PRINTED IN U.S.A.

INVENTORY LIST

QTY.	ARTICLES	QTY.	APPLIANCES	QTY.	PROSTHETIC DEVICES	ACQUIRED AFTER ADMISSION	
						Date	Item
	Belts		T.V. - Ser. #:		Dentures: ☐ Upper		
	Blouses		Radio - Ser. #:		☐ Lower ☐ Partial		
	Coats		Hair Dryer		Eye Wear		
	Dresses		Electric Razor		Cane		
	Gloves				Walker - Ser. #:		
	Hats				W/chair - Ser. #:		
	Housecoats - Robes		JEWELRY		Brace		
	Jackets		Ring (Describe)				
	Nightgowns - Pajamas						
	Purses		Watch (Describe)		OTHER		
	Shaving Kit						
	Shoes		Other				
	Shorts						
	Slacks						
	Slippers						
	Slips		FURNITURE				
	Socks/Hose						
	Suitcases						
	Suits				VALUABLES RELEASED FROM SAFE		
	Sweaters						
	Ties						
	Undershirts						
	Underwear						

(Left margin label: ON DISCHARGE)

I received on discharge in satisfactory condition the above articles and a copy of this list.
Disposition of belongings: _____

▶ _____ _____   ▶ _____ _____
Signature of Patient/Resp. Party   Date   Signature of Facility Representative   Date

NOTE ▶ Patient/Responsible Party is responsible for assuring that all personal belongings are properly marked. All items brought in after admission are added to this inventory at the request of Patient/Responsible Party.

QTY.	ARTICLES	QTY.	APPLIANCES	QTY.	PROSTHETIC DEVICES	ACQUIRED AFTER ADMISSION	
						Date	Item
1	Belts (black)		T.V. - Ser. #:		Dentures: ☐ Upper		
2	~~Blouses~~ Shirts (polo)		Radio - Ser. #:		☐ Lower ☐ Partial		
	Coats	1	Hair Dryer		Eye Wear		
	Dresses		Electric Razor		Cane		
	Gloves				Walker - Ser. #:		
	Hats				W/chair - Ser. #:		
1	~~Housecoats~~ - Robes (red)		JEWELRY		Brace		
	Jackets	1	Ring (Describe)				
	Nightgowns - Pajamas		Yellow metal wedding band				
	Purses	1	Watch (Describe)		OTHER		
	Shaving Kit		Timex silver metal	1	Bible		
1 pr	Shoes (black laced)		Other	8	handkerchiefs, white		
	Shorts						
2	Slacks (knit, black, grey)						
1 pr	Slippers (brown felt)						
	Slips		FURNITURE				
6 pr	Socks/~~Hose~~ (black)						
	Suitcases						
	Suits				VALUABLES LOCKED IN SAFE		
	Sweaters						
	Ties						
6	Undershirts (white T)						
6	Underwear (white jockey)						

(Left margin label: ON ADMISSION)

I certify that this is a correct list of my clothes and belongings which I wish to retain in my possession and for which I take ENTIRE RESPONSIBILITY. I have received a copy of this list.

▶ *Joseph Cervanti*   1/25/2002   ▶ *Della Sheeling*   1/25/2002
Signature of Patient/Resp. Party   Date   Signature of Facility Representative   Date

If the patient is unable to sign, state reason: _____
▶ Signature of Witness: _____

PATIENT NAME—LAST	FIRST	MIDDLE	HOSP. NO.	ROOM NO.
Cervanti	Joseph	—		203B

Form 883/2 BRIGGS, Des Moines, Iowa 50306
PRINTED IN U.S.A.

INVENTORY LIST

FIGURE 20-4 The personal inventory lists and describes all items that the resident brings into the facility. (Reprinted with permission of Briggs Corporation, Des Moines, IA 50306; 800-247-2343)

The items listed are also described. Be careful in your descriptions. For example, do not describe a ring as a "diamond in a gold setting." The correct description is "clear stone in a yellow metal setting." This is done because the staff is not qualified to determine whether the stone is a diamond or whether it is glass. After the inventory is completed, sign the form. The resident or a family member also signs the form. Residents are discouraged from keeping large sums of money or valuable items in their rooms. Facilities are required to provide accounts for residents so they can deposit and withdraw money as it is needed. Other valuable items can be placed in the facility safe.

Helping the Resident Adapt to the Facility

Remember that living in the long-term care facility is a very different experience for the resident. It will take the resident time to adapt to the environment, the routine, and the caregivers. Some residents may have a temporary period of confusion and disorientation until they become familiar with the facility. Residents may feel overwhelmed by the amount of information they are expected to remember. Be patient in repeating and reinforcing the information.

Introduce the resident to other residents and caregivers. Take time to talk with new residents so they feel safe and secure in their new home. Fire drills and other routine procedures may be frightening. Explain what is happening and guide the resident through the process. If the new admission is a teenager or young adult, be sure to introduce him or her to other residents in the same age group.

Welcome the family and consider them members of the care team. Follow your facility policies regarding such issues as:

- Family members taking residents outside the facility
- Family members feeding residents or providing other types of care

TRANSFERRING THE RESIDENT

There are two types of resident transfers:

- Within the facility, transferring the resident from one room or nursing unit to another
- Outside the facility to another health care agency

There are several reasons why a resident may be transferred within the facility:

- The resident's condition changes, requiring a different level of care
- Residents in the same room do not get along
- Resident requests a different room

When a transfer within the facility occurs, all items go with the resident to the new room or unit (Figure 20-5).

- Clothing and all personal items belonging to the resident
- Items in the bedside stand
- Chart, care plan, other medical records, and medications if resident is moving to another unit
- Medications

A resident may be transferred out of the facility to another health care agency because the resident needs:

- The services of an acute care hospital
- Evaluation and treatment for psychiatric problems

If the resident is transferred outside the facility, personal possessions, medical records, and personal care items remain in the facility. The only item that goes with the resident is a transfer record. The transfer record contains information for the receiving facility (Figure 20-6).

FIGURE 20-5 All items go with the resident when she is transferred to another room in the same facility.

Comp.#1874 Page 1, Film 1, One Color, Punches on Left

SUGGESTIONS FOR COMPLETING FORM
1. The purpose of this form is to insure continuity of care in transfer from a skilled care facility to an acute care facility or another skilled care facility.
2. The form is not intended to supply information of long-term nature.
3. Original should accompany resident with transfer. Carbon copy should be retained in resident's record.

INSTRUCTIONS:
This form has two sides. After completing front side, pull out carbon; turn form over; reinsert carbon face down. When writing, press firmly.

RESIDENT TRANSFER FORM
(INTER-AGENCY REFERRAL)
(Reference tags: F203 - F205)

RESIDENT'S LAST NAME	FIRST NAME	MI	SEX ☐M ☐F	SOCIAL SECURITY NUMBER

RESIDENT'S ADDRESS (Street, City, State, Zip)	DATE OF BIRTH	RELIGION

DATE OF THIS TRANSFER	FACILITY NAME AND ADDRESS TRANSFERRING TO	PHYSICIAN IN CHARGE AT TIME OF TRANSFER

Will this physician care for resident after admission to new facility? ☐ YES ☐ NO

DATES OF STAY AT FACILITY TRANSFERRING FROM
ADMISSION   DISCHARGE

PAYMENT SOURCE FOR CHARGES TO RESIDENT
A. ☐ SELF OR FAMILY
B. ☐ PRIVATE INSURANCE
C. ☐ BLUE CROSS BLUE SHIELD
D. ☐ EMPLOYER OR UNION
E. ☐ PUBLIC AGENCY (Give name)
F. ☐ OTHER (Explain)

NAME AND ADDRESS OF FACILITY TRANSFERRING FROM

NAME AND ADDRESSES OF ALL HOSPITALS AND EXTENDED CARE FACILITIES FROM WHICH RESIDENT WAS DISCHARGED IN PAST 60 DAYS.

CLINIC APPOINTMENT SCHEDULED	DATE	TIME	☐ CLINIC APPOINTMENT CARD ATTACHED	DATE OF LAST PHYSICAL EXAMINATION	DATE OF LAST BOWEL MOVEMENT

RELATIVE OR GUARDIAN (Name, Address, Phone Number, Relationship to Resident)	WAS THIS PERSON NOTIFIED REGARDING THIS TRANSFER? ☐ YES ☐ NO	WAS THIS PERSON (OR WAS THE RESIDENT) GIVEN INFORMATION ON HOW TO CONTACT THE STATE OMBUDSMAN? ☐ YES ☐ NO

DIAGNOSES AT TIME OF TRANSFER

(a) PRIMARY

EMPLOYMENT RELATED: ☐ YES ☐ NO

(b) SECONDARY

VITALS AT TIME OF TRANSFER: Ht. _____ Wt. _____

T _____ P _____ R _____ B/P _____

REASON FOR TRANSFER

CHECK ALL THAT APPLY

DISABILITIES
☐ Amputation
☐ Paralysis
☐ Contracture(s)
☐ Pressure Ulcer

INCONTINENCE
☐ Bladder
☐ Bowel
☐ Saliva

IMPAIRMENTS
☐ Mental
☐ Speech
☐ Hearing
☐ Vision
☐ Sensation

ACTIVITY TOLERANCE LIMITATIONS
☐ None ☐ Moderate ☐ Severe

RESIDENT KNOWS DIAGNOSIS?
☐ Yes ☐ No

POTENTIAL FOR REHABILITATION
☐ Good ☐ Fair ☐ Poor

DIET, DRUGS, AND OTHER THERAPY
at Time of Discharge

Diet Order:
Therapy:

Current Medications	Strength & Frequency	Time Last Dose	Amt. Sent

IMPORTANT MEDICAL INFORMATION
(State allergies if any)

☐ May **NOT** use generic substitutes
*(Physician or nurse must sign below - See verification of meds.)

ADVANCE DIRECTIVES
☐ Yes ☐ Attached ☐ None

BED HOLD POLICY
Given to resident ☐ Yes ☐ No
Attached ☐ Yes ☐ No, reason:

TB Test   Date _____ Type _____ Result _____
Chest X-Ray Date _____ Result _____
C.B.C.   Date _____ Result _____
Biochem   Date _____ Result _____
Urinalysis   Date _____ Result _____

SUGGESTIONS FOR ACTIVE CARE

BED

Position in good body alignment and
change position every_____ hrs.
Avoid _____ position.
Prone position _____ times/day as tolerated.

SITTING

_____ hr(s)._____ times/day.

WEIGHT BEARING
☐ Full ☐ Partial ☐ None
on _____ leg.

EXERCISES
Range of motion _____ times/day
to _____ by
☐ resident ☐ nurse ☐ family.
Stand_____ minutes_____ times/day.

LOCOMOTION
Walk _____ times/day.
(distance)   (no.)

SOCIAL ACTIVITIES
Encourage: (☐ group ☐ individual) activities
(☐ within ☐ outside) home.

Transportation: ☐ Ambulance ☐ Car
☐ Car for handicapped ☐ Bus

VERIFICATION OF MEDS
*Signature of Physician or Nurse X _____   Date __/__/__

CFS 2-4/2P © 1992 Briggs Corporation, Des Moines, IA 50306 (800) 247-2343
R195   Printed in U.S.A.

RESIDENT TRANSFER FORM
☐ Continued on Reverse

FIGURE 20-6 The transfer record goes with the resident from one facility to the next. (Reprinted with permission of Briggs Corporation, Des Moines, IA 50306; 800-247-2343) *(continues)*

Comp.#1874 Page 2, Film 1, One Color, Backer

RESIDENT TRANSFER FORM (continued)

SELF CARE STATUS
(Check level of ability. Write S in space if needs supervision only. Draw line across if inapplicable.)

		Independent	Needs Assistance	Unable To Do
Bed Activity	Turns			
	Sits			
Personal Hygiene	Face, Hair, Arms			
	Trunk & Perineum			
	Lower Extremities			
	Bladder Program			
	Bowel Program			
Dressing	Upper Extremities			
	Trunk			
	Lower Extremities			
	Appliance, Splint			
Feeding				
Transfer	Sitting			
	Standing			
	Tub			
	Toilet			
Loco-motion	Wheelchair			
	Walking			
	Stairs			

BED ☐ Low   Mattress: ☐ Firm ☐ Reg.

Other _____

Side Rails: ☐ Yes ☐ No

BEHAVIOR ☐ Cooperative ☐ Oriented X_____

☐ Disruptive ☐ Belligerent ☐ Combative

☐ Senile ☐ Suspicious ☐ Withdrawn

MENTAL STATUS

☐ Alert ☐ Forgetful ☐ Confused

COMMUNICATION ABILITY	Yes	No
Able to make needs known		
Can speak		
Can hear		
Can write		
Understands speaking		
Understands writing		
Understands gestures		
Understands English		

If no, state language spoken or understood: _____

_____

DIET

☐ Regular ☐ Low Salt ☐ Diabetic ☐ Bland

☐ Low Residue ☐ Other _____

☐ Feeds Self ☐ Needs Help

☐ Partial Assist ☐ Total Assist

RESIDENT USES

☐ Appliance

☐ Catheter (date of last change____ /____ /____

☐ Colostomy ☐ Cane ☐ Crutches ☐ Prosthesis

☐ Walker ☐ Chair ☐ Hearing Aid

☐ Dentures (Specify _____)

OTHER EQUIPMENT

ADDITIONAL PERTINENT INFORMATION
(Explain necessary details of care, diagnosis, medications, treatments, prognosis, teaching, habits, preferences, etc. Therapists and social workers add signature and title to notes.)

SOCIAL INFORMATION
(Adjustment to disability, emotional support from family, motivation for self-care, socializing ability, financial plan, family health problem, etc.)

PERSON COMPLETING THIS FORM: Signature/Title _____   Date ____ /____ /____

RESIDENT TRANSFER FORM

FIGURE 20-6 *(continued)*

PROCEDURE 71

Transferring the Resident

1. Find out if the resident is to be transferred within the facility or out of the facility.
2. If within the facility, find out if the resident will be moved by wheelchair or in the bed.
3. If out of the facility, find out if the resident will be taken to the exit by wheelchair to a car or if the resident will be transferred by ambulance.
4. Carry out each beginning procedure action.
5. For transfer within the facility, the following items will be moved with the resident:
   - Resident's belongings
   - Personal care items from bedside table
   - Supplies or equipment used for resident's care
   - Medical records, care plan, and medications (if moving to another unit)
6. Help resident dress if necessary.
7. Move resident to new unit as indicated.
8. Help resident get settled in new room.
9. Introduce resident to staff and other residents.
10. Tell the resident good-bye and wish him well.
11. Carry out each procedure completion action.

If resident is being transferred out of facility:

1. If resident is going by car, make sure the resident is well groomed and dressed appropriately for the weather, then assist into wheelchair and take to exit. Assist in transferring into car.
2. If resident is going by ambulance, follow nurse's instructions.
3. The nurse will give appropriate records and transfer form to family or ambulance drivers.
4. Tell the resident good-bye.
5. Carry out each procedure completion action.

DISCHARGING THE RESIDENT

Discharging of residents from the long-term care facility has become a common occurrence. Residents are discharged because they:

- Have improved enough to go home
- Do not need the high-level services of the facility but can function in a less restrictive environment such as an assisted living facility
- Require care that can be provided by another long-term care facility

The discharge procedure is usually simple if the resident is going to another facility. The social worker and nurse relay information to the receiving facility. The resident's belongings are sent to the new facility.

Discharge to the resident's home is more complicated and requires a number of actions called **discharge planning**. Discharge planning is a cooperative procedure that involves all members of the interdisciplinary health care team. The social worker is the coordinator for discharge planning and is responsible for arranging for **community services**. Community services may include intermittent services of a:

1. Registered nurse for ongoing assessment, monitoring, supervision of other caregivers, planning of care, teaching, and implementation of treatments
2. Home health aide for personal care including bathing, positioning, passive range of motion exercises, taking vital signs, and doing simple treatments
3. Rehabilitation staff for physical therapy, occupational therapy, and speech therapy
4. Homemaker for completing routine household chores such as light cleaning, laundry, cooking, and grocery shopping
5. Home-delivered meals. These are delivered for the noon meal and meet the nutritional requirements of the resident. Meals for persons on diabetic, low-salt, low-fat, and low-cholesterol diets can usually be arranged.

PROCEDURE
72 · Discharging the Resident

1. Check with the nurse to be sure the resident has an order to be discharged.
2. Carry out each beginning procedure action.
3. Collect equipment:
   - Wheelchair
   - Cart to transport items to exit
4. Help the resident to dress if necessary.
5. Collect the resident's personal belongings.
   - Check them against the admission inventory list.
   - Help resident pack.
   - Check bathroom, closets, dressers, and bedside table for overlooked items.
6. Check with nurse to see if there are other items such as records, unused supplies, or medications that will go home with the resident.
7. Help resident into wheelchair and take resident to exit.
   - Help resident transfer into car.
   - Be sure all items go with resident.
   - Be gracious as you say good-bye.
8. Return wheelchair.
9. Return to resident's room.
   - Strip bed. Dispose of soiled linens.
   - Discard disposable items.
10. Notify housekeeping so room can be cleaned.
11. Record discharge according to facility policy.
    - Time
    - Method of transport
    - Person(s) accompanying resident
    - Resident's reaction
    - Signature
12. Report completion of procedure to nurse.

Factors to Consider Before Discharge

Before discharge planning proceeds, the interdisciplinary team must consider several factors:

1. Does the resident have the potential to regain enough independence to go home?
2. Is there a person (spouse, family member, or friend) willing to serve as a liaison (go-between) for the resident when he or she goes home? The person living alone will usually need someone to call or check on him, run errands, help with money management, and oversee the household management.
3. Are adequate community services available? If the resident needs continuing physical therapy, for example, there must be an agency that provides this service. In some areas of the country there are not enough therapists to meet the demand.
4. Does the resident need 24-hour-a-day supervision or care? Medicare and private insurance will not pay for this type of care. Most people could not afford to pay for it themselves. (Continuous care may cost several hundreds of dollars per day.)
5. Will the structure of the resident's home allow the resident to function adequately and safely? For example, is there a bedroom and bathroom on the same floor?

These factors are especially critical if the resident will be living alone. If the resident, the family, and the care team determine that discharge is a reasonable expectation, then planning proceeds.

1. The interdisciplinary team will prepare a discharge plan of care. This plan provides information to the resident and caregivers (family, friends, or community service providers) on how to help the resident maintain health (Figure 20-7).
2. The social worker arranges for the community services.
3. The physical therapist or a rehabilitation nurse may take the resident home for a short visit to evaluate the resident's ability to function in the home setting. The therapist will make recommendations, if necessary, that may include:
   - Rearranging rooms (for example turning the living room into the bedroom)

Comp.#1872 Page 1, Film 1, One Color, Punches on Left

POST-DISCHARGE PLAN OF CARE
(Reference tags: F203, F204; Cross reference tags: F157, F284)

The following discharge information is to help you maintain your health and independence.

You are being discharged : ☐ home ☐ to a residential care facility (see facility name and address below).

Facility _____ Phone _____

Address _____ City/State/Zip _____

THE FOLLOWING COMMUNITY RESOURCES ARE AVAILABLE TO MEET YOUR INDIVIDUAL NEEDS ▶

State Ombudsman _____ Phone _____

Address _____ City/State/Zip _____

Visiting Nurse _____ Phone _____

Address _____ City/State/Zip _____

Other Agency _____ Phone _____

Address _____ City/State/Zip _____

COMMUNITY RESOURCES AND SERVICES PLANNING ▶

Nursing needs: _____

Personal care: _____

Transportation: _____

Meals: _____

Housekeeping: _____

Social support/Family system/Special requests: _____

Financial status/needs: _____

Financial access/Payment for services: _____

Therapy services: _____

Other: _____

Person completing this section: _____ / _____ / _____
Signature and title   Date

SCHEDULED APPOINTMENTS ▶

Appointment With	Date	Purpose	Telephone

NAME—Last	First	Middle	Attending Physician	Chart No.

CFS 2-2/2P © 1992 Briggs Corporation, Des Moines, IA 50306 (800) 247-2343
Printed in U.S.A.

POST-DISCHARGE PLAN OF CARE
☐ Continued on Reverse

FIGURE 20-7 Care plan for the resident who is to be discharged home. (Reprinted with permission of Briggs Corporation, Des Moines, IA 50306; 800-247-2343) *(continues)*

Comp.#1872 Page 2, Film 1, One Color

POST-DISCHARGE PLAN OF CARE (continued)

DIETARY AND NUTRITIONAL NEEDS ▶

Suggested food/fluids: _____

Special instructions: _____

Avoid: _____

☐ Copy of diet given   ☐ Diet explained to resident/caregiver   ☐ Restrictions explained (if applicable)

Person completing this section _____   ___/___/___
Signature and title   *Date*

ACTIVITIES AND LEISURE PURSUITS ▶

Suggested activities: ☐ T.V./Movies   ☐ Radio   ☐ Reading   ☐ Senior Center   ☐ Talking books

☐ Volunteer Work   ☐ Other_____

Special instructions: _____

Activities to avoid: _____

Person completing this section _____   ___/___/___
Signature and title   *Date*

MEDICATIONS ▶

Medication	Dose and Frequency	Purpose and Special Instructions	Amount Sent With Resident	Prescription Sent With Resident	Prescription Called To Pharmacy

Person completing this section _____   ___/___/___
Signature and title   *Date*

WOUND CARE, TREATMENTS, THERAPY ▶ Procedures you should do

Procedure	Purpose	Frequency

Person completing this section _____   ___/___/___
Signature and title   *Date*

IMPORTANT NAMES AND PHONE NUMBERS ▶

Physician _____   Phone _____
Name and address

Pharmacy _____   Phone _____
Name and address

These discharge instructions have been reviewed with me in a language I understand. All questions have been answered to my satisfaction. I have received the medications or written prescriptions as indicated above.

Signature **X**_____   ___/___/___
Resident / Caregiver   *Date*

Please contact us if you have further questions.

Facility_____   Telephone _____

NAME—Last	First	Middle	Attending Physician	Chart No.

POST-DISCHARGE PLAN OF CARE

FIGURE 20-7 *(continued)*

- Building a ramp from the outside entrance
- Installing a telephone that is accessible to the resident
- Renting equipment such as a seat for the shower or tub
- Suggesting safety measures, such as the removal of throw rugs and electrical cords on the floor

4. The interdisciplinary health care team will determine what the resident and family need to learn before discharge and who will be responsible for teaching. Some examples follow. Not all residents need all of these, and some residents will need teaching not included here.

- The physical therapist will teach the resident how to transfer in and out of bed, how to ambulate with an artificial leg (prosthesis), how to walk up and down stairs (Figure 20-8).
- The occupational therapist will teach the resident how to dress and undress, how

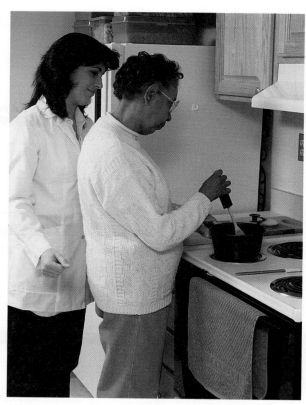

FIGURE 20-9 The occupational therapist teaches the resident how to manage the activities of daily living before she goes home.

FIGURE 20-8 The physical therapist teaches the resident how to go up and down stairs in preparation for going home.

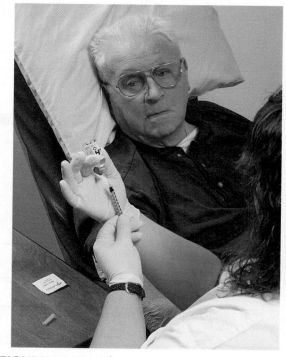

FIGURE 20-10 The nurse teaches the resident how to inject his insulin.

to use the telephone, or how to cook (Figure 20-9).

5. The dietitian will teach the resident and family the basics of planning and preparing diabetic meals.

6. The nursing staff will teach the resident how to give his own insulin (Figure 20-10), how to check his blood sugar, how to

recognize signs and symptoms of complications, or how to change a colostomy or wound dressings.

A discharge date will be arranged and all members of the team, including the resident and family, will strive to meet the goals that will enable the resident to return home.

LESSON SYNTHESIS: Putting It All Together

*Y*ou have just completed this lesson. Now go back and review the Clinical Focus. Try to see how the Clinical Focus relates to the concepts presented in the lesson. Then answer the following questions.

1. Would you expect Mr. Tyler to feel anxiety on admission to the long-term care facility? What is a likely reason for this anxiety? How may the interdisciplinary team help Mr. Tyler to overcome this anxiety?

2. How can you make him feel more comfortable and secure in his new environment?

3. What information would you want to learn about Mr. Tyler's present condition? How will you do this?

4. How will the nursing staff use the information that you obtain in formulating a care plan that is appropriate for this resident?

REVIEW

A. Select the one best answer for each of the following.

1. Most residents are admitted to long-term care facilities because
   (A) their families no longer want to deal with them
   (B) the resident no longer wants the responsibility of keeping up a home
   (C) the resident is tired and needs rest
   (D) the resident requires health care services

2. Residents admitted to long-term care facilities may need all but
   (A) specialized treatments
   (B) 24-hour-a-day care and supervision
   (C) rehabilitation services
   (D) laundry services

3. The length of hospital stays for acute illness is limited because
   (A) of staff shortages
   (B) of the inconvenience to the family
   (C) of diagnosis-related groups
   (D) the resident wants to go home

4. Before admission, the family will need to
   (A). choose a facility if the resident is unable to do so
   (B) draw the resident's money out of the bank
   (C) sell the resident's home
   (D) try to care for the resident at home

5. The members of the interdisciplinary health care team will obtain assessments of new residents for the purpose of
   (A) starting the plan of care
   (B) keeping the resident busy

(C) making the family think the staff is attentive

(D) determining the cost of the resident's stay

6. When a new resident is admitted, the nursing assistant will do all but
   (A) take the resident's vital signs
   (B) weigh and measure the resident
   (C) help the resident put away personal possessions
   (D) charge the resident for the care

7. When a resident is transferred from one nursing unit to another within the facility, the nursing assistant will
   (A) move the resident's belongings to the new room
   (B) give the resident any medication that is due before moving
   (C) call the resident's family for permission before moving the resident
   (D) move all the furniture in the room to the new room

8. Residents may be discharged because they
   (A) have improved enough to go home
   (B) have complained to the administrator
   (C) want special items for breakfast every day
   (D) are difficult to care for

9. Community services include all but
   (A) services of a registered nurse
   (B) home-delivered meals
   (C) services of a home health aide
   (D) taking the resident to the movies

10. Community services are usually coordinated and arranged for by the
    (A) administrator
    (B) family
    (C) director of nursing
    (D) social worker

11. A young adult may be admitted to a long-term care facility for all of the following reasons except
    (A) a chronic disease such as multiple sclerosis

(B) injuries received in an accident
(C) a need for 24-hour nursing care
(D) violations of the law

B. Answer each statement true (T) or false (F).

12. T F The discharge planner selects the long-term care facility for patients who need that service.

13. T F The family may need to apply for Medicaid if the resident has exhausted his funds.

14. T F Copies of the Residents' Rights are only given to residents who are able to read and understand them.

15. T F The physician makes out the personal inventory after the resident is admitted.

16. T F Residents are advised not to bring any personal possessions with them to the long-term care facility.

17. T F A resident may be transferred to another room because of friction between roommates.

18. T F Some admissions to long-term care facilities are considered permanent.

19. T F Families are discouraged from visiting residents.

20. T F Most families have concerns about admitting a family member to a long-term care facility.

21. T F First impressions of the family and resident are extremely important.

Warm and Cold Applications

Clinical Focus

Think about the reasons for warm and cold applications and the safety precautions to observe when they are carried out as you study this lesson and meet:

*M*rs. Lipskin, who is assigned to your care. She tires easily and is returned to her bed for rest in the afternoon. As she was getting into bed, she slipped and hit her forearm against the side of the bed. To counteract pain and swelling from the injury, a disposable cold pack is ordered and applied to her arm.

OBJECTIVES

After studying this lesson, you should be able to:

- Define and spell vocabulary words and terms.
- State the effects of warm and cold applications.
- Give reasons why warm and cold applications may be ordered.
- Describe precautions in carrying out warm and cold application procedures.
- Demonstrate the following:
    Procedure 73 Applying an Aquamatic K-Pad®
    Procedure 74 Applying a Disposable Cold Pack
    Procedure 75 Applying an Ice Bag
    Procedure 76 Assisting with the Application of a Hypothermia Blanket

VOCABULARY

Aquamatic K-Pad® (*ack-kwah-MAT-ick KAY-pad*)

asepto syringe (*ay-SEP-toh sih-RINJ*)

diathermy (*DIE-ah-ther-mee*)

hypothermia (*high-poh-THER-mee-ah*)

ice bag (*ise bag*)

thermal blanket (*THER-mal BLAN-kit*)

vasoconstriction (*vas-oh-kon-STRICK-shun*)

vasodilation (*vas-oh-die-LAY-shun*)

warm soak (*warm sohk*)

wet compress (*wet KOM-press*)

Warm and cold applications require a physician's order. Some facilities permit only licensed care providers to perform warm and cold applications. In other facilities, nursing assistants are permitted to carry out these procedures under the supervision of the nurse. All warm and cold applications must be performed carefully to prevent injury to the resident. *Be sure you know and follow the policy of your facility and are adequately prepared and supervised.*

Older people have less sensitivity to changes in temperature. They may not realize when an application is too hot or cold. If the temperature is too high, burns may result. Other types of tissue damage may occur if the temperature is too cold. Warm and cold applications that are left on too long can also cause damage.

SAFETY

The older resident has less sensitivity to pain and is at greater risk for injury. *Note: Heat is especially dangerous.* When using warm or cold applications on older residents, it is very important that you:

- Frequently check the area that is being treated.
- Report unusual changes. You should check for excessive redness, blanching (whitening), or other discoloration. Report any complaints of discomfort or pain.
- Do not rely on the resident's ability to inform you of any problems; check carefully yourself. The resident may not be aware that a problem exists.
- Follow facility policy for discontinuing the treatment.

Applications of warm and cold may be either moist or dry (Figure 21-1). Moisture makes both heat and cold more penetrating. Therefore,

---

FIGURE 21-1 Warm and cold applications

Dry Warm Applications
Aquamatic K-Pad®
Disposable warm pack

Moist Warm Applications
Warm soaks
Compresses
Tub bath
Sitz bath

Dry Cold Applications
Ice cap
Ice bag
Disposable cold pack
Aquamatic K-Pad®
Hypothermia blanket

Moist Cold Applications
Compresses
Soaks

---

moist heat or moist cold is more likely to cause injury. Extra care must be taken to protect the resident when moist treatments are used. Be sure you know:

- Exact method to be used
- Correct temperature and placement
- Proper length of time the warm or cold application is to be performed
- How often to check the area being treated

COMMERCIAL PREPARATIONS

Easy-to-use commercial warm and cold packs are available for dry applications. For one type of pack, a single blow to the pack before application activates the heat or cold. The pack is discarded after one use.

Reusable packs are also available, but infection control issues make them less desirable.

USE OF WARM APPLICATIONS

Warm applications are ordered to:

- Relieve muscle spasms
- Reduce pain
- Promote healing
- Combat local infection
- Improve mobility before exercise periods
- Soothe the resident

The value of heat treatments (**diathermy**) lies in the fact that heat dilates or increases the size of blood vessels (**vasodilation**). This brings more blood to the area to promote healing. Warmth is very soothing when there is pain.

There must be a specific order for a warm application. Some groups of people require extra care when they receive warm applications (Figure 21-2).

Cautions

Follow these cautions when working with residents.

- Constant warmth must be carefully monitored.
- Moisture intensifies the effect of warmth. Use extra caution.
- Never allow a resident to lie on a constant heat unit, because heat may be trapped and build up to dangerous levels.
- Temperature of a constant heat unit should be between 95° and 100°F.

FIGURE 21-2   Use caution when applying warm and cold treatments.

Caution: Consider the age and condition of the resident when using warm or cold treatments.

Proceed with caution with:
- Elderly residents
- Uncooperative residents
- Unconscious residents
- Paralyzed residents
- Residents with tissue damage
- Residents with poor circulation

- Always use a bath thermometer to check solution temperatures.
- Always remove the body part being soaked before adding warm solution.
- Always stay with the resident during the treatment.
- Protect areas not being treated from excessive exposure.
- Warmth is not applied to the head because it could cause blood vessels in the area to dilate, resulting in headaches.
- Rubber or plastic should never touch the resident's skin. Be sure all appliances are covered with cloth.

Dry Warm Applications

The **Aquamatic K-Pad®** is commonly used to provide dry warmth. It consists of a plastic pad with fluid-filled coils and a control unit that maintains a constant temperature of the fluid.

The fluid in the pad is distilled water that is supplied from a reservoir in the control unit. The control unit is placed on the bedside stand and is plugged into an electrical outlet. In most facilities, the temperature is preset by the central supply department. The temperature is usually set at 95° to 100°F. See Procedure 73.

Moist Warm Applications

Remember: Moisture intensifies heat and you must use extra care. For each of the warm treatments, follow the facility policy for:

- Method of applying the treatment
- Length of time treatment is to be applied
- How often resident is to be checked for condition of skin in the treatment area and general response to the treatment
- Signs that treatment should be discontinued

Moist warm treatments include:

- **Warm soaks**—The resident, or the part of the resident's body that is being treated, is immersed in a tub filled with water at a specific temperature, usually 105°.

On the Job

The resident who has back pain cannot benefit from an Aqua K-Pad® that is lying on the floor.

Applying an
Aquamatic K-Pad®

1. Carry out each beginning procedure action.
2. Assemble equipment:
   - K-Pad® and control unit
   - Distilled water
   - Covering for pad
3. Check the cord for frayed or damaged insulation. Also check that the tubing between the control unit and the pad is intact.
4. Place the control unit on the bedside stand (Figure 21-3).
5. Remove the cover of the control unit and check the level of the distilled water. If it is low, fill the unit two-thirds full or to the fill line using distilled water. Tilt the unit back and forth gently to clear the tubing of air.
6. Screw the cover in place and loosen it one-quarter turn.
7. If the temperature was not preset, check with the nurse for the proper setting before turning on the unit. Remove the key after setting the temperature.
8. Plug in the unit.
9. Cover pad with an appropriate cover, according to facility policy or as specified by the manufacturer of the unit. Do not use pins to hold the cover in place.
10. Expose the area of the resident to be treated. Place the covered pad on the resident and note the time.

    - Be sure the tubing between the control unit and the pad does not hang over the side of the bed. It should be coiled on the bed to promote the flow of liquid.

FIGURE 21-3 The disposable Aquamatic K-Pad® and control unit (reusable) maintain an even temperature.

11. Following facility policy, periodically check the skin under the pad.
12. Check the level of the water in the control unit. Refill if necessary to the fill line.
13. Remove the pad after the prescribed amount of time.
14. Carry out each procedure completion action.

- **Wet compresses**—Wet compresses are moistened with a solution and placed on the affected area.
    - An **asepto syringe** may be used to add water to the compresses to keep them moist.

- The compresses can be kept warm by covering them with an Aquamatic K-Pad®.
- Each time the pad is removed and replaced, be careful to reposition the protective covering.

USE OF COLD APPLICATIONS

Applications of cold are given only with a physician's order. The application of cold:

- Constricts or decreases the size of blood vessels (**vasoconstriction**) and reduces swelling
- Decreases sensitivity to pain
- Reduces temperature
- Slows inflammation
- Reduces itching

Cautions

Remember, moisture intensifies the effect of cold just as it does heat. Caution must be used in the application of moist cold.

- Excessive cold can damage body tissues.
- Report color changes such as blanching (turning white) or cyanosis (becoming bluish).
- Report feelings of numbness or discomfort experienced by resident.
- Stop the cold treatment if shivering develops. Cover resident with blanket and report immediately to the nurse. Cold applications may be dry or moist.

Dry Cold Applications

Several methods exist for applying therapeutic cold. For the elderly, careful attention to the application is required to prevent injury.

- **Disposable cold pack**—This single-use commercial pack can be stored until needed. Reusable commercial packs are also available (for both warm and cold applications). The pack remains effective for approximately 15 to 30 minutes. If the cold pack must be activated, follow the manufacturer's instructions exactly. When activating the pack, do not hold it in front of your face. If a leak occurs, the chemicals inside the pack may splash. Check the area being treated every 10 minutes.
- **Ice bag**—This reusable waterproof canvas container can be filled with ice to provide temporary local cold. An ice bag is never placed directly on the affected area because the weight of the bag will cause the resident discomfort.
- **Thermal blanket**—This is a large, fluid-filled blanket that is placed over or around the resident. The temperature of the fluid in the blanket may be raised or lowered. The blanket is

---

PROCEDURE 74 Applying a Disposable Cold Pack

1. Carry out each beginning procedure action.
2. Assemble equipment:
   - Disposable commercial cold pack
   - Cloth covering (towel, warm water bag cover, or other cover specified by the facility)
   - Tape or rolls of gauze
3. Expose area to be treated. Note condition of area.
4. Place cold pack in cloth covering.
5. Strike or squeeze cold pack to activate chemicals. (Follow manufacturer's instructions.)
6. Place covered cold pack on proper area and cover with a towel (Figure 21-4). Note time of application.

FIGURE 21-4 Once the cold pack is in place, cover the entire application with a towel.

(continues)

PROCEDURE 74 *(continued)*

7. Secure cover with tape or gauze, if necessary, to hold in place.
8. Leave resident in comfortable position with signal cord within easy reach.
9. Return to bedside every 10 minutes. Check area being treated for discoloration or numbness. If these signs and symptoms occur, discontinue treatment and report them to your supervisor.
10. If no adverse symptoms occur, remove pack in 30 minutes, or after amount of time given in your instructions. Note condition of area. Continuous treatment requires application of a fresh pack.
11. Remove pack from cover and discard according to facility policy. Return unused gauze and tape.
12. Put cover in laundry hamper.
13. Carry out each procedure completion action.

PROCEDURE 75 Applying an Ice Bag

1. Carry out each beginning procedure action.
2. Assemble equipment:
   - Ice bag
   - Cover (usually cotton, such as a towel, or cover specified by your facility)
   - Paper towels
   - Spoon or similar utensil
   - Ice cubes or crushed ice
3. Prepare ice bag as follows:
   a. Fill ice bag with cold water and check for leaks.
   b. Empty the bag.
   c. If ice cubes are used, rinse them in water to remove sharp edges. The use of crushed ice gives more flexibility to the bag and is more comfortable for the resident.
   d. Fill ice bag half full, using ice scooper, paper cup, or large spoon (Figure 21-5). Avoid making ice bags too heavy. Do not allow scoop to touch ice bag.
   e. To remove air from ice bag:
      - Rest ice bag flat on a paper towel on a flat surface.
      - Put top in place, but do not screw on.
      - Press bag until air is removed.

FIGURE 21-5 Fill ice bag half full.

   f. Fasten top securely.
   g. Test for leakage.
   h. Wipe dry with paper towels. Place in cloth cover.

Note: As an alternative, a gel pack stored in the freezer can be used for cold applications. These packs can be refrozen and reused if this is the facility policy.

4. Apply ice bag to the affected part.
5. Refill ice bag before all ice is melted.
6. Check skin area under the ice bag every 10 minutes. Report to supervising nurse

(continues)

PROCEDURE 75 *(continued)*

immediately if skin is discolored or white or if resident reports skin is numb.

7. Continue the cold application for the amount of time specified by your supervisor. If the resident feels cold, cover with a blanket, but do not cover the area being treated.
8. Carry out each procedure completion action.
9. When the treatment is complete. wash the bag with soap and water, rinse,

dry completely, and then screw top on. Wipe with a disinfectant if this is your facility policy. Leave air in ice bag to prevent sides from sticking together.
10. If a reusable cold pack is used, wash it thoroughly with soap and water or wipe with a disinfectant, according to facility policy. Return pack to the refrigerator. Discard a disposable pack.

PROCEDURE 76 Assisting with the Application of a Hypothermia Blanket

Note: Applying a hypothermia blanket and monitoring a resident receiving a hypothermia treatment is a professional nursing responsibility. The nurse will supervise the procedure and monitor the resident throughout the treatment. The nurse will check the specific gravity of the resident's urine, vital signs, and nervous system response. The nursing assistant may be asked to assist in setting up equipment, positioning the resident and the thermal blanket, observing the resident during the treatment, and keeping the resident comfortable. In addition, the nursing assistant may be asked to transport equipment to and from the central supply service.

1. Wash hands, collect equipment, and take equipment to bedside.
2. Assemble equipment:
   - Disposable gloves
   - Hyperthermia/hypothermia control unit
   - Fluid for control unit
   - Thermometer probes (rectal or skin)
   - Adhesive tape
   - Sphygmomanometer
   - Stethoscope

   - Hyperthermia/hypothermia blanket (disposable or reusable), one or two as ordered
   - Bath blanket or sheet, one or two as ordered
   - Lanolin-based skin cream
3. Follow manufacturer's directions for setting up the equipment. Check equipment for safety. Be sure the control unit is grounded.
4. Connect blanket(s) to control unit and set control.
5. Turn on control unit and add liquid.
6. Allow blanket(s) to precool as you prepare resident.
7. Carry out each beginning procedure action.
8. Place resident in hospital-type gown with ties.
9. Measure vital signs and record.
10. Place hyperthermia/hypothermia blanket on bed and cover with sheet. Position resident on the sheet-covered thermal blanket in the recumbent position, with head on pillow that does not touch blanket.
11. Wash hands. Put on gloves.

(continues)

PROCEDURE *76* *(continued)*

12. Insert rectal thermometer probe into rectum (unless contraindicated) and tape in place. (Alternatively, place skin probe into axilla and secure in place with tape.)
13. Plug end of probe into proper jack on control panel.
14. Place second sheet over resident and place second thermal blanket over sheet, if ordered.
15. Apply lanolin-based cream to resident's skin where it contacts the blanket.
16. Remove gloves. Discard according to facility policy. Wash hands.
17. Monitor vital signs, neurologic response, and intake and output every 5 minutes until desired body temperature is reached, and then every 15 minutes as ordered.
18. Report color changes in skin or excessive shivering.
19. Resident should be repositioned every 30 minutes to 1 hour. Reapply skin cream as necessary. Covering sheets should be changed if they become moist. Put on gloves each time you care for resident. At the end of care, remove gloves, discard according to facility policy, and wash hands.
20. At completion of treatment, follow manufacturer's instructions for turning off unit, disconnecting blanket(s), and returning to storage.
21. Put on gloves. Continue to monitor resident as you remove the equipment.
22. Replace any damp bedding or garments and cover resident. Continue to monitor resident every 30 minutes for 2 hours or until stable, whichever is longer.
23. Clean thermometer probe and store according to facility policy.
24. Remove gloves and discard according to facility policy.
25. Carry out each procedure completion action.

used to lower or raise the resident's body temperature. However, it is most often used in care facilities to lower the body temperature. This process is called **hypothermia**. A licensed professional usually monitors the use of this type of blanket.

Moist Cold Application

- **Wet compresses**—The same cautions apply to cold as to warm compresses. They may be kept wet with an asepto syringe and cold by placing a covered ice bag against the area that is affected.

   Follow facility policy for:
- Method of applying the treatment
- Length of time treatment is to be applied
- How often resident is to be checked for condition of skin in the treatment area and general response to the treatment
- Signs that treatment should be discontinued

LESSON SYNTHESIS: Putting It All Together

You have just completed this lesson. Now go back and review the Clinical Focus. Try to see how the Clinical Focus relates to the concepts presented in the lesson. Then answer the following questions.

1. How was the disposable cold pack activated?

2. How might it have been secured in place?

3. Is the pack placed directly on the area of the body to be treated?

4. How often should you check the area in contact with the pack?

5. What signs or symptoms should be reported to the nurse during the treatment?

REVIEW

A. Write the definition for each of the following terms.

1. diathermy

2. hypothermia

3. vasoconstriction

4. vasodilation

5. ice bag

B. Answer each statement true (T) or false (F).

6. T F Warm and cold treatments are part of the job description for all nursing assistants.

7. T F The elderly are usually more sensitive to warm and cold treatments.

8. T F A physician's order is required for all warm and cold applications.

9. T F Moisture increases the effect of both warm and cold treatments.

10. T F Heat may be applied to the head because it causes vasoconstriction and relieves headache.

11. T F All heat or cold appliances must be covered with cloth so that rubber or plastic never touches the skin.

12. T F Residents should not be left alone when receiving a heat treatment.

13. T F Always place a filled ice bag on top of the area being treated.

C. Select the one best answer for each of the following.

14. Which resident is at greatest risk for injury during a heat treatment?
    (A) resident who is conscious
    (B) resident who is cooperative
    (C) resident who is paralyzed
    (D) resident who has warm pink skin

15. The control unit of the Aquamatic K-Pad® is filled
    (A) to the top
    (B) ⅔ full
    (C) ½ full
    (D) ¾ full

16. The tubes of the Aquamatic K-Pad®
should be
(A) allowed to hang below bed level
(B) coiled on the bedside stand
(C) pinned to the headboard of the bed
(D) coiled on the bed

17. The highest temperature an Aquamatic
K-Pad® should be set at is
(A) 100°F
(B) 98°F
(C) 95°F
(D) 110°F

18. Ice bags are
(A) filled to the top
(B) partially filled with air before
adding ice
(C) filled with the largest ice cubes
(D) tested for leaks before filling

D. Clinical Situations

19. Mrs. Maupin has an order for an
Aquamatic K-Pad® to be applied
for back pain. Shauna, the nursing
assistant, notes that her lower back
has become discolored and is more
painful. What action should Shauna
take?

20. Shauna's supervisor tells her to apply
cold to Mrs. Bronson's injured ankle.
Shauna replies that she needs more
information to give proper care to
Mrs. Bronson. What information does
Shauna need?

SECTION 7

Introduction to Restorative Care

LESSONS

22 Restorative/
Rehabilitative Care
of the Resident

23 Restoring Residents'
Mobility

Restorative/Rehabilitative Care of the Resident

Clinical Focus

Think about the care you would give to residents with disorders for which restorative care is appropriate as you study this lesson and meet:

*M*rs. Murphy, who was admitted to the facility while you were on your day off. She is 5 feet, 9 inches tall, with a heavy frame. She is 78 years old and had a stroke 2 months ago. She is unable to use her left arm or leg. Mrs. Murphy is relearning mobility skills and how to perform the activities of daily living. You are assigned to care for her and must assist her in these tasks.

OBJECTIVES

After studying this lesson, you should be able to:

- Define and spell vocabulary words and terms.
- List the complications associated with inactivity.
- Describe the reasons why some residents have self-care deficits.
- Describe the principles of restorative care.
- Explain the benefits of restorative care.
- Describe the responsibilities of the nursing assistant for implementing restorative care.
- State the guidelines for doing passive range of motion exercises.
- State the guidelines for positioning residents in bed and chair.
- Describe the purpose of an orthosis.
- List the reasons for implementing bowel and bladder programs.
- Describe the responsibilities of the nursing assistant for implementing bowel and bladder programs.
- Use correct body mechanics in carrying out all procedures in this lesson.
- Demonstrate the following:
  Procedure 77 Passive Range of Motion Exercises
  Procedure 78 Moving the Resident in Bed
  Procedure 79 Turning the Resident to the Side

OBJECTIVES

Procedure 80 Logrolling the Resident onto the Side
Procedure 81 Supine Position
Procedure 82 Semisupine or Tilt Position
Procedure 83 Lateral (Side-Lying) Position
Procedure 84 Lateral Position on the Affected Side
Procedure 85 Semiprone Position
Procedure 86 Fowler's Position
Procedure 87 Chair Positioning
Procedure 88 Repositioning a Resident in a Wheelchair
Procedure 89 Wheelchair Activities to Relieve Pressure
Procedure 90 Assisting with Independent Bed Movement

VOCABULARY

active assistive range of motion (*ACK-tiv ah-SIS-tiv rainj of MOH-shun*)

active range of motion (*ACK-tiv rainj of MOH-shun*)

activities of daily living (ADL) (*ack-TIV-ih-tees of DAY-lee LIV-ing*)

adaptive devices (*ah-DAP-tiv dih-VICE-es*)

amputation (*am-pyou-TAY-shun*)

arthritis (*are-THRIGH-tis*)

atrophy (*AT-roh-fee*)

body alignment (*BAH-dee ah-LINE-ment*)

chronic disease (*KRON-ick dih-ZEEZ*)

contracture (*kon-TRACK-shur*)

deconditioned (*dee-kon-DISH-und*)

disability (*dis-ah-BILL-ih-tee*)

dislocation (*dis-loh-KAY-shun*)

disorientation (*dis-oh-ree-en-TAY-shun*)

embolus (*EM-boh-lus*)

flaccid (*FLASS-id*)

footboard (*FOOT-bord*)

functional ability (*FUNK-shun-al ah-BILL-ih tee*)

goniometer (*gah-nee-AH-meh-ter*)

hemiplegia (*hem-ee-PLEE-jee-ah*)

incontinence (*in-KON-tin-ens*)

instrumental activities of daily living (IADL) (*in-strew-MEN-tal ack-TIV-ih-tees of DAY-lee LIV-ing*)

interdisciplinary health care team (*in-ter-DISS-ih-plin-air-ee helth kair teem*)

lateral (*LAT-er-al*)

mobility skills (*moh-BILL-ih-tee skills*)

orthosis (*or-THOH-sis*)

osteoporosis (*oss-tee-oh-poh-ROH-sis*)

paralysis (*pah-RAL-ih-sis*)

paraplegia (*pair-ah-PLEE-jee-ah*)

passive range of motion (*PASS-iv rainj of MOH-shun*)

perceptual deficit (*per-SEP-tyou-al DEF-ih-sit*)

pneumonia (*new-MOH-nee-ah*)

postural support (*POS-chur-al sup-PORT*)

pressure ulcer (*PRESH-ur UL-sir*)

progressive mobilization (*proh-GRESS-iv moh-bill-ih-ZAY-shun*)

prone (*prohn*)

protraction (*proh-TRACK-shun*)

quadriplegia (*kwahd-rih-PLEE-jee-ah*)

rehabilitation (*ree-hah-bill-ih-TAY-shun*)

residual limb (*rih-ZID-you-al lim*)

restorative care (*ree-STOR-ah-tiv kair*)

retraction (*ree-TRACK-shun*)

self range of motion (*self rainj of MOH-shun*)

sensory deprivation (*SEN-soh-ree deh-prih-VAY-shun*)

sensory stimulation (*SEN-soh-ree stim-you-LAY-shun*)

shearing (*SHEER-ing*)

sling (*sling*)

spasticity (*spas-TIS-ih-tee*)

splint (*splint*)

strengths (*strenths*)

subluxation (*sub-luck-SAY-shun*)

supine (*SOO-pine*)

task segmentation (*task seg-men-TAY-shun*)

thrombus (*THROM-bus*)

turning sheet (*TURN-ing sheet*)

RESTORATIVE CARE AND THE INTERDISCIPLINARY HEALTH CARE TEAM

Restorative care is a process in which the **interdisciplinary health care team** assists the resident to reach an optimal level of ability.

Several sections of OBRA refer to restorative care. The Residents' Rights state that the residents' independence must be promoted. The section on nursing assistant training requires that all nursing assistant courses include basic restorative skills. These include:

- Training of the resident in self-care according to the resident's abilities
- Assisting residents in transferring, ambulating, eating, and dressing
- Maintenance of range of motion
- Proper turning and positioning in bed and chair
- Bowel and bladder training
- Care and use of prostheses and orthoses

The Minimum Data Set (MDS) 2.0 includes a section on physical functioning and structural problems (Figure 22-1). The nurse is responsible for collecting these data, but the nursing assistants can provide valuable information about the resident's abilities.

Restorative care and rehabilitation are similar and in many cases identical. Some of the differences are that:

- **Rehabilitation** involves the skills of therapists including any or all of these individuals: physical therapist, occupational therapist, speech/language pathologist.
- Rehabilitation is more intense and is time-limited. That means the resident is working harder to meet a goal with a definite time limit. Medicare covers the cost of the therapists' services for a specified period of time.
- Rehabilitation nurses coordinate the care and services of the residents in rehabilitation programs. They work with the therapists to see that the programs are carried out consistently 24 hours a day.

FIGURE 22-1 Physical functioning and structural problems are evaluated on the MDS 2.0. (Courtesy of the Health Care Finance Administration. Reprinted with permission of Briggs Corporation, Des Moines, IA 50306; 800-247-2343)

- Rehabilitation is a specialized health care service. Many skilled care facilities now employ full-time therapists and other rehabilitation staff to meet the needs of residents. As a nursing assistant, you may be given additional training to work with the professionals in the rehabilitation department.
- Restorative care is a nursing responsibility with assistance from other members of the interdisciplinary health care team. Nurses assess the residents and plan restorative programs. The nursing assistants implement the programs.

Restorative care is successful when members of the team:

- Have a positive attitude about the residents and their capabilities
- Have confidence in their own abilities as care providers
- Are willing to learn from other care providers, residents, and their families
- Learn to think creatively to increase residents' quality of life
- Cooperate with other staff as team members
- Realize that "ideal" working situations seldom exist, but attempt to bring "ideal" and "real" closer together
- Continually learn and acquire new skills by participating in educational programs

PURPOSES OF RESTORATIVE/ REHABILITATIVE CARE

All nursing care should be considered restorative care. The interdisciplinary health care team is concerned with:

- Increasing the resident's physical abilities. This may include **mobility skills** (the ability to move from one place to another) and the ability to care for oneself (Figure 22-2)
- Preventing complications that result from mental and physical inactivity
- Maintaining the resident's current abilities
- Helping the resident adapt to limitations imposed by a **disability** (the inability to perform certain activities because of a physical or mental impairment)
- Increasing the resident's quality of life

Most of the residents receiving rehabilitation will be discharged from the facility. Some of the residents receiving restorative care will also be able to go home.

Some of the residents living in long-term care facilities will never be able to return to their

FIGURE 22-2 This resident is using an adaptive device to increase her independence.

homes. For this reason, the staff may feel it is pointless to try to improve their abilities.

When residents are admitted to long-term care facilities, "good care" does not mean that the health care providers will do everything for the residents. In a short period of time, this approach will result in residents becoming helpless. In other words:

- Residents are stripped of all motivation for independence. They have no reason to act independently.
- Muscles weaken, circulation slows down, and all body systems gradually lose the ability to function. Both mind and body deteriorate.
- When residents are placed in positions of dependency, they also lose their self-esteem. They no longer see themselves as people of value.
- Residents become disinterested in what is happening around them. Life has little meaning.

People need hope and quality in their lives, even when they are living with a **chronic disease** (a disease or condition that is permanent). If residents are forced to be dependent and are not allowed to make decisions, then there is little reason for living.

Restorative care provides hope and quality by empowering the resident, that is, encouraging and allowing the resident to be as independent as possible. There may be reasons why some residents really cannot do things for themselves. In these cases, the team must do for residents what they are unable to do for themselves. However, the residents should still be allowed to make decisions regarding their care. If residents are no longer mentally competent to make decisions, the team will be responsible for all aspects of their care.

Principles for Restorative/ Rehabilitative Care

The following principles provide the foundation for restorative care:

1. **Begin treatment as soon as possible.** This means that plans for maintaining or increasing the resident's level of independence are made as soon as the resident is admitted to the facility.
2. **Stress the resident's ability, not disability.** The resident's **strengths** are used to help the resident adapt to any limitations. This means that care providers think in terms of what the resident can do, not what the resident cannot do.

3. **Activity strengthens and inactivity weakens.** Complications result from physical and mental inactivity. These can cause further disability or even be life-threatening.
4. **Treat the whole person.** It is important to attend to the residents' emotional and mental health needs as well as their physical well-being. The interdisciplinary team also works with the residents' families. Families directly influence the emotional and mental health of the residents.

PREVENTING COMPLICATIONS FROM INACTIVITY

Restorative/rehabilitative care attempts to prevent the complications that result from inactivity. These complications can affect elderly people more quickly than younger people because of the changes that are taking place in their bodies. Refer to Table 22-1 for a summary of possible complications and preventive nursing assistant actions.

TABLE 22-1 Complications Resulting from Inactivity	
Complications by Body System	**Prevention**
Musculoskeletal System	
• Muscles become weak and **atrophy**. This means that muscles that are not used shrink and become useless.	• Carry out exercise programs planned for the residents' capabilities.
• **Contractures** can develop, making movement impossible. The joints become stiff when they are not moved. In a short time the tissue around the joints also stiffens. Soon the joint cannot be moved at all (Figure 22-3).	• Do range of motion exercises. • Use correct positioning techniques. • Use splints and other devices to maintain the proper joint position.

FIGURE 22-3 Contractures are a complication of immobility.

(continues)

TABLE 22-1 Complications Resulting from Inactivity *(continued)*

Complications by Body System	Prevention
Musculoskeletal System • **Osteoporosis** develops with nonuse. When the legs do not bear weight, calcium begins to leave the bones and enter the bloodstream. This causes brittle bones; fractures may occur without reason.	• Offer the resident opportunities to stand and bear weight on the legs, for example, during transfer procedures.
Integumentary System • **Pressure ulcers** develop over pressure areas. If a resident sits or lies in one spot, blood cannot circulate to that area. The cells in the skin and tissue begin to die, causing an ulcer to develop (Figure 22-4). 	• Reposition the resident every 1 or 2 hours. • Do range of motion exercises twice a day. • Provide adequate nutrition and fluids. **FIGURE 22-4** Pressure ulcers are also a complication of immobility.
Cardiovascular System • The heart becomes **deconditioned**. The heart is a muscle and weakens when the body is inactive. In its weakened state, the heart takes longer to return to a normal pace after activity. If this happens, the resident must rest between physical activities. • Blood does not circulate as efficiently. This can lead to **embolus** and **thrombus**. A thrombus is a blood clot that forms in a blood vessel. If the thrombus breaks loose and moves through the circulatory system, it is called an embolus.	• Follow all instructions for assisting the resident with ambulation (walking) and exercise programs. • Follow all instructions for ambulation and exercise.
Respiratory System • The lungs do not expand as efficiently when a resident is immobile. Secretions collect in the lungs and bacteria grow in the secretions, causing **pneumonia**, an infection of the lungs.	• Provide the resident with fluids to drink. • Position the resident so the lungs can expand. • Encourage the resident to take deep breaths. *(continues)*

TABLE 22-1 Complications Resulting from Inactivity (continued)

Complications by Body System	Prevention
Gastrointestinal System • Without exercise or activity, the appetite decreases, causing weight loss. • Risk of pressure ulcers increases with weight loss and lack of nutrition. • Peristalsis slows down, causing indigestion and constipation (the inability to move the bowels).	• Tell the nurse if the resident likes or dislikes certain foods. • Encourage resident to drink adequate fluids. • Assist the resident with ambulation and exercise. • Assist the resident to develop a bowel elimination schedule. Provide privacy for toileting.
Urinary System • The bladder does not always empty completely if a person is not able to sit properly on the toilet or commode. This increases the risk of bladder infection. • Incontinence can result from inability to get to the bathroom. • Urinary stones may develop from the calcium in the bloodstream resulting from osteoporosis.	• Encourage adequate fluid intake. • Assist the resident to the toilet regularly and provide privacy.
Psychosocial Reactions • Depression can occur from physical and mental inactivity. Depression is an emotional condition that causes the resident to be slow, unresponsive, and sad. • Inactivity and **sensory deprivation** can lead to **disorientation**. Sensory deprivation occurs when there is a lack of stimulation to the senses—vision, hearing, smelling, tasting, and touching. A person who is disoriented is confused about time, place, and who he or she is.	• Cooperate with activities department to provide **sensory stimulation** programs. These are activities that increase the resident's awareness of the surroundings.

ACTIVITIES OF DAILY LIVING

One purpose of restorative care is to increase the resident's physical abilities. This includes mobility skills and the ability to carry out **activities of daily living (ADL)**. These are the tasks that adults do throughout a day to meet their basic needs. The ADL are:

• Bathing
• Grooming—hair care, nail care, oral care, shaving, and applying makeup
• Dressing and undressing
• Eating
• Toileting
• Mobility (the ability to move about)

The ADL are taught to people when they are children. Healthy adults do these tasks automatically. If the resident cannot complete any or all of the ADL, a self-care deficit exists. A self-care deficit may be due to:

• Diseases such as multiple sclerosis, arthritis, Parkinson's disease, or Alzheimer's disease
• A stroke or injuries that have damaged the brain or spinal cord
• Vision impairment
• Emotional illness

Problems can result from these conditions that limit the resident's ability to do self-care. Examples of these problems are:

- Decreased strength
- Lack of endurance
- Limited range of motion
- **Paralysis**
- **Perceptual deficits**
- Depression
- Disorientation

Paralysis occurs because of damage to the brain or spinal cord. It means the resident cannot move one or more of the extremities. Brain damage from a stroke frequently causes **hemiplegia,** which means paralysis on one side of the body. Spinal cord injuries can cause **quadriplegia** (paralysis from the neck down) or **paraplegia** (paralysis from the waist down).

Perceptual deficits usually occur because of damage to the brain from disease or injury. Examples of perceptual deficits include the inability to:

- Organize a task. ADL cannot be completed unless the resident is able to prepare for the task, get the necessary items together, and then do the task.
- Sequence a task. A resident with this inability may put on a dress before the slip or shoes before the socks.
- Exercise judgment. This deficit may be noted if a resident puts on a wool coat in hot weather, when appropriate clothing is available.
- Identify common objects such as eating utensils and grooming items. When this occurs, the resident may look at a fork, but not know what it is.
- Use common items. The resident may be able to identify an item such as a comb or toothbrush, but be unable to pick it up and use it, even though there is no physical reason for the problem.
- Initiate or start a task without assistance.

Instrumental Activities of Daily Living

Higher-level tasks are called **instrumental activities of daily living** or **IADL**. These include skills that adults need to function independently. Examples of IADL include:

- Managing money
- Managing a household
- Driving a car

In some situations the adult may not be able to physically complete these tasks but is able to competently direct others to do so.

SETTING UP RESTORATIVE PROGRAMS

Residents with self-care deficits are evaluated by therapists and nurses. The results of the evaluation will determine whether a resident's **functional ability** (ability to do ADL) can be increased. In other words, can the interdisciplinary team help this resident to relearn an ADL?

- This is discussed with the resident and the family. If the resident, family, and staff agree that the resident's physical abilities can be increased, then a restorative program is planned by the interdisciplinary team.
- The members of the interdisciplinary team meet together at the care plan conference. Methods for solving the resident's problems are discussed with the resident and family.

When the resident is unable to do any ADL independently, it is generally best to concentrate on relearning just one ADL at a time. The first step is to find out what the resident wants to work on first. The interdisciplinary team then works with the resident and family to plan the process. They will:

- Establish goals.
  - Each ADL consists of several steps. This is called **task segmentation** (Table 22-2).
  - The resident will not be able to do all steps right away. Some residents may never be able to do all of the steps.
  - Goals, therefore, are very small. For example, if the resident is in a restorative program for eating, the first goal for the resident may be to hold a glass, bring it to her mouth, and drink from it.

    All goals are functional (purposeful). For example, instead of saying the resident will walk 30 feet, the goal will state: resident will walk to the dining room for breakfast.
- Plan approaches.
  - Approaches include the techniques and procedures carried out by care providers to assist resident to relearn the ADL.

The resident may participate in other physical or occupational rehabilitation programs. These programs are planned to help the resident acquire skills needed to complete a task. For example, exercises may be done that will increase range of motion, strength, or endurance.

Table 22-2 Task Segmentation			
ADL	**Steps of Activity**	**ADL**	**Steps of Activity**

Grooming	• Washes, brushes, combs hair
	• Brushes teeth
	  • Gets equipment ready
	  • Places paste on brush
	  • Brushes teeth
	  • Rinses mouth
	  • Cleans and puts equipment away
	• Shaves
	  • Gets equipment ready
	  • Shaves face
	  • Cleans/puts equipment away
	• Nail care
	  • Gets equipment ready
	  • Cleans nails
	  • Trims nails
	  • Cleans/puts equipment away
		Dressing/ Undressing (cont'd)	• Manages buttons, snaps, ties, zippers
			• Puts on/takes off skirt/pants
			• Buckles belt
			• Puts on/takes off shoes/socks

		Eating	• Gets to table • Uses spoon, fork, knife appropriately • Opens/pours • Brings food to mouth • Chews, swallows • Uses napkin
		Toileting	• Gets to commode/toilet • Manipulates clothing • Sits on toilet • Eliminates in toilet • Cleans self • Flushes toilet • Gets clothing in place • Washes hands
Bathing	• Gathers supplies • Gets to tub/sink/shower • Undresses • Regulates water • Washes/rinses upper body • Washes/rinses lower body • Dries body • Puts away supplies	**Mobility**	• Gets self to side of bed • Maintains upright position • Comes to standing position • Places self in position to sit in chair • Locks wheelchair brakes • Turns body to sit • Lowers self into chair • Propels wheelchair • Repositions self in chair • Raises self from chair • Places self in position to sit on edge of bed • Walks alone/with assistance • Uses assistive device
Dressing/ Undressing	• Obtains/selects clothing • Puts on/takes off slipover top • Puts on/takes off cardigan-style top		

Approaches Used in Restorative Programs

• Setup
  • Residents with self-care deficits cannot set up or prepare for ADL. You may need to provide the setup (Figure 22-5). *Example:* The setup for mealtime includes bringing the tray to the resident and assisting with uncovering food, opening containers, removing eating utensils from package, and preparing food, if necessary.
• Verbal cues
  • Verbal cues are short, simple phrases to prompt the resident to do something. *Example:* Give the resident a prepared washcloth and then say, "Please wash your face."

FIGURE 22-5 Many residents can complete the activities of daily living if you set up the articles they need.

- Hand-over-hand technique
  - For this technique, your hand is placed over the resident's hand to guide it (Figure 22-6). *Example:* For eating program, place a spoon with food in the

FIGURE 22-6 The nursing assistant is using hand-over-hand technique to help the resident regain eating skills.

resident's hand. Place your hand over the resident's hand. Guide the spoon to the resident's mouth. Eventually, the resident will be able to do this without assistance.

- Demonstration
  - "Act out" what you want the resident to do. *Example:* Before giving the resident a toothbrush, make the motions of brushing your teeth with the toothbrush.

The care plan will indicate the approach to be used. The decision is made by the physical therapist, occupational therapist, or restorative nurse.

Adaptive devices are sometimes used to simplify ADL (Figure 22-7A–C). An adaptive device is an ordinary item that is changed in some way so that it can be used by individuals with specific disabilities. These devices allow people to do things they may not otherwise be able to do. If adaptive devices are ordered, be sure they are used each time the ADL is carried out.

Guidelines for mobility programs and toileting are presented later in this lesson.

Not all residents have potential for restorative programs. For those who do not, the goals are concerned with preventing complications and maintaining current abilities as long as possible. Restorative programs may remain in place after the resident reaches the highest goal possible. This is done to be sure that the resident does not lose the skill. Some residents with progressive diseases such as Alzheimer's reach the point where even maintenance is difficult. Preventing complications such as pressure ulcers and contractures is then the major goal.

THE RESTORATIVE/REHABILITATIVE ENVIRONMENT

A restorative environment is not only for residents in restorative programs. The staff can provide an environment and act in such a manner that all residents will benefit. The interdisciplinary team can help promote this environment:

- Give residents a sense of control and the opportunity to make decisions.
- Remember that mental and physical activity are essential to the residents' well-being. Opportunities for physical exercise and various types of activities must be offered to residents.

A. TOOTHBRUSH HOLDER TO APPLY TOOTHPASTE WITH ONLY ONE HAND

B. LONG-HANDLED SPONGE

C. LONG-HANDLED BRUSH AND COMB

D. COMBINATION NAIL CLIPPER AND FILE FOR ONE-HANDED USE

E. AEROSOL CAN ADAPTER WITH TRIGGER TO PUSH BUTTON

F. GROOMING AIDS WITH BUILT-UP HANDLES FOR EASIER GRIPPING

FIGURE 22-7 A. Adaptive devices used for grooming and bathing

A. LONG-HANDLED SHOEHORN

B. SHOE GRABBER AND SHOE HORN

C. STOCKING AID

D. TROUSER AID

E. DRESSING STICK

F. BUTTON LOOP

G. ZIPPER AID

FIGURE 22-7 B. Dressing aids

A. FOOD BUMPER SNAPS OVER A DINNER PLATE TO KEEP THE FOOD ON THE PLATE

B. PLATES WITH INNER LIP TO KEEP FOOD ON PLATE

C. PLATE WITH HIGH CURVED EDGE TO HELP PUSH FOOD ON FORK OR SPOON

D. FEEDING CUP

E. CUTLERY WITH BUILT-UP HANDLES FOR EASIER GRIPPING; MOVABLE GRIP RINGS ADJUST FOR COMFORT

F. ANGLED CUTLERY FOR PEOPLE WITH LIMITED ARM AND WRIST MOVEMENT

HAND CLIP FOR PEOPLE WHO CANNOT GRIP HANDLES

G. GRIPPER FOR PEOPLE WHO CANNOT GRIP STANDARD OR BUILT-UP HANDLES

FIGURE 22-7 C. Adaptive devices used for eating

*G*uidelines for

Nursing Assistant Responsibilities in General Restorative Program

General

1. Know the cause of the resident's self-care deficit.
2. Know the resident's goals as stated on the care plan.
3. Be consistent. Read the care plan and follow the specific approaches each time you work with the resident.
4. Keep your directions simple but not childish when you are helping the resident relearn an activity.
5. Avoid distractions. Do the ADL in a private, quiet area. Restorative programs are incorporated into the resident's daily care. For example, if the resident is in a grooming program to relearn how to comb her hair, then the program is carried out when the hair would usually be combed.
6. Use adaptive devices consistently and correctly.
7. Do not show impatience. Be encouraging and give praise.
8. Treat the resident with dignity at all times.
9. Realize that the resident's progress may be uneven and inconsistent. A resident may do better one day than another.

Grooming

1. A grooming program may be for combing/brushing hair, applying makeup, doing nail care, shaving, or oral care.
2. The resident should sit in a comfortable chair that supports the resident's body.
3. Place the necessary items on the overbed table. Place the table in front of the resident and adjust it to the appropriate height so the resident can reach every item.
4. Avoid putting too many items on the table at once. Do not put the items close together or the resident may have trouble picking the correct item.

Bathing

1. Residents in bathing programs should also be allowed to:
   - Wash their hands after toileting
   - Wash their face and hands after eating

   - Follow the program for AM and PM care as well as for bathing
2. A setup is usually needed:
   - Prepare the water (basin, tub, or shower).
   - Obtain all the necessary items (towels, washcloths, soap).
   - Help the resident choose clothing to put on after the bath.

Eating

1. Assist the resident to go to the bathroom.
2. Provide opportunity for handwashing.
3. Be sure the resident has dentures in if needed and that the mouth is clean.
4. Seat the resident in a regular dining chair at a dining table.
5. Avoid distractions. Turn off televisions and radios.
6. Prepare the tray: open cartons, butter the bread, cut the meat, add seasonings as the resident wishes, and pour liquids. The resident may eventually be able to do these things independently.

Dressing/Undressing

The following adaptations will make the program more likely to succeed:

1. Use loose-fitting styles or clothing one size larger.
2. Encourage the family to bring clothing that fastens in front rather than in back. Velcro® closings are usually easier to manipulate than zippers, buttons, or snaps.
3. Suggest garments with large buttons rather than small ones. It is easier to match buttons with the right buttonholes if the resident starts to button from the bottom of a shirt or blouse rather than the top.
4. Suggest that elastic thread be used for cuff buttons so they do not need to be undone each time.
5. Encourage the resident to wear slip-on shoes or shoes with Velcro® closings.

FIGURE 22-8 All residents should be assisted to look attractive and well groomed.

- Encourage and assist residents to be well dressed and well groomed at all times (Figure 22-8).
- Use touch freely in appropriate ways with residents (Figure 22-9).
- Provide cues for orientation throughout the building such as large clocks, calendars, pictures, and color codes.
- Respect the resident's identity, individuality, and privacy at all times.
- Respect and understand the resident's sexuality and need for intimacy.
- Give residents opportunities to help others. All people need to feel useful.
- Encourage and assist residents to remain a part of the community and encourage the community to be a part of the facility.

FIGURE 22-9 Touching residents is important for restorative care.

- The environment should be safe, serene, and colorful.

PROGRESSIVE MOBILIZATION

Progressive mobilization is a process used to increase a resident's mobility skills. Mobility includes:

- Moving in bed
- Changing position in bed
- Moving to and coming to a sitting position on the edge of the bed
- Coming to a standing position
- Transferring into a bathtub, shower, and car or out of bed and into a chair
- Ambulating or moving about in a wheelchair

Not all residents are able to complete every step of progressive mobilization. All residents should be given the opportunity to reach their own potential. Progressive mobilization, like all restorative programs, must begin at the simplest level. A resident may not be able to do any of these skills independently but may be able to do each skill with assistance.

RANGE OF MOTION

Exercise is a basic physical need. Residents who are unable to do active exercises are exercised through passive range of motion exercises by the care provider. The physical or occupational therapist may order additional exercises to increase specific abilities or to strengthen certain muscles.

Range of motion exercises are one technique used to prevent the formation of contractures (see Figure 22-3). It is the responsibility of each person on the health care team to recognize risks for contracture formation and to implement preventive therapy. The therapists and professional nurses are trained to use a special instrument called a **goniometer** to assess the resident for the presence of contractures, to determine how a potential contracture affects the resident's functional capacity, and to set rehabilitation goals and interventions.

There are four stages of contracture development:

- Stage I has an onset of 0–4 days and within 2 weeks has a 0–15 degree loss in range of motion
- Stage II advances in one to two more weeks through 15-45 degrees loss in range of motion

---

Guidelines for

Passive Range of Motion Exercises

1. Always tell the resident what you are doing and why. Have the resident help you if possible.
2. Passive exercises of the neck are not generally done on elderly people. Arthritis is a common problem and passive exercises can injure the neck. Instead, encourage the resident to move the head independently.
3. Move each joint to its fullest range. Remember that the maximum range in an elderly person may be small.
4. Never force movement or cause pain. If the resident cannot speak, watch the face for signs of pain.

5. Use gentle, physical contact. Support the extremities at the joints. Use the palms of your hands to cup the joints.
6. Do each motion at least five times. The exercises should be done at least twice a day. Do each joint unless you have been instructed to omit specific joints or a specific movement for a joint.
7. Do each motion slowly, smoothly, gently, and rhythmically. A resident's stiff joints may gradually loosen as you continue the exercises.
8. Come to a complete stop at the end of each movement before starting the next movement.

- Stage III has a 45-90 degree loss
- Stage IV has a 90+ degree loss of range of motion

A *fixed contracture* is one that allows the resident no range of motion. The only treatment is surgery, which is expensive and not appropriate for all residents.

Contractures are painful, much like a continuous, severe cramp in the muscle. In the presence of contractures, blood flow is impeded and pressure ulcers can form. It is imperative that the appropriate range of motion exercises be completed when ordered:

- **Passive range of motion**
  The care provider moves the joints for the resident.
- **Active assistive range of motion**
  The care provider supports the joints and assists in the movement while the resident attempts to do independent movement.
- **Active range of motion**
  The resident is able to move the joints without assistance.
- **Self range of motion**
  The resident uses the strong extremity to move the affected extremity. *Example:* A resident with a stroke may use the strong arm to passively move the paralyzed arm.

Nursing assistants in long-term care facilities may do passive range of motion exercises with residents several times a day.

Definitions of Joint Movements

Specific terms describe joint movements. Not all joints are capable of the same movements.

1. Flexion—bending a joint; decreasing the angle of the joint (Figure 22-10)
   - Palmar flexion—bending the hand down toward the wrist
   - Dorsiflexion—bending the hand back or bending the foot back

FIGURE 22-10 Flexion—bending a joint

FIGURE 22-11 Extension—straightening a joint

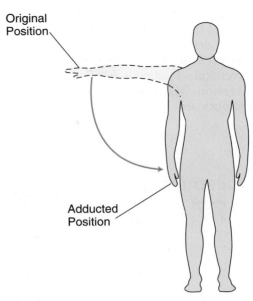

FIGURE 22-13 Adduction—moving an extremity back to the body

- Plantar flexion—bending the foot forward toward the sole
2. Extension—the opposite of flexion—to straighten the joint out; increasing the angle of the joint (Figure 22-11)
3. Abduction—moving an extremity away from the body (Figure 22-12)
    - Horizontal abduction—bringing the arm out so the elbow is parallel to shoulder
4. Adduction—the opposite of abduction—moving the extremity back to the body (Figure 22-13)

- Horizontal adduction—bringing the arm up and crossing it over the chest
5. Rotation—turning around an axis (Figure 22-14)
    - Internal rotation—turning toward the median line
    - External rotation—turning outward from the median line
6. Pronation—turning the forearm so the palm is facing downward
7. Supination—the opposite of pronation—turning the forearm so the palm is facing upward

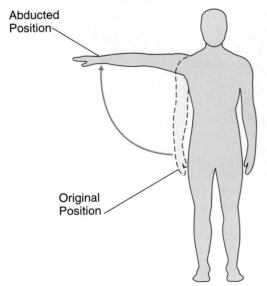

FIGURE 22-12 Abduction—moving an extremity away from the body

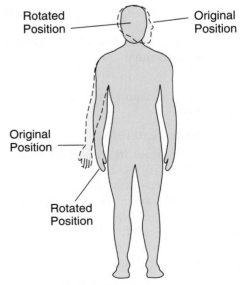

FIGURE 22-14 Rotation

8. Radial deviation—lateral movement of wrist toward thumb side of hand
9. Ulnar deviation—lateral movement of wrist toward little finger side of hand
10. Inversion—turning inward
11. Eversion—the opposite of inversion—turning outward

12. Opposition—bringing palmar surface of thumb to the finger joint

It is important that you review the section on body mechanics in Lesson 9. You will need to use your muscles correctly as you help residents with their mobility. This will help prevent painful and costly injuries to both you and the residents.

PROCEDURE 77 Passive Range of Motion Exercises

1. Carry out each beginning procedure action.
2. Position the resident in good **body alignment**. This means the resident's spine is straight and the resident's extremities are straight in relation to the body. The body is straight in the bed. Bring the resident close to your side of the bed.
3. Place a bath blanket over the covers. Then bring the covers to the foot of the bed. Expose only the extremity that you are working on.
4. Remember to use correct body mechanics to avoid straining your back.
5. Lower the side rail. Do the exercises on the arm and leg on that side. Raise the side rail. Go to the other side of the bed. Do the exercises on the arm and leg on that side.
6. When all four extremities have been exercised, carry out procedure completion actions.
7. Report any unusual resident reactions or problems to the nurse.

Shoulder
Support the elbow and wrist during all shoulder exercises.

1. Flexion and extension
   • With shoulder in adduction, flex the resident's elbow and raise entire arm over the head (flexion) (Figure 22-15). *Note:* This movement is flexing the resident's elbow as well as the shoulder.
   • Bring arm back down parallel to body (extension) (Figure 22-16). *Note:* This

FIGURE 22-15 Shoulder flexion: Flex elbow and raise entire arm over head.

FIGURE 22-16 Supporting the upper arm and wrist, straighten elbow.

movement is extending the resident's elbow as well as the shoulder.
Repeat flexion and extension five to seven times.

(continues)

PROCEDURE 77 *(continued)*

FIGURE 22-17 Shoulder abduction and adduction: Supporting elbow and wrist, bring the entire arm out at right angle from the body.

2. Abduction and adduction
   - Bring entire arm out at right angle to body (abduction) (Figure 22-17).
   - Return arm to position parallel with body (adduction) (Figure 22-18).

   Repeat abduction and adduction five to seven times.
3. Horizontal adduction and horizontal abduction

FIGURE 22-18 Return arm to position parallel to body.

- With arm parallel to body, bring arm up and cross it over chest (horizontal adduction) (Figure 22-19).
- Bring arm back so elbow is parallel to shoulder (horizontal abduction) (Figure 22-20).

Repeat horizontal adduction and horizontal abduction five to seven times.
4. External rotation and internal rotation
   - With elbow parallel to shoulder, place forearm in up position with palm of hand up (external rotation) (Figure 22-21).
   - Bring forearm down with elbow and shoulder remaining stationary (internal rotation) (Figure 22-22).

Repeat external rotation and internal rotation five to seven times.

FIGURE 22-19 Horizontal adduction of shoulder

FIGURE 22-20 Horizontal abduction of shoulder

(continues)

PROCEDURE 77 *(continued)*

FIGURE 22-21 External rotation of shoulder

FIGURE 22-22 Internal rotation of the shoulder

Elbow

Support the resident's wrist during the elbow exercises.

1. Flexion and extension
   - With arm parallel to body and palm up, bend elbow (flexion) (Figure 22-23).
   - Return arm to position parallel with body and palm up (extension) (Figure 22-24).

   Repeat flexion and extension of elbow five to seven times.

2. Supination and pronation
   - Place your hand in resident's hand as if to shake hands. Turn resident's hand with yours so the palm is down (pronation).

- Without moving your hand, turn resident's hand with yours so resident's palm is up (supination) (Figure 22-25).

Repeat supination and pronation five to seven times.

FIGURE 22-23 Flexion of the elbow: Bring lower arm toward upper arm.

FIGURE 22-24 Extension of the shoulder and elbow

FIGURE 22-25 Supination: Grasp resident's hand as if to shake hands; turn hand so resident's hand is palm up.

(continues)

PROCEDURE *77* *(continued)*

Wrist

Support the forearm during wrist exercises. The elbow and shoulder will rest on the bed.

1. Flexion (palmar flexion), extension (dorsiflexion)
- Bend wrist forward (flexion, palmar flexion) (Figure 22-26).
- Straighten wrist so hand is even with forearm (extension) (Figure 22-27).

Repeat flexion and extension five to seven times.

FIGURE 22-26 Wrist flexion and extension: Place hand over resident's hand while supporting wrist and bend wrist.

FIGURE 22-27 Supporting arm above wrist and hand, straighten wrist.

2. Ulnar and radial deviation
- Move hand toward little finger side (ulnar deviation) (Figure 22-28).
- Move hand toward thumb side (radial deviation) (Figure 22-29).

Repeat ulnar and radial deviation five to seven times.

FIGURE 22-28 Ulnar deviation of the wrist

FIGURE 22-29 Radial deviation of the wrist

Fingers

Support the wrist and forearm during the finger and thumb exercises.

1. Flexion and extension
- Curl the fingers together (flexion) (Figure 22-30).

FIGURE 22-30 Finger flexion: Supporting wrist with one hand, cover resident's fingers and curl them to make a fist.

(continues)

PROCEDURE *77* *(continued)*

- Straighten the fingers out (extension) (Figure 22-31).

Repeat flexion and extension of the fingers five to seven times.

2. Abduction and adduction
   - Spread each finger apart from the one next to it (abduction) (Figure 22-32).
   - Bring each finger back (adduction) (Figure 22-33).

Repeat abduction and adduction five to seven times.

FIGURE 22-31 Finger extension: Slip fingers over resident's flexed fingers and straighten the fingers.

FIGURE 22-32 Abduction of the fingers

FIGURE 22-33 Adduction of the fingers

Thumb
1. Flexion and extension
   - Bend the thumb forward (flexion).
   - Straighten the thumb out (extension).

Repeat flexion and extension of the thumb five to seven times.

2. Abduction and adduction
   - Move the thumb away from the other fingers (abduction) (Figure 22-34).
   - Move the thumb back toward the other fingers (adduction).

Repeat abduction and adduction five to seven times.

3. Opposition
   - Move the thumb to the base of each finger and then back (Figure 22-35).

Repeat opposition five to seven times. *Note:* Opposition is an exercise for the thumb, not the fingers. It is important that the thumb receive the movement.

FIGURE 22-34 Abduction and adduction of thumb: Supporting hand, draw thumb toward and away from extended fingers.

FIGURE 22-35 Thumb opposition: Supporting the hand, touch each finger with the thumb.

(continues)

PROCEDURE 77 *(continued)*

Hips

Support the knee and ankle during hip exercises.

1. Abduction and adduction
- Place the palm of your hand under the resident's knee and the other hand under the heel.
- Move the entire leg away from the body (abduction) (Figure 22-36).
- Move the entire leg back toward the body (adduction) (Figure 22-37).

Repeat abduction and adduction of the hip five to seven times.

FIGURE 22-38 Hip and knee flexion: Supporting resident's knee and ankle, flex knee and hip.

FIGURE 22-36 Abduction of the hip: Supporting resident's knee and ankle, move entire leg away from body.

FIGURE 22-37 Adduction of hip: Supporting leg, return to center of body.

2. Flexion and extension
- Place one hand under the resident's knee. Place your other hand under the heel with the resident's foot resting against your forearm.
- Bend the resident's knee and hip toward the resident's trunk (flexion) (Figure 22-38).

Note: You are flexing the knee at the same time as the hip.

- Straighten the knee and hip (extension). Be sure to support the knee so it does not "flop" down (Figure 22-39).

FIGURE 22-39 Knee extension: Supporting knee and ankle, straighten knee.

Note: You are extending the knee at the same time as the hip. Repeat flexion and extension of the hip and knee five to seven times.

3. Internal rotation and external rotation
- Place one hand on the resident's leg just above the knee. Place the other hand on the resident's lower leg just above the ankle.
- With the resident's leg extended, roll the leg back and forth. Rolling the leg inward is internal rotation. Rolling the leg outward is external rotation (Figure 22-40).

Repeat internal rotation and external rotation of the hip five to seven times.

Knee

Flexion and extension are the only knee movements. These were done with the hip.

(continues)

PROCEDURE 77 (continued)

FIGURE 22-40 External and internal rotation of hip

Ankle

1. Plantar flexion and dorsiflexion

   * Bend resident's knee slightly and support lower leg with your forearm and hand.
   * With your other hand, bend resident's foot downward (plantar flexion) (Figure 22-41).
   * Then gently bend resident's foot backward (dorsiflexion, hyperextension) (Figure 22-42).

   Repeat plantar flexion and dorsiflexion five to seven times.

2. Inversion and eversion

   * Place both hands on the resident's foot. Move the foot inward (inversion) (Figure 22-43).
   * With your hands still on the resident's foot, move the foot outward (eversion) (Figure 22-44).

FIGURE 22-41 Plantar flex the ankle by drawing the foot in a downward position.

FIGURE 22-42 Dorsiflexion: Grasp the resident's heel with one hand, using your upper arm to support the foot. Dorsiflex the ankle by bringing toes and foot toward the knee.

FIGURE 22-43 Ankle inversion: Grasp resident's foot and gently turn it inward.

FIGURE 22-44 Foot eversion: Grasp resident's foot and gently turn it outward.

Repeat inversion and eversion five to seven times.

Toes

1. Flexion and extension

   * Bend (flexion) and straighten (extension) each toe.

   Repeat flexion and extension of the toes five to seven times.

(continues)

PROCEDURE *77* *(continued)*

2. Abduction and adduction
  • Move each toe away from the next toe, one at a time (abduction) (Figure 22-45).
  • Move each toe toward the next toe, one at a time (adduction) (Figure 22-46).

Repeat abduction and adduction five to seven times.

Additional exercises can be done with the resident in the prone (lying on the abdomen)

FIGURE 22-46   Toe adduction: Move each toe toward the next toe.

FIGURE 22-45   Toe abduction: Move each toe away from the next toe, one at a time.

position. However, many residents cannot lie in this position. Your facility may not include these exercises. Check with your supervisor and be sure you receive instruction before doing the additional exercises.

Carry out procedure completion actions. Report to the nurse any pain or change in range of motion of the resident's joints. Position resident comfortably.

SELF RANGE OF MOTION EXERCISES

Self range of motion exercises are done by the resident. The resident can use a strong extremity to move a paralyzed or weak extremity (Figure 22-47). The physical therapist or restorative nurse will give you instructions if you are to assist a resident with self range of motion exercises.

ACTIVE RANGE OF MOTION EXERCISES

Residents can do many exercises independently that involve movement of the joints. Many long-term care facilities have health and fitness trails within the facility that have several stations and instructions for the resident. Active range of motion exercises can also be done by residents in wheelchairs.

FIGURE 22-47   The resident is using her stronger arm to raise her weak arm.

POSITIONING THE RESIDENT

Residents who cannot move themselves about in bed need to be repositioned frequently. As a nursing assistant, you will carry out these procedures several times a day. Three basic positions are: **supine** (lying on the back), **prone** (lying on the abdomen), and **lateral** (lying on either side). Each of these positions has variations.

Positioning procedures have several steps:

- Moving the resident's body so it is in correct body alignment
  - You may need to move the resident toward the head of the bed, the foot of the bed, or either side of the bed.
- Turning the resident to the desired position
  - To either the right or left side from the side, the back, or the abdomen
  - To the back from either side or the abdomen
  - To the abdomen from the back or other side
- Placing pillows or other supportive devices to maintain the position

Purposes of Positioning

Positioning is done to:

- Improve circulation and respiratory function
- Maintain the resident's body alignment and good posture
- Prevent contractures, skin breakdown, pain, discomfort, thromboses, pneumonia, and edema
- Increase sensory stimulation. The sense of touch is stimulated when the assistant moves the resident. The sense of vision is stimulated when the resident is turned and sees a different part of the environment.

*G*uidelines for

Positioning

1. A firm mattress helps to maintain correct body alignment.
2. Lock the wheels of the bed before beginning the positioning procedure.
3. Raise the bed to a comfortable working height. Remember to lower the bed when the procedure is finished.
4. Raise the side rail on the other side of the bed unless there is another person helping you.
5. Use safety devices appropriately and *never* tie them to the side rails or bed frame. Tie them to the part of the bed supporting the mattress.
6. Handle the resident's body gently during mobility activities. Use the palms of your hands rather than your fingertips to support the extremities.
7. Incorporate range of motion exercises into positioning procedures. These exercises are in addition to those carried out routinely.
8. Encourage the resident's independence. Provide the assistance that is needed but avoid "overhelping."
9. Turn the resident at least every 2 hours. Inspect the skin for signs of breakdown each time. Gently massage around reddened areas with lotion. Rubbing over the area may cause further skin damage.
10. Use a turning sheet to move a dependent resident in bed. This avoids friction and **shearing** the skin. Shearing occurs when the resident's body slides across the sheets; the skin moves in one direction as deeper tissues move in the opposite direction.
11. Support paralyzed extremities in extension. Prevent prolonged overstretching of weakened muscles. **Flaccid** paralysis means the extremity is limp and incapable of independent movement. **Spasticity** occurs in some paralyzed limbs. Spasticity can cause involuntary movements. It may cause the joints to assume positions of flexion. Contractures can happen easily in spastic limbs.
12. Avoid dependent positions of extremities. The wrists and feet should never hang. This will cause edema (swelling).
13. Check incontinent residents each time you move them. If they have soiled the bed, cleanse them thoroughly. Change the sheets. Change clothing if soiled.

(continues)

Guidelines (continued)

14. Tighten the sheets frequently. Wrinkles cause pressure areas on the resident's skin.

15. Items used for positioning are used only for a specific resident. Send sheets, pillows, and other washable items to the laundry as necessary. Do not let these items touch the floor.

16. Remember the privacy of the resident when completing all positioning procedures.

Supportive Equipment

Supportive equipment may be needed to position the resident. The procedure must be adapted for residents with catheters or other tubes. You may need further instructions from the nurse for positioning residents with contractures.

Postural supports are devices to help maintain the resident in good posture and body alignment. Examples of postural supports include:

- Trochanter rolls
- Bath blankets
- Pillows of various sizes and shapes
- Bath towels
- Footboards
- Splints or slings, if ordered
- Turning sheet

Other postural supports are prescribed for specific residents for specific purposes (Figure 22-48). Be sure you know how to apply these devices correctly.

A trochanter roll is used to prevent external rotation of the hip. It is put in place when the resident is in supine (on the back) position. If the hip contracts in this position, the resident will be unable to move the leg. You can make a trochanter roll with a bath blanket:

- Fold the blanket in thirds, lengthwise. The roll should be 12 to 14 inches wide.
- The blanket is placed lengthwise under the resident's hips. Roll the end that is on the affected side *under* until it is firmly against the resident's body. It should extend from above the hip to just above the knee (Figure 22-49).

Footboards are sometimes ordered to prevent plantar flexion of the feet. This causes contracture of the ankle.

- The footboard should be well-padded, smooth, and firm.
- The footboard must extend 2 inches above the toes. This will prevent skin breakdown on the toes.

FIGURE 22-48 Supports help position residents and maintain body alignment. (Courtesy of J. T. Posey Co., Inc., Arcadia, CA)

FIGURE 22-49 Trochanter roll in place to prevent external rotation of hip

• The bottoms of the feet rest against the foot-board to maintain position.

A folded pillow placed between the soles of the feet and the foot of the bed can take the place of a footboard. In some cases, a footboard may be harmful. For example, if spasticity is present in the legs, a footboard against the soles of the feet will stimulate spasticity and possibly cause skin breakdown from the rubbing of the

feet against the footboard. Special shoes worn in bed are sometimes used to maintain the feet in correct alignment (Figure 22-50). In most cases, ankle contractures can be avoided by doing passive range of motion exercises consistently.

• A bed cradle (Figure 22-51) is placed on the bed over the resident's legs. The bed covers are placed over the bed cradle. This keeps the weight of the covers off the resident's legs and feet. It prevents the covers from forcing the feet into plantar flexion, which could cause a contracture.

A device called an **orthosis** can also be used to maintain position of an extremity. The correct use of these devices prevents contracture

FIGURE 22-50 Special foot supports worn in bed prevent contractures of the ankle. (Bunny boot foot support is provided by Sammons Preston, Inc., a Bissell® HealthCare Company. Reprinted with permission.)

FIGURE 22-51 A bed cradle prevents pressure on the foot from the top covers.

formation. Orthoses are also called splints. Figures 22-52A–D are examples of orthoses for the upper extremities.

- The splint must be applied correctly. Follow the manufacturer's directions for each splint.
- Keep the splint clean. If it becomes soiled, check with the nurse to see how it should be cleaned.

The physician may also order splints or orthoses for the lower extremities. A common type is called the ankle stirrup (Figure 22-53). The stirrup provides support for an unstable ankle. The stirrup is applied to the lower leg before the shoe is put on.

When using splints:

- The splint may be ordered to be on and off the extremity at various times throughout the day. Be sure you know the correct procedure and schedule.
- Check the splint to be sure there are no pressure areas against the resident's skin.

- Folded washcloths should *never* be placed in the resident's hand. The rough surface of the cloth increases spasticity and the risk of contractures.

Slings are sometimes used to prevent a paralyzed arm from hanging. The force of gravity pulls on the weight of the arm, causing subluxation. This occurs when the shoulder joint separates (a dislocation). It is a permanent and painful condition. A sling is not usually worn constantly because it forces the upper arm into a position of adduction and the elbow into flexion. If you apply a sling, remember:

- Read the manufacturer's instructions for application.
- Position the hands and fingers at about heart level.
- Support the hand and fingers with the sling. Avoid palmar flexion of the wrist.

FIGURE 22-52 A. This orthosis maintains the wrist and hand in neutral position. (Neutral Position® wrist/hand orthosis is provided by Sammons Preston, Inc., a Bissell® HealthCare Company. Reprinted with permission.) B. This is a cock-up wrist splint. (Cock-up wrist splint is provided by Sammons Preston, Inc., a Bissell® HealthCare Company. Reprinted with permission.) C. A soft, foam orthosis encourages and maintains normal extension of the wrist, fingers, and thumb joints. (Foam wrist/hand orthosis is provided by Sammons Preston, Inc., a Bissell® HealthCare Company. Reprinted with permission.) D. The antispasticity ball splint reduces spasticity by maintaining hand, fingers, and wrist in correct position. (Antispasticity ball splint is provided by Sammons Preston, Inc., a Bissell® HealthCare Company. Reprinted with permission.)

FIGURE 22-53 This ankle stirrup reduces instability of the ankle. (Aircast® ankle stirrup is provided by Sammons Preston, Inc., a Bissell® HealthCare Company. Reprinted with permission.)

- Check the sling for foreign bodies that may produce pressure spots.
- Position the sling to provide adequate support at the elbow so the shoulder is in good position.
- Apply the sling properly to prevent it from pulling on the resident's neck (Figure 22-54).

FIGURE 22-54 When properly applied, a sling supports the wrist and does not pull on the resident's neck.

TURNING THE DEPENDENT RESIDENT WITH A TURNING SHEET

A **turning sheet** is used to move a dependent resident in bed. Using a regular flat bed sheet:

- Fold the sheet in half, end to end.
- Place this on the resident's bed when the bed is made. Change it as needed.
- Place the folded side toward the head of the bed. Let the ends hang freely over the sides of the bed.
- Place it on the bed so that it extends from the resident's shoulders to knees.

PROCEDURE
78 Moving the Resident in Bed

Note: A turning sheet should always be used to move dependent residents in bed. This avoids injury to the resident and the caregivers. *Always use the principles of good body mechanics to avoid injury to your back.*

1. Carry out each beginning procedure action.

Remember to use disposable gloves if there may be contact with open lesions, wet linens, or body fluids.

2. Be sure the turning sheet is in place on the bed.
3. Two people are needed, standing on opposite sides of the bed. Three or four people may be needed if the resident is

(continues)

PROCEDURE *78* *(continued)*

very heavy or has many restrictions (tubing, traction devices, etc.).

4. Before beginning this procedure:
   - The bed must be flat.
   - Raise it to a comfortable working height.
   - Fanfold the top covers to the foot of the bed. Do not expose the resident's bare body.
   - Remove all supportive devices from the bed.
   - Put the resident in supine position.
   - Cross the resident's arms over the chest or abdomen.
   - If the resident lacks head control, position the turning sheet to extend up under the head.
   - Remove the pillow under the resident's head and prop it against the headboard.
   - Keep your feet separated, your back straight, and your knees and hips flexed as you complete these procedures to avoid back injuries.

   These directions apply to all assistants who are helping with this procedure. There are one or two assistants on each side of the bed, depending on the size of the resident.

5. Grasp the turning sheet at the level of the resident's shoulders and hips.
   - Using an overhand grasp, roll or gather the sheet until your hands touch the resident's body. Pull the sheet taut.

6. If the resident lacks head control, grasp the sheet at a level that allows you to maintain stability of the resident's head.

7. If you are moving the resident to the head of the bed, face *the foot of the bed* with your feet about 12 inches apart and your outer foot forward (Figure 22-55). If you are moving the resident down in bed, face *the head of the bed* with your feet about 12 inches apart and your outer foot

forward. These positions allow you to flex your elbows and move the resident toward you, following the principles of body mechanics.

8. Before moving, place your weight on the forward foot.
   - As you move, shift your weight to the other foot. (Avoid twisting. Move smoothly.)

9. If moving the resident to *the side of the bed*, the persons on the side of the bed to which the resident will be moved should:
   - Place one foot forward (maintaining a broad base of support). Body weight is on this foot.
   - As the resident is moved, body weight is shifted to the other foot.

10. The assistant(s) on the other side of the bed grasp the turning sheet to avoid dragging the resident's body. The person on this side does very little actual lifting.

11. One person gives the signal by counting to three
    - All persons move on the count of three, flexing their elbows and moving the sheet toward the head of the bed.

12. Position the resident according to directions and carry out procedure completion actions.

FIGURE 22-55 Moving a resident up in bed with a turning sheet

PROCEDURE 79 Turning the Resident to the Side

Note: Directions are given for turning the resident onto the right side. Reverse directions for positioning a resident on the left side.

1. Carry out each beginning procedure action.
2. Follow procedure for moving the resident to the head of the bed if necessary (Procedure 78). *Remember:* Keep your feet about 12 inches apart. Bend your knees and keep your back straight. Get as close to the bed and resident as possible.
3. Now move the resident to the left side of the bed. Assistants on both sides face the bed.
4. Move the resident's right arm away from the body.
   - Place the resident's left arm across the abdomen.
5. Cross the resident's left leg over the right leg.
6. To turn the resident without the turning sheet (turning the resident away from you):
   - The assistant on the resident's left side places the right hand so it cups the resident's left shoulder.
   - The other hand is placed so the palm is against the resident's hip (Figure 22-56).

Note: To turn the resident toward you, stand on the right side of the bed and place your hands as indicated (Figure 22-57).

7. If the resident is large, the assistant on the other side can place both hands beside the hands of the other assistant. On the count of three, turn the resident onto the right side.
8. To turn the resident with the turning sheet:
   - The assistant on the resident's left side grasps the turning sheet at the shoulders and hips.

FIGURE 22-56 Turning the resident away from you

FIGURE 22-57 Turning the resident toward you

FIGURE 22-58 Turning the resident onto the side using a turning sheet

(continues)

PROCEDURE 79 *(continued)*

- The other assistant reaches across the resident and grasps the turning sheet at the knees and waist.

9. The assistant on the right side bends elbows to pull the sheet so the resi-

dent is turned. The other assistant grasps the sheet to assist in the turn (Figure 22-58).

10. Complete positioning procedure (see Procedure 80).

PROCEDURE 80 Logrolling the Resident onto the Side

Note: This procedure is used when the resident's spinal column must be kept straight. This technique may be used after spinal surgery or spinal injury. Directions are given for turning the resident onto the left side.

1. Carry out each beginning procedure action. Remember to use disposable gloves if there may be contact with open lesions, wet linens, or body fluids.

2. This procedure takes two or more people, depending on the size of the resident.
   - If the resident is small, two people can stand on the side to which the resident will be turning.
   - If the resident is large, another person can stand on the other side of the bed.

3. The bed is always kept flat for residents who need logrolling.
   - Elevate the bed to a comfortable working height.
   - Lower the side rails.

4. Make sure the turning sheet is in place under the resident. If the resident has poor head and neck control, the sheet should be wide enough to come up under

the back of the head.

5. Place a pillow lengthwise between the resident's legs.
   - Fold the resident's arms over the chest.
   - The resident's back and legs must be straight throughout the procedure.

6. The assistant(s) on the left side reaches across the resident and grasps the turning sheet. The sheet should be folded until the assistant's hands are close to the resident's body (Figure 22-59).
   - They gently pull the sheet toward themselves until the resident is lying on the left side (Figure 22-60).
   - If the resident is large and there is an assistant on the other side:
     - The assistant places one hand under the resident's right shoulder. The other hand is placed under the resident's right hip. As the other assistants move the resident onto the left side, this assistant helps by supporting the resident during the move.

(continues)

PROCEDURE 80 *(continued)*

7. Support the resident's body with pillows as needed. Be sure to maintain good body alignment.

8. Carry out procedure completion actions.

FIGURE 22-59 Begin logrolling the resident by grasping the turning sheet on the opposite side.

FIGURE 22-60 Pulling together, turn resident to side in one smooth movement.

POSITIONING THE DEPENDENT RESIDENT

Special Points for the Resident with Arthritis

Residents with **arthritis** (disease of the joints) are at risk for developing contractures. Be sure you avoid positions of flexion as much as possible.

1. Use a small, flat pillow under the head extending down to the shoulders.
2. Do not place pillows under the knees in supine position.
3. Prone position helps prevent flexion contractures of the hips and knees and should be considered for residents with arthritis.

PROCEDURE
81   Supine Position

Note: This procedure should be used to position a resident who is paralyzed on one side of the body (hemiplegia). The instructions would apply to the paralyzed side. The resident should be encouraged to move the strong side. These directions are also appropriate for anyone in the supine position.

1. Carry out each beginning procedure action.
2. Refer to previous procedures for turning the resident onto the back and moving to the head of the bed. Head of bed may be slightly elevated.
3. Center a flat pillow under the resident's head. It should come down to the resident's shoulders. This will prevent too much neck flexion.
4. If the resident's leg(s) tend to fall into external rotation, place a trochanter roll under the affected hip or both hips, as directed under the section on supportive equipment.
5. Place a folded towel or small, flat pillow under each shoulder. Place the shoulders in slight abduction.
6. Place the shoulders and elbows in extension. (The arms will be straight.)
   - The forearm is pronated. (The palm of the hand is against the bed.)
7. Place a pillow under each arm that extends from the elbow to the ends of the fingers.
   - The wrist and the fingers should be extended with the fingers in slight abduction (separated).

- The hand, wrist, elbow, and shoulder on each side should be about the same distance from the bed.
8. Place a pillow under each leg, extending from the knee to the ankle. This prevents pressure on the heel.
9. Place a folded pillow between the end of the bed and the soles of the resident's feet (Figure 22-61).
10. Make sure the top covers are not pressing on the tops of the resident's feet.
11. Carry out each procedure completion action.

FIGURE 22-61 Supine or dorsal recumbent position. Resident is flat on back. Bed is flat or head is slightly raised. Pillows are placed under resident's head, shoulders, arms/hands, calves, and ankles. Foot alignment is maintained. Trochanter rolls or rolled pillows placed along hips/thighs prevent external rotation.

PROCEDURE 82 — Semisupine or Tilt Position

OBRA

Note: Directions are given for the resident lying on the left side. This position prevents pressure on the sacrum, coccyx, and hip.

1. Carry out beginning procedure actions.
2. Gather equipment:
   - Pillows
3. Start with the resident in supine position. Roll the resident's trunk and shoulder away from you so that there is a 45° angle between the resident's back and the bed.
4. Place a pillow behind the resident's back for support.
5. Bring the resident's left shoulder forward. Flex the elbow of the left arm and place the lower left arm palm up on a pillow.
6. Flex the elbow of the right arm and bring the forearm across the chest with palm down.

7. Extend both legs. Place right leg a little behind left leg. Support right leg with two pillows. Pillows extend from groin to ankle (Figure 22-62).
8. Carry out procedure completion actions.

FIGURE 22-62 Semisupine or tilt position. In this position, the resident is supported on the side with weight distributed across the shoulders. This position takes pressure off the sacrum, coccyx, and hip.

PROCEDURE 83 — Lateral (Side-Lying) Position

Note: Directions are given for positioning a resident on the right side. Use the same guidelines for positioning on the left side. It is especially important that this procedure be followed when a resident with hemiplegia is positioned on the unaffected side.

1. Carry out each beginning procedure action.
2. Follow previous procedures for moving the resident in bed (Procedure 78) and turning the resident to the side (Procedure 79).

(continues)

PROCEDURE *83* *(continued)*

3. Place a flat pillow under the resident's head. It should extend 3 to 4 inches beyond the resident's face.
4. When the resident is on his side, the bottom shoulder and hip should be in **protraction** (brought forward). This means you should not pull the shoulder and hip back. To do so will place the shoulder in **retraction** and eventually will cause contracture of those joints.
5. The right shoulder should be slightly abducted and can be in a position of internal or partial external rotation, or extension. For partial external rotation, it will have to be supported on pillows.
   * Use the position that is most comfortable for the resident.
   * Be sure the wrist and fingers are extended and fingers slightly abducted.
6. Slightly flex the right knee.
7. Support the left arm on pillows so that the resident's elbow and wrist are supported.
   * The left shoulder is protracted.
   * The elbow is very slightly flexed.
   * The hand is pronated (palm down).
   * The wrist and fingers are extended with fingers slightly abducted.
   * The shoulder, elbow, and wrist should be about the same height from the bed.

8. Support the left leg on pillows that extend from the knee to the foot.
   * Place the hip and knee in slight flexion. The hip is protracted.
   * The ankle, knee, and hip should all be about the same distance from the bed.
9. If the resident tends to fall back, place a pillow against the resident's back for support (Figure 22-63).
10. Place the top covers loosely over the resident.
11. Carry out each procedure completion action.

Note: The right (top) foot and hand should not dangle over the ends of the pillows.

FIGURE 22-63   Lateral (side-lying) position. In this position, the resident's shoulders and pelvis are maintained in proper alignment.

PROCEDURE *84*   Lateral Position on the Affected Side

1. Follow Steps 1 through 4 in Procedure 83.
2. The affected (bottom) shoulder is protracted with elbow extended and forearm pronated.
3. The affected hip is protracted with hip and knee slightly flexed.
4. The unaffected side can be positioned as described in Procedure 83, *or*

5. If resident will be in this position only a few minutes, omit the pillows and encourage the resident to actively move these strong extremities.
6. Carry out each procedure completion action.

PROCEDURE 85 Semiprone Position

This position relieves pressure on the iliac crest and the greater trochanter. Directions are given for the resident lying on the left side.

1. Carry out beginning procedure actions.
2. Gather equipment:
   * Sheepskin
   * Pillows
   * Two foam blocks, each 3 × 6 × 18 inches
3. Place the sheepskin under the resident so it reaches from the shoulders to the knees.
4. Place the left arm in extension and tuck it slightly beneath the resident's body.
5. Place a pillow in front of and at right angles to the resident's chest.
6. Flex the resident's right knee and hip. Support with pillows that are parallel to the leg.
7. Grasp the resident's left arm from the back of the resident. Turn the resident onto the chest facing away from you. Gently pull the left arm toward you and push on resident's hip.
8. Extend the right arm upward and toward the head of the bed. Place it on the head pillow with the fingers and palm against the bed.

9. Flex the upper arm on a pillow.
10. Lift up the sheepskin and place a foam block under the sheepskin above the iliac crest.
11. Place the other foam block under the sheepskin just below the iliac crest (Figure 22-64). You should be able to slide your hand between the hip and the bed.
12. Carry out procedure completion actions.

FIGURE 22-64 Semiprone position. The resident is lying on a full sheepskin for pressure relief. The resident is almost lying on his stomach. Foam blocks under the sheepskin help to relieve pressure on the iliac crest and greater trochanter.

PROCEDURE 86 Fowler's Position

Fowler's position is a variation of supine position. In the semi-Fowler's position, the back rest of the bed is raised 30° from the horizontal position. For the Fowler's position, the back rest is raised 45° to 60° from the horizontal position. In the high Fowler's position, the back rest is at 90° from the horizontal position.

Note: A resident at risk for skin breakdown along the lower spine and buttocks should not have the back rest elevated more than 30° (unless there is a nasogastric or gastrostomy tube in place or for 30 minutes after eating). A higher position causes shearing of the skin over the lower spine and buttocks.

(continues)

PROCEDURE 86*(continued)*

This position is used most often for residents who have trouble breathing.

1. Carry out each beginning procedure action.
2. Use the turning sheet to move the resident's body into good alignment.
3. Raise the back rest to the desired level.
4. Place one, two, or three pillows behind the resident's head and shoulders.
5. The knees may be slightly flexed and supported with small pillows. This will prevent the resident from sliding down in bed.
6. A pillow can be placed between the resident's feet and the end of the bed.
7. Pillows may be placed under each arm. These should extend from the elbows to fingertips to support the shoulders (Figure 22-65).

8. Place top covers loosely over resident.
9. Carry out each procedure completion action.

FIGURE 22-65 Fowler's position. The head of the bed is elevated at a low angle of 30° or 45° or at a high angle of 90°.

Special Points for the Resident with Lower Extremity Amputation

Hip flexion contractures can develop easily after a resident has a leg **amputation** (removal of a limb). Knee flexion contractures may develop in residents with below-the-knee amputations. To prevent these:

1. Avoid placing pillows under the **residual limb** (stump).

FIGURE 22-66 Avoid placing pillows under the resident's residual limb. The nursing assistant will place the residual limb flat on the bed.

2. Keep the residual limb flat on the bed with knees extended (Figure 22-66).
3. Keep hips flat on surface of bed.
4. Keep legs adducted.

Special Points for the Resident with Paralysis

1. If the affected extremities tend to go into flexion, use extension as much as possible when positioning.
2. If the affected extremities tend to go into extension, use flexion when positioning.
3. When paralysis is present in any resident (stroke, spinal cord injury, multiple sclerosis, etc.), use smooth, slow movements. This will avoid causing spasms.

Bridging

Bridging is a technique that prevents pressure on a specific area by the placement of pillows or cushions.

1. Trochanter area
   * Place pillows under trunk and lower extremities when resident is on side, leaving trochanter area free from pressure.

2. Ankle
   * Support foot and lower leg, leaving ankle area suspended.
3. Heels
   * Support entire lower legs with pillows. Maintain good alignment of feet.
4. Sacrum
   * Support both sides of trunk and pelvis, leaving sacral area free from pressure.

Positioning the Resident in a Chair or Wheelchair

Correct positioning for dependent residents sitting in chairs is just as important as it is when they are in bed. The resident's hips and knees should be at 90° angles. The feet should be flat on the floor (Figure 22-67). Pressure ulcers and contractures can occur just as readily in the chair. Wheelchairs are for transportation; they are not designed to be used for long periods of sitting. If this is unavoidable, be sure that the resident is allowed to stand and move about at intervals.

FIGURE 22-67 Correct chair position maintains the elbows, hips, knees, and ankles at 90°.

PROCEDURE
87 Chair Positioning

 OBRA

1. Carry out each beginning procedure action.
2. Head and spine should be erect and in alignment.
3. The resident's arms should rest on the arms of the chair or in the resident's lap. If the shoulders appear to be pushed upward:
   * Place a cushion on the chair seat. This raises the resident's body and allows for proper placement of the arms.

   If the shoulders appear to be hanging:
   * Place pillows or pads under the resident's lower arms.
4. The back of the wheelchair or other similar chair should come to the level of the resident's shoulder blades. If the back is too high:
   * Place a cushion on the chair seat to elevate the resident's body.

   If the back is too low:
   * Ask the nurse if an extension can be placed on the back of the chair to make it higher.
5. The back and buttocks should be back in the chair. The back and hips form a 90° angle.
   * A postural support may be needed to keep the hips back in the chair. Special flat pads can be placed between the resident's clothing and the chair to prevent sliding.

(continues)

PROCEDURE 87 *(continued)*

6. The upper and lower leg should form a 90° angle. The front edge of the seat should be about two fingers' width away from the back of the knees. If the seat is touching the back of the resident's knees:
   - Place a cushion between the resident and the back of the chair. This will bring the resident forward.

7. The feet and ankles also form 90° angles. If the resident's feet do not touch the floor:
   - Place a footstool under the feet. This prevents plantar flexion of the ankle.
   - Place resident's feet on footrests of wheelchair.

8. Carry out each procedure completion action.

PROCEDURE 88

Repositioning a Resident in a Wheelchair

Residents who slide down in a wheelchair will need to be moved back and up. You will need another assistant to help you. One stands in back of the wheelchair and one stands in front of the wheelchair.

1. Carry out each beginning procedure action.
2. Use good body mechanics: separate your feet and knees, bend your knees, and keep your back straight.
3. The assistant in back places both arms around the resident's waist.
   - He crosses his own arms in front of the resident's waist.
   - He grasps the resident's left forearm with his right hand and the resident's right forearm with his left hand.
4. The assistant in front places both arms around the resident's knees (Figure 22-68).
5. On the count of three, both assistants lift and raise the resident up and back in the chair.
6. Carry out each procedure completion action.

Note: It is helpful to place a lifting sheet (turning sheet) in the seats of chairs for residents who are very frail or heavy. With an assistant on each side, the sheet can be grasped to move the resident.

FIGURE 22-68   Residents may need to be repositioned in their wheelchairs.

PROCEDURE 89 Wheelchair Activities to Relieve Pressure

OBRA

Residents who are in a wheelchair for longer than 1 to 2 hours need to relieve the pressure on the hips and buttocks. Teach them to do these activities. You may need to help dependent residents to do these.

Leaning
1. Lock the wheels.
2. Have resident lean slightly forward. (Do not let resident fall out of chair.)
3. Have resident lean from side to side, getting as much weight as possible off each hip.

Wheelchair Pushups
1. Raise the foot pedals. Make sure the resident does not stand on the pedals. Lock the wheels.
2. Tell the resident to place the palms of the hands on the arms of the chair. Then tell the resident to flex (bend) the elbows.
3. Have the resident lean forward, put the feet back, and spread the knees.

4. Tell the resident to lift the buttocks off the chair by pushing down with the hands and straightening the knees (Figure 22-69).

FIGURE 22-69 Residents in wheelchairs can relieve pressure by doing wheelchair pushups.

FIGURE 22-70 The geriatric chair is designed to allow position changes while maintaining body alignment and comfort. (Photo courtesy of Hill-Rom® Long Term Care Division)

Some long-term care facilities use geriatric chairs. These allow the resident's position to be changed (Figure 22-70).

Cardiac chairs are also frequently used for residents. These are similar to recliners. The resident may be placed in different positions. Pillows can be used to relieve pressure on the shoulders, arms, and hips (Figure 22-71).

FIGURE 22-71 Correct positioning in a chair is just as important as positioning in bed.

INDEPENDENT BED MOVEMENT —

The next step in progressive mobilization is to teach the resident how to move independently in bed. This provides exercise and prepares the resident to learn how to move into position to transfer out of bed.

The directions given here are for residents with hemiplegia. These directions can be used with any resident. You should not implement these procedures without instructions from the physical therapist or nurse.

PROCEDURE 90

Assisting with Independent Bed Movement

1. Carry out each beginning procedure action.
2. Make sure the resident understands what you are going to do.
3. These directions are for moving to the head of the bed.
   - Instruct the resident to place his affected arm over his abdomen. Have resident grasp the side rail with his strong hand.
   - Have resident place his strong foot under his weak leg and then slide his strong foot down under his weak ankle. The weak leg will be supported by the stronger leg.
   - Tell the resident to flex the knee of his strong leg and push that foot against the mattress to help him lift his hips.
   - Have the resident raise his head and pull up with his strong arm and leg, pushing himself toward the head of the bed. (If resident is unable to support his weak leg, hold the leg off the bed while the resident moves. This avoids shearing and friction of the weak leg against the sheet.)
4. Moving to the foot of the bed
   - Reverse procedure in Step 3.
5. Moving toward affected side, to side of bed
   - The resident moves segments of his body in sequence; legs and hips, head and shoulders. Order may be reversed.

   - Instruct the resident to place his affected arm over his abdomen.
   - Tell the resident to place his strong foot under the knee of his affected leg and slide it down under the affected ankle. Lift his affected leg and move it toward edge of bed on affected side.
   - Have the resident remove his strong foot and flex the knee of the strong leg. Now have the resident place his foot firmly on the bed and push down, raising his hips and moving them toward his affected side.
   - Tell the resident to raise his head and shoulders and move them toward his affected side by pushing against the mattress or side rail with his strong side. The resident can use his strong arm to push against the mattress to assist in the move.
6. Moving toward strong side, to side of bed
   - Follow above procedure, moving to strong side.
   - Resident can use the strong arm to grasp side rail to assist in move.
7. Turning onto the side for lateral position.
   - If the resident is going to lie on the affected side, follow directions for moving to the *strong side first.*
   - Then have the resident use his strong arm to reach toward the opposite side rail to bring himself onto his side.

(continues)

PROCEDURE 90 *(continued)*

- If the resident is going to lie on the strong side, follow directions for moving to *affected side first.* Have resident grasp his weak hand with his strong hand and raise his arms up with elbows extended. Then have resident use strong arm to "swing" body onto strong side.

8. When the procedure is completed, position the resident according to your instructions.

9. Carry out each procedure completion action.

On the Job

Unfortunately, you may work with a person who will put forth little effort in carrying out some of these very important procedures. The resident will eventually suffer from shortcuts taken by staff. Always let your conscience be your guide and perform all tasks to the very best of your ability.

CONTINUING WITH PROGRESSIVE MOBILIZATION

It is important to complete passive range of motion exercises and positioning procedures correctly. This will prevent contractures and other complications that can prevent the resident from making progress in mobilization.

Transfer and ambulation activities are the next steps in progressive mobilization. Instructions for these procedures are in Lesson 23.

BOWEL AND BLADDER PROGRAMS

Bowel and bladder programs are considered restorative/rehabilitation procedures. These programs are implemented for residents who are incontinent. **Incontinence** is the inability to control the bowel or the bladder (or both).

Incontinence is not a disease and it is *never* a normal consequence of aging. There are a number of reasons why residents in the long-term care facility may be incontinent:

- The resident may be unable to get to the bathroom. This could be because of:
  - Disorientation
  - Impaired mobility
  - Physical environment—bathroom is too far away
- The resident may have a spinal cord injury.
- The resident may have problems holding urine in the bladder when coughing or laughing. This can be caused by:
  - Multiple childbirths
  - Obesity
  - Hormone deficiencies
- The resident may be unable to void and the bladder becomes full, causing it to "overflow."

Incontinence causes many physical and psychological problems. It is embarrassing and may cause the resident to withdraw from all activities. Incontinence can quickly cause skin breakdown and urinary tract infections. It is difficult to avoid unpleasant odors when residents are incontinent. It is better to prevent incontinence than to try and deal with the consequences. Many different types of programs can be used for incontinence.

Reasons for Implementing Bowel and Bladder Management Programs

1. To avoid incontinence
2. To reduce the resident's anxiety, fear, and embarrassment related to incontinence
3. To restore self-respect and dignity, which encourages the resident to participate more fully in facility activities

4. To prevent overfilling of the bladder and complications

5. To prevent urinary tract infections and skin problems

*G*uidelines for

Bowel and Bladder Programs

Before beginning a bowel and bladder program, the nurse will complete an assessment and then plan the program. A bladder retraining assessment form is shown in Figure 22-72. As a nursing assistant, you can help in the following ways:

1. Carry out all instructions accurately and on a timely basis.
2. Avoid the use of incontinent panties or pads during a retraining program.
3. Be consistent in carrying out the program.
4. Assist the resident to be well groomed and appropriately dressed at all times. This increases motivation to succeed.
5. Remember that comfort and privacy are important during all toileting procedures.

It may take several days for the assessment to be completed. Your responsibilities may be to:

1. Record the resident's daily fluid intake.
2. Check the resident for continence at least every 2 hours between 7:00 AM and 10:00 PM and every 4 hours during the night.
3. Record bowel eliminations and the amount of all voidings.
4. Record observations of symptoms that may indicate the reasons for the incontinence. This may include such problems as disorientation and inability to ambulate.

After the assessment is completed, the nurse will determine the type of program best suited to that resident. Program selection is based on the cause of the incontinence and the resident's:

- Mobility skills
- Orientation
- Motivation

In most cases, you will need to continue with the actions you carried out during the assessment. Different methods are used for each program. The programs may:

1. Restore a normal pattern of voiding by increasing the time between voiding.
2. Avoid incontinence by taking the resident to the bathroom according to the resident's habits. Positive reinforcement (giving praise) is important.
3. Avoid incontinence by taking the resident to the bathroom on a fixed voiding schedule, usually every 2 hours.

Other techniques are incorporated into each program. Your facility will have specific procedures to follow. It is important that all team members understand the procedures and the reasons for doing them faithfully.

Incontinence is not an inevitable problem in long-term facilities. Not all residents can be "retrained" but, in most cases, incontinence can be avoided. Catheters are not an alternative to incontinence except in very rare circumstances.

(continues)

$\mathcal{G}$**uidelines** (*continued*)

BLADDER RETRAINING ASSESSMENT
(Reference tags: F315, F316)

CURRENT RESIDENT STATUS

DIAGNOSIS_____ RESIDENT'S AGE_____

RECENT SURGERY? ☐ Yes ☐ No If Yes, date _____ / _____ / _____ and type_____

CURRENT MEDICATIONS (i.e., Diuretics, Psychotropics, etc.)_____

_____

_____

Mental Status and Ability to Communicate	Mobility Status	Vision Status	Right	Left
☐ Alert	☐ Independent	Adequate	☐	☐
☐ Aphasic	☐ Transfer/standing ability	Adequate w/aid	☐	☐
☐ Oriented x_____	☐ Wheelchair bound	Poor	☐	☐
☐ Disoriented	☐ Bed rest	Blind	☐	☐
☐ Depressed	☐ Contractures	**Hearing Status**	**Right**	**Left**
☐ Cooperative	☐ Other_____	Adequate	☐	☐
☐ Uncooperative	_____	Adequate w/aid	☐	☐
☐ Slow comprehension	_____	Poor	☐	☐
☐ Other_____	_____	Deaf	☐	☐

BLADDER ASSESSMENT

1. **LENGTH OF INCONTINENCE:** _____ Days _____ Months _____ Years

2. **REASON FOR INCONTINENCE (if known):** _____
   CATHETER: ☐ Yes ☐ No If Yes, specify type and size _____
   Date inserted _____ / _____ / _____ Reason for catheter _____

3. **USUAL VOIDING PATTERN:** Frequency_____ Amt./voiding _____ cc: /24 hrs. _____ cc
   Pattern: ☐ Upon arising ☐ After meals ☐ No apparent pattern ☐ Night time only
   ☐ Other (specify) _____

4. **SYMPTOMS:** (Check all that apply)
   ☐ Voids often in small amounts ☐ Difficulty stopping stream ☐ Urgency
   ☐ Fills bladder/voids large amount ☐ Dribbles constantly ☐ Burning/Pain
   ☐ Unable to void ☐ Dribbles after voiding ☐ Edema
   ☐ Difficulty starting stream ☐ Dribbles while coughing ☐ Other (specify)_____

5. **HISTORY OF:** ☐ Urinary Disorders ☐ Bladder Disorders ☐ Kidney Disease ☐ Prostate Problems
   ☐ Neurological Disorders ☐ Fecal Impactions ☐ Other (specify)_____

6. **RELIEF AFTER VOIDING:** ☐ Complete ☐ Continued desire to void

7. **BLADDER DISTENDED:** ☐ Yes ☐ No **EMPTIED BY EXTERNAL STIMULI:** ☐ Yes ☐ No
   If Yes, Check: ☐ Kegel Exercises ☐ Warm water over perineum
   ☐ Other (specify) _____

8. **RESIDUAL URINE:** ☐ Yes ☐ No If Yes, Amount: _____ cc

9. **PERCEPTION OF NEED TO VOID:** ☐ Present ☐ Diminished ☐ Absent

10. **WELL HYDRATED:** ☐ Yes ☐ No **AVERAGE FLUID INTAKE (24 HRS)** _____ cc
    AVERAGE FLUID OUTPUT (24 HRS) _____ cc
    Fluids Preferred _____

NAME—Last	First	Middle	Attending Physician	Chart No.

CFS 6-10HH © 1992 Briggs Corporation, Des Moines, IA 50306 (800) 247-2343
Printed in U.S.A.

BLADDER RETRAINING ASSESSMENT
☐ Continued on Reverse

FIGURE 22-72 Bladder retraining assessment form (Reprinted with permission of Briggs Corporation, Des Moines, IA 50306; 800-247-2343)

(continues)

Guidelines (continued)

EVALUATION FOR BLADDER RETRAINING POTENTIAL

☐ **ABLE TO PARTICIPATE IN RETRAINING**   EVALUATION PERIOD:_____ TO _____

PLAN:_____

_____

PROVIDE FLUIDS: **FLUIDS SHOULD BE SPACED AS FOLLOWS:**

_____ cc every 24 Hrs	☐7AM	☐11	☐3PM	☐7	☐11PM ☐3
_____ cc 7-3 shift	☐8	☐12N	☐4	☐8	☐12MN ☐4
_____ cc 3-11 shift	☐9	☐1PM	☐5	☐9	☐1AM ☐5
_____ cc 11-7 shift	☐10	☐2	☐6	☐10	☐2 ☐6

OFFER NO FLUIDS AFTER _____ **PM   TOILET FOR VOIDING EVERY** ____ Hrs (Day and Evening) ____ Hrs (Night)
(Except as needed for medications)
RECORD RESULTS ON BLADDER RETRAINING RECORD.

☐ **UNABLE TO PARTICIPATE IN RETRAINING**

REASON: _____

_____

REEVALUATION DATE: _____

COMPLETED BY: _____   ___/___/___
                         Signature/Title   Date

BLADDER RETRAINING PROGRESS NOTES OR REEVALUATION NOTES

DATE	TIME	NOTES - ALL ENTRIES MUST BE SIGNED WITH NAME AND TITLE

NAME—Last	First	Middle	Attending Physician	Chart No.

BLADDER RETRAINING NOTES

FIGURE 22-72   *(continued)*

LESSON SYNTHESIS: Putting It All Together

You have just completed this lesson. Now go back and review the Clinical Focus. Try to see how the Clinical Focus relates to the concepts presented in this lesson. Then answer the following questions.

1. Why will you encourage Mrs. Murphy to do as much of her own care as possible?

2. If range of motion activities are not carefully and regularly carried out with her left arm and leg, what serious complication could develop?

3. When not being exercised, what is the proper position for Mrs. Murphy's affected arm and leg?

4. Before attempting to move Mrs. Murphy, what actions should the nursing assistant take?

REVIEW

A. Select the one best answer for each of the following.

1. Restorative care is the responsibility of the
   (A) physician
   (B) nursing staff
   (C) physical therapist
   (D) occupational therapist

2. "Activity strengthens and inactivity weakens" is a principle of restorative care and means that
   (A) complications result from physical and mental inactivity
   (B) residents should receive several hours of bed rest each day
   (C) residents are not encouraged to move about
   (D) inactivity is not harmful

3. "Treat the whole person" is a principle of restorative care and means that it is important to
   (A) attend to the physical needs of the resident
   (B) attend to the emotional needs of the resident
   (C) attend to the mental needs of the resident
   (D) provide for the physical, emotional, and mental needs of the resident

4. Contractures can be prevented by all but
   (A) doing range of motion exercises regularly
   (B) using correct positioning techniques
   (C) correctly applying splints
   (D) encouraging bedrest

5. An example of an instrumental activity of daily living is
   (A) feeding oneself
   (B) managing a household
   (C) swimming
   (D) riding a bicycle

6. A self-care deficit may be due to all but
   (A) paralysis
   (B) perceptual deficits
   (C) depression
   (D) being active

7. The first step in progressive mobilization is teaching the resident to
   (A) come to a standing position
   (B) change position in bed
   (C) move in bed
   (D) move about in a wheelchair

8. Passive range of motion means
   (A) the care provider moves the joints for the resident

(B) the care provider supports the joints and assists in the movements while the resident attempts independent movement

(C) the resident is able to move the joints without any assistance

(D) the resident uses the strong extremity to move the affected extremity

9. An orthosis is (a, an)
   (A) artificial body part
   (B) sling
   (C) splint
   (D) cane

10. The purpose of an orthosis is to
    (A) replace a missing body part
    (B) simplify an activity of daily living
    (C) help a person ambulate
    (D) support a joint in correct position

11. The main purpose of bowel and bladder programs is to
    (A) save time for the nursing staff so they do not have to change incontinent residents
    (B) increase the resident's self-esteem and dignity
    (C) save money on incontinent pads
    (D) save on laundry costs

B. **Match each term (items a.–j.) with the proper definition.**

   a. flexion   f. pronation
   b. extension   g. supination
   c. abduction   h. inversion
   d. adduction   i. eversion
   e. rotation   j. opposition

12. _____ bringing palmar surface of thumb to the finger joint

13. _____ bending a joint

14. _____ moving an extremity away from the body

15. _____ turning the forearm so the palm is facing downward

16. _____ straightening a joint

17. _____ turning inward

18. _____ moving an extremity back to the body

19. _____ turning around an axis

20. _____ turning the forearm so the palm is facing upward

21. _____ turning outward

C. **Answer each statement true (T) or false (F).**

22. T F It is a resident's right to have the staff do everything for him or her.

23. T F OBRA requires that restorative care be included in nursing assistant courses.

24. T F One purpose of restorative care is to help the resident adapt to limitations imposed by a disability.

25. T F Successful restorative care means that the resident always regains his or her functional abilities.

26. T F Restorative care generally involves training from physical therapists and occupational therapists.

27. T F Long-term inactivity can cause the heart to become deconditioned.

28. T F Restorative care is only important for residents who are planning to return to their homes.

29. T F Correct positioning can prevent pressure ulcers and contracture formation.

30. T F Incontinence is not considered a normal change of aging.

LESSON 23

Restoring Residents' Mobility

Clinical Focus

Think about the special precautions you must take to safeguard a resident during periods of mobility as you study this lesson and meet:

*M*s. Peabody, who, although ambulatory with a walker since her hip surgery, is unsteady and needs assistance.

OBJECTIVES

After studying this lesson, you should be able to:

- Define and spell vocabulary words and terms.
- List the guidelines for transfer procedures.
- State the contraindications to using a transfer belt.
- Describe the factors that are considered in determining the correct method of transfer.
- List the guidelines for ambulation procedures.
- Describe the purpose of assistive devices used in ambulation.
- Describe safety measures when using assistive devices.
- Demonstrate the following:

  Procedure 91   Using a Transfer Belt (Gait Belt)
  Procedure 92   Bringing the Resident to Sitting Position at the Edge of the Bed
  Procedure 93   Assisted Standing Transfer
  Procedure 94   Transferring the Resident from Chair to Bed
  Procedure 95   Assisted Standing Transfer/Two Assistants
  Procedure 96   Wheelchair to Toilet and Toilet to Wheelchair Transfers
  Procedure 97   Transferring to Tub Chair or Shower Chair
  Procedure 98   Transferring a Nonstanding Resident from Wheelchair to Bed
  Procedure 99   Transferring Resident with a Mechanical Lift
  Procedure 100 Sliding Board Transfer
  Procedure 101 Ambulating a Resident
  Procedure 102 Assisting Resident to Ambulate with Cane or Walker

VOCABULARY

ambulate *(AM-byou-late)*

aneurysm *(AN-you-rizm)*

assistive device *(ah-SIS-tiv dih-VICE)*

colostomy *(koh-LAHS-toh-mee)*

gait *(gayt)*

gait belt *(gayt belt)*

gait training *(gayt TRAYN-ing)*

mechanical lift *(mih-KAN-ih-kul lift)*

non-weight bearing *(NON-wayt BAIR-ing)*

pacemaker *(PAYS-may-ker)*

paraplegia *(pair-ah-PLEE-jee-ah)*

partial weight bearing *(PAR-shul wayt BAIR-ing)*

sliding board *(SLYD-ing bord)*

transfer *(TRANS-fer)*

transfer belt *(TRANS-fer belt)*

weight bearing *(wayt BAIR-ing)*

Many residents in long-term care facilities have impaired mobility. *Mobility* means movement. Restorative care includes assisting dependent residents with mobility and helping residents regain independent mobility.

In Lesson 22 you learned how to help residents regain independence in activities of daily living. You also learned how to perform procedures that will prevent the complications caused by immobility. The next step is to help residents get out of bed, to transfer, and to **ambulate** (walk).

Remember that restorative care is a team effort. While you are helping residents on the nursing unit, other departments are working with the residents to help them reach their goals for increasing their abilities (Figure 23-1).

FIGURE 23-1 Staff in occupational therapy direct the residents in activities that will help them regain the use of their hands.

TRANSFERS

The word **transfer** means to move a resident from one place to another. Transfers are used to:

- Move a resident out of bed and into a chair
- Move a resident from a chair and into bed
- Move a resident from a wheelchair to a toilet or commode
- Move a resident from a toilet or commode into a wheelchair
- Move a resident from a chair into a car and back
- Move a resident from a chair into a tub lift or shower chair and back into the chair

The nurse or physical therapist determines the method of transfer. The method selected depends on:

1. The resident's physical condition, including:
   - Paralysis of any extremity
   - Absence of an extremity due to amputation
   - Recent hip surgery
2. The resident's strength, endurance, and balance. These abilities may be affected by:
   - Respiratory disease
   - Cardiac disease
   - Neurologic disease
   - Ability to stand on one or both legs. This is called **weight bearing**. For example, a resident may not be able to bear weight on a paralyzed leg. After hip surgery the physician may order the resident to be **non-weight bearing** or to be only **partial weight bearing**.
3. The resident's mental condition. Can the resident understand instructions?
4. The resident's size

There are two basic types of transfer: standing and sitting. For a standing transfer, the resident must be able to stand and have weight bear-

*G*uidelines for

Transfers

Note: Always use the correct transfer method as directed by the nurse or physical therapist. Disregarding these instructions can result in injury to the resident or to you. If you have difficulty transferring a resident by the indicated method, consult with the nurse.

1. If the transfer requires two people, do not try to do it alone. You risk injuring yourself and the resident.
2. Use correct body mechanics for all transfers.
3. *Residents should never place their hands on your body during a transfer.* This is a dangerous practice. A resident who is disoriented or frightened can cause you to lose your balance. A resident who loses balance during transfer can pull you down. If a resident's arms are around your neck, any sudden movement can injure you.
4. *Never place your hands under a resident's arms.* Remember that residents' bones are fragile. This practice can fracture ribs and dislocate shoulders.
5. Use a transfer belt for standing transfers unless it is contraindicated (see Procedure 91).
6. The resident should wear sturdy, well-fitting shoes with nonslip soles for all standing transfers and ambulation.
7. Give the resident only the assistance needed.
8. Stand close to the resident when transferring. If the resident has a weak or paralyzed leg, brace that knee with your knee or leg.
9. Always transfer toward the resident's strongest side.
10. Allow the resident to see the surface to which the resident is being transferred. Encourage the resident to keep the head up.
11. Always explain to the resident what you are doing and how the resident can help.

ing on one leg. Examples of sitting transfers are those done with a mechanical lift or sliding board.

Several steps are involved in transferring a resident from bed to chair:

- Bringing the resident to a sitting position on the edge of the bed
- Bringing the resident to a standing position
- Moving the resident to the chair
- Seating the resident

PROCEDURE 91

Using a Transfer Belt (Gait Belt)

A **transfer belt** is a webbed belt 1½ to 2 inches wide. It is 54 to 60 inches long. It is an assistive and safety device used to transfer or ambulate residents who need help. When the belt is used to assist a resident with ambulation, it is called a **gait belt**.

1. Carry out each beginning procedure action.

2. Show the resident the transfer belt and explain that it is a safety device. Assure the resident that the belt is used only for a short time during the actual transfer or ambulation exercise.

3. The belt should never be placed over bare skin. If it is used to transfer a resident to a shower seat or tub lift, place a

(continues)

PROCEDURE 91 *(continued)*

towel around the resident's waist and then apply the belt over it.

4. Keep the belt at the resident's waist level.
5. Buckle the belt in front—not at the back or the side (Figure 23-2A).
6. Thread the belt through the teeth side first and place belt through both openings to ensure a safe closure (Figure 23-2B).

FIGURE 23-2A Buckle the transfer belt in front.

FIGURE 23-2B Thread the belt through the teeth side of the buckle first.

7. Use an *underhand* grasp when holding the belt (Figure 23-3).
8. The belt should be snug but you should be able to get your fingers under it. This will prevent the belt from riding up under the breasts, rib cage, or axillae.

FIGURE 23-3 Both of the patient's hands should be on the arms of the chair.

9. Check female residents to be sure breasts are not under the belt.
10. Avoid overusing the belt by pulling the resident up with too much force. *Remember:* The belt is not a lifting device—it is used for support and stability.
11. Transfer resident using the correct method.
12. Carry out each procedure completion action.

Note: The transfer belt may be contraindicated for these conditions:

1. **Colostomy** located in the upper abdomen. This is a surgical opening created for the evacuation of feces.
2. **Pacemaker** located in the abdomen. This is a device used to maintain a normal heart rate.
3. Recent abdominal surgery.
4. Recent back or rib fractures.
5. Advanced cardiac disease.
6. Advanced lung disease.
7. Abdominal **aneurysms**. An aneurysm is a weak spot in an artery wall.

Note: Do not use the pants/slacks belt as a transfer or gait belt when transferring or ambulating residents. Upward movement of the belt can cause male residents severe pain in the scrotum.

PROCEDURE 92
Bringing the Resident to Sitting Position at the Edge of the Bed

1. Carry out each beginning procedure action.

Note: You may be asked to check the resident's pulse before beginning any activity. If so, take the pulse now.

2. If you will be transferring the resident into the chair:

- Have the chair ready to receive the resident. If it is a wheelchair, lock the brakes. Put the foot pedals up or remove them if possible. If the arm of the chair is removable, it is easier to work with it off.
- Have the resident's clothing and shoes ready.
- Have the transfer belt ready if it is to be used.

Note: If the resident is to transfer out of the bed, the bed must be in the low position. *Remember to use correct body mechanics.*

3. Begin with the resident lying in supine position in the center of the bed.

4. Have the resident cross arms over the abdomen or chest.

5. Cross the resident's farthest leg over the leg nearest you.

6. Stand facing the bed with your thigh that is nearest the resident's head braced against the bed. *Bend your knees and hips. Assume a broad base of support. Get close to the resident.*

7. With one hand on the resident's far shoulder and one on the far hip, turn the resident onto the side, facing you (Figure 23-4).

8. Flex the resident's hips and knees.

9. With your arm that is closest to the resident's legs, reach across the top leg and secure both legs with your arm.

10. Place your other arm so that your forearm supports the resident's shoulders. The resident's neck and head are cradled by your elbow.

11. As you shift your weight from your front to back leg, lower the resident's legs over the edge of the bed. At the same time, bring the resident's head and shoulders to upright position (Figure 23-5).

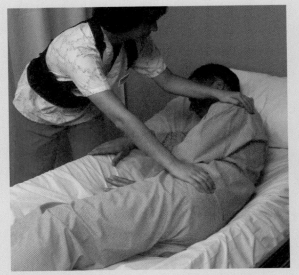

FIGURE 23-4 Help the resident turn to the side before sitting on the edge of the bed.

FIGURE 23-5 Help the resident to a sitting position on the edge of the bed.

(continues)

PROCEDURE 92 *(continued)*

Note: If the resident is able to, ask the resident to use the lower arm to support the upper body. Ask the resident to use the upper arm to push into the mattress to raise the upper body.

12. Carry out transfer as indicated in the next procedures.

PROCEDURE 93 Assisted Standing Transfer

Note: The bed should be in the low position when you transfer a resident into or out of bed. You must use good body mechanics—keep your back straight, bend from the knees and hips, and maintain a broad base of support.

1. Carry out each beginning procedure action.
2. The chair is placed on the resident's strong side. Place it at the foot or the head of the bed and parallel to the bed.
3. If you are using a wheelchair, lock the brakes. The front casters of the chair should be straight. Put the foot pedals up or remove them from the chair.
4. Lock the wheels of the bed.
5. Check the resident's pulse if instructed to do so. Bring the resident to a sitting position on the edge of the bed as directed in Procedure 92. Allow resident to sit for a few seconds to stabilize.
6. Put a transfer belt around the resident's waist.
7. Put shoes and socks on the resident.

Note: If you are unsure of the resident's balance, you can put the transfer belt on while the resident is lying down. You can also put the shoes and socks on at that time.

8. Tell the resident what to do to help.
9. Assist the resident to assume the transfer position:
   • Ask the resident to lean forward ("nose over toes").

   • Have resident separate the knees for a broad base of support.
   • Have resident move the feet back.

Note: Be sure to check the resident's feet before transferring. Some residents are unable to tell what position their feet are in.

   • Ask the resident to place the palms of the hands against the edge of the mattress. This will help the resident to "push off."

10. Place yourself in front of the resident. If the resident has a weak or paralyzed leg, brace that knee with your knee.
11. Place your other leg several inches back.
12. Place your hands in the transfer belt (underhand grasp) with one hand on each side of the resident's body.
13. If the resident has a weak or paralyzed arm, do not let it hang or dangle during the transfer.
    • If the resident has a sling, put this on before the transfer.
    • If there is no sling, the hand can be placed in the pants pocket or the resident can cradle the weak arm with the strong arm.
14. Before moving the resident, make sure both you and the resident are ready to move.
15. Tell the resident that on the count of three she will:
    • Use the hands (if able) to press into the mattress.

(continues)

PROCEDURE 93 *(continued)*

- Straighten the elbows.
- Straighten the knees and come to a standing position.

16. At the same time, you will use the transfer belt to gently assist the resident to stand—do not lift the resident with the belt.
    - Remember, the resident should not grasp your neck, arms, or any part of your body. You should not use your hands and arms on the resident's body.

17. If the resident cannot take any steps:
    - Have resident pivot around to the front of the chair until the chair touches the back of the resident's legs.

18. Instruct resident to place hands on the arms of the chair and then gently lower resident into the chair (Figure 23-6).

19. If you took the resident's pulse before the activity, recheck it now. If there is a significant difference, report this to the nurse.

20. Position the resident comfortably. Place the signal light within easy reach. Be sure the resident has access to drinking water and any other items that may be needed.

21. Carry out each procedure completion action.

FIGURE 23-6 Instruct the resident to place her hands on the arms of the chair and then gently lower resident into chair.

PROCEDURE 94 Transferring the Resident from Chair to Bed

Note: Use good body mechanics—keep your back straight, bend from the knees and hips, and maintain a broad base of support with your feet.

1. Reverse Procedure 93.
2. If the resident has a weak or paralyzed side, place the wheelchair so that the resident can transfer to the strong side. Lock the brakes on the wheelchair and remove the footrests.
3. Lock the wheels on the bed.
4. Place the transfer belt around the resident's waist.
5. Have resident assume the transfer position as described in Procedure 93.
6. Follow Steps 10 through 14 in Procedure 93.
7. Tell the resident to place the hands on the arms of the wheelchair or chair.
8. On the count of three, have resident straighten both elbows and knees to come to a standing position.

(continues)

PROCEDURE 94 *(continued)*

9. Pivot around to the bed. When the resident feels the bed against the backs of the legs, have resident slowly sit down on the edge of the bed.
10. Remove the transfer belt and the resident's shoes and socks. If balance is questionable, this can be done after the resident is lying down.
11. Place your arm closest to the head of the bed around the resident's shoulders. Place your other arm around the resident's knees (Figure 23-7).
12. Guide the resident to a supine position. Position the resident comfortably.
13. Carry out each procedure completion action.

FIGURE 23-7   Assist the resident to lie down.

PROCEDURE 95

Assisted Standing Transfer/Two Assistants

Note: This procedure is for a resident who is heavier, taller, has impaired balance, or only partial weight-bearing ability.

Follow your instructions when you are told that two people are required to move or transfer a resident. Disregarding instructions can result in serious injury to you and the resident. *Remember: Use good body mechanics*—keep your back straight, bend from the knees and hips, and maintain a broad base of support with your feet.

1. Carry out each beginning procedure action.

This procedure is carried out the same as a one-person transfer except:

2. Both assistants stand in front of and to each side of the resident.
3. Both assistants put both hands in the transfer belt. Each assistant has one

hand in the front of the belt and one in the back of the belt (Figure 23-8).

FIGURE 23-8   Some residents need the help of two nursing assistants. The nursing assistants have both hands in the transfer belt.

(continues)

PROCEDURE 95 *(continued)*

4. If the resident has a paralyzed leg, one assistant blocks that leg with her knee against the resident's knee.

It is important that both assistants and the resident clearly understand the direction of the move.

5. On the count of three, both assistants and the resident pivot around to the chair.
6. Continue procedure as with one assistant.
7. Carry out each procedure completion action.

PROCEDURE 96
Wheelchair to Toilet and Toilet to Wheelchair Transfers

Remember: Use good body mechanics—keep your back straight, bend from the hips and knees, and maintain a broad base of support with your feet.

1. Carry out each beginning procedure action.
2. You may need to adapt the procedure to the physical arrangement of the bathroom.

- Grab bars should be placed securely on the wall or attached to the toilet seat (Figure 23-9). *Towel bars are not safe to use as grab bars.*

FIGURE 23-9   Grab bars provide safety.

3. Most toilets are 16 inches high. Some residents may have difficulty coming to a standing position from this level. A raised toilet seat can be added, which will raise it to 20 inches.
4. Follow all the guidelines for transfers. Use the transfer belt.
5. Place wheelchair at a right angle to the toilet. Lock the brakes. Be sure the foot pedals are up or off.
6. While the resident is still sitting, loosen clothing.
7. Bring resident to a standing position as described earlier.

- Ask the resident to lean forward.
- Have the resident separate knees for a broad base of support.
- Have the resident move the feet back.
- Have resident place palms of the hands on the wheelchair arms to help "push off."
- On the count of three, help the resident to a standing position (Figure 23-10).

8. Encourage the resident to stand erect. Pivot to toilet seat.
9. Have resident use the grab bars for support while you manipulate the clothing. If the resident's balance is questionable, you will need another assistant to do this while you help the resident stand.

(continues)

PROCEDURE *96* (continued)

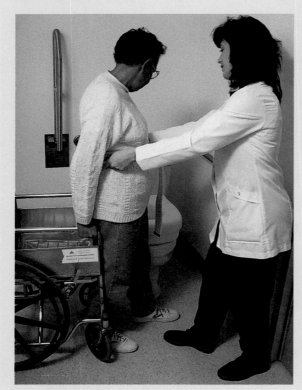

FIGURE 23-10 Help the resident to a standing position.

10. With your hands in the transfer belt, assist the resident to sitting position on the toilet.
11. Remove transfer belt. Provide privacy, but remain close by.

When resident is finished toileting:

12. Position wheelchair at a right angle to toilet. Lock the brakes. Be sure the foot pedals are up or off. If possible, place wheelchair on resident's strong side.
13. Have toilet tissue ready.
14. Put on gloves.
15. Bring resident to standing position. Have resident use grab bars while you clean resident's buttocks and genitalia.

    - If resident is able, provide support while the resident performs this task.

16. Arrange clothing while resident is still using the grab bars for support.
17. Assist the resident to pivot to the wheelchair.

    - Have resident put hands on the arms of the chair.
    - When resident feels the edge of the seat against the back of the legs, have the resident slowly sit in the chair.
    - Your hands are still in the transfer belt so you can provide assistance.

18. Wheel the chair to the lavatory. Assist the resident in washing and drying hands.
19. Remove your gloves. Wash and dry your hands.
20. Carry out each procedure completion action.

PROCEDURE *97* Transferring to Tub Chair or Shower Chair

Remember: Use good body mechanics—keep your back straight, bend from the hips and knees, and maintain a broad base of support with your feet.

The procedure for transferring a resident from a wheelchair to a tub chair or shower chair is carried out in the same manner as a transfer from a wheelchair to toilet or chair, with added considerations.

1. Carry out each beginning procedure action.

(continues)

PROCEDURE *97* *(continued)*

FIGURE 23-11 Transport the resident to the shower or tub room by wheelchair.

2. Transport the resident to the shower or tub room by wheelchair (Figure 23-11).
3. Lock wheelchair. Remove footrests.
4. Remove the resident's top clothing while resident is seated in the wheelchair.
5. Leave the resident's shoes on until the resident has transferred to the shower or tub chair.
   - Place a large towel around the resident's shoulders to avoid chilling and exposure.
   - Place a towel around the resident's waist before applying transfer belt. Apply transfer belt.
   - Assist the resident to stand.

- Have resident pivot around or take a step to the shower or tub chair.
- Loosen and bring underwear and slacks down below resident's hips.

6. Have resident sit down in shower chair or tub chair. Remove underwear, slacks, shoes, and socks.
7. Place towel over resident's lap.
8. Remove transfer belt. When shower/bath is completed, reverse procedure.
9. Dry resident while seated in tub or shower chair.
10. Help resident put on upper body clothing while seated in tub or shower chair. Then apply transfer belt.
11. Put resident's underwear and slacks on.
    - Pull up to the hips.
    - Put on socks and shoes.
12. Assist resident to stand. Pull up underwear and slacks.
13. Assist resident to pivot or step to wheelchair.
    - When the resident feels the wheelchair against the back of the legs, have resident place hands on arms of wheelchair.
    - Then have resident slowly seat self in wheelchair.
14. Carry out each procedure completion action.

PROCEDURE 98

Transferring a Nonstanding Resident from Wheelchair to Bed

OBRA

This procedure is used for residents who are unable to stand. The resident must be able to follow directions. This is not an appropriate transfer for a resident who is large. The procedure requires two assistants. It should only be done when the wheelchair has removable arms and removable footrests.

Remember: Use good body mechanics—keep your back straight, bend from the hips and knees, and maintain a broad base of support with your feet.

1. Carry out each beginning procedure action.

(continues)

PROCEDURE 98 *(continued)*

2. Lock wheels of bed. Put bed in lowest horizontal position.
3. Remove arms from wheelchair. Remove footrests from wheelchair. Place wheelchair at head of bed facing foot of bed. Wheelchair should be parallel to bed.
4. The first assistant stands behind the wheelchair. The second assistant stands in front of the wheelchair.
5. The first assistant places arms around resident's trunk. This assistant crosses arms and grasps the resident's left forearm with assistant's right hand. The resident's right forearm is grasped with the assistant's left hand.
6. The second assistant stands beside resident's legs, facing bed. This assistant places both arms under resident's legs.
7. Remember to use good body mechanics. On the count of three, the resident is lifted out of the chair and into bed.
8. Position resident as necessary.
9. Carry out each procedure completion action.

USING MECHANICAL LIFTS

A **mechanical lift** may be needed to transfer certain residents. This device is used to move residents who are unable to bear weight, are heavy, or have poor trunk control. Remember these precautions when using a mechanical lift:

- *Two people are required for this procedure.*
- Be sure both people have been instructed in the correct procedure before attempting to use a mechanical lift with residents.
- The procedure may vary depending on the manufacturer of the equipment.
- Be sure the equipment is in good working order.

PROCEDURE 99 Transferring Resident with a Mechanical Lift

1. Carry out each beginning procedure action.
2. Get another assistant or nurse to help you. One person operates the lift. The other person guides the sling and resident.
3. Check sling and straps for frayed areas or poorly closing clasps.
4. Place a wheelchair or other chair parallel to bed, facing the head of the bed.
5. Lock the bed. Lock the wheelchair or other chair wheels.
6. Position the sling under the resident's body by rolling him first onto his left side. Place the folded sling against his body (Figure 23-12).

FIGURE 23-12 Position sling under the resident's body by rolling him first onto his left side. Place folded sling against his body.

(continues)

PROCEDURE *99* *(continued)*

7. Roll resident onto his right side and straighten the sling (Figure 23-13).
8. Make sure that the sling reaches from his shoulders to his knees (Figure 23-14).
9. Position the lift over the bed and attach the hooks to the sling (Figure 23-15). Make sure that the open end of each hook is turned away from the resident's body (Figure 23-16).
10. Raise the lift following the directions for the specific type of lift used at your facility. Gently swing the resident to the chair. One nursing assistant can support the resident's legs (Figure 23-17).

FIGURE 23-15 Position the lift over the bed and attach the hooks to the sling.

FIGURE 23-13 Roll resident onto his right side and straighten the sling.

FIGURE 23-16 Make sure that the open end of each hook is turned away from the resident's body.

FIGURE 23-14 Make sure that the sling reaches from his shoulders to his knees.

11. Lower the lift and seat the resident in the chair. Unhook suspension straps and move lift out of the way. The sling may be left under the resident until he is ready to be lifted back into bed (Figure 23-18).
12. Position resident as necessary. Place signal light, drinking water, and other items as needed within resident's reach. Make sure resident is covered and warm.
13. Carry out each procedure completion action.

(continues)

PROCEDURE *99* *(continued)*

FIGURE 23-17 Raise the lift following the directions for the type of lift used at your facility. Gently swing resident into chair.

FIGURE 23-18 Lower the resident into the chair. Unhook suspension straps and move the lift out of the way. The sling may be left under the resident until he is ready to be lifted back into bed.

SLIDING BOARD TRANSFER

A **sliding board** (Figure 23-19) is used for a sitting transfer. The board should be smooth and waxed to ease movement. This procedure is used for residents who are paralyzed in both legs (**paraplegia**) or who have had both legs amputated. It can be used for other residents who are non-weight bearing as designated by the nurse or physical therapist. The resident must have stability of the upper body for this type of transfer.

FIGURE 23-19 Sliding boards are used for some types of transfers.

Guidelines for
Sliding Board Transfers

1. The two transfer surfaces should be at the same level.
2. The wheelchair must have removable, swing-away, or lift-off footrests and removable armrests.
3. Residents with adequate upper body strength may eventually be able to do this transfer independently.
4. The resident must be dressed for this transfer so that the buttocks and backs of the upper legs are completely covered. Never attempt to transfer a resident across the sliding board if there is a possibility that bare skin will contact the board.
5. Position wheelchair so resident can transfer toward strong side.
6. Place a transfer belt around resident's waist.
7. Lock the wheelchair and the bed.

PROCEDURE
100 Sliding Board Transfer

1. Carry out each beginning procedure action.
2. Place wheelchair at slight angle next to bed. Remove armrest and footrest on side next to bed.
3. Bring resident to sitting position on edge of bed as described in Procedure 92. Apply transfer belt.
4. Position sliding board so one end is on wheelchair and the other end is just under the resident's buttocks. *The beveled side of the sliding board is facing up.*
5. Stand in front of the resident. Assume a broad base of support with your knees and hips flexed and your back straight.
6. Using an underhand grasp, grasp the belt on each side of the resident.
7. Slide the resident across the board and into the chair.
8. Remove the board from under the resident. Remove the transfer belt.
9. Replace the armrest and footrest.
10. Reposition resident in wheelchair if necessary. Make sure signal light and any items the resident may need are within reach.
11. Carry out each procedure completion action. To return resident to bed, reverse the procedure.

AMBULATION

Ambulation is the process of walking. It is good exercise for the resident. The weight bearing on the legs helps prevent or delay the onset of disuse osteoporosis. Walking increases the resident's independence and provides more opportunities for socializing and activities.

The term **gait** refers to the way in which a person walks. There are many disorders that can affect a person's gait, such as:

- Stroke—one side of the body is paralyzed (hemiplegia).
- Multiple sclerosis—one or both legs are weakened and balance may be disturbed.

- Huntington's disease—the resident has involuntary movements that disturb balance.
- Parkinson's disease—the resident has stiffness and slowness of movements, causing shuffling.
- Arthritis—resident has pain and stiffness in joints.

Evaluation by the Nurse or Physical Therapist

Before an ambulation program is started, the nurse or physical therapist will evaluate the resident's:

- Tolerance to movement in bed
- Ability to participate in active (as opposed to passive) exercise
- Ability to transfer safely with minimal assistance
- Ability to stand and bear weight
- Strength, endurance, and balance

- Mental state to determine if the resident can follow directions
- Ability to walk alone (is the assistance of a person or equipment needed?)

Normal Gait Pattern

There are two phases to a normal gait (walking). The leg is on the floor during the first phase and the leg is brought forward during the second phase. Walking begins with the ankle in dorsiflexion and the heel striking the floor first (Figure 23-20), rolling onto the ball of the foot. The resident must be able to stand straight on this leg while bringing the other leg forward. The arms normally have slight swinging movement during walking. Each arm moves in the same direction as the opposite leg (Figure 23-21). To walk safely, the resident must have adequate joint motion in the hips and knees and strength in the muscles of the hips, buttocks, and legs. The

FIGURE 23-20 Walking begins with the ankle in dorsiflexion. The heel strikes the floor first.

FIGURE 23-21 Each arm moves in the same direction as the opposite leg during walking.

FIGURE 23-22 The physical therapist will teach some residents how to manipulate stairs.

FIGURE 23-23 All assistive devices have rubber tips on the bottoms and rubber handgrips.

physical therapist may work with the resident on exercises to promote movement and strength before the resident starts walking.

Gait Training

The physical therapist may work with the resident on **gait training** (teaching the resident to walk).

The physical therapist will teach the resident how to:

- Walk correctly
- Walk on different surfaces, such as linoleum floors, carpet, grass, gravel
- Manipulate stairs (Figure 23-22)
- Get in and out of a chair
- Use an assistive device if one is ordered

Assistive Devices

An **assistive device** is often prescribed. These devices include crutches, canes, and walkers. An assistive device can help compensate for problems the resident has with walking. Several

types of crutches, canes, and walkers are used. The needs of the resident and the cause of the problem are factors in selecting the device. The nurse or physical therapist will adjust the device to fit the resident. The gait used with the device is determined by the resident's abilities, the cause of the impairment, and the type of assistive device. The nurse or physical therapist will select the appropriate gait. You should know the gaits that have been selected. When you walk with the resident you can then observe to make sure the resident is using the device correctly.

Safety Guidelines for Using Assistive Devices

All canes, crutches, and walkers have rubber tips on the bottoms and rubber handgrips. (Figure 23-23). These must be replaced if the ridges are cracked, loose, or worn down. If the ridges are filled with debris, use alcohol and cotton swabs to clean them. Replace any loose or cracked handgrips. Check screws, nuts, and bolts for tightness. Do not use any device that appears unsafe. Report the problem according to facility policy.

Use of Crutches. Standard crutches (Figure 23-24) are seldom recommended for older adults. They can be hard to handle and require balance and two strong arms. Metal forearm or Canadian crutches may be used by residents who have weakness of both legs. The cuff of the

FIGURE 23-24 Standard crutches are seldom recommended for older adults. (Courtesy of Lumex Medical Products, Bay Shore, NY)

FIGURE 23-25 Forearm crutches will remain in place when the handle is released. (Courtesy of Lumex Medical Products, Bay Shore, NY)

FIGURE 23-26 Platform crutches permit weight bearing on the forearms, creating stability. (Courtesy of Lumex Medical Products, Bay Shore, NY)

FIGURE 23-27 Several types of canes are available. (Courtesy of Lumex Medical Products, Bay Shore, NY)

crutch encloses the forearm so the resident can release that hand without dropping the crutch (Figure 23-25).

Forearm crutches with platforms permit weight bearing on the forearms, which provides stability. During use, the elbows are in a constant 90° angle to the shoulder (Figure 23-26). The resident may need assistance in attaching the arm straps of the platforms. If you care for residents with crutches, you will be taught the gaits the resident is to use.

Use of Canes.   Quad canes and tripod canes provide a wide base of support. Pyramid canes are four-pronged devices with a broad base and are narrower at the top. Single-prong canes with T-handles or J-handles have straight handles with a handgrip and are easier to hold than half-circle handled canes (Figure 23-27). Canes are recommended for aiding balance rather than for providing support. The cane is always held by the arm on the *strong* side of the body.

Use of Walkers.   Walkers also come in a variety of styles (Figure 23-28). Walkers are recommended for individuals who have general weakness of both legs, partial weight bearing on one leg, or mild balance problems.

FIGURE 23-28   Walkers come in a variety of styles. (Courtesy of Lumex Medical Products, Bay Shore, NY)

---

*G*uidelines for
Ambulation

1. Always use a transfer (gait) belt if the resident has problems with balance, coordination, or endurance.
2. If the resident's endurance is questionable, ask another person to follow behind with a wheelchair. Have the resident sit in the chair if weakness occurs.
3. If resident has balance problems, two people should ambulate the resident to provide counterbalance.
4. The resident should wear sturdy, well-fitting shoes with nonslip soles.
5. Check clothing to be sure shoelaces or slacks are not inhibiting safe ambulation.
6. Know whether the resident needs an assistive device. An assistive device is anything the resident uses during ambulation, such as canes, walkers, and crutches.

PROCEDURE *101*
Ambulating a Resident

1. Carry out each beginning procedure action.
2. Place the bed in lowest position.
3. Bring the resident to a sitting position on the edge of the bed.
4. Put the gait belt around the resident's waist.
5. Using an underhand grasp on the gait belt, assist the resident to a standing position.
6. Stand on the resident's weak side. Place your hand closest to the resident in the back of the gait belt, using an underhand grasp.
7. Place your other hand in front of the resident's shoulder.
8. Walk with the resident, coordinating your steps. Watch the resident for signs of weakness or faintness.
9. Encourage the resident to walk erect. Encourage normal arm swing.
10. Stop the activity before the resident becomes fatigued.
11. Assist the resident back into chair or bed.
12. Carry out each procedure completion action.

PROCEDURE *102*
Assisting Resident to Ambulate with Cane or Walker

1. Carry out each beginning procedure action.
2. Get walker or cane as directed.
3. Check walker or cane for worn areas or loose parts. Be sure rubber tips and handgrips have adequate tread. If these are cracked or worn, they should be replaced.
4. Place bed in lowest horizontal position.
   - Assist resident to sitting position on edge of bed.
   - Apply transfer (gait) belt if needed.
   - If resident is sitting in a wheelchair, lock the brakes and be sure footrests are up or off. Apply gait belt if needed.
5. Place walker or cane within reach.

Note: Canes and walkers are not transfer devices. Never allow residents to use either device while they are getting up from the chair or bed.

6. Help resident to come to a standing position.
7. Place cane or walker within resident's reach.

Ambulating with a Cane
Note: A cane is *always* held on the strong side (Figure 23-29). For example, a person who has hemiplegia (paralysis on one side) on the right side would hold the cane with the left hand. A person who has had hip surgery on the right side would hold the cane on the left side.

1. For a three-point gait, resident advances the cane 10 to 18 inches. Then resident brings the weaker leg forward and then the stronger leg.
2. For a two-point gait, resident advances the cane and weak leg at the same time. Then resident brings the strong leg forward.
3. If resident has a gait belt on, stand slightly in back of the resident on resident's weak
(continues)

PROCEDURE *102*   *(continued)*

FIGURE 23-29 The cane is held on the strong side of the body.

side, with your hand closest to resident in the gait belt.

4. After ambulating, return resident to bedside or chair.
   - Have resident walk within a step of bed or chair.
   - Place cane to one side and assist resident to turn around.
   - When resident feels the bed or chair touching the back of the legs, have resident reach for the arm of the chair or mattress of bed and lower self into chair or bed.
5. Carry out each procedure completion action.

Ambulating with a Walker

Note: There are many different types of walkers. The directions given here are for a standard walker.

1. Have resident advance walker 10 to 18 inches. *All four points of the walker should strike the floor at the same time.*
2. The resident then brings weaker leg forward into walker, followed by stronger leg.
3. After ambulating, return resident to bedside or chair.
   - Have resident walk within a step of bed or chair.
   - Place walker to one side and assist resident to turn around.
   - When resident feels the bed or chair touching the back of the legs, have resident reach for arm of chair or mattress of bed and lower self into chair or bed.
4. Carry out each procedure completion action.

USING A WHEELCHAIR

Many residents who are unable to ambulate can gain some independence with the use of a wheelchair. A wheelchair should fit the person using it. Correct fit and body alignment will prevent contractures. An appropriate wheelchair will have:

- About 4 inches between the top of the back upholstery and the resident's axillae
- Armrests that support the arms without pushing the shoulders up or forcing them to hang
- Two to three inches clearance between the front edge of the seat and the back of the resident's knee
- Enough space between the resident's hip and the chair to slide your hand between the resident's hips on each side and the side of the wheelchair; the right amount of space avoids internal or external rotation of hips.

FIGURE 23-30 The wheelchair should fit the resident correctly.

- Two inches between the bottom of the footrests and the floor
- The feet at 90° angles to the legs, whether they are on the footrests or on the floor (when the footrests have been removed) (Figure 23-30)

If the wheelchair does not fit the resident, check with the nurse or physical therapist to see how you can use pads or other devices to adapt the chair to the resident.

Wheelchair Safety

Observe residents in wheelchairs. Remind them to:

- Place the casters in forward position for balance and stability. To do this, go forward and then back up so the casters swing to the forward position.
- Keep the wheelchair locked when not moving.
- Lift footrests out of the way when getting in or out of the wheelchair.
- Not attempt to pick up an object off the floor. If there is satisfactory trunk stability and balance, the resident may be taught to do so, but instruct resident to:
  - Remember to avoid shifting weight in the direction of the reach
  - Not move forward in the seat
  - Not reach down between the knees

The safest method is to ask for help in picking up an object from the floor. Otherwise, position the chair beside the object with casters in forward position. Lock the chair and reach only as far as the arm will extend. The resident may have an assistive reaching device that can be used to pick up objects.

The following procedures for wheelchair maneuvers are rarely implemented in a long-term care facility. However, residents may go outside

the facility or be discharged. In these situations, the skills will be required. The caregiver should be evaluated on the ability to carry them out.

SPECIAL MANEUVERS WITH WHEELCHAIRS

Certain situations will require special maneuvers to be made with residents in wheelchairs. Do not attempt to use the following procedures unless you have been instructed to do so.

Tilting a Wheelchair Backward

1. This procedure is used for curbs, single steps, ramps, and doorsills. Do not use this procedure with an indoor wheelchair.
2. Before proceeding, make sure the resident understands what you are doing. Check to see that arms, hands, fingers, and legs are in safe position. Use good body mechanics to avoid injury. Have an assistant with you the first few times you do this.
3. The purpose of the procedure is to rotate the wheelchair around the axles of the rear wheels until it reaches the balance point.
4. With your foot on the tipping lever, apply a pushing force down and under the chair while pulling back and down on the handgrip (Figure 23-31).

FIGURE 23-31 With your foot on the tipping lever, apply a pushing force down and under the chair while pulling back and down on the handgrip.

FIGURE 23-32 You can maneuver the chair on the rear wheels when you have reached the balance point.

5. Tilt back until little or no effort is required to stabilize the chair. This is the balance point, about 30°. You can now maneuver the chair on the rear wheels (Figure 23-32).
6. To return the wheelchair to the upright position, keep your foot on the tipping lever. Lower the chair, reversing the procedure. Do this slowly and smoothly and do not let the chair drop (Figure 23-33).

Manipulating Ramps and Inclines

1. Push the resident up a ramp or incline, facing forward, with the trunk slightly forward, with or without an attendant.

FIGURE 23-33 Reverse the procedure to lower the chair.

2. To go down, the resident faces forward but does not lean forward.
3. It is safer if you help the resident going down the ramp. Position yourself behind the chair, place it in balance position, and slowly move it down the ramp.
4. Keep your back straight and knees bent throughout the procedure.

Manipulating Curbs

1. To go up, place the chair in balance position. Move forward until the front casters are on top of the curb and the rear wheels are touching the curb (Figure 23-34).
2. Lower the front of the chair to the sidewalk, making sure the wheelchair does not roll backward (Figure 23-35).
3. With your body close to the wheelchair, use one single smooth movement to lift the chair by the handles, rolling it up over the curb and pushing it forward (Figure 23-36).
4. After the wheelchair is safely on the sidewalk, step up onto the curb (Figure 23-37).
5. To go down, turn the wheelchair around and pull it to the edge of the curb.
6. Stand below the curb and allow the large wheels to slowly roll down onto the lower level.
7. After the large wheels are on the lower level, tilt the chair to its balance point while lifting the front casters off the curb.
8. When the wheelchair is on the lower level, move backward until you can safely turn the

FIGURE 23-34 Move forward until the front casters are on top of the curb and the rear wheels are touching the curb.

FIGURE 23-35 Make sure the wheelchair does not roll backward.

chair around. A second assistant is needed if the curb or step is high.

Going Up and Down Stairs

Attempt this procedure only if necessary and an elevator is not available. Never use a wheelchair on escalators. At least two people are needed who are strong enough to carry the procedure

FIGURE 23-36 Use one single smooth movement to lift the chair by the handles, rolling it up over the curb.

FIGURE 23-37 Step up onto the curb after the wheelchair is on the sidewalk.

out to its completion. Check the position of the resident's extremities and inspect the handgrip for good fit on the chair.

1. To go upstairs, place the wheelchair in backward position with the rear wheels touching the first step. The strongest assistant is at the rear of the chair, standing on the second step.
2. The assistant in front grasps the chair frame on either side of the resident's lower legs, taking care not to grasp a removable part.
3. The rear assistant tilts the wheelchair to its balance point.
4. Working together, the assistants lift and roll the chair up onto the next step, keeping it at the balance point, moving themselves up with the chair (Figure 23-38).
5. This procedure is continued until the top step is reached.
6. With the chair still at the balance point, the rear assistant rolls the chair back until the assistant(s) in front are off the steps.
7. The rear assistant turns the chair around and gently returns it to upright position.
8. To go downstairs, the front assistant(s) stands on the third step from the top.
9. The rear assistant tilts the chair to the balance point and rolls it to the edge of the top step. This person is in charge of the procedure.

FIGURE 23-38 The assistants lift and roll the chair up and onto the next step, keeping it at the balance point.

10. With the front assistant firmly grasping the wheelchair frame, the chair is lowered one step by rolling the large wheels over the edge of the step. All assistants move down one step (Figure 23-39).
11. Repeat the process until the chair reaches the bottom of the stairs. The rear assistant

gently returns the wheelchair to the upright position.

POSITIONING THE DEPENDENT RESIDENT IN THE WHEELCHAIR

The dependent person may slide down in the wheelchair, requiring assistance to regain body alignment. Several procedures can be implemented to correct the dependent resident's position in the wheelchair.

Method 1: Stand in front of the resident and make sure the feet are in alignment and arms are on the armrests. Help resident lean forward and push with the hands and legs as you push against the resident's knees (Figure 23-40).

Method 2: An alternate method is to place a soft towel or small sheet under the resident's buttocks. Use this as a pull sheet to move the resident up in the chair. This requires two people (Figure 23-41).

Method 3: This method also requires two people. Place the transfer belt around the

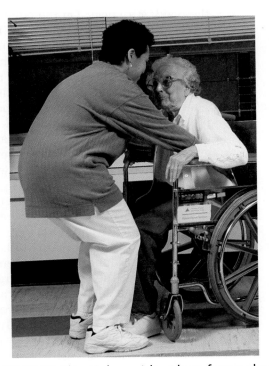

FIGURE 23-40 Help resident lean forward and push with the hands and legs as you push against the resident's knees.

FIGURE 23-39 All assistants move down one step.

FIGURE 23-41 A lifting sheet may be used to move the resident up in the wheelchair.

FIGURE 23-42 A transfer belt may be used to move a lighter resident up in the wheelchair.

resident's waist. One caregiver stands in back of the wheelchair and grasps the transfer belt with one hand on each side of the resident. The other one stands in front of the resident and places her hands and arms under the resident's knees. On the count of three this caregiver supports the lower extremities while the other one moves the resident back in the chair (Figure 23-42). This method is not recommended for a heavy resident.

Method 4: This method also requires two people. One assistant stands in back of the wheelchair and a second caregiver stands in front of the resident. Both caregivers work with knees and hips bent and backs straight. You are the caregiver behind the chair. Lean forward with your head over the resident's shoulder. Instruct the resident to fold the arms. Place your arms around the resident's trunk. Grasp the resident's right wrist with your left hand and grasp the resident's left wrist with your right hand. The other caregiver encircles the resident's knees with hands and arms. On the count of three, both caregivers lift and move the resident up (Figure 23-43).

Method 5: One person can do this procedure. The resident must be oriented and able to follow directions. Stand in front of the resident. Flex your knees and hips and keep your back straight. Position your feet, one on each side of the resident's feet. Brace your knees against the resident's knees. Have the resident lean forward. Lean forward over the resident's right shoulder with the resident's head

FIGURE 23-43 On the count of three, both assistants lift and move the resident up.

FIGURE 23-44   Encircle your arms around the resident's trunk.

FIGURE 23-45   Wheelchair pushups relieve pressure from sitting.

under your right arm. Encircle your arms around the resident's trunk. The resident's arms are folded together (Figure 23-44). Rock resident forward and on the count of three, when resident's weight is over the legs, push against the resident's knees to move back in the chair.

If the resident can bear weight, it is easier and more beneficial to assist the resident to stand and then sit back down, getting the hips to the back of the chair. Wedge cushions placed in the wheelchair will prevent the resident from sliding forward.

WHEELCHAIR ACTIVITY

Pressure over the ischia is greatly increased when the resident is sitting. Teach the resident (and provide assistance if necessary) to periodically relieve the pressure by shifting weight every 15 minutes. *Be sure wheelchair is locked before beginning any activities involving the resident's movement in the chair.*

Wheelchair Pushups

1. Teach the resident to place one hand on each armrest, keeping both elbows bent.
2. Then have resident lean forward slightly, pushing on the armrests and straightening the elbows while lifting the buttocks off the seat of the wheelchair. Have resident hold this position to the count of five if possible (Figure 23-45).

Leaning

1. Teach the resident who cannot do pushups to place the hands on the armrests or thighs and lean forward slightly, and then to lean to each side to relieve pressure on buttocks (Figure 23-46). Monitor the resident with balance problems to avoid falling out of the chair.

FIGURE 23-46   Leaning forward is another method for relieving pressure.

LESSON SYNTHESIS: Putting It All Together

You have just completed this lesson. Now go back and review the Clinical Focus. Try to see how the Clinical Focus relates to the concepts presented in the lesson. Then answer the following questions.

1. Why is it important for the person doing the transfer always to maintain a wide base of support?

2. Why are *specific instructions* written about how a resident is to be transferred?

3. The person doing the transfer should never place his or her hands under the resident's arms. Explain the reasons for this.

4. Explain why a transfer should always be toward the resident's strongest side.

REVIEW

A. Select the one best answer for each of the following.

1. The method used for transferring a resident depends on all but the resident's
   (A) size
   (B) physical condition
   (C) strength, endurance, balance
   (D) method of payment

2. A transfer belt should never be used on residents who
   (A) have an abdominal aneurysm
   (B) need assistance in transferring
   (C) are tall
   (D) cannot walk

3. During a transfer, the resident should never
   (A) be allowed to help in the move
   (B) place his hands on your body
   (C) wear shoes
   (D) be allowed to stand

4. When transferring a resident, you should never place your hands under a resident's arms because
   (A) the resident may not want you to stand so close
   (B) the resident cannot see where he is going
   (C) the resident's bones are fragile
   (D) the resident may be ticklish

5. Using a mechanical lift requires that
   (A) there always be two persons to do the procedure
   (B) the resident be able to assist in the move
   (C) the resident be mentally alert
   (D) the resident be very small

6. A sliding board transfer is useful for residents who
   (A) are paraplegic
   (B) have cardiac problems
   (C) have had a stroke
   (D) have diabetes

7. A resident's gait may be affected by all but
   (A) a stroke
   (B) Parkinson's disease
   (C) multiple sclerosis
   (D) incontinence

B. Answer each statement true (T) or false (F).

8. T F During a transfer, a resident should place his or her hands on the nursing assistant's shoulders.

9. T F A transfer belt should always be used when ambulating a resident, unless contraindicated.

10. T F Always transfer toward the resident's strong side.

11. T F During a transfer, the nursing assistant should place his or her hands around the resident's trunk.

12. T F Always explain what the transfer person is doing and what the resident can do to help.

13. T F Towel bars are not safe to use as grab bars.

14. T F Always hold a cane on the weak side.

15. T F When using a walker, the front two tips of the walker should strike the floor first and then the back two tips should strike the floor.

SECTION 8

Residents with Specific Disorders

LESSONS

24 **Caring for Residents with Cardiovascular System Disorders**

25 **Caring for Residents with Respiratory System Disorders**

26 **Caring for Residents with Endocrine System Disorders**

27 **Caring for Residents with Reproductive System Disorders**

28 **Caring for Residents with Musculoskeletal System Disorders**

29 **Caring for Residents with Nervous System Disorders**

LESSON 24

Caring for Residents with Cardiovascular System Disorders

Clinical Focus

Think how you might assist a resident with cardiovascular disorders as you study this lesson and meet:

*W*alter Rabinowitz, who has congestive heart failure and poor circulation in his feet. He sits in a cardiac chair that supports him in an upright position comfortably. He is always complaining that his feet are cold. He has an order for elasticized stockings. During morning care, he asks for a hot water bag to put on his feet. Nursing assistants know there are safer methods of providing the comfort he needs.

OBJECTIVES

After studying this lesson, you should be able to:

- Define and spell vocabulary words and terms.
- Identify the parts and function of the cardiovascular system.
- Review changes in the cardiovascular system as they relate to the aging process.
- Describe common cardiovascular disorders affecting the long-term resident.
- List observations to make when caring for residents with cardiovascular disorders.
- Describe the care given by the nursing assistant to residents with cardiovascular disorders.
- Correctly apply elasticized stockings.
- Demonstrate the following:
  Procedure 103 Applying Elasticized Stockings

VOCABULARY

anastomose *(ah-NAS-tah-mohz)*
anemia *(ah-NEE-mee-ah)*

angina pectoris *(an-JYE-nah or AN-jih-nah PECK-tor-is)*

VOCABULARY

aorta *(ay-OR-tah)*

arteriosclerosis *(are-ter-ree-oh-skleh-ROH-sis)*

artery *(ARE-ter-ee)*

ascites *(ah-SIGH-teez)*

atherosclerosis *(ath-er-oh-skleh-ROH-sis)*

atrium (plural: atria) *(AY-tree-um; pl. AY-tree-ah)*

capillary *(KAP-ih-lair-ee)*

cardiac cycle *(KAR-dee-ack SIGH-kul)*

cardiovascular *(kar-dee-oh-VAS-kyou-lar)*

congestive heart failure *(kon-JES-tiv hart FAIL-your)*

dementia *(dee-MEN-she-ah)*

deoxygenated *(dee-ock-sih-jen-AY-ted)*

diaphoresis *(die-ah-foh-REE-sis)*

diastole *(die-AS-toh-lee)*

dyspnea *(DISP-nee-ah)*

edema *(eh-DEE-mah)*

electrocardiogram (ECG or EKG) *(ee-leck-troh-KAR-dee-oh-gram)*

erythrocytes *(eh-RITH-roh-sights)*

heart attack *(hart ah-TACK)*

heart block *(hart block)*

hemoptysis *(hee-MOP-tih-sis)*

hypertension *(high-per-TEN-shun)*

hypoxia *(high-POCK-see-ah)*

infarction *(in-FARK-shun)*

inferior vena cava *(in-FEER-ee-or VEE-nah KAY-vah)*

ischemia *(is-KEE-mee-ah)*

leukemia *(loo-KEE-mee-ah)*

leukocytes *(LOO-koh-sights)*

lumen *(LOO-men)*

lymph *(limf)*

lymph node *(limf nohd)*

myocardial infarction *(my-oh-KAR-dee-al in-FARK-shun)*

nitroglycerin *(nigh-troh-GLIS-er-in)*

orthopnea *(or-thop-NEE-ah)*

orthopneic position *(or-thop-NEE-ick poh-ZISH-un)*

oxygenated *(ock-sih-jen-AT-ted)*

pacemaker *(PAYS-may-ker)*

peripheral vascular disease *(peh-RIF-er-al VAS-kyou-lar dih-ZEEZ)*

phlebitis *(fleh-BYE-tis)*

plaque *(plak)*

plasma *(PLAZ-mah)*

platelet *(PLAYT-let)*

pulmonary artery *(PULL-moh-nair-ee ARE-ter-ee)*

pulmonary veins *(PULL-moh-nair-ee vains)*

serum *(SEER-rum)*

stroke *(strohk)*

superior vena cava *(soo-PEER-ee-or VEE-nah KAY-vah)*

syncope *(SIN-koh-pe)*

systole *(SIS-toh-lee)*

TED hose *(TED hohs)*

thrombocyte *(THROM-boh-sight)*

thrombophlebitis *(throm-boh-fleh-BYE-tis)*

transient ischemic attack (TIA) *(TRAN-see-ent is-KEE-mick ah-TACK)*

valve *(valv)*

varicose veins *(VAIR-ih-kohs vains)*

vasodilator *(vas-oh-die-LAY-tor)*

vein *(vain)*

ventricle *(VEN-trih-kul)*

venule *(VEN-youl)*

INTRODUCTION

The **cardiovascular** system is the transportation system of the body. It carries substances from where they are formed to where they may be used or eliminated. The cardiovascular system consists of the:

- Heart—a central pump
- Blood vessels—a closed circuit of arteries that lead from the heart to capillaries and then to veins that lead back to the heart
- Blood—a collection of various cells, each with a special job to perform

FIGURE 24-1 Changes in the cardiovascular system caused by aging

- Vascular walls become less flexible.

- Vascular lumens narrow.

- Blood pressure increases.

- Cardiac output decreases.

- System cannot adapt to sudden or intense changes or demands.

- Capillaries become more fragile.

- Heart rate decreases.

Cardiovascular disease is the most common cause of death in the United States. Many residents in your care will suffer from disabilities caused by cardiovascular disease. Cardiovascular disease is responsible for changes that reduce the blood flow to the body tissues and result in

- Heart attack
- Peripheral vascular disease
- Hypertension (high blood pressure)
- Stroke

Reduced blood flow is called **ischemia**. Ischemia means that less oxygen is delivered to tissues, leading, eventually, to death of the tissues (**infarction**). Changes in the cardiovascular system caused by aging are summarized in Figure 24-1.

- Lymphatic vessels and **lymph nodes**—filter tissue fluid and return it as **lymph** back to the bloodstream

The bloodstream, spleen, liver, and bone marrow make some of the blood cells and destroy them when they are worn out.

THE HEART

The heart is a muscular organ that pumps the blood in a continuous flow through the blood vessels of the body. It is separated into a right and left side (Figure 24-2).

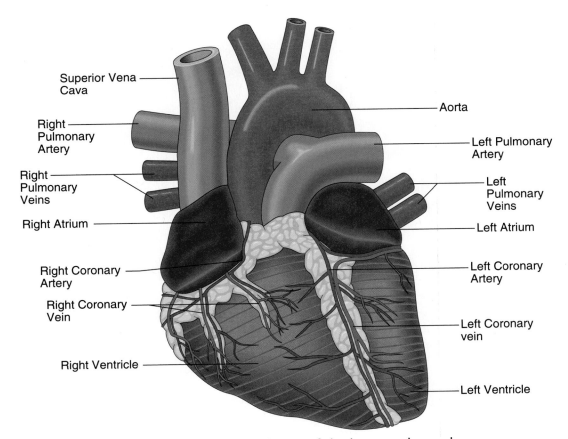

Superior Vena Cava

Right Pulmonary Artery

Right Pulmonary Veins

Right Atrium

Right Coronary Artery

Right Coronary Vein

Right Ventricle

Aorta

Left Pulmonary Artery

Left Pulmonary Veins

Left Atrium

Left Coronary Artery

Left Coronary vein

Left Ventricle

FIGURE 24-2 External view of the heart and vessels

Structure and Function

The *right side* of the heart:

- Receives blood from the body
- Sends blood to the lungs where carbon dioxide is removed and oxygen is picked up (Figure 24-3)

The *left side* of the heart:

- Receives blood from the lungs by way of the pulmonary veins
- Sends blood out to the body, where the oxygen is given up to the cells and the waste product carbon dioxide is picked up

Each side of the heart is divided into upper and lower parts (chambers) by **valves**. The valves permit blood flow in one direction only. The *upper chambers* are called the right **atrium** and left atrium. The *lower chambers* are the right and left **ventricles**.

The two upper chambers contract first, forcing the blood through the open valves into the two lower chambers. The ventricles fill and the valves close. The ventricles then contract, squeezing the blood up through the large blood vessels.

Blood Vessels of the Heart

The major blood vessels of the heart are the:

- **Superior vena cava** (SVC)—returns blood to the right atrium from the upper part of the body
- **Inferior vena cava** (IVC)—returns blood to right atrium from the lower part of the body
- **Pulmonary artery**—carries blood to the lungs from the right ventricle
- **Pulmonary veins**—return blood to the left atrium from the lungs
- **Aorta** (a large artery)—carries blood to the body from the left ventricle
- Coronary arteries—nourish the heart muscle with fresh blood

Valves at the base of the pulmonary artery and aorta close as the blood moves forward, preventing backflow of blood into the ventricles between contractions.

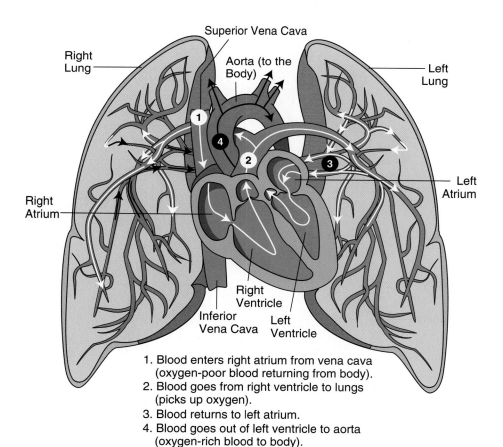

1. Blood enters right atrium from vena cava (oxygen-poor blood returning from body).
2. Blood goes from right ventricle to lungs (picks up oxygen).
3. Blood returns to left atrium.
4. Blood goes out of left ventricle to aorta (oxygen-rich blood to body).

FIGURE 24-3 Flow of blood from the heart to the lungs, back to the heart, to the body, and back to the heart to begin the cycle again

Cardiac Cycle

The contractions and relaxations of the heart muscle are called the **cardiac cycle**. The cardiac cycle is controlled by special nerve tissues within the heart and by two sets of nerves:

- One set of nerves carries messages to increase the heart rate.
- The other set of nerves carries messages to slow the heart rate.

Electrical impulses passing through the nerve tissue make the muscle contract:

- **Systole** is the term meaning heart *contraction.*
- **Diastole** is the term meaning heart *relaxation.*

For a short time, the heart rests completely between beats. The pulse you feel at the radial artery corresponds to ventricular contraction. The sounds you hear when listening to the heart and when taking a blood pressure are the sounds made by the closing of the valves during the cardiac cycle.

An **electrocardiogram**, called an ECG or an EKG, is a test that traces the electrical impulses of the heart. Heart disease may be detected with this test.

Blood Vessels

There are three kinds of blood vessels:

- **Arteries**
- **Capillaries**
- **Veins**

Arteries

Arteries carry blood away from the heart (Figure 24-4). The blood contains oxygen picked up in the lungs. The blood is **oxygenated** and is needed to keep the body cells alive and functioning. The arteries get smaller and finally form tiny networks of vessels called capillaries.

Capillaries

Nutrients and oxygen in the blood are exchanged through the walls of the capillaries for carbon dioxide and waste products. The capillaries form larger vessels called **venules** to begin the journey back to the heart.

Veins

Many venules join to form larger vessels called veins (Figure 24-5). The largest veins, the supe-rior vena cava and the inferior vena cava, return the blood to the right atrium. This blood has less oxygen and more carbon dioxide and is called **deoxygenated** blood.

The cardiovascular system is a closed system, with the gases and other substances passing into and out of the bloodstream as the blood passes throughout the body.

Blood vessels frequently take their names from bones nearby. For example, the radial artery and radial vein are found close to the radius, which is one of the forearm bones.

Lymph

Lymph is fluid that is drained from the tissues. It passes into lymphatic vessels through masses of cells called lymph nodes. Eventually, the fluid returns to the general circulation. The lymph nodes act as filters, removing harmful substances picked up in the tissues before they reach the general circulation.

The Blood

The blood is a red body fluid that carries the nutrients, chemicals, and waste products of the body. The average quantity of blood in the body is about 4 to 6 liters (or 4 to 6 quarts). The blood consists of two portions:

- Plasma
- Blood cells

Plasma

The liquid part of the blood, called **plasma**, carries:

- Water
- Nutrients
- Wastes
- Proteins that help blood to clot
- Proteins that fight infection and help to move materials in and out of the bloodstream

Serum is the fluid that is left after the cells and some of the proteins have been removed.

Blood Cells

Three kinds of blood cells are:

1. **Erythrocytes** (red blood cells)—carry oxygen and a small amount of carbon dioxide
2. **Leukocytes** (white blood cells)—protect the body by fighting infection

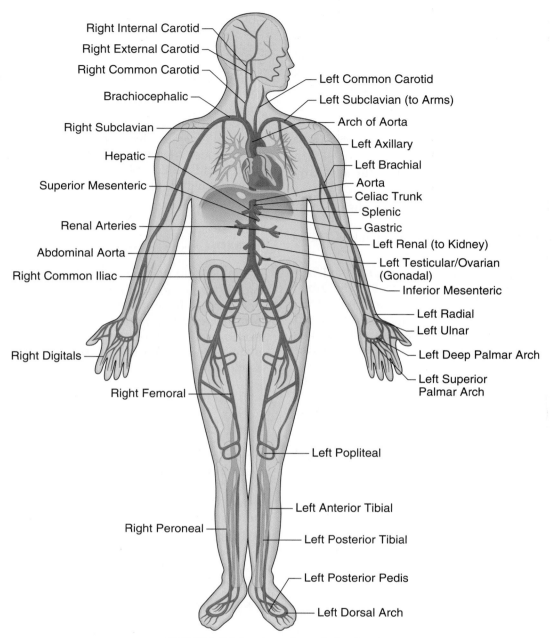

Right Internal Carotid
Right External Carotid
Right Common Carotid
Brachiocephalic
Right Subclavian
Hepatic
Superior Mesenteric
Renal Arteries
Abdominal Aorta
Right Common Iliac
Right Digitals
Right Femoral
Right Peroneal

Left Common Carotid
Left Subclavian (to Arms)
Arch of Aorta
Left Axillary
Left Brachial
Aorta
Celiac Trunk
Splenic
Gastric
Left Renal (to Kidney)
Left Testicular/Ovarian (Gonadal)
Inferior Mesenteric
Left Radial
Left Ulnar
Left Deep Palmar Arch
Left Superior Palmar Arch
Left Popliteal
Left Anterior Tibial
Left Posterior Tibial
Left Posterior Pedis
Left Dorsal Arch

FIGURE 24-4 Arteries of the body

3. **Platelets** or **thrombocytes**—pieces of cells that contain a chemical important to blood clotting

DISORDERS OF THE BLOOD

Blood abnormalities commonly seen in the elderly include:

- Cancer
- Anemia

Cancer

Cancers of the blood include forms of **leukemia** In leukemia:

- Excessive numbers of white blood cells are formed.
- Too few platelets and red blood cells are produced.

The person with leukemia:

- Tires easily
- Is subject to infections and anemia
- Is apt to bleed

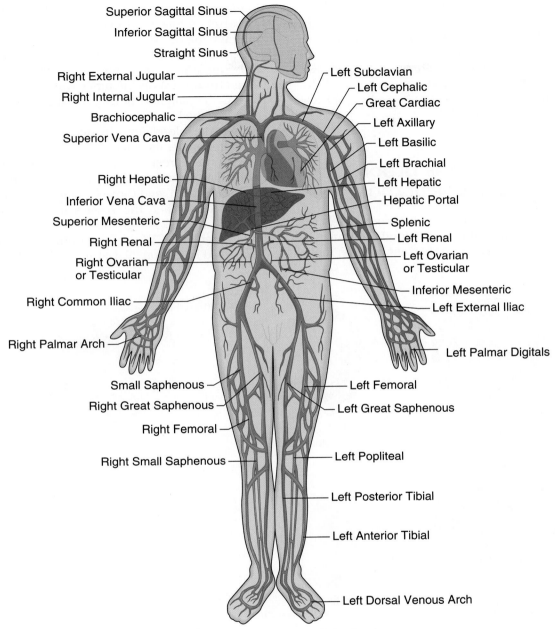

FIGURE 24-5   Veins of the body

These conditions are normally treated with radiation or drugs.

Anemia

Anemias are the result of a decrease in (1) the quantity or quality of red blood cells and (2) their ability to carry oxygen. People suffering from anemia have little energy. They:

- Are usually pale or jaundiced (skin is yellow)
- Complain of light-headedness
- Feel cold
- Experience dizziness
- Have an increased respiratory rate
- Suffer from poor digestion

Special Care

Residents who have cancer or anemia require special care. You must:

- Check vital signs.
- Encourage rest and a good diet.
- See that resident avoids unnecessary exertion.
- Handle resident very gently.
- Give special mouth care because the mouth and tongue become sensitive.

- Be sure to report any signs of bleeding, such as bruises or discolorations, because further blood loss makes the condition worse.
- Keep resident warm.
- Protect resident from falls that may result from dizziness or weakness.
- Change the resident's position often—at least every 2 hours.

DISORDERS OF THE BLOOD VESSELS AND CIRCULATION

Several changes can occur in blood vessels that will affect the flow of blood (circulation) through the vessels. **Arteriosclerosis** means hardening of the arteries. When this happens, the arteries lose their elasticity. It is then more difficult for the blood to flow through the vessels. **Atherosclerosis** occurs when deposits of fatty materials and calcium form roughened areas (**plaques**) on the inner walls of the arteries. As the plaques thicken, the space within the arteries (the **lumen**) narrows (Figure 24-6). This causes the blood flow to decrease. When this happens, ischemia can occur.

Arteriosclerosis and atherosclerosis are especially dangerous when they affect the arteries of the brain, heart, and those leading from the body to the legs. When the vessels in the brain are affected, the risk is high for **stroke** (cerebral vascular accident, CVA, or brain attack). Stroke is discussed in Lesson 29. Before a stroke happens,

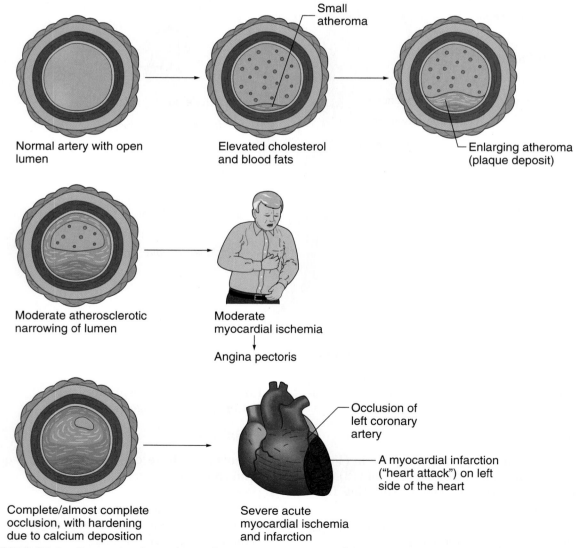

Normal artery with open lumen

Elevated cholesterol and blood fats

Small atheroma

Enlarging atheroma (plaque deposit)

Moderate atherosclerotic narrowing of lumen

Moderate myocardial ischemia
↓
Angina pectoris

Complete/almost complete occlusion, with hardening due to calcium deposition

Severe acute myocardial ischemia and infarction

Occlusion of left coronary artery

A myocardial infarction ("heart attack") on left side of the heart

FIGURE 24-6 Cross-sections through a coronary artery showing progressive arteriosclerosis and atherosclerosis the person may have a transient ischemic attack (TIA). The person may also get a form of **dementia** (confusion and disorientation) when the brain cells do not receive adequate oxygen. Dementia is discussed in Lesson 30.

When the vessels of the heart are affected, the person may have a heart attack (**myocardial infarction**). When the vessels in the legs are affected, the person has **peripheral vascular disease**. When the arteries are diseased, hypertension (high blood pressure) may occur (Figure 24-7).

The veins can also cause problems. **Varicose veins** form when the valves in the veins in the legs become weakened (Figure 24-8). This means the blood does not flow through the veins as it should. The veins then become distended and visible through the skin. The veins may become inflamed (**phlebitis**). A blood clot may form (**thrombophlebitis**). Report the signs of these disorders:

- Pain or aching in the area
- Signs of inflammation (warmth and redness)

NEVER rub or massage the area.

Transient Ischemic Attack

Transient ischemic attack (TIA) is a temporary interruption of the blood flow to part of the brain. The resident may experience:

- Weakness or paralysis of any extremity or the face
- Vision problems
- Difficulty with speech
- Difficulty with swallowing

These symptoms come on quickly and may last from just a few minutes to 24 hours. There are

AFFECTED SITE   COMPLICATION

- Stroke
- Cerebral Arteries
- Carotid Arteries
- Atherosclerotic Carotid Artery
- Stroke
- Aorta — Aneurysm
- Coronary Arteries — Angina, Myocardial Infarction
- Renal Arteries — Hypertension
- Iliac Arteries — Peripheral Vascular Disease
- Femoral Arteries — Peripheral Vascular Disease
- Tibial Arteries — Peripheral Vascular Disease

FIGURE 24-7 Atherosclerosis and arteriosclerosis can cause disease in many parts of the body.

FIGURE 24-8 Veins contain valves to prevent the backward flow of blood. A. External view of the vein shows wider area of valve. B. Internal view with the valve open as blood flows through. C. internal view with the valve closed. D. Vein with weakened valve causing a varicose vein.

no permanent effects. However, a TIA is usually a warning that a stroke will occur at some time. If a resident has any of these symptoms, you should report them to the nurse immediately.

Peripheral Vascular Disease

Peripheral vascular disease may be caused by:

- Diseases of the arteries (arteriosclerosis and atherosclerosis)
- Abnormalities of the veins (varicose veins)

The signs and symptoms of peripheral vascular disease include:

- Burning pain during exercise
- Hair loss over feet and toes
- Thick and rigid toenails
- Dusky red skin or cyanotic, brownish skin
- Dry and scaly or shiny skin
- Chronic edema of the feet and legs
- Cool skin temperature of feet and legs
- Difficulty with ambulation

When the arteries are affected, the blood flow may be seriously interrupted. This condition requires immediate medical treatment. Vascular ulcers may occur. These are sores that start because of the poor circulation of the blood in the legs. These ulcers are difficult to treat and may take months to heal.

When residents have peripheral vascular disease, it is important that:

- Circulation is maintained. Complications such as ulcers may then be prevented.
- The feet and legs receive excellent skin care

Hypertension

Hypertension means elevated blood pressure. Hypertension may have an unknown origin or follow disease of the:

- Blood vessels
- Kidneys
- Liver

---

*G*uidelines for

Caring for Residents with Peripheral Vascular Disease

1. Elevate the feet when the resident is sitting in a chair for prolonged periods of time. When the feet are not elevated, make sure that the resident's feet are flat on the floor. If they are not, support the feet with a footstool. Discourage the resident from crossing the legs when sitting.

2. Discourage the resident from using circular garters.
3. Discourage smoking because it interferes with circulation.
4. Avoid using the knee gatch on the bed.
5. Avoid the use of heating pads or hot water bottles. The resident may not feel temperatures that are too hot.

(continues)

Guidelines (continued)

6. Maintain body warmth. Make sure the resident has warm clothes, including well-fitting socks. Provide blankets for the bed.
7. Prevent injury to the feet:
   - Instruct the resident to wear shoes when out of bed.
   - Check to see that the shoes are in good repair and that they fit well.
   - Avoid pressure to the legs and feet from any source.
8. Inspect the feet carefully when you bathe the resident or if the resident complains of any discomfort in the feet. Promptly report any signs of inflammation, injury, or circulatory problems (Figure 24-9).
   - Broken skin
   - Color change—redness, white, or cyanotic
   - Heat or coldness
   - Cracking between toes
   - Corns or calluses
   - Swelling
   - Pain
   - Loss of function
   - Drainage

9. Bathe the feet regularly.
   - Dry thoroughly and gently between the toes.
   - Use a moisturizing lotion to the feet and legs if the skin is dry.
10. Do not cut the toenails of residents with peripheral vascular disease without instructions from the nurse.

FIGURE 24-9 Signs that may indicate peripheral vascular disease
• Broken skin
• Coldness or heat
• Color change
• Cracking between toes
• Corns or callouses
• Pain
• Loss of function
• Drainage
• Swelling

Diseases of the blood vessels increase the overall blood pressure. When blood vessels are narrowed due to disease, the heart attempts to make up for the resistance in the vessels by enlarging. Over a period of time, the heart eventually fails. Hypertension further increases the rate at which disease progresses in the vessels.

Elderly people usually have a somewhat higher pressure than younger people. The normal blood pressure for young adults is 120/80, but in the elderly, the norm is higher, with the highest level of normal being 140/90 mm Hg. Above this level, the probability of stroke and heart attack increases dramatically. Hypertension is dangerous because often there are no symptoms. It may be detected during a routine blood pressure check. Report any blood pressures when the systolic is over 140 or the diastolic is over 90.

Control of Hypertension. Control of hypertension is essential. Steps can be taken to bring the hypertension under control to avoid the serious consequences of stroke and heart attack. These steps include:

- Drugs to lower the pressure
- Weight reduction
- Dietary restrictions, such as limiting salt intake
- Discouraging smoking
- Regular exercise

Report immediately any signs or symptoms of hypertension:

- Flushed face
- Dizziness
- Nose bleeds
- Headaches
- Changes in speech patterns
- Blurred vision

HEART DISEASE

Many residents have some form of heart disease. Heart disease often makes self-care difficult because the resident tires easily, and residents become depressed and frustrated by their limitations. Heart disease may sometimes be due to an infection, but most heart disease develops because of changes in the blood vessels. The space inside the vessels becomes smaller. These changes make it harder and harder for the heart to do its job of pumping blood.

Preventative Measures

Individuals can take positive steps in managing their own life-styles to avoid the risk factors that contribute to heart and artery disease. These risk factors include:

- Cigarette smoking
- Obesity
- Physical inactivity
- Hypertension
- Abnormally high levels of high blood cholesterol
- Excessive emotional stress and depression

These factors are especially important when there is a history of diabetes or a family history of coronary artery disease at an early age. Several diagnostic tests that provide information leading to diagnoses of cardiac disorders are listed in Figure 24-10.

FIGURE 24-10   Diagnostic tests
• **Electrocardiogram (ECG or EKG)—** a measurement of the electrical activity of the heart.
• **Ultrasonography**—noninvasive test that in acute disease shows decreased blood flow distal to the occlusion.
• **Blood serum marker blood tests—** test that looks for chemicals that are released when heart muscle is damaged.
• **Radionuclide imaging**—a test that uses radioactive isotopes to detect areas of poor blood flow in the heart, using a scanning technique.
• **Coronary angiography**—Introduction of a dye within the coronary arteries, which can be seen on x-ray to show areas of blockage.

Heart Attack

A **heart attack** occurs when the heart is not able to function properly. There are different kinds of attacks, and some have more serious effects than others. However, every attack is serious, and each requires some form of treatment (therapy). A heart attack is often referred to as an MI (myocardial infarction).

In myocardial infarction the normal flow of blood to the heart is decreased. Narrowing of the coronary (heart) blood vessels that supply blood to the heart may occur slowly over a period of years, allowing some new circulation to develop. However, when the heart attack occurs, the flow of blood has diminished so much that not enough blood reaches the heart and the heart muscle may die. This lack of blood flow is known as ischemia.

Sometimes the flow of blood is cut off abruptly because a blood clot lodges in a coronary artery.

Acute Myocardial Infarction

An acute MI is a serious medical emergency. The blood flow to the myocardium is cut off suddenly. The closure of a large vessel can result in death (infarction) of that part of the heart muscle not being supplied with blood. If too much of the heart muscle dies, the resident cannot survive.

Survival depends largely on how quickly proper medical intervention occurs (Figure 24-11). You must recognize the signs and symptoms of this type of heart attack and report to the nurse immediately.

Signs and Symptoms.   These include:
- Crushing chest pain, spreading down the arms and up into the neck and jaw; sometimes described as "severe indigestion"
- Clammy, ashen, or pale skin
- Excessive sweating (**diaphoresis**)
- Nausea
- Vomiting (sometimes)
- Anxiety and weakness
- Weak pulse
- Low blood pressure
- Shock
- Shortness of breath
- **Syncope** (fainting)
- Restlessness

Nursing Assistant Care.   You can help by:
- Staying with the resident
- Using the intercom or call bell to summon help
- Staying calm

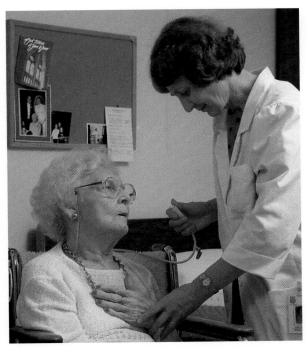

FIGURE 24-11 If you suspect the resident is having a heart attack, summon help immediately and do not leave the resident.

FIGURE 24-12 Myocardial infarct therapies
• **Bypass graft:** Blood flow is diverted through an **anastamosed** graft to bypass the thrombosed arterial segment.
• **Embolectomy:** A balloon-tipped catheter is used to remove thrombolytic material from an artery.
• **Laser surgery:** A hot-tip laser obliterates the blood clot and plaque by vaporizing it.
• **Percutaneous transluminal coronary angioplasty (PTCA):** The nonsurgical technique uses a tiny balloon catheter that is inserted into the narrowed vessels to open them up and allow the blood to flow.
• **Reperfusion therapy:** Medical therapy that uses blood clot-dissolving drugs or a mechanical therapy for the same purpose.
• **Thromboendarterectomy:** The artery is opened and the obstructing thrombus and medial layer of the arterial wall are removed.

The resident will usually be transferred immediately to the intensive care unit (ICU) or coronary care unit (CCU) of an acute care hospital. Early treatment is designed to reverse the shock, relieve the pain, and keep the heart functioning. Choice of therapy depends on how quickly care is started and the stability of the resident's condition. Several therapies are described in Figure 24-12.

Angina Pectoris

Angina pectoris is a condition in which there is decreased blood flow to the heart. Signs and symptoms of an angina heart attack that you should immediately report include:

- Pain when exercising or under stress. Stress causes a need for an immediate increase in the coronary circulation. The pain is described as dull, with increasing intensity. It is usually centered under the breast bone (sternum) spreading to the left arm and up into the neck.
- Pale or flushed face
- Resident freely perspiring

Signs and symptoms may differ with individual residents, but the symptoms are usually the same each time that a resident experiences an attack. You may assist the resident with angina pectoris by:

- Helping the resident to avoid unnecessary emotional or physical stress
- Encouraging the resident not to smoke
- Reporting any signs and symptoms of an attack to the nurse at once

Residents with a history of angina pectoris take medication called a **vasodilator** to keep the blood vessels open. **Nitroglycerin** is one type of vasodilator. It is usually administered in a patch. The nitroglycerin patch is secured to the resident's chest and the medication is absorbed slowly over a 24-hour period.

Heart Failure

Many residents have a condition in which the heart functions less efficiently. The resident is said to be in heart failure (also called **congestive heart failure**) when certain symptoms are present, including:

- Cough
- **Dyspnea** (difficulty breathing)

- **Orthopnea** (difficulty in breathing unless sitting upright)
- Cyanosis
- **Hemoptysis** (spitting up blood)
- Fluid retained in the lungs and throughout the body
- **Edema** (fluid in the tissue spaces)
- **Ascites** (fluid collecting in the abdomen)
- Neck veins swell
- Fatiguing easily
- **Hypoxia** (inadequate oxygen levels)
- Confusion
- Irregular and rapid pulse

Nursing Assistant Care.   Acute heart failure is an urgent situation requiring expert care. You will assist in this care. Watch the resident carefully and report any increase in signs and symptoms at once.

Nursing care may include:

- Positioning. The resident is usually more comfortable either sitting up in bed, in an **orthopneic position** or high Fowler's position, supported by pillows, or supported in a chair. The position must be changed frequently, but changes in position should be made slowly. Padded footboards help keep the weight of the bedding off the toes.
- Application of elasticized stockings or **TED hose**. TED hose are elastic antiembolism stockings. TED hose and Ace bandages help channel blood to the deeper vessels. They must be checked often and reapplied every 6 to 8 hours. Check the extremities carefully

for adequate circulation. The skin should be pink and warm.

- Give attention to general hygiene. Complete bathing is tiring, but partial baths can stimulate circulation and provide comfort. Special attention must be given to the skin because the combination of position, edema, and poor circulation contributes to tissue breakdown.
- Assist with oxygen therapy. Oxygen therapy may be provided either by face mask or nasal cannula. Because cardiac residents often breathe through the mouth, the mouth tends to be very dry. Special mouth care may be needed. (For oxygen safety, refer to Lesson 8.)
- Provide for elimination. A bedside commode is convenient. The use of a commode is less tiring for the resident than using a bedpan for elimination.
- Encourage adequate nutrition. Small, easily digested meals should be encouraged. You may need to assist in feeding the resident to prevent fatigue.
- Monitor and record fluid intake. Residents with acute heart failure may be given drugs that increase the output of urine and alter the heart rate. Measuring the intake and output and taking daily weights are ways of determining if fluid is being retained. These procedures are part of the care you will give.
- Regularly check vital signs. Sometimes the force of heart contraction, which propels the blood forward into the blood vessels, does not have enough strength to make the vessels expand.

PROCEDURE
_103_ Applying Elasticized Stockings

1. Carry out each beginning procedure action.
2. Assemble equipment:
   - Elasticized stockings of proper length and size
3. With resident lying down, expose one leg at a time.
4. Grasp stocking with both hands at the top and roll toward toe end (Figure 24-13).
5. Adjust over toes, positioning opening at base of toes (unless toes are to be covered) (Figure 24-14). Remember that the raised seams should be on the outside.

(continues)

PROCEDURE *103*   *(continued)*

6. Apply stocking to leg by rolling upward toward body (Figure 24-15).
7. Check to be sure stocking is applied evenly and smoothly and there are no wrinkles (Figures 24-16 and 24-17).
8. Repeat procedure on other leg.
9. Carry out each procedure completion action.

FIGURE 24-15   Draw stocking smoothly toward knee.

FIGURE 24-13   Grasp stocking with both hands at stocking top, gather, and slip over toes.

FIGURE 24-16   Check to be sure stocking has no wrinkles.

FIGURE 24-14   Position opening on top of foot at base of toes.

FIGURE 24-17   Check material on toes to be sure it is not too tight.

Chronic Heart Failure

Residents can live for years with some level of chronic heart failure. A resident with chronic heart failure needs a calm environment with planned activity that promotes mobility but not fatigue. Visiting should be limited to one or two visitors because too many visitors at one time can be tiring.

The basic care given to residents in chronic failure includes:

- Measuring fluid intake and output
- Taking apical and radial pulse
- Assisting when necessary to prevent fatigue and maintain mobility
- Reporting any change in signs and symptoms
- Reporting unusual behavior or responses

This condition requires the use of medications for long periods of time. This results in a tendency for drug levels in the body to build. Elderly people are more sensitive to drugs. Therefore, you must be alert to unusual responses or behavior that may indicate a drug reaction. Report anything unusual about the residents in your care to your supervisor.

Heart Block

Heart block is a condition that develops due to interference in the electrical current through the heart. (The flow of electrical current through the heart muscle makes the normal cardiac cycle possible.)

An electronic device called a **pacemaker** (Figure 24-18) is implanted under the chest muscles or in the abdomen. An electrode carries electrical current from the pacemaker directly into the heart muscle to replace the lost control. The electrical current signals the heart to contract. Some pacemakers send messages only if normal messages carried by the conduction system are delayed. This type of pacemaker is called a demand pacemaker. Other pacemakers send regular signals to keep the heart contracting. The rate of signals is preset.

When caring for a resident who has a pacemaker:

- Count and record the pulse rate.
- Report any irregularities or changes below the present rate.
- Report any discoloration over the implant site.
- Report hiccoughing because this may indicate problems.
- Keep resident away from microwave ovens and cellular phones because they may disrupt the function of the pacemaker.

Residents usually function very well with pacemakers so long as they are adequately monitored.

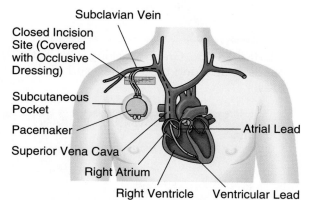

Subclavian Vein

Closed Incision Site (Covered with Occlusive Dressing)

Subcutaneous Pocket

Pacemaker

Superior Vena Cava

Right Atrium

Right Ventricle

Atrial Lead

Ventricular Lead

FIGURE 24-18 The electronic pacemaker sends electrical impulses to the heart muscle, causing it to contract. A. A typical pacemaker. B. The pacemaker inserted under the skin with electrode placed inside the heart, resting on the heart muscle (Courtesy of Medtronic, Inc.)

LESSON SYNTHESIS: Putting It All Together

*Y*ou have just completed this lesson. Now go back and review the *Clinical Focus. Try to see how the Clinical Focus relates to the concepts presented in the lesson. Then answer the following questions.*

1. Explain how a cardiac chair contributes to Mr. Rabinowitz's comfort and improved functioning of his cardiovascular system.

2. What actions can you take to increase Mr. Rabinowitz's warmth without using a hot water bag?

3. How do elasticized stockings assist the circulation in the legs?

4. What precautions should be taken when applying the elasticized stockings?

REVIEW

A. Select the one best answer for each of the following.

1. The cardiovascular system includes the
   - (A) liver
   - (B) lungs
   - (C) heart, blood, and blood vessels
   - (D) spleen

2. Which of the following is not a possible result of an inadequate blood supply?
   - (A) dementia
   - (B) myocardial infarction
   - (C) pneumonia
   - (D) stroke

3. The structures of the heart that permit blood flow in one direction only are called
   - (A) valves
   - (B) ventricles
   - (C) atria
   - (D) myocardium

4. The major artery is called the
   - (A) vena cava
   - (B) aorta
   - (C) pulmonary vein
   - (D) pulmonary artery

5. All of the following are functions of the lymph system except
   - (A) manufacturing new red blood cells
   - (B) transporting oxygen
   - (C) filtering out harmful substances before they reach the general circulation
   - (D) inhibiting bleeding

6. Red blood cells are responsible for
   - (A) delivery of oxygen to all body cells
   - (B) protecting the body by fighting infection
   - (C) the blood clotting process
   - (D) making lymph fluid

7. One effect of aging on the cardiovascular system is to
   - (A) increase cardiac output
   - (B) increase heart rate
   - (C) enlarge vascular lumens
   - (D) increase blood pressure

8. The formation of plaque on the inner walls of the arteries is called
   - (A) atherosclerosis
   - (B) arteriosclerosis
   - (C) varicose veins
   - (D) peripheral vascular disease

9. When the valves in the veins of the legs become weakened, the result is
   - (A) dementia
   - (B) stroke
   - (C) varicose veins
   - (D) heart failure

10. When caring for persons with peripheral vascular disease, all of the following are required except
    (A) regularly inspecting the feet and legs
    (B) maintaining appropriate hygiene of the feet and legs
    (C) preventing injury to the feet and legs
    (D) allowing person to cross legs when sitting

11. A symptom of heart attack or MI is
    (A) crushing chest pain
    (B) dry skin
    (C) high blood pressure
    (D) strong pulse

12. Persons with heart failure are more comfortable in the
    (A) orthopneic position
    (B) supine position
    (C) side-lying position
    (D) prone position

13. Which of the following actions is not appropriate when caring for a resident who has a pacemaker?
    (A) counting, recording, and reporting the pulse rate
    (B) reporting hiccoughing
    (C) reporting any discoloration over the implant site
    (D) allowing resident to use a cellular phone

B. **Match each term (items a.–i.) with the proper explanation.**

    a. edema
    b. myocardial infarction
    c. ventricles
    d. ischemia
    e. radial artery
    f. atria
    g. valves
    h. atherosclerosis
    i. arteries

14. _____ upper heart chambers

15. _____ fluid in the tissue spaces

16. _____ vessels that carry blood away from the heart

17. _____ located close to the radius

18. _____ lower heart chambers

19. _____ form of vascular disease in which plaques are formed in the walls of arteries

20. _____ diminished blood flow

C. **Answer each statement true (T) or false (F).**

21. T F The elderly heart muscle is less effective.

22. T F The person with orthopnea has difficulty breathing in an upright position.

23. T F The anemic person must be handled very gently.

24. T F Leukemias are an example of a blood abnormality.

25. T F Diabetes is not a risk factor for coronary artery disease.

LESSON 25

Caring for Residents with Respiratory System Disorders

Clinical Focus

Think about the special care needed by residents with respiratory disorders as you study this lesson and meet:

*M*ary Calcetas, who is 60 and has been a cigarette smoker for many years. Emphysema has taken its toll and now the very act of breathing is an effort. Walking the length of the corridor to the day room requires two rest periods along the way. Smoking is only permitted under supervision in the day room; so, difficult as it is, she slowly makes her way there early each morning. When an infection occurs, she requires nasal oxygen and orthopneic positioning. The nurse assigns you to collect a sputum specimen this morning.

OBJECTIVES

After studying this lesson, you should be able to:

- Define and spell vocabulary words and terms.
- Identify the parts and function of the respiratory system.
- Review changes in the respiratory system as they relate to the aging process.
- Describe common respiratory conditions affecting the long-term care resident.
- Give proper care to residents in respiratory distress and receiving respiratory therapy.
- Demonstrate the following:
  Procedure 104 Collecting a Sputum Specimen
  Procedure 105 Refilling the Humidifier Bottle

VOCABULARY

allergen *(**AL**-er-jen)*

alveoli *(al-**VEE**-oh-lee)*

aspiration *(**ass**-pih-**RAY**-shun)*

asthma *(**AZ**-mah)*

bronchi *(**BRONG**-kee)*

bronchioles *(**BRONG**-kee-ohls)*

bronchitis *(brong-**KEYE**-tis)*

cannula *(**KAN**-you-lah)*

carbon dioxide *(**KAR**-bon dye-**OCK**-side)*

chronic obstructive pulmonary disease (COPD) *(**KRON**-ick ob-**STRUCK**-tiv **PULL**-moh-nair-ee dih-**ZEEZ**)*

dyspnea *(disp-**NEE**-ah)*

emphysema *(**em**-fih-**SEE**-mah)*

endotracheal tube *(**en**-doh-**TRAY**-kee-al toob)*

expectorate *(eck-**SPECK**-toh-rayt)*

high Fowler's position *(high **FOW**-lerz poh-**ZISH**-un)*

influenza *(**in**-flew-**EN**-zah)*

larynx *(**LAR**-inks)*

orthopneic position *(or-thop-**NEE**-ick poh-**ZISH**-un)*

oxygen *(**OCK**-sih-jen)*

oxygen mask *(**OCK**-sih-jen mask)*

pharynx *(**FAR**-inks)*

phlegm *(flem)*

pleura *(**PLOOR**-ah)*

pneumonia *(new-**MOH**-nee-ah)*

regurgitate *(ree-**GUR**-jih-tayt)*

sputum *(**SPEW**-tum)*

tachypnea *(**tack**-ip-**NEE**-ah)*

thorax *(**THOR**-acks)*

trachea *(**TRAY**-kee-ah)*

tracheostomy *(**tray**-kee-**OS**-toh-mee)*

ventilation *(ven-tih-**LAY**-shun)*

vocal cords *(**VOH**-kal kords)*

INTRODUCTION

The respiratory system exchanges gases to meet the body's metabolic needs. The two gases are:

- **Oxygen** (O_2)
- **Carbon dioxide** (CO_2)

Oxygen is brought into the lungs and carried to the cells to produce energy.

Carbon dioxide is a waste product that is carried to the lungs from the cells for excretion.

There is a close connection between the respiratory and circulatory systems. Cells depend on the bloodstream to carry gases to and from the lungs.

THE RESPIRATORY ORGANS

The respiratory organs are shown in Figure 25-1.

Upper Respiratory Tract

The upper respiratory tract consists of the:

- Nose
- **Pharynx** (throat)
- **Larynx** (voice box)
- **Trachea** (windpipe)
- **Bronchi**

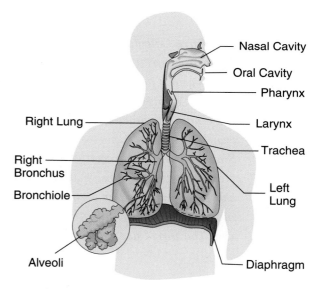

FIGURE 25-1 The respiratory system

The Lungs

There are two lungs, each surrounded by a double-walled membrane called the **pleura**. Between the layers of the pleura is a small amount of fluid that reduces friction as the lungs alternately expand and contract, filling with and then expelling air. The air is warmed,

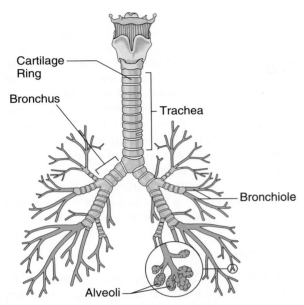

FIGURE 25-2 Ventral view of the structures of the lower respiratory tract

filtered, and moistened as it passes over the vascular mucous membrane that lines the respiratory tract, from nose to alveoli.

The bronchi join the upper respiratory tract to the lungs. Within the lungs, the bronchi branch into smaller and smaller divisions called **bronchioles**. The **alveoli** are tiny air sacs that extend from the bronchioles. The alveoli, bronchioles, and the important pulmonary blood vessels form the lungs (Figure 25-2). The way in which oxygen and carbon dioxide are exchanged between the alveoli and the capillaries is shown in Figure 25-3.

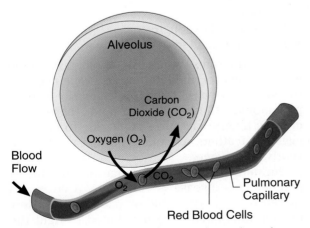

FIGURE 25-3 Oxygen and carbon dioxide are exchanged between the capillaries and each of the alveoli.

The Act of Respiration

The lungs are located in the **thorax**. The size of the thorax depends on the contraction of the diaphragm and intercostal muscles. As the muscles contract, the thorax enlarges, expanding the lungs. Air carrying oxygen enters the lungs. When the muscles relax, the thorax resumes its normal size and the lungs recoil. Air carrying carbon dioxide leaves the lungs and is breathed out.

- *Inspiration* is the act of drawing air into the lungs.
- *Expiration* is the act of expelling air.
- **Ventilation** is the combination of these two actions.

VOICE PRODUCTION

The larynx, or voice box, is part of the respiratory tract. It is important in voice production. Two membranes called the **vocal cords** stretch across the inside of the larynx. As air passes upward through the larynx, it moves through an opening in the vocal cords. Changes in the shape of the vocal cords and the size of the opening permit controlled amounts of air to reach the mouth, nasal cavities, and sinuses, where—formed by the teeth, lips, and tongue—specific speech sounds are made.

CHANGES IN THE RESPIRATORY SYSTEM CAUSED BY AGING

Refer to Figure 25-4. With aging, the following changes occur:

- Breathing capacity drops by one-half.
- The alveoli enlarge and lose elasticity, making recoil less effective.
- The respiratory rate increases.
- The diaphragm and intercostal muscles lose strength, so gaseous exchange is less efficient.
- Changes in the larynx make the voice higher pitched and weaker.
- Cough mechanism is less effective.

INTRODUCTION TO PATHOLOGY

The respiratory system is affected by the same kinds of pathologies as other systems. Two of the most common pathologies are:

- Malignancies
- Infections

FIGURE 25-4 Changes in the respiratory system as a result of aging

- Lung tissue loses elasticity
- Slower rate of gas exchange
- Breathing capacity diminished
- Diaphragm less efficient
- Rate of breathing increases
- Larynx changes make voice weaker and higher pitched
- Less efficient cough

Malignancies

Malignant tumors can develop in any part of the respiratory tract. Although the exact causes of malignancy are not fully understood, cigarette smoking and exposure to other cancer-producing agents in the environment are known to be contributing factors. Lung cancers are treated by surgery, radiation, or chemotherapy, or a combination of all three therapies.

Cancer of the Larynx

Cancer of the larynx may require removal of the larynx, resulting in loss of the voice. The resident breathes through an artificial opening in the neck and trachea. The permanent opening is called a **tracheostomy** and is a permanent stoma.

Loss of voice is a major trauma for anyone. Just think for a moment of how frustrated you would feel if you could no longer use your voice to communicate your thoughts, feelings, wants, and needs to others.

Postsurgical care is given in the acute care hospital. At this time, writing is the major form of communication available to patients. Later, the resident may be taught new ways to speak through:

- Esophageal speech
- Electronic speech

Esophageal Speech. The resident learns to swallow air and then bring it back up (**regurgitate**) through the esophagus into the mouth. Here it is formed by the teeth and tongue into words as it would be if it were being exhaled from the lungs. Esophageal speech is difficult to learn, but motivated residents can succeed.

Electronic Speech. Residents who cannot use esophageal speech may be able to use an electronic artificial larynx to create speech. Some residents may use a combination of both techniques.

Residents with laryngectomies (removal of larynx) need patience and understanding from all health care providers. Communication is possible, but the voice does not sound normal. More time is needed by the resident to formulate the sounds. A difficult psychological adjustment must be made by the resident. The loss of one's voice requires an adjustment similar to that experienced when grieving for the loss of a loved one. Expect periods of depression, anger, and hostility.

Infections

The respiratory tract is exposed to many pathogens in the environment. Respiratory infections are common in the elderly because of reduced resistance and can be life-threatening.

Upper respiratory tract infections such as colds or sore throats are caused by viruses or bacteria. These infections are usually self-limiting and are treated by rest, fluids, and antibiotics (if caused by bacteria). Two common infections are influenza and pneumonia. Both can be life-threatening to the elderly and those with compromised immune systems.

Influenza. **Influenza** (flu) is a viral respiratory infection. There is usually a sudden onset of signs and symptoms, including:

- Chills
- Fever
- Muscle pain
- Weakness
- Fatigue
- Laryngitis
- Hoarseness
- Nonproductive cough
- Runny nose and eyes

The symptoms usually last 3 to 5 days. In the elderly, however, the fatigue and cough may last for several weeks. Influenza can also lead to pneumonia. Elderly people and those with chronic illness who are not allergic to chicken, eggs, or feathers are encouraged to receive a yearly flu vaccine.

Influenza can be very dangerous to elderly people. This disease is caused by a virus and therefore is not treatable with antibiotics. New medications have been developed to fight the virus, but it is too early to determine their effectiveness.

Vaccines are available to prevent the disease. The virus that causes influenza changes each year. This means that the vaccine must be modified each year. Long-term care facilities give the vaccine annually to residents unless a resident refuses or there are other reasons not to administer it. Employees working in health care should also receive the vaccine annually.

Pneumonia. **Pneumonia** is a serious infection of the lungs that causes the alveoli to fill with fluid, affecting the exchange of gases. Pneumonia is the sixth leading cause of death in the United States; 45,000 people die of pneumonia each year. It is difficult to determine the exact cause. Possible causes of pneumonia include:

- Viruses
- Bacteria
- **Aspiration** of food and liquids (accidentally taking food and liquids into the trachea instead of the esophagus)
- Immobility, which allows fluid to accumulate in the lungs

The resident may have chills, fever, chest pain, and a productive cough (produces sputum). **Sputum** or **phlegm** is matter that is brought up (**expectorated**) from the lungs. Sputum varies in color and character. Respiration may be labored and cyanosis may be present. Treatment includes bed rest, oxygen, and positioning to relieve breathing. Antibiotics are given for bacterial pneumonia. Drugs are also given to relieve chest pain. Residents are encouraged to take fluids. A pneumonia vaccine is available for immunization.

Residents are better able to resist respiratory tract infections when they take in adequate fluids and remain active.

Effect of Age on the Response to Infections

As people age, their bodies may not respond as strongly to infections as those of younger people. The signs and symptoms of infection may not be as pronounced. Be sure to report:

- Changes in rate or rhythm of respirations
- Cough
- Elevated temperature
- Persistant fatigue
- Difficulty breathing (**dyspnea**)
- Rapid, shallow, or noisy breathing (**tachypnea**)
- Confusion
- Restlessness
- Changes in color of secretions
- Cyanosis
- Pallor
- Shortness of breath (SOB)

Infections are treated vigorously with:

- Rest
- Antibiotics (for bacterial infections)
- Oxygen therapy
- Drugs to keep air passageways clear
- Supportive care

Always practice standard precautions when caring for residents with respiratory infections. Remember that these infectious organisms are often airborne and found in droplets of respiratory secretions. Transmission-based precautions may be required in addition to standard precautions.

Collecting a Sputum Specimen

You may need to collect a sputum specimen from the resident. A culture of the specimen identifies the cause of the infection.

You must be sure that the specimen comes from the lungs and is not saliva from the mouth.

If the resident cannot expectorate sputum, suctioning may be needed to obtain the specimen. (The nurse usually performs this procedure.) It is easier to collect the specimen when the resident wakes up in the morning and after taking two or three deep breaths.

PROCEDURE
104 Collecting a Sputum Specimen

1. Carry out each beginning procedure action.
2. Assemble equipment:
   - Disposable gloves
   - Disposable mask

- Container and cover for specimen
- Glass of water
- Label, including:
  - Resident's full name
  - Room number

(continues)

PROCEDURE *104* *(continued)*

- Resident number
- Date and time of collection
- Physician's name
- Examination to be done
- Other information as requested
- Tissues
- Emesis basin
- Biohazard specimen transport bag
- Laboratory requisition

3. Wash hands and put on disposable mask and gloves.
4. Ask the resident to rinse mouth with water and spit into emesis basin.
5. Ask resident to breathe deeply and then cough deeply to bring up sputum. The resident spits the sputum into the container.

   - While coughing, have resident cover mouth with tissue to prevent spread of infection.

   - Collect 1 to 2 tablespoons of sputum unless otherwise ordered.
   - Do not contaminate the outside of the container.

6. Remove gloves and discard according to facility policy.
7. Wash your hands. Remove and discard mask.
8. Cover container tightly and attach completed label.
9. Place specimen container into biohazard transport bag and attach laboratory requisition.
10. Carry out each procedure completion action.
11. Follow facility policy for transport of specimen to laboratory.

CHRONIC OBSTRUCTIVE PULMONARY DISEASE

Chronic obstructive pulmonary disease (COPD) is also called chronic obstructive lung disease (COLD). This term refers to conditions resulting from a prolonged impairment in the exchange of gases in the respiratory system. Several conditions can lead to COPD, including:

- Tuberculosis
- Frequent pneumonia
- Chronic asthma
- Chronic bronchitis
- Emphysema

Asthma

Asthma is a breathing disorder resulting from:

- Constriction of the muscles of the bronchioles
- Swelling of the respiratory membranes
- Production of large amounts of mucus that fill the narrowed passageways

A person having an asthma attack has labored breathing and frequent coughing. An attack may result when the person contacts an **allergen** or is under emotional stress. Common allergens are:

- Pollen
- Medications
- Dust
- Feathers
- Foods such as chicken, eggs, or chocolate

If a resident has known allergies (hypersensitivity to specific items), they should be marked in the resident's health record. Long-term treatment consists of determining the allergen and eliminating it. To relieve the attack, the resident is given medication to decrease the swelling and dilate the bronchioles. Low levels of oxygen are also given.

Chronic Bronchitis

Chronic **bronchitis** is prolonged inflammation in the bronchi due to infection or irritants. Signs and symptoms include:

- Swollen and red bronchial tissues, resulting in narrowed bronchial passageways
- Persistent cough, which may or may not produce sputum
- Respiratory distress

Treatment, in general includes:

- Antibiotics to fight the infection
- Drugs to loosen the phlegm (secretions) deep in the respiratory tract
- Techniques to improve ventilation and drainage

Emphysema

Emphysema develops after chronic obstruction of the airflow to the alveoli. The air sacs:

- Become distended
- Lose their elasticity and recoil ability
- Finally become nonfunctional
- Lose ability to exchange gases

The resident can bring air into the lungs, but it becomes more difficult to expel air from the lungs. As a result, there is less and less room for air to reenter.

Several factors contribute to emphysema, including:

- Air pollutants, such as cigarette smoke, auto exhaust fumes, and insecticides
- Genetic predisposition to emphysema
- Recurrent infections, such as pneumonia and bronchitis
- Chronic asthma

People with emphysema are at greater risk for infections such as pneumonia. They experience:

- Chronic oxygen shortage and fatigue
- Increasing breathing difficulty (requires greater and greater effort)
- Productive coughing that may bring up large amounts of heavy mucous secretions (phlegm), or nonproductive coughing
- Dizziness and restlessness as carbon dioxide levels rise in the bloodstream
- Loss of appetite and weight loss
- Strain on the heart and blood vessels

TREATMENT AND CARE OF RESIDENTS WITH COPD

The goals of treatment of the resident with COPD are to:

- Loosen and thin phlegm
- Improve ventilation
- Improve gaseous exchange
- Prevent infections

Special techniques are used to loosen the phlegm and make it easier to bring up. Removing phlegm from the passageways makes breathing

Clinical Focus:

Compare Mrs. Calcetas's symptoms with the changes in the respiratory system that are a result of aging. Think about how one condition affects the other.

easier. Some procedures will be carried out by the nurse or respiratory therapist. You may assist in:

- Positioning the resident for better ventilation
- Breathing exercises to improve respiratory efficiency
- Caring for the resident during oxygen therapy to improve gaseous exchange

Positioning for Better Ventilation

Two positions are used to improve ventilation:

- High Fowler's position
- Orthopneic position

In the **high Fowler's position**, the resident is sitting almost upright, with the knees flexed. The resident must be supported in proper alignment with pillows.

In the **orthopneic position**, an overbed table is positioned in front of the resident (Figure 25-5). The resident leans forward with arms on the table. A pillow on the overbed table supports the head. The arms may be positioned on

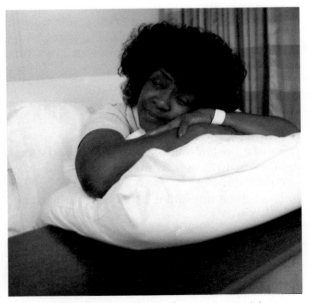

FIGURE 25-5 The orthopneic position

Clinical Focus:
Practice the breathing exercises and think about how they could help Mrs. Calcetas.

or around the pillow. Additional pillows are used to support the resident's body and maintain proper alignment.

Most residents with COPD who are ambulatory breathe best when sitting in a chair and leaning forward with the elbows on the arms of the chair or on their legs.

Exercises

Residents can be taught breathing exercises that improve respiration and general respiratory muscle tone. Breathing exercises stress the expiration phase of respiration. The resident is first taught the basic breathing pattern, which is to:

- Breathe in through the nose to the count of one, allowing the abdomen to rise.
- Purse the lips to the count of two and three as the abdominal wall is contracted and air is forced out of the lungs.

Oxygen Therapy

Residents with COPD benefit by breathing low levels of oxygen. Oxygen therapy may be administered by:

- **Cannulas**—small tubes placed in the resident's nostrils and held in place by straps (Figure 25-6).
- **Oxygen mask**—placed over the resident's nose and mouth and secured in place (Figure 25-7)
- Nasal catheter—a small plastic or latex tube that is inserted into the nose

The nurse will set up the oxygen equipment and will start the oxygen flow. You observe the resident for the following:

- Proper position of the catheter, cannula, or mask and the elastic band—snug but not constricting
- Signs of irritation from straps, catheter, cannula, or mask
- The tubing not kinked, pinched, or restricted in any way
- Flowmeter registers volume of oxygen flow properly in liters
- Oxygen moisturized
- Resident's face free of secretions
- Safety precautions being followed (review Lesson 8)

FIGURE 25-6 This resident is receiving oxygen through a cannula attached to the oxygen source.

Source of Oxygen. Oxygen may be piped into the resident's room, but in long-term care facilities, tanks of oxygen may be used (Figure 25-8). If a tank is used, be sure that:

- "No Smoking" signs are in place.
- There is sufficient oxygen in the tank. Check the gauge each time you visit the resident.
- An additional tank is available.
- Empty tanks are marked and stored according to facility policy.
- The tank is upright and secure on the carrier or in the stand.
- The oxygen is moisturized.

Oxygen does not explode, but when it is present, burning is more intense and rapid. Everyone must follow oxygen safety measures. If there is a fire, sound the alarm and move the resident to safety, following facility policy.

FIGURE 25-7 The mask is placed over the resident's nose and mouth to deliver oxygen.

FIGURE 25-8 Oxygen is usually piped directly to each resident unit.

Oxygen Concentrator

An oxygen concentrator takes in room air and removes impurities and gases other than oxygen, allowing the oxygen to become concentrated in the unit. The air delivered to the resident from the concentrator is more than 90% oxygen. It is delivered by tubing attached to a nasal cannula or mask. The flow rate is usually 2 liters per minute (L/min). A humidifier bottle may be attached to the concentrator to offset the drying effect of the oxygen.

General Oxygen Concentrator Precautions. Be sure to follow these precautions when a concentrator is used to supply oxygen to a resident:

- Concentrator is placed at least 5 feet away from a heat source and at least 4 inches from the wall.
- Smoking is not permitted in the same room.
- Be sure the unit is plugged in and grounded.
- Do not use an extension cord with the concentrator.
- Never change the flowmeter setting.
- Notify the nurse if the alarm sounds.
- Be sure the fluid level in the humidifier (if used) is adequate.
- Wipe cannula or mask daily with a damp cloth (do not use alcohol- or oil-based products).
- Clean concentrator surfaces using a damp cloth only.
- Remove filter weekly. Wash in warm soapy water, rinse, squeeze dry, and replace.

Special Mouth Care

Breathing through the mouth and breathing oxygen are drying to the mucous membranes of the mouth and the nasal passages. The resident may complain that sputum has a bad taste. Make sure that the resident rinses his or her mouth frequently and that you provide special mouth care. This attention adds greatly to the resident's comfort. Encourage fluid intake because adequate fluids help decrease the thickness of secretions.

PROCEDURE 105 Refilling the Humidifier Bottle

1. Carry out each beginning procedure action.
2. Remove mask or cannula from resident or connect it to a temporary oxygen source if constant oxygen is required.
3. Turn oxygen concentrator off.
4. Remove the lid from the humidifier bottle.
5. Remove the bottle and discard any remaining water.
6. Rinse bottle well with warm water. Shake dry.
7. Refill jar with distilled water to the fill line.
8. Replace bottle and reattach lid.
9. Turn on unit.
10. Position mask or cannula on resident.
11. Wash hands.
12. Carry out procedure completion actions.

Ineffective Cough

If cough is ineffective, it may be necessary to intubate the resident. An **endotracheal tube** is placed directly into the trachea through an opening (tracheotomy) in the throat. Both oxygen delivery and suctioning can take place through the tube. The tracheotomy may be made into a permanent tracheostomy.

A machine that delivers oxygen under pressure at a preset rate may be needed to assist ventilation. This technique is known as intermittent positive pressure breathing (IPPB). The machine may be attached directly to the endotracheal tube. When a resident is receiving assisted ventilation, you will check for:

- Change of color
- Signs of congestion
- Changes in vital signs
- Indications of respiratory distress

LESSON SYNTHESIS: Putting It All Together

You have just completed this lesson. Now go back and review the Clinical Focus. Try to see how the Clinical Focus relates to the concepts presented in the lesson. Then answer the following questions.

1. Why does Mrs. Calcetas have to rest so often when she tries to walk to the day room?

2. Why would smoking make Mrs. Calcetas's condition more difficult?

3. Why should Mrs. Calcetas rinse her mouth and then cough deeply to obtain a sputum specimen?

4. Why should the person collecting the specimen wear gloves?

5. What nursing care techniques could you use to help improve Mrs. Calcetas's breathing?

REVIEW

A. Select the correctly spelled word and then write its definition using the word in the definition.

1. xpectorate   expectorate   espectarate

2. experation   xpiration   expiration

3. thorax   tharox   thorix

4. flegm   flem   phlegm

B. Complete each statement by filling in the missing information.

5. Another name for the windpipe is the _____.

6. As a person ages, breathing capacity diminishes by _____.

7. Changes in the larynx make the voice _____ and _____.

8. List three changes that occur in the respiratory system as a person ages.

_____   _____   _____

9. When collecting a sputum specimen, the assistant should wear _____.

10. State the two positions used to assist a resident in respiratory distress.

_____   _____

C. Select the one best answer for each of the following.

11. Rapid and shallow breathing is known as
    (A) apnea
    (B) emphysema
    (C) pleura
    (D) tachypnea

12. The technique of swallowing air, regurgitating it, and forming words with the teeth and tongue is called
    (A) nasal speech
    (B) esophageal speech
    (C) electronic speech
    (D) sinus speech

13. Sputum is matter from the
    (A) lungs
    (B) nose
    (C) mouth
    (D) sinuses

14. An asthma attack may occur when a sensitive person
    (A) contacts an allergen
    (B) washes hands regularly
    (C) sleeps soundly
    (D) eats nonallergenic foods

15. What is the name given to the position in which the resident is sitting almost upright with the knees flexed?
    (A) orthopneic
    (B) upright
    (C) high Fowler's
    (D) left Sims'

16. Breathing exercises for residents with COPD stress
    (A) inspiratory phase
    (B) expiratory phase
    (C) resting phase
    (D) inhalation phase

17. When a resident receives oxygen from a tank through a nasal cannula, the nursing assistant must be sure that
    (A) the flowmeter registers the proper moisture content
    (B) oxygen is being administered with humidification
    (C) there is no irritation from the strap or cannula
    (D) tank leans against the wall

D. Identify and write the name of each structure shown in the figure.

18. _____
19. _____
20. _____
21. _____
22. _____

E. Clinical Experience
Fill in the blanks by selecting the correct word from the list.

adjustment	gloves
anger	normal
burned	patience
common	report
cover	sputum
depression	strongly

23. Mr. Drummond had a laryngectomy. He is new to your unit. He uses esophageal speech. What characteristics might you expect of him?
    a. His speech will not sound _____.
    b. He had to make a great psychological _____ to his condition.
    c. He will experience periods of _____ and _____.
    d. His care will require much _____ from staff members.

24. Mrs. Burton, who is 87, is one of the residents you care for. She said she does not have "much energy" this morning. She seems a little confused and has a slight cough. Her temperature is elevated only slightly.
    a. You know that influenza and pneumonia are _____ complications of the aging process.
    b. You also remember that as people age, they do not respond to infection as _____ as younger people.
    c. You will _____ your findings promptly.

25. Mr. Ornsteen has a respiratory infection and is confined to bed. You are assigned to care for him. What do you need to remember to protect yourself?
    a. Use _____ when handling respiratory or nasal secretions.
    b. Instruct him to _____ his nose and mouth when coughing or sneezing.
    c. Do not contaminate the outside of the specimen container when obtaining a _____ specimen.

Caring for Residents with Endocrine System Disorders

Clinical Focus

Think about the special observations and care the resident with endocrine disorders needs as you study this lesson and meet:

*M*r. McFarland, who is an insulin-dependent diabetic assigned to your care. He has had a cold. This morning he seems very restless and less responsive than usual. He grows increasingly confused. His 11:00 am glucometer reading shows hyperglycemia. Certain actions must be taken immediately.

OBJECTIVES

After studying this lesson, you should be able to:

- Define and spell vocabulary words and terms.
- Identify the parts and function of the endocrine system.
- Review changes in the endocrine system as they relate to the aging process.
- Recognize reportable signs and symptoms of hypoglycemia and hyperglycemia.

VOCABULARY

adrenal glands *(ah-DREE-nal glands)*
adrenaline *(ah-DREN-ah-lin)*
cortisone *(KOR-tih-sohn)*
diabetes mellitus *(die-ah-BEE-teez MEL-ih-tus)*

diabetic coma *(die-ah-BET-ick KOH-mah)*
diabetic ketoacidosis (DKA) *(dye-ah-BET-ick kee-toh-ah-sih-DOH-sis)*
endocrine gland *(EN-doh-krin gland)*
estrogen *(ES-troh-jen)*

VOCABULARY

gangrene   (*GANG-green*)

glucagon   (*GLOO-kah-gon*)

glucose   (*GLOO-kohs*)

glycosuria   (*gligh-koh-SOO-ree-ah*)

goiter   (*GOY-ter*)

gonad   (*GOH-nad*)

hormone   (*HOR-mohn*)

hyperglycemia   (*high-per-gly-SEE-mee-ah*)

hyperthyroidism   (*high-per-THIGH-roy-dizm*)

hypoglycemia   (*high-poh-gly-SEE-mee-ah*)

hypothyroidism   (*high-poh-THIGH-roy-dizm*)

insulin   (*IN-soo-lin*)

insulin-dependent diabetes mellitus (IDDM)   (*IN-soo-lin dee-PEN-dent die-ah-BEE-teez MEL-ih-tus*)

insulin shock   (*IN-soo-lin shock*)

islets of Langerhans   (*EYE-lets of LANG-ger-hans*)

ketones   (*KEE-tohns*)

metabolism   (*meh-TAB-oh-lizm*)

non–insulin-dependent diabetes mellitus (NIDDM)   (*non–IN-soo-lin dee-PEN-dent die-ah-BEE-teez MEL-ih-tus*)

ovaries   (*OH-vah-rees*)

pancreas   (*PAN-kree-as*)

parathormone   (*pair-ah-THOR-mohn*)

parathyroid glands   (*pair-ah-THIGH-royd glands*)

pineal body   (*PIN-ee-al BAH-dee*)

pituitary gland   (*pih-TOO-ih-tair-ee gland*)

polydipsia   (*pol-ee-DIP-see-ah*)

polyphagia   (*pol-ee-FAY-jee-ah*)

polyuria   (*pol-ee-YOU-ree-ah*)

progesterone   (*proh-JES-teh-rohn*)

scrotum   (*SKROH-tum*)

testes   (*TES-teez*)

testosterone   (*tes-TOS-teh-rohn*)

thyroid gland   (*THIGH-royd gland*)

thyroxine   (*thigh-ROCK-sin*)

INTRODUCTION

The endocrine system (Figure 26-1), consists of:
- **Endocrine glands**, some of which are in pairs
- Clusters of cells

The seven distinct endocrine glands are:
- Pituitary gland
- Pineal body
- Adrenal glands
- Gonads—ovaries (women); testes (men)
- Thyroid gland
- Parathyroid glands
- Islets of Langerhans (pancreas)

The endocrine tissues are located throughout the body. They have the following functions and properties:
- Produce chemical messengers (**hormones**)
- Directly enter the bloodstream
- Regulate body activities and body chemistry

Some endocrine glands secrete more than one hormone. Hormone-producing cells may be found as part of organs that carry on other functions. For example:
- The thyroid gland produces two hormones:
  - Thyrocalcitonin
  - Thyroxine
- The **pancreas** produces two hormones:
  - Glucagon
  - Insulin

The pancreas also produces enzymes that are important in the digestive process.

ENDOCRINE GLANDS

Pituitary Gland

The **pituitary gland** is found under the brain and secretes more than one hormone. It is sometimes called the master gland. The hormones secreted by this gland control:
- Growth
- Urine production

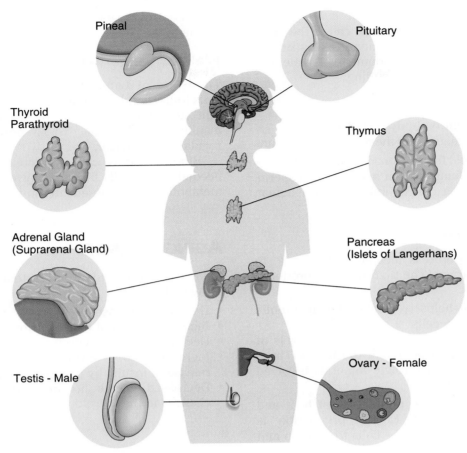

FIGURE 26-1 The endocrine system

- Activity of most of the other glands
- Reproductive activity
- Blood chemistry

Pineal Body

The **pineal body** is a small gland that is also located in the skull beneath the brain. It is thought to delay sexual maturity until the rest of the body is ready for reproduction. It grows smaller as we age.

Adrenal Glands

There are two **adrenal glands**. One gland is located on top of each of the two kidneys. Each gland has two portions that secrete separate hormones. Two of these hormones, **adrenaline** (epinephrine) and **cortisone**, are often prescribed medications. In general, the adrenal hormones:

- Control the release of energy to meet emergencies
- Control water and electrolyte balance in the body

- Secrete small amounts of male and female sex hormones

Gonads

The term **gonads** refers to the sex glands.

- Female gonads = ovaries
- Male gonads = testes

Symbols are used to indicate the different sexes:

- ♀ indicates female (woman)
- ♂ indicates male (man)

Ovaries (♀). The paired **ovaries** are located within the pelvis on either side of the uterus. When stimulated by the pituitary gland, they produce the hormones:

- **Progesterone**—helps to maintain pregnancy
- **Estrogen**—responsible for the development of female characteristics such as:
  - Enlargement of the female reproductive organs
  - Appearance of pubic and axillary hair
  - Enlargement of the breasts
  - Onset and regulation of menstruation

Testes (♂). The paired **testes** are located outside of the body in a pouch called the **scrotum**. They produce the hormone **testosterone**, which regulates the development of male secondary characteristics, including:

- Muscular development
- Deepening voice
- Growth of hair on body and face
- Growth and maturity of the reproductive organs

The male and female gonads also produce special cells, the female ovum and the male sperm, that unite during conception to form a human embryo.

Thyroid Gland

The **thyroid gland** is located in the neck, in front of the larynx. The thyroid gland produces two hormones:

- **Thyroxine**—helps regulate the metabolic rate of all body cells
- Thyrocalcitonin—helps regulate the levels of calcium and phosphates in the blood. These are two of the electrolyte minerals involved in electrolyte balance.

Metabolism is the production of heat and energy by the cells. Energy production is related to the ability of the cells to take up and use oxygen.

Disorders of the thyroid gland include:

- **Hyperthyroidism** (exophthalmic **goiter** or toxic goiter) results from overproduction of thyroxine. The resident shows:
    - Irritability and restlessness
    - Nervousness
    - Rapid pulse
    - Increased appetite
    - Weight loss
    - Sensitivity
- **Hypothyroidism** results from underproduction of thyroxine. The lack of iodine can result in a low thyroxine production. This is known as simple goiter. A severe lack of thyroxine results in a condition called myxedema. The resident with hypothyroidism shows:
    - Slow responses
    - Lethargy
    - Weight gain
    - Slow pulse

Parathyroid Glands

The **parathyroid glands** are several tiny glands embedded in the back of the thyroid gland. They produce the hormone **parathormone** that also helps control the use of calcium and phosphorus by the body.

Islets of Langerhans

The **islets of Langerhans** are small groups of cells found within the pancreas. Two very important hormones produced by these cells are insulin and glucagon. These hormones help regulate blood sugar.

Blood sugar is called **glucose**. Glucose is needed by all cells for *all* body work. Glucose metabolism is discussed later in this lesson.

AGING CHANGES

Changes in the endocrine system caused by aging include:

- Decreased glucose tolerance
- Increased levels of parathormone
- Decreased vaginal secretions
- Increased blood sugar level due to slower release of insulin by pancreatic cells
- Decreased metabolic rate resulting from changes in the thyroid

GLUCOSE METABOLISM

Glucose is the primary energy source for all of the work done by the body. The level of glucose is an important factor in proper functioning. Various hormones and enzymes maintain this level and help the body to use (metabolize) glucose for energy. Two of these hormones are:

- **Glucagon**—raises the blood sugar level by converting stored sugar (glycogen) to glucose.
- **Insulin**—lowers the blood sugar level by causing glucose to move from the bloodstream into the cells. It also helps to convert glucose to glycogen (stored sugar).

Abnormal blood sugar levels are called:

- **Hyperglycemia**—the blood sugar level is too high.
- **Hypoglycemia**—the blood sugar level is too low.

Diabetes mellitus is a major disorder of carbohydrate, fat, and protein metabolism. It is usually caused by:

- Insufficient insulin in the body
- Inability of the cells to use the available insulin

DIABETES MELLITUS

In **diabetes mellitus** the body cannot use glucose normally to meet the energy needs of the body. This disease is common in older people. In fact, in people over age 65, one of every 20 requires treatment for diabetes.

The two forms of diabetes are:

- **Insulin–dependent diabetes mellitus (IDDM) (Type 1).** Insulin is produced by beta cells in the pancreas. In Type 1 diabetes, the beta cells are damaged, resulting in decreased or no production of insulin. Insulin is required for the metabolism of glucose. With too little insulin released by the pancreas, abnormal amounts of glucose accumulate in the bloodstream, because it cannot be absorbed by body cells where it is used for energy.
- **Non–insulin-dependent diabetes mellitus (NIDDM) (Type 2).** In Type 2 diabetes, insufficient insulin is produced or the body ignores the insulin. As a result, glucose builds up in the bloodstream and is not absorbed by body cells.

Both forms may be seen in older people, but the non–insulin-dependent form is more common.

Insulin-Dependent Diabetes Mellitus (Type 1)

IDDM is more often seen in younger people. Signs and symptoms include:

- Abrupt onset
- Excess thirst (**polydipsia**)
- Excess urine elimination (**polyuria**)
- Excessive hunger (**polyphagia**)
- Sugar in the urine (**glycosuria**)
- Excess blood sugar (hyperglycemia)

This form of diabetes is more difficult to control. Diabetic persons may experience periods of hypoglycemia (**insulin shock**) or hyperglycemia (**diabetic coma**). These people require:

- Regular injections of insulin to balance their blood sugar
- Regulation of food intake
- Planned exercise (which uses sugar for energy) as part of the treatment program

Non–Insulin-Dependent Diabetes Mellitus (Type 2)

NIDDM is also known as old-age diabetes. The older the person, the more likely that diabetes will develop. This form of diabetes is more sta-

FIGURE 26-2 Signs of diabetes mellitus
• Polyuria (excessive urine)
• Polydipsia (excessive thirst)
• Polyphagia (excessive hunger)
• Weight loss
• Blurring of vision
• Complaints of itching
• Burning on urination
• Redness or tenderness at injection site
• Slow healing of infections or injuries

ble than IDDM, with fewer incidents of diabetic coma or insulin shock.

Signs and Symptoms.   Often only one or two symptoms appear in the elderly person. The person is usually overweight and may have constant fatigue or a sore or infection that takes an unusually long time to heal. About half of those with diabetes show the obvious signs (Figure 26-2). The rest have less well-defined symptoms such as:

- Fatiguing easily
- Skin infections
- Slow healing
- Itching
- Burning on urination
- Pain in fingers and toes
- Vision changes

Therapy consists of:

- Diet control
- Weight reduction
- Exercise
- Oral hypoglycemic agents

Complications of Diabetes

Complications, which can be severe and nonreversible in the elderly, include:

- Renal disease
- Vision changes
- Cardiovascular damage
- Hyperglycemia
- Hypoglycemia

Vision Changes.   This is particularly common in long-term diabetes. Serious vision changes are often thought to be due to general aging. However, they may really be related to diabetes. Complications include:

- Glaucoma
- Cataracts
- Retinitis proliferans
- Blindness

Cardiovascular Damage. The consequences of hypoglycemia (insulin shock) or hyperglycemia (diabetic coma) can be severe in the elderly resident and may include:

- Heart attacks
- Strokes
- Peripheral vascular disease
- Amputation

Because injuries heal poorly, an ingrown toenail or improperly cut nails can lead to serious problems. Vascular changes can interfere with the normal circulation to the legs and feet. Damage may be so extensive that the tissues of the toes, feet, and legs may die. As a result, they have to be removed (amputated). **Gangrene** (death of tissue) (Figure 26-3) followed by amputation is a common problem for the older resident with diabetes. Careful observations and care can help prevent this serious condition.

Hyperglycemia. This condition occurs when too little insulin is available for metabolic needs. Sugar and acid compounds (**ketones**) build up in the blood. The condition is known as **diabetic ketoacidosis (DKA)** and can lead to death. Sugar and ketones then spill over into the urine.

A sudden, unexpected need for insulin brought about by stress, illness, injury, or curtailed activity may bring on DKA. It usually develops slowly, sometimes over a 24-hour period. The first symptoms may be headache, drowsiness, and confusion. The resident seems less respon-sive, irritable, confused, and drowsy and may slip slowly into unconsciousness (coma).

Signs and symptoms of hyperglycemia include:

- Thirst
- Blurred vision
- Nausea and vomiting
- A sweet odor to the breath
- Dry, flushed skin

It is important to note these signs early so that treatment can begin right away. Learn the signs and symptoms of diabetic coma (Figure 26-4). If these signs are noted in a resident, report them immediately. The treatment for hyperglycemia is insulin and fluids, which will be given intravenously by the nurse.

Hypoglycemia. Hypoglycemia or low blood sugar is far less common when oral antidiabetic agents are given than when insulin is given by injection. When hypoglycemia results from an overdose of insulin, it is known as *insulin reaction* or insulin shock. Hypoglycemia can be brought on by:

- Not eating planned snacks or eating less food (as a result of decreased appetite)
- Unusual activity
- Stress

FIGURE 26-3 Gangrene of the toes and feet often results in amputation.

FIGURE 26-4 Signs and symptoms to be reported for diabetes coma and insulin shock	
Diabetic Coma (Hyperglycemia)	**Insulin Shock (Hypoglycemia)**
Gradual onset	Sudden onset
Drowsiness	Nervousness
Deep, difficult breathing	Shallow breathing
Nausea	Hunger
Hot, flushed, dry skin	Moist, pale skin
Mental confusion	Mental confusion Vision disturbance
Loss of consciousness	Loss of consciousness
Sweet odor to breath	

- Vomiting
- Diarrhea
- Interaction of oral drugs with other medications being taken

In contrast to DKA, which develops slowly, hypoglycemia may occur rapidly.

Signs and symptoms of hypoglycemia include:

- Hunger
- Sweating
- Dizziness
- Drowsiness
- Blurred vision
- Erratic behavior
- Staggering gait
- Mental confusion
- Disorientation
- Pale and moist skin

Learn the signs and symptoms of hypoglycemia (see Figure 26-4). Report immediately to the nurse if you observe them in a resident.

The resident with hypoglycemia is treated with sugar in some form. A food containing sugar is given orally if the resident is conscious. If the resident is unconscious, glucagon (a hormone) may be given by injection. Orange juice or other easily absorbed sources of sugar are usually kept on the unit where they are easily accessible for the nurse to use in an emergency. Every staff member should be aware of the storage location.

Treatment of Diabetes

For people with diabetes living independently, control of the disease depends on self-care. For a resident with diabetes, self-care is assisted. Residents should be encouraged to take part in their own care as much as possible.

The goals for the care of the person with diabetes, whether at home or in a facility, are the same:

- Maintain a proper metabolic balance
- Prevent complications

Although uncommon, the less stable form of diabetes (IDDM) may appear in later years. If you notice any of the acute signs, they should be reported at once. A few elderly diabetic residents are insulin dependent. The treatment is then the same as for any insulin-dependent person. Some people who have had diabetes since youth will continue to require regular insulin injections.

Three factors must be balanced in each diabetic's life:

- Diet
- Exercise
- Drugs

Note that some people with diabetes are able to manage the disease by diet and exercise and do not require drug therapy.

Diet. Most residents with diabetes receive specially balanced diabetic meals. Your responsibilities include:

- Checking trays carefully to be sure the correct diet is given
- Serving the trays
- Assisting in feeding
- Noticing and recording how much and what food was eaten
- Returning trays after meals
- Informing the nurse if food is not eaten
- Giving supplemental foods as ordered

If concentrated sugars such as jellies or jams are on the tray, be sure to check with the nurse before feeding the resident (concentrated sugars usually are never permitted in a diabetic diet). You must know what is allowed for each resident with diabetes in your care.

Exercise. The more a person exercises, the more sugar is needed for energy. The increased need for sugar usage increases the need for insulin. Less exercise decreases the need. A resident's activity will influence the need for both food and insulin. Be sure to report unusual activity or unusual inactivity.

Drugs. Drugs used in the treatment of diabetes are called antidiabetic drugs. Some of these may be taken by mouth (oral hypoglycemics). Insulin must be injected. The nurse will administer the drugs, but you also have some responsibilities. For oral hypoglycemics, be sure to report if the drugs are not taken. For example, if a pill is given to the resident and then is spit out after the nurse leaves the room, report this to the nurse immediately.

If the resident is receiving insulin, check the injection site and report:

- Redness
- Pain
- Itching

Nursing Assistant Responsibilities

Residents who experience emotional stress or have an infection of any kind are at greater risk for imbalance. They need to be monitored with extra care and attention. When providing routine care for the resident with diabetes you must:

- Know the signs of insulin shock and diabetic coma.

- Be alert for the signs of diabetic coma or insulin shock and report them immediately to the nurse.
- Know the storage location of juice or other easily absorbed carbohydrates.
- When food trays are delivered, check that the resident receives the proper diet.
- Give extra nourishments only as ordered.
- Keep a record of the food consumed on the resident's chart.
- Report uneaten meals to the nurse.
- Give special attention to the care of the diabetic resident's feet.
  - Wash daily, carefully drying between toes.
  - Inspect feet closely for any breaks or signs of irritation.
  - Report any abnormalities to the nurse.
  - Do not allow moisture to collect between toes.
  - Apply lotion to dry feet.
  - Toenails of a diabetic are cut only by a podiatrist or an RN who is a specialist in foot care.

- Shoes and stockings should be clean, free of holes, and fit well. Anything that might injure the feet or interfere with the circulation must be avoided.
- Do not allow the resident to go barefoot.
- Prevent pressure over the toes and feet by not tucking in bedding tightly.
- Inspect the skin regularly for signs of infection.
- Avoid very warm or cold applications to the skin.

Testing to Monitor Control of Diabetes

Drugs for hypoglycemia and insulin are prescribed according to how well the body uses sugar for energy. For this reason, blood tests for sugar are performed regularly and treatment is adjusted as necessary. This is a licensed nursing procedure.

LESSON SYNTHESIS: Putting It All Together

You have just completed this lesson. Now go back and review the Clinical Focus. Try to see how the Clinical Focus relates to the concepts presented in the lesson. Then answer the following questions.

1. How might Mr. McFarland's cold have affected his condition?

2. Explain what is meant by the fact that the resident is demonstrating hyperglycemia.

3. What action should the nursing assistant take after noting the change in Mr. McFarland's behavior?

4. What actions might the nurse decide would be appropriate?

5. What general actions should the nursing assistant take when caring for the resident with diabetes mellitus?

REVIEW

A. Match each term (items a.–j.) with the proper definition.

a. thyroxine
b. hypoglycemia
c. gonads
d. polyuria
e. glycosuria

f. hormone
g. obesity
h. hyperglycemia
i. glucose
j. gangrene

1. _____ internal secretion produced by glands

2. _____ death of tissue

3. _____ low blood sugar

4. _____ sugar in the urine

5. _____ reproductive glands

6. _____ blood sugar

7. _____ produced by the thyroid gland

8. _____ excessive urine output

9. _____ overweight

10. _____ excessive blood sugar

B. Provide brief answers for each of the following.

11. List three changes in the endocrine system due to aging.

12. Describe the role of thyroxine in the body.

13. What two chemical electrolytes are influenced by the levels of parathormone?

14. List the names of the two forms of diabetes mellitus.

15. What is the most common form of diabetes mellitus?

16. List four signs of insulin–dependent diabetes mellitus.

17. List four signs of non–insulin-dependent diabetes mellitus.

18. List three factors that must be balanced for the resident with diabetes.

C. Select the one best answer for each of the following.

19. Endocrine glands
(A) release secretions into tubes that reach the body surface
(B) are all located in the abdomen
(C) each secrete one hormone only
(D) release secretions directly into the bloodstream

20. Hormones produced by the ovaries help
(A) urine production
(B) enlarge breasts
(C) control electrolyte balance
(D) regulate the levels of calcium

21. Which of the following is the male gonad?
(A) pituitary gland
(B) ovary
(C) testes
(D) thyroid

22. What sign or symptom is most often seen in a person with IDDM?
(A) abrupt onset
(B) skin infections
(C) itching
(D) pain in fingers and toes

23. What sign or symptom may be shown by an elderly person with NIDDM?
(A) excessive hunger
(B) burning on urination
(C) abrupt onset
(D) excessive thirst

24. The nursing assistant entered Mr. Lanzo's room and noted that he did not seem well. His skin was dry and flushed and he said he was thirsty. She reported to the nurse right away. What other symptom did she note that made her suspect the resident was hyperglycemic?
(A) complaint of hunger
(B) disorientation
(C) sweet odor to his breath
(D) pale, moist skin

25. When taking care of residents who have diabetes mellitus, the nursing assistant must remember to
    (A) administer insulin on time
    (B) wash the feet only occasionally so they will not get too dry
    (C) avoid applying lotion to the feet
    (D) make sure to serve the proper diet

26. If a resident with diabetes is receiving insulin, the nursing assistant should check the injection site for
    (A) redness or itching
    (B) blueness
    (C) coldness
    (D) puncture marks

27. The nursing assistant notices that a resident with diabetes has long toenails. Her proper action is to
    (A) cut the nails
    (B) let the resident cut his own nails
    (C) report to the nurse so the podiatrist can be called to cut the nails
    (D) ignore the matter because the resident wears shoes to protect his feet

D. Clinical Experience

28. Mrs. Barker, a diabetic, has not eaten all the food on her tray. She is on a diabetic diet. What action should the nursing assistant take?
    (A) Ignore it because it is not important.
    (B) Insist the resident eat every spoonful.
    (C) Report and record the amount of food eaten.
    (D) Throw the food away so no one knows.

29. Mr. Samuels, a diabetic, has a darkened area on the little toe of his left foot. The nursing assistant reports this because she knows that a complication of diabetes is
    (A) glaucoma
    (B) renal disease
    (C) cataracts
    (D) gangrene

30. Mr. Lorenzo, who has IDDM, has an unpleasant visit with his daughter and her husband and now seems very upset. The nursing assistant will watch him closely for signs of hyperglycemia including
    (A) shallow breathing
    (B) gradual onset
    (C) moist, pale skin
    (D) hunger

Caring for Residents with Reproductive System Disorders

Clinical Focus

Think about the special care required by residents with disorders of the reproductive system as you study this lesson and meet:

*B*essie Shutt, who is the mother of seven and grand-mother to 23 children and 14 great-grandchildren. She suffers from congestive heart failure and chronic obstructive pulmonary disease. She has a prolapsed uterus and complains of itching in the vaginal area. She is also occasionally incontinent of urine.

OBJECTIVES

After studying this lesson, you should be able to:

- Define and spell vocabulary words and terms.
- Identify the parts and functions of the male and female reproductive systems.
- Review changes in the reproductive systems of men and women caused by aging.
- Describe conditions of the reproductive tract affecting long-term residents.
- Identify and describe common sexually transmitted diseases.

VOCABULARY

benign prostatic hypertrophy *(bee-**NINE** pros-**TAT**-ick high-**PER**-troh-fee)*

chlamydia *(klah-**MID**-ee-ah)*

climacteric *(kligh-**MACK**-ter-ick)*

clitoris *(**KLIT**-or-is)*

Cowper's glands *(**KOW**-perz glands)*

ejaculatory duct *(ee-**JACK**-you-lah-**toh**-ree dukt)*

endometrium *(en-doh-**MEE**-tree-um)*

epididymis *(**ep**-ih-**DID**-ih-mis)*

VOCABULARY

estrogen *(ES-troh-jen)*

foreskin *(FOR-skin)*

genitalia *(jen-ih-TAY-lee-ah)*

gonorrhea *(gon-or-REE-ah)*

hysterectomy *(his-teh-RECK-toh-mee)*

labia majora *(LAY-bee-ah mah-JOR-ah)*

labia minora *(LAY-bee-ah mih-NOR-ah)*

menopause *(MEN-oh-pawz)*

menstruation *(men-stroo-AY-shun)*

ovulation *(oh-vyou-LAY-shun)*

ovum (plural: ova) *(OH-vum; plural: OH-vah)*

penis *(PEE-nis)*

perineum *(pair-ih-NEE-um)*

progesterone *(proh-JES-ter-ohn)*

prostate *(PROS-tayt)*

pruritus *(prew-RYE-tus)*

puberty *(PYOU-ber-tee)*

scrotum *(SKROH-tum)*

seminal vesicles *(SEM-ih-nal VES-ih-kuls)*

sperm *(spurm)*

syphilis *(SIF-ih-lis)*

testes *(TES-teez)*

testicles *(TES-tih-kuls)*

testosterone *(tes-TOS-teh-rohn)*

transurethral prostatectomy *(trans-you-REE-thral pros-tah-TECK-toh-mee)*

trichomonas vaginitis *(trick-oh-MOH-nas vaj-ih-NIGH-tis)*

urethra *(you-REE-thrah)*

uterine tubes *(YOU-ter-in toobs)*

uterus *(YOU-ter-us)*

vagina *(vah-JYE-nah)*

vaginitis *(vaj-ih-NIGH-tis)*

vas deferens *(vas DEF-er-ens)*

venereal warts *(vee-NEE-ree-al warts)*

vulva *(VUL-vah)*

INTRODUCTION

The male and female reproductive systems share some features. They:

- Consist of gonads, tubes, and accessory structures
- Contribute to the reproductive process
- Provide the sex hormones
- Bring pleasure

Remember, human sexuality is the interaction between the physical and emotional needs of an individual. Sexuality is intimately involved with the individual's sense of identity. You may wish to return to Lesson 13 and review human sexuality.

THE MALE REPRODUCTIVE SYSTEM

The male reproductive system consists of the primary organs (**genitalia**) and the accessory glands (Figure 27-1).

The primary organs are the:

- Penis
- Testes
- Epididymis
- Vas deferens
- Ejaculatory duct

The accessory glands include the:

- Seminal vesicles
- Prostate
- Cowper's glands

Penis

The male **penis** is the organ used for sexual intercourse (also called coitus or copulation). When the special tissues of which the penis is made become filled with blood, the penis becomes enlarged and firm. The outer portion of the glans of the penis is covered by a loose skin fold called the **foreskin**.

The male **urethra** serves two purposes. It carries:

- Reproductive fluid during intercourse
- Urine during voiding

The two activities cannot occur at the same time because they are under the control of different parts of the nervous system.

Testes

The **testes (testicles)** are found in a pouch-like structure called the **scrotum**, which is located outside the body. The testes produce **sperm** throughout life and the male hormone **testosterone**. Testosterone is responsible for the male characteristics.

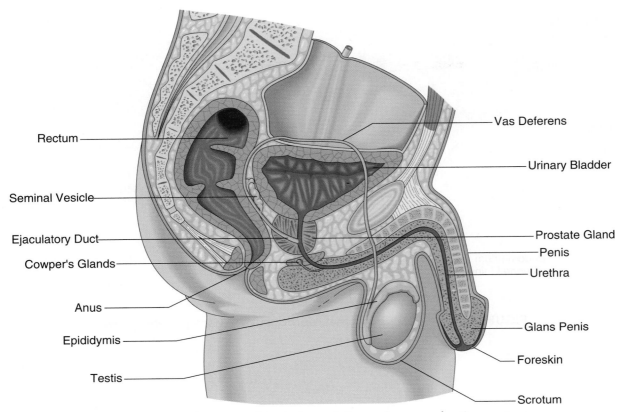

FIGURE 27-1   Cross-sectional view of the male reproductive system

Epididymis

The **epididymis** is a tube 20 feet long coiled on the back of each testis, which stores the sperm. The epididymis is the beginning of a pathway that moves the sperm upward and out of the body. This pathway includes the:

- Epididymis
- Vas deferens
- Ejaculatory duct
- Urethra

Vas Deferens

The **vas deferens** that transports the sperm passes behind the urinary bladder, joining with the ejaculatory duct and entering the urethra.

Ejaculatory Duct

The **ejaculatory duct** carries the fluid produced in the **seminal vesicles**. Fluids are added as the sperm are propelled forward. The sperm and fluid form the seminal fluid or ejaculate. The fluid contains nutrients and other substances needed by the sperm.

Glands that contribute to the seminal fluid are the:

- Seminal vesicles—the ejaculatory duct carries the fluid from the vesicles into the urethra.
- **Prostate** gland—surrounds the neck of the bladder and adds its secretions to the fluid.
- **Cowper's glands**—two small glands located beside the urethra. They produce mucus for lubrication.

Accessory Glands

The seminal fluid or ejaculate is released as the result of a rhythmic series of muscular contractions. These force the fluid through the urethra to the outside. The process is called ejaculation and occurs during sexual intercourse. Ejaculation may also occur spontaneously at other times.

THE FEMALE REPRODUCTIVE SYSTEM

The female reproductive system consists of the internal organs (Figures 27-2A and 27-2B) and the external genitalia (the **vulva**) (Figure 27-3). The internal organs are the:

- Ovaries
- Fallopian (uterine) tubes

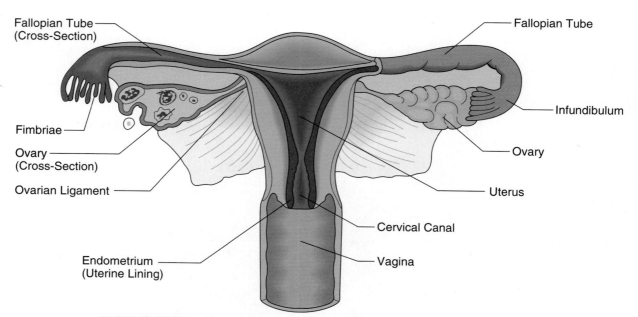

FIGURE 27-2A Female internal reproductive organs (anterior view)

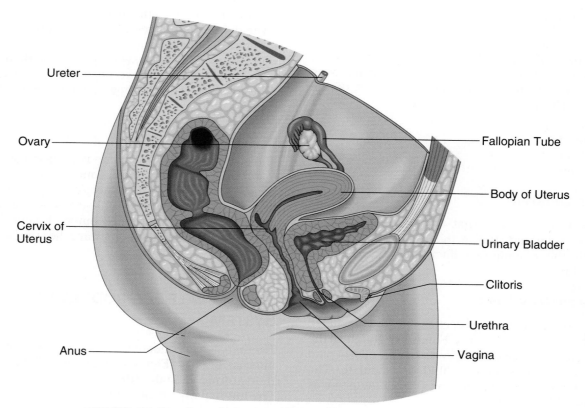

FIGURE 27-2B Female internal reproductive organs (lateral view)

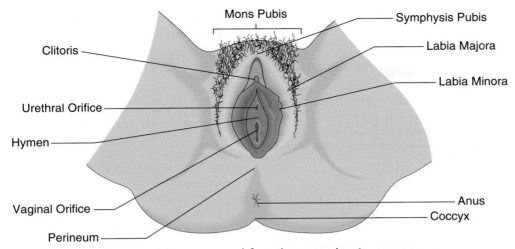

FIGURE 27-3 External female reproductive organs

- Uterus
- Vagina

Vulva

The outside of the vulva is made up of two folds called the **labia majora** (see Figure 27-3). The labia majora:

- Are covered with hair
- Surround the openings of the female urethra and vagina
- Enclose two hairless lips, the **labia minora**

The area between the vagina and anus is called the **perineum**.

Clitoris. The **clitoris** is an organ similar to the male penis. It:

- Is found near the union of the labia
- Is a sensitive structure
- Functions during sexual stimulation to begin the rhythmic series of contractions associated with female climax, or orgasm

Ovaries

The two ovaries, which are the female gonads, produce the egg (**ovum**) and the hormones progesterone and estrogen. **Estrogen** is needed in the development of female characteristics. **Progesterone** is the hormone that maintains pregnancy.

Fallopian Tubes

The fallopian tubes (**uterine tubes** or oviducts) carry the ovum toward the uterus.

Uterus

The **uterus** (or womb) is a hollow muscular organ about 3 inches long. It is lined with a special membrane, the **endometrium**, that:

- Is shed periodically unless pregnancy occurs
- Nourishes the growing fetus (unborn infant in the uterus) during pregnancy

Vagina

The **vagina** is a muscular tube that serves as the output (excretory duct) for the menstrual flow and receives the penis during sexual intercourse.

MENSTRUAL CYCLE

The menstrual cycle (female sexual cycle) begins at **puberty**. Puberty occurs in girls between the ages of 9 and 17. The cycle varies in length, usually between 25 and 30 days. The average is 28 days, which is why it is considered a monthly cycle.

During the menstrual cycle, a mature egg, or ovum (plural, **ova**):

- Is released from one of the ovaries
- Travels from the ovary to one of the fallopian tubes
- May be fertilized by a male sperm

At the same time that the ovum is being matured and expelled from the ovary (**ovulation**), the lining of the uterus (endometrium) is:

- Being built up
- Made ready to receive the fertilized ovum

If fertilization does not occur, the endometrium is:

- No longer needed
- Carried out of the body as the menstrual flow

This process is known as **menstruation**.

It is interesting that, unlike the sperm cells, all the special cells that will become the ova exist at the time a woman is born. When the last ova are released, the menstrual cycle ceases and **menopause** begins.

MENOPAUSE

As women age, the menstrual cycle becomes irregular and gradually ceases altogether. This is called the:

- Menopause
- **Climacteric**
- Change of life

Menopause usually occurs around the age of 55 and involves a natural series of changes that stops the menstrual cycle. These changes are not abrupt, but usually take place over a period of years. Because the ova are no longer being matured and released, pregnancy cannot occur.

Some women may undergo menopause earlier in life after surgical removal of the uterus.

CHANGES IN THE REPRODUCTIVE SYSTEM AS A RESULT OF AGING

Changes occur in both male and female reproductive organs with aging. However, the need for sexual pleasure and sensual satisfaction does not stop.

Changes in the Male Reproductive System

As men age, these changes occur:

- Sexual response is slower.
- Ejaculation is delayed.
- The number of sperm decreases (but number is still adequate for reproduction).
- Testosterone levels gradually decrease.
- The prostate gland may enlarge causing difficult urination.
- The scrotum becomes less firm.
- Seminal fluid thins.
- The size of the testes decreases.
- Note that usually the sex drive (libido) remains unchanged.

Changes in the Female Reproductive System

During and after menopause, these changes occur:

- Estrogen levels decrease.
- Tissue of vulva and vaginal walls thins.
- Lubrication of vagina decreases (because of this, elderly women are more prone to vaginal infections).
- Breast tissues and muscles weaken (sagging of breasts).
- Egg production ceases.
- Ovulation and the menstrual cycle cease.
- Again, the libido remains unchanged.

RELATED CONDITIONS

Malignancy

Malignancies of the male and female reproductive organs are common. Be sure to report any bleeding or discharge from the reproductive tract.

In women, frequent sites for cancer development include the:

- Uterine wall
- Ovaries
- Cervix
- Breasts

In men, malignancies are often found in the:

- Prostate gland
- Testes

Radiation, surgery, and chemotherapy may be used alone or in combination to treat malignancies.

Any condition that affects the reproductive organs threatens the individual's self-concept and sense of sexual identity. In addition to the fear resulting from the diagnosis of a malignancy, the resident also fears that he or she will lose the ability to function fully as a sexual human being.

You must provide emotional support to those who are diagnosed with a malignancy of the reproductive system.

Breast tumors develop in men and women, both old and young. They are most common among mature women.

Breast tumors are often first found during self-examination or through *mammography* (x-ray examination). Most of these masses are benign tumors. The self-examination procedure should be:

- Performed by all adult women
- Carried out each month on the last day of the menstrual flow
- Carried out on one selected day of the month, after menopause
- Carried out using a procedure recommended by the American Cancer Society

Prolapsed Uterus

Prolapsed uterus is a condition that may be experienced by women who have had:

- Repeated pregnancies
- Injuries to the pelvic organs
- Injury to the muscles of the pelvic floor
- Weakening of the supportive pelvic structure due to aging

When prolapsed uterus occurs:

- The uterus drops down from its normal position, causing pressure in the vagina.
- There is a feeling of weight in the pelvic area.
- Urinary incontinence or retention occurs.
- The person is predisposed to urinary infections.

Prolapsed uterus is treated by repositioning the uterus or removing it (**hysterectomy**). Both treatments require surgery in an acute care facility.

Rectocele and Cystocele

Rectoceles and cystoceles are hernias. They usually occur at the same time and are frequently seen in older women.

- A rectocele is a weakening of the wall between the vagina and rectum. This hernia frequently causes constipation and hemorrhoids (varicose veins of the rectum).
- A cystocele is a weakening of the muscles between the bladder and vagina. Cystoceles cause urinary incontinence.

These conditions are corrected by a surgical procedure that tightens the vaginal walls. It is performed in an acute care facility.

Vaginitis

Vaginitis is a fairly common condition in older women because of the decrease in protection resulting from the thinner vaginal wall. This type of infection tends to be chronic and difficult to control.

A fungus infection caused by *Candida albicans* often results in vulvovaginitis. When infection is present:

- There may be a thick, white, cheesy vaginal discharge.

- Inflammation and itching are intense.
- Douches are not given for this condition.
- Special drugs and creams are prescribed to fight the infection.

Senile vaginitis responds to estrogen therapy, vaginal suppositories, and mild douches to wash out the canal. Each treatment requires a physician's order.

Pruritus

Itching (**pruritus**) of the vulva and anus is a common complaint of older women. Continual irritation can cause tissue breakdown and permit bacteria to enter and cause infection. Many factors can contribute to pruritus. A search must be made for the cause and steps taken to correct the condition. For example:

- If soaps are irritating, they should not be used.
- If incontinence allows acid urine to irritate the tissues, regular perineal care can often eliminate the problem.

Benign Prostatic Hypertrophy

Benign prostatic hypertrophy is a common problem for elderly men. It is a nonmalignant enlargement of the prostate gland. Recall that the urethra passes through the center of this gland. Thus, as the gland enlarges it closes off the flow of urine.

Residents with this condition may have difficulty starting and stopping the stream of urine. They may not be able to empty their bladder completely, leading to bladder infections. Observe for the following:

- Frequency of urination
- Nocturia
- Poor urinary control such as dribbling

To release the obstruction, a surgical procedure can be performed by entering through the urethra. This is called a **transurethral prostatectomy** (TURP). Although some surgical procedures on the prostate gland can cause impotence, this is not a complication of the transurethral approach.

SEXUALLY TRANSMITTED DISEASES

Sexually transmitted diseases (STDs) affect both men and women. Although most STDs can be treated and cured, people do not develop immunity to repeated infections. In the elderly, an STD may indicate sexual abuse. The organisms causing STDs can be transmitted from:

- Mucous membrane to mucous membrane such as from genitals to mouth or genitals
- Mucous membrane to skin, such as genitals to hands
- Skin to mucous membrane, such as hands to genitals

Any disease that is transmitted mainly in this way is an STD. There are many STDs. Some are seen more commonly than others. Contact precautions should be used when caring for residents with STDs.

A complete discussion of STDs is presented here for your protection because these diseases pose a risk for health care workers as well as the people being cared for.

The most common STDs are gonorrhea, herpes simplex II, and syphilis. Other STDs are caused by chlamydia, human papilloma virus, human immuno deficiency virus, and the *Trichomonas* parasite.

It is important to realize that people may:

- Not always be aware that they have been infected
- Be too embarrassed to talk about the problem
- Not realize the serious damage these infectious diseases can do to the body

Sexually transmitted diseases are as easily transmitted between older persons as between younger.

Trichomonas Vaginitis

Trichomonas vaginitis is caused by a parasite, *Trichomonas vaginalis*. This condition:

- Is sexually transmitted
- May affect the male reproductive tract with no signs and symptoms
- In women, causes a large amount of white, foul-smelling vaginal discharge called leukorrhea
- Can be controlled with medication
- Requires that both sex partners receive treatment

Gonorrhea

Gonorrhea is a serious STD caused by the bacterium *Neisseria gonorrheae*. The disease causes an acute inflammation.

- In men:
  - Greenish yellow discharge appears from the penis within 2 to 5 days after contact.

- There is a burning on urination.
- The disease can spread throughout the reproductive tract, causing sterility (inability to reproduce).
- In women:
  - Eighty percent of women infected may have no signs or symptoms until after the disease spreads.
  - Pelvic inflammatory disease can lead to formation of abscesses and sterility.
  - The disease can be spread before a woman is aware of being infected.
  - All sex partners must be treated with antibiotics.
  - When a pregnant woman has gonorrhea, her baby's eyes may be permanently damaged if they are contaminated by the disease during birth. As a preventive measure, all babies' eyes are routinely treated with silver nitrate drops or antibiotics shortly after birth.

Syphilis

Syphilis is caused by the microorganism *Treponema pallidum*. Both sexes show the same effects of the disease. It is treated with antibiotics. If untreated, the disease may pass through three stages.

1. First stage—a sore (chancre) develops within 90 days of exposure. The chancre heals without treatment. Because it is not painful, it may go entirely unnoticed.
2. Second stage—a rash, sore throat, or other mild symptoms suggestive of a viral infection may occur. Again, the signs and symptoms disappear without treatment. The disease is infectious during the first and second stages and may be transmitted to a sexual partner. By this time, the microorganisms have entered vital organs such as the heart, liver, brain, and spinal cord.
3. Third stage—the stage in which permanent damage is done to vital organs. It may not appear for many years or at all.

If an infected woman is pregnant the microorganisms can attack the fetus, causing it to die or be seriously deformed.

Herpes

Herpes simplex II (genital herpes) is an infectious disease caused by the herpes simplex virus. It is transmitted primarily through direct sexual contact. The person who has herpes:

- May develop red, blister-like sores on the reproductive organs
- Has sores that are associated with a burning sensation
- Usually has sores that heal in about 2 weeks
- Must remember that the fluid in the blisters is infectious
- May shed organisms even when an outbreak is not present

People infected with herpes may have only one episode or repeated attacks. In many cases, repeated attacks are milder. Other consequences of a herpes infection include:

- A greater incidence of cancer of the cervix and miscarriages in infected women compared to women who are not infected.
- Newborn children can be infected during the birth process.
- The mother with an active case of herpes simplex II usually delivers by cesarean section.

Treatment with the drug acyclovir reduces the discomfort and degree of communicability. There is no cure at the present time.

Venereal Warts

Venereal warts are caused by a virus. Characteristics of the infection include:

- Lesions on the genitals on both skin and mucous membranes
- Cauliflower-shaped, raised, and darkened warts
- Warts may be removed by ointments or surgery but often recur.
- Venereal warts may cause discomfort during intercourse and may cause bleeding when dislodged.
- They predispose to development of cancerous changes.
- The infection rate for venereal warts is the most rapidly growing for all STDs.

Chlamydia Infection

Chlamydia are small infectious organisms that invade mucous membranes of the body. These organisms are:

- Introduced into the eyes infecting the conjunctiva. This causes inflammation (conjunctivitis) and a more serious condition called trachoma. Trachoma can lead to blindness.
- Sexually transmitted and commonly cause infections of the reproductive tract
- The cause of pelvic inflammatory disease with scarring and systemic infections. The scarring can result in sterility.
- Responsible for signs and symptoms similar to those of gonorrhea, except that the discharge is usually yellow to whitish in color
- Treated with antibiotics

People with pelvic infections are usually checked for gonorrhea. If they test negative for gonorrhea, they are frequently diagnosed with nonspecified urethritis because many different organisms may cause the infection. However, chlamydia organisms are the most common cause.

Personal Precautions

An individual can practice certain actions to lessen the risk of contracting STDs. These include:

- Abstaining from sex
- Knowing your sexual partner well before engaging in sexual activity
- Limiting the number of sexual partners
- Using a latex condom throughout sexual contact
- Washing well following sexual intercourse
- Using approved germicides that can be applied to the vagina, penis, and condom
- Providing to your partner and being provided with a negative test result covering the 3-month period before sexual activity

LESSON SYNTHESIS: Putting It All Together

*Y*ou have just completed this lesson. Now go back and review the *Clinical Focus. Try to see how the Clinical Focus relates to the concepts presented in the lesson. Then answer the following questions.*

1. What change occurs in the lubrication of the vagina in the aging woman?

2. What increased risk does this change pose for Mrs. Shutt?

3. Do Mrs. Shutt's periods of incontinence contribute to her pruritus?

4. What special care can you give to make Mrs. Shutt more comfortable?

5. If Mrs. Shutt does not tell you of her discomfort, how may you be alerted to her problem?

6. Which of Mrs. Shutt's diagnoses might contribute to her incontinence?

REVIEW

A. Match each term (items a.–e.) with the proper definition.

a. chlamydia   d. pruritus
b. climacteric   e. vaginitis
c. hysterectomy

1. _____ itching

2. _____ small infectious organisms

3. _____ menopause

4. _____ inflammation of the vagina

5. _____ removal of the uterus

B. Select the one best answer for each of the following.

6. The male organ used for intercourse is the
(A) vas deferens
(B) testis
(C) penis
(D) prostate

7. The male gland that may become enlarged and obstruct the flow of urine is the
(A) prostate
(B) seminal vesicles

(C) Cowper's glands
(D) penis

8. The female gonads are the
(A) uterus
(B) ovaries
(C) vagina
(D) perineum

9. As men age,
(A) ejaculation is more rapid
(B) sperm count increases
(C) testosterone levels decrease
(D) sexual response is more rapid

10. One characteristic of female menopause is
(A) loss of egg production
(B) reduced libido
(C) regular menstrual periods
(D) thickening of vaginal walls

C. Fill in the blanks by selecting the correct word or phrase from the list.

abuse   testes
cystocele   vulva
genitalia

11. The primary sexual organs are known as the _____.

12. An STD in the elderly may be a sign of sexual _____.

13. The female external genitalia is called the _____.

14. The male glands that produce the sperm are called the _____.

15. A weakening of the wall between the vagina and bladder is called a _____.

D. Brief Answers

16. List three functions of both the male and female reproductive systems.

17. List three changes resulting from aging for the male reproductive system and three changes for the female reproductive system.

18. List five common STDs.

19. List four precautions to take to avoid getting an STD when caring for residents with an STD.

E. Clinical Experience

20. Mr. Fazzio is acting very withdrawn this morning. When Starr, the nursing assistant, reports to her supervisor she learns that the physician has told Mr. Fazzio that he has a "lump" in his prostate gland that must be treated.
    a. Could this knowledge explain Mr. Fazzio's behavior?
    b. What fears may Mr. Fazzio be feeling?
    c. How can you help Mr. Fazzio at this time?

21. Mrs. Wells was admitted to your facility this morning. She has a diagnosis of mild confusion, malnutrition, congestive heart failure, and pelvic inflammatory disease. A culture was ordered to determine the cause of her infection. What type of precautions should be used with this resident?

Caring for Residents with Musculoskeletal System Disorders

Clinical Focus

Think of the special challenges in providing nursing assistant care to a resident with disorders of the musculoskeletal system as you study this lesson and meet:

*E*ssie Branch, who suffers from osteo-arthritis and osteoporosis. These conditions affect both her ability to provide self-care and to enjoy full mobility. Her osteoporosis has caused compression fractures of her spine so she is no longer able to hold her head erect easily.

OBJECTIVES

After studying this lesson, you should be able to:

- Define and spell vocabulary words and terms.
- List the functions of the voluntary muscles.
- List the functions of the bones.
- Describe the changes of aging that affect the musculoskeletal system.
- Identify the symptoms related to common musculoskeletal system disorders.
- Describe the appropriate nursing care for residents with musculoskeletal disorders.

VOCABULARY

amputation   (*am*-pyou-***TAY***-shun)

arthritis   (are-***THRY***-tis)

atrophy   (***AT***-roh-fee)

bursae   (***BUR***-see)

VOCABULARY

bursitis   (bur-**SIGH**-tis)

cartilage   (**KAR**-tih-lij)

cast   (kast)

contracture   (kuhn-**TRAK**-tyoor)

external fixation   (eks-**TER**-nal fix-**AY**-shun)

fracture   (**FRACK**-shur)

joint   (joynt)

kyphosis   (kigh-**FOH**-sis)

ligament   (**LIG**-ah-ment)

open reduction/internal fixation (ORIF)—
    (**OH**-pen ree-**DUCK**-shun/in-**TER**-nal fiks-**AY**-shun)

osteoarthritis   (**os**-tee-oh-are-**THRY**-tis)

osteoporosis   (**os**-tee-oh-poor-**OH**-sis)

phantom pain   (**FAN**-tom payn)

podiatrist   (poh-**DYE**-ah-trist)

prosthesis   (pros-**THEE**-sis)

rheumatoid arthritis   (**REW**-mah-toyd are-**THRY**-tis)

tendon   (**TEN**-don)

traction   (**TRACK**-shun)

THE MUSCULOSKELETAL SYSTEM

The musculoskeletal system is composed of:

• Bones
• Skeletal muscles
• Joints
• Tendons
• Ligaments
• Bursae

The bones form a framework for the body that is called a *skeleton*. The muscles are formed of tissue that has the ability to contract and relax and allow movement. The muscles lie over the bones. Together, the bones and muscles have many functions, including:

• Giving shape and form to the body
• Protecting and supporting vital body organs such as the brain and heart
• Permitting movement
• Producing some of the red blood cells
• Storing calcium and phosphorus

Bones

The human body has 206 bones (Figure 28-1). All of the bones are not alike. Some are:

• Longer bones—bones of the arms and legs
• Short bones—bones of the fingers and toes
• Irregular bones—bones that form the spinal column
• Flat bones—pelvic bones and shoulder blades

Each bone has a name. Many other body structures take their names from that of the nearby bone. For example, the radius is a bone in the forearm. Close by are the:

• Radial nerve
• Radial artery
• Radial vein

Learning the names of the bones is not difficult. Draw a line down the center of the skeleton in Figure 28-1, dividing it in half. Note that the bones on one side of the line are matched by bones in the other side.

Muscles

The body contains more than 500 muscles (Figure 28-2). They work in groups to bring about body movement. There are three types of muscles:

• Cardiac muscle—found only in the heart wall
• Skeletal muscles—also called voluntary muscles because you can control their actions of contraction and relaxation
• Visceral or smooth muscles—also called involuntary muscles because we do not usually control them consciously

Involuntary muscles make up the walls of organs like the stomach and guard body openings like those of the digestive and urinary tracts. A special part of the brain controls involuntary muscles automatically.

Muscles are named by location, shape, or action. The quadriceps femoris, for example, is located near the femur (thigh bone). Muscles have three parts:

• Origin, or beginning
• Body, or middle part
• Insertion, or ending

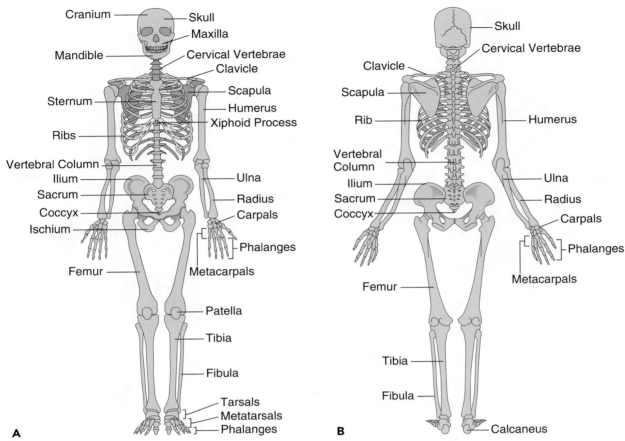

FIGURE 28-1   The human skeleton: A. anterior view, B. posterior view

The origin and body of a muscle are found on one side of a joint and the insertion is attached to the other side. Skeletal muscles are attached to the bones by tough, fibrous bands called **tendons**.

When the muscle shortens (contracts), it pulls the point of insertion toward the point of origin, changing the position of the bone (Figure 28-3).

This relationship between muscles and bones permits movements such as walking, sitting, or holding a pencil.

Muscles that are not used will **atrophy**. This means they become weaker and smaller. Lack of joint movement may cause a **contracture** to form. The muscle shortens, causing the joint to become fixed, making further movement difficult or impossible.

Joints

Two bones meet or come together (articulate) at a **joint**. The elbows, knees, and hips are joints. **Ligaments** are fibrous bands that help support the points of articulation.

The ends of movable bones are covered with a protective substance called **cartilage**. The bones of the skull are not movable. The joints of the skull bones are called suture lines.

Joint movements depend on the way in which the joint is formed. Elbows and knees, for example, are hinge joints. The hip and shoulder are ball joints (Figure 28-4).

Joints are enclosed in a capsule lined with synovial membrane. The membrane secretes small amounts of fluid called synovial fluid (Figure 28-5). Small sacs of synovial fluid called **bursae** are located around joints and help reduce friction during joint movement.

CHANGES IN THE MUSCULOSKELETAL SYSTEM CAUSED BY AGING

The aging process causes several changes in the musculoskeletal system:

- The bones become more brittle because of calcium loss.

FIGURE 28-2 Principal skeletal muscles of the body: A. anterior view, B. posterior view

- The joints become less flexible. The range through which the joints can be moved (range of motion) decreases.
- Muscles may become smaller because of less regular exercise. This may limit the person's strength and endurance.

- The body tends to become more flexed. It is important to avoid flexion, if possible, when positioning residents. This increases the flexion that is naturally occurring. Flexion makes movement more difficult.

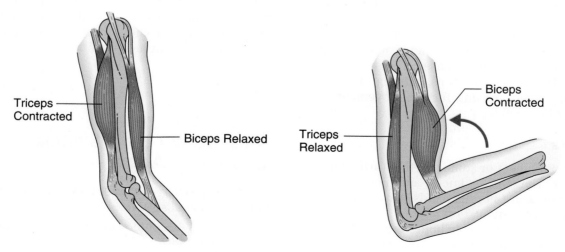

FIGURE 28-3 Coordination of muscles

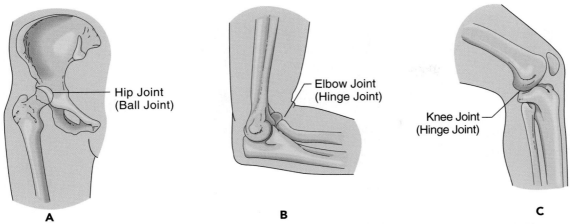

FIGURE 28-4   Types of joints: A. Ball joint. B and C. Hinge joints

Because of these changes, older adults are at risk for falling. Maintain a safe environment to prevent falls. Closely monitor residents who have a history of falling. When an older person falls, the bones may easily fracture because they are more brittle.

CONDITIONS AFFECTING THE MUSCULOSKELETAL SYSTEM

Residents with diseases or problems of the musculoskeletal system receive special care that is known as orthopedic care.

Sometimes a bursa becomes inflamed. This is called **bursitis**. The bursa is painful and movement may be reduced. Bursitis may be due to infection or excessive pressure or movement placed on the area.

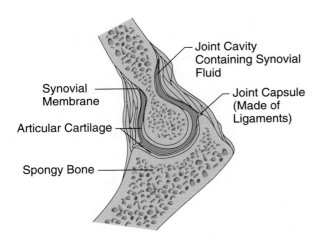

FIGURE 28-5   Parts of a joint

Osteoporosis

Osteoporosis may develop because of a lack of mobility or as a result of aging. It affects primarily women due to lack of the hormone estrogen following menopause. As osteoporosis develops, the bones lose calcium and become brittle.

The vertebrae in the spine of a person with osteoporosis may collapse without warning, resulting in a curvature of the spine called **kyphosis** (hunched back).

Fractures are common in people with osteoporosis because the bones lack strength. It is important to carry out all safety measures to prevent falls. Care must be used when moving and lifting the residents. Unsafe handling can damage the resident's joints and bones.

Fractures

A **fracture** is a break or loss of continuity in a bone (Figure 28-6). The break may be completely through the bone *(complete fracture)* or only partially through the bone *(incomplete fracture)*. All fractures are either closed or open:

- Closed fracture
  - The bones do not protrude through the skin and are in good alignment after the fracture.

Clinical Focus:
Review safety measures for Mrs. Branch that are most important for preventing fractures.

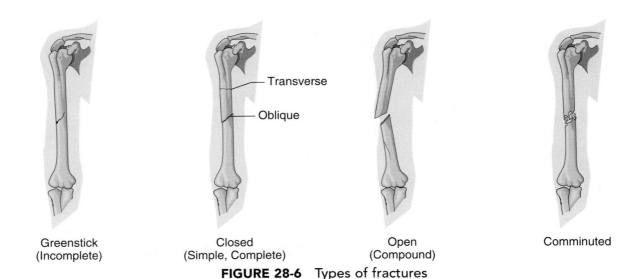

Greenstick (Incomplete)   Closed (Simple, Complete)   Transverse   Oblique   Open (Compound)   Comminuted

FIGURE 28-6 Types of fractures

- Open fracture
    - Fragments of broken bone protrude through the skin.

Fractures are also identified according to the type of break in the bone:

- Comminuted fracture
    - The bone is broken into many pieces.
- Compression fracture
    - The internal spongy part of the bone is crushed but the hard outer covering of the bone is not broken. This type of fracture occurs most often in the vertebrae.
- Spiral fracture
    - The bone is broken in a twisted manner.

To promote the healing of fractures, the bone must be:

- In correct alignment
- Kept immobile

Treatment of Fractures with a Cast. A cast or splint to support the area may be all that is needed to treat a closed fracture of the arm or lower leg. A **cast** is made by applying a wet substance to the extremity, in layers. The substance is molded and shaped as it is applied so it will fit the extremity. If a resident in the facility breaks a bone, the resident may be taken to a hospital to have a cast applied. The resident may then return to the facility. After a cast is applied, follow these special precautions:

- Allow the wet cast to air dry.
- Do not put pressure on the wet cast. Any pressure can leave permanent indentations that can press against the resident's skin, causing it to break down. Use the palms of your hands, not your fingers, to move the casted extremity.

- Keep the casted extremity elevated and uncovered until it is dry.
- Check the skin area around the cast frequently for signs of circulatory impairment: blue color (cyanosis), cold to touch, swelling (edema), odor, drainage, and complaints of pain or tingling in the area. Report any of these signs immediately.
- Closely observe skin areas around the cast edges for signs of irritation.
- After an arm cast dries, a sling may be needed for support. Residents with a leg cast may need a wheelchair for support.

Treatment of Fractures with Traction. **Traction** is used to treat some fractures. This means the broken ends of the bone are pulled into normal alignment. In *skin traction* a belt or strap is applied to the body and weights are attached to the ropes (Figure 28-7). *Skeletal traction* involves the insertion of a metal pin into the bone. Weights are then attached by ropes to the pin (Figure 28-8). Traction may be used until the bone heals or it may be used only until surgery is performed or a cast is applied. When caring for a resident in traction:

- Review the placement of pulleys, ropes, and weights with the nurse so you know the purpose and correct placement of each.
- Do not disturb the weights or permit them to swing, drop, or rest on any surface.
- Keep the resident in good alignment and ensure that the body is acting properly as countertraction.
- Check under belts or straps for areas of pressure or irritation.
- Make sure that straps and belts are smooth, straight, and properly secured.

Water
Weight Bag

FIGURE 28-7 Buck's traction is an example of skin traction sometimes used for a fractured hip.

Treatment of Fractures with External Fixation.

External fixation devices are sometimes used to manage fractures of the tibia (large bone in lower leg) (Figure 28-9). These devices are inserted into the bone to maintain alignment. The external part allows the orthopedic surgeon to adjust the device as necessary to promote healing.

Fractured Hip

The most common fracture seen in residents of long-term care facilities is a fractured hip. This term refers to any break involving the upper third of the femur (upper leg bone) (Figure 28-10). A fractured hip may occur spontaneously as a result of osteoporosis. The resident is walking and, without warning, the bone breaks, causing

FIGURE 28-8 Skeletal traction immobilizes a body part by attaching weights directly to the resident's bones with pins, screws, wires, or tongs.

the resident to fall. In other cases, the resident falls, causing the bone to break. Signs and symptoms of a fractured hip include:

- Pain in the hip sometimes radiating to the knee
- Feeling of pressure on the hip
- Shortening and turning outward of the leg on the injured side
- Bruising and swelling of the hip, groin, and thigh
- The resident may have heard a "snap" just before or after the fall.

If you suspect a fractured hip, *NEVER* attempt to move the resident without instructions from the nurse. The resident will be taken by ambulance to the hospital for x-rays of the affected joint and bones. If a fracture has occurred, the resident will be admitted to the hospital for repair of the fracture.

Open Reduction/Internal Fixation. Fractured hips are usually repaired by **open reduction/internal fixation (ORIF)**. This method may also be used for fractures of other large bones. The resident is given a general anesthetic and is asleep during surgery. An incision is made, the surgeon aligns the broken ends of the bone, and a nail, pin, or screw is inserted to maintain alignment. The device is usually permanent. The resident will stay in the hospital for several days and then convalesce in the long-term care facility.

Caring for Residents with ORIF. Residents who have had an ORIF usually have physical therapy for several weeks after. The physical

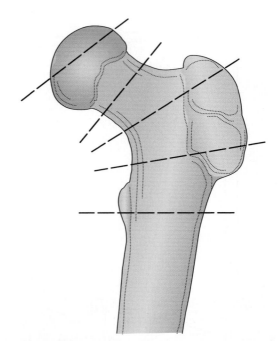

FIGURE 28-10 The lines indicate where fractures usually occur in the femur.

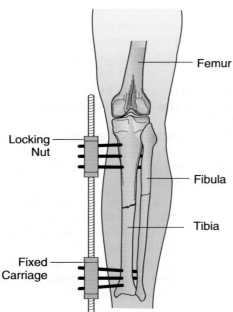

FIGURE 28-9 External fixation devices are sometimes used for fractures of the tibia.

therapist starts a program of progressive mobilization and teaches the resident to:

- Move independently in bed
- Transfer from bed to chair without bearing weight on the involved leg
- Stand and hold onto a bar while doing active range of motion exercises with the involved leg without weight bearing (Figure 28-11).
- Start weight bearing by standing and balancing, then walking through the parallel bars
- Walk with cane or walker

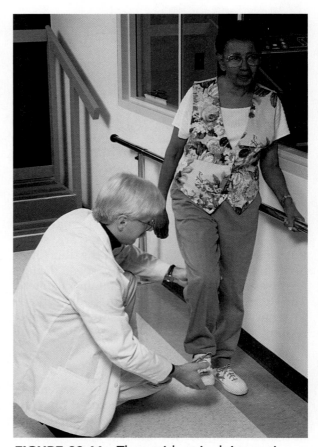

FIGURE 28-11 The resident is doing active range of motion exercises without weight bearing on the affected side.

FIGURE 28-12 Orthopedic problems in older adults

Condition	Disease Process	Treatment	Special Care
Osteoarthritis	Breakdown (degeneration) of joints. Weight-bearing joints such as ankles, knees, and hips are most commonly involved. Movement is painful and condition is progressive.	Medication to relieve pain; physiotherapy to maintain mobility; light massage and heat; ambulatory aids to reduce pressure in joints; weight reduction; surgery in selected cases.	Give positive, emotional support; carry out heat treatments, massage, and ROM exercises, as ordered.
Osteoporosis	Defective bone formation and maintenance. Bones become brittle and are easily broken. Complications: fractures, kidney stones, and loss of height and posture. More common in females than males.	Keep resident as active as possible; diet adequate in protein and vitamins C and D, and calcium; maintain adequate fluid intake; hormone therapy.	Encourage food and fluid intake. Assist in exercise. Report pain; apply support as needed. Emotional support must not be overlooked.
Rheumatoid Arthritis	Inflammation of joint lining (synovium). Joint changes cause painful muscle spasms, flexion, and deformities. Signs and symptoms may temporarily disappear (remission). Flareups may be related to emotional stress.	Drugs to reduce pain and inflammation; heat treatments for comfort; exercise when inflammation subsides; surgery in selected cases.	Provide emotional support. Provide self-help devices such as long shoe horns and grab bars. Carry out heat treatments and ROM exercises, as ordered.

When you care for a resident with ORIF, you must:

- Know whether there are any restrictions for positioning the resident in bed
- Know whether the resident is allowed to bear weight on the affected leg
- Know how to transfer the resident if the resident is non-weight bearing or partial weight bearing
- Know whether you should do passive range of motion exercises on the affected leg
- Encourage the resident to do activities of daily living as independently as possible
- Encourage involvement in activities away from the nursing unit
- Report:
  - Complaints of pain
  - Changes in vital signs
  - Signs of bleeding, inflammation (redness, heat, swelling), or drainage from the incision
- Signs of disorientation or confusion (common after hip surgery and usually temporary)

Arthritis

Arthritis is a common problem in the elderly. The conditions and care are described in Figure 28-12. Many forms of arthritis exist, but the two most common forms are:

- Osteoarthritis
- Rheumatoid arthritis

Osteoarthritis is due to the "wear and tear" of the joints. The cartilage at the ends of the bones wears away with movement. It begins during middle age and can be very painful. This form of arthritis does not usually cause severe disability. However, for some individuals, it can limit their mobility. The joints, especially hip joints, may require replacement with an artificial joint (**prosthesis**) (Figure 28-13).

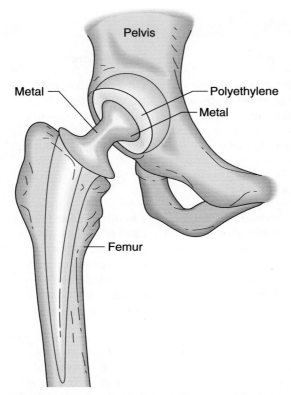

FIGURE 28-13 A damaged hip joint can be replaced with an artificial joint (prosthesis).

Caring for Residents with a Hip Prosthesis. The physician usually places the resident on hip precautions for a minimum of 6 weeks after surgery. These precautions may include:

- Turn to back and unaffected hip only.
- Keep affected leg in neutral position when in bed and during activities.
- Place abductor splint (Figure 28-14) or at least two pillows between the legs when turning. Keep hips abducted when in wheelchair.
- Use an elevated toilet seat to avoid hip flexion when rising.
- Report any signs or symptoms of:
  - Swelling of affected leg
  - Redness or discoloration of hip

Clinical Focus:
Think of how the osteoarthritis affects Ms. Branch's ability to carry out ADL. How can you help her without increasing her dependency?

FIGURE 28-14 Residents often use the abduction pillow upon their return to the facility following hip surgery. The pillow prevents the resident from crossing the ankles, and holds the hip in proper alignment, preventing contractures.

- Pain at the hip, groin, or thigh
- Drainage or bleeding from incision
- Chest pain (a blood clot in the lungs is sometimes a complication of hip surgery)
- Do not allow the resident to:
  - Adduct the legs (cross affected leg over midline) (Figure 28-15)
  - Flex legs past 90°
  - Flex hip when in side-lying position
  - Bend forward at hip during transfers or other activities or when sitting up in bed (Figure 28-16)
  - Sit for long periods of time
  - Internally rotate affected leg (Figure 28-17)

Rheumatoid arthritis can begin at any age and sometimes occurs in children. This disease can be mild or progressive until it destroys the

FIGURE 28-15 The resident with a new hip prosthesis should never cross the affected leg over the midline of the body.

FIGURE 28-17   The resident with a new hip prosthesis should never internally rotate the hip on the affected side.

Lower Extremity Amputation

You may care for residents who have had one or both feet or legs surgically removed (amputated). When an elderly person has an **amputation**, it is usually because of circulatory

FIGURE 28-16   The resident with a new hip prosthesis should never flex the affected hip more than 90°.

joints. In either case, severe pain is a symptom. Hand deformities from rheumatoid arthritis are shown in Figure 28-18.

The most important aspect of care for residents with arthritis is to balance activity with rest. Too much activity at one time may increase the pain. Too much rest results in stiffness and can lead to contractures. When you touch the resident's body, remember to be gentle.

FIGURE 28-18   Joint deformities as a result of rheumatoid arthritis

problems. These problems may be due to changes in the blood vessels or because of diabetes. Gangrene may develop (the tissues die) and amputation is needed.

It is common for people to experience **phantom pain** after the removal of a limb. Residents may feel pain or tingling where the limb used to be. These feelings may persist for months. The pain is real, although it is difficult to explain.

After an amputation, some people are fitted with a prosthesis (an artificial limb). They have to learn how to walk and sit when the prosthesis is worn. If you are responsible for helping a resident put on a prosthesis, be sure you know how to attach and secure it.

Residents who have had amputations need to be positioned correctly. This is explained in Lesson 22.

Foot Problems

As people age, foot and toenail problems develop. If these problems are not corrected, they may affect the person's ability to walk. Many people require the services of a **podiatrist** for treatment of the feet and toenails. Nursing assistants provide foot care as follows:

1. Clean the resident's feet thoroughly during the bathing procedure.
   - Wash, rinse, and dry carefully between each toe.
   - Clean the toenails.
2. Observe the feet for:
   - Bluish color
   - Swelling
   - Breaks in the skin
3. Report any changes to the nurse.
4. Protect the resident's feet.
   - Be sure the resident wears properly fitting shoes and socks when up.
   - Avoid bumping or hitting the resident's feet as you do positioning and range of motion procedures.
   - Loosen the covers over the resident's feet.
5. Do not allow the resident's feet to dangle. If the feet do not touch the floor when sitting in a chair, provide a footstool.
6. Know your facility's policy for cutting toenails.

LESSON SYNTHESIS: Putting It All Together

*Y*ou have just completed this lesson. Now go back and review the Clinical Focus. Try to see how the Clinical Focus relates to the concepts presented in this lesson. Then answer the following questions.

1. What factors contribute to Essie Branch's flexed posture?

2. Why are women more prone to osteoporosis in later years compared to men?

3. Because the bones of this resident have less strength, what special precautions must be included in her care?

REVIEW

A. **Select the one best answer for each of the following.**

1. The musculoskeletal system performs all of the following, except
   (A) gives shape and form to the body
   (B) produces hormones
   (C) produces red blood cells
   (D) permits movement

2. Skeletal muscles are attached to the bones by
   (A) ligaments
   (B) tendons
   (C) cartilage
   (D) bursae

3. Small sacs of synovial fluid are located around joints. They sometimes become inflamed, causing
   (A) bursitis
   (B) arthritis
   (C) tendinitis
   (D) osteoporosis

4. When a resident develops osteoporosis all of the following occur, except
   (A) the bones become brittle and porous
   (B) the bones fracture easily
   (C) kyphosis may develop
   (D) the bones become stronger

5. When a resident has a new cast, signs and symptoms indicating circulatory impairment include all of the following, except
   (A) pink toes
   (B) cold to touch
   (C) complaints of pain and tingling
   (D) swelling

6. Skin traction involves
   (A) application of a belt or strap to the body and attachment of weights
   (B) insertion of a metal pin into the bones and attachment of weights
   (C) application of a splint
   (D) application of an external fixation device

7. When a resident has had an ORIF, you must know
   (A) whether the resident can bear weight
   (B) what type of device was installed
   (C) how long the surgery took
   (D) how the fracture occurred

8. When a resident has had a hip prosthesis inserted, you must discourage the resident from
   (A) doing activities of daily living independently
   (B) being out of bed
   (C) adducting the legs
   (D) participating in activities

9. A resident with rheumatoid arthritis may have all of the following, except
   (A) no joint deformity
   (B) inflammation of the joint lining
   (C) painful muscle spasms and flexion
   (D) temporary remissions

10. Osteoarthritis is
    (A) due to wear and tear of the joints
    (B) common in children
    (C) a cause of severe disability
    (D) not painful

11. With any type of arthritis, the most important aspect of care is to
    (A) encourage the resident to remain in bed as much as possible
    (B) encourage the resident to exercise as much as possible
    (C) balance rest and activity
    (D) perform all activities of daily living for the resident

12. Amputation of a lower extremity may cause phantom pain. Phantom pain is
    (A) due to the resident's imagination
    (B) due to the resident's need for attention
    (C) a type of surgical pain
    (D) real and may persist for months

B. Answer each statement true (T) or false (F).

13. T   F   As one ages, the joints become more flexible.

14. T   F   Movements in a joint depend on the way in which the joint is formed.

15. T   F   When a person has osteoporosis, the vertebrae may collapse without warning.

16. T   F   Gangrene can be treated successfully with medication.

Caring for Residents with Nervous System Disorders

Clinical Focus

Think of the special challenge presented in providing nursing assistant care to a resident with neurologic disorders as you study this lesson and meet:

*T*homas Raye, who suffers from Parkinson's disease. This is a neurologic disorder that affects his ability to control and coordinate his voluntary movements. Although able to move, Mr. Raye cannot stop and start activities smoothly. He walks with small, shuffling steps and stands with a characteristic bent frame.

OBJECTIVES

After studying this lesson, you should be able to:

- Define and spell vocabulary words and terms.
- List the functions of the nervous system.
- List the structures of the nervous system.
- Recognize the changes of aging that affect the nervous system.
- Describe the sensory deficits caused by disease.
- Identify the symptoms related to common nervous system disorders.
- Describe the nursing care for residents with nervous system disorders.
- Demonstrate the following:
  Procedure 106 Care of Eyeglasses
  Procedure 107 Applying and Removing In-the-Ear or Behind-the-Ear Hearing Aids

VOCABULARY

age-related macular degeneration (*ayj-ree-**LAY**-ted **MAH**-kyou-lar **dee**-jen-er-**AY**-shun*)

aneurysm (***AN**-you-rizm*)

aphasia (*ah-**FAY**-zee-ah*)

atherosclerosis (*ath-er-oh-skleh-**ROH**-sis*)

auditory nerve (***awe**-dih-**TOH**-ree nurv*)

brain stem (*brayn stem*)

cataract (***KAT**-ah-ract*)

central nervous system (***SEN**-tral **NUR**-vus **SIS**-tem*)

cerebellum (*ser-eh-**BELL**-um*)

cerebrospinal fluid (*ser-eh-broh-**SPY**-nal **FLEW**-id*)

cerebrovascular accident (CVA) (***ser**-eh-broh-**VASS**-kyou-lar **ACK**-sih-dent*)

cerebrum (***SER**-eh-brum*)

choroid (***KOH**-royd*)

conjunctiva (***kon**-junk-**TIGH**-vah*)

cornea (***KOR**-nee-ah*)

dementia (*dee-**MEN**-she-ah*)

diabetic retinopathy (***die**-ah-**BET**-ick **ret**-ih-**NOP**-ah-thee*)

embolus (***EM**-boh-lus*)

emotional lability (*ee-**MOH**-shun-al lah-**BILL**-ih-tee*)

equilibrium (***ee**-kwih-**LIB**-ree-um*)

genetic disease (*jeh-**NET**-ick dih-**ZEEZ***)

glaucoma (*glaw-**KOH**-mah*)

hemianopsia (***hem**-ee-an-**OP**-see-ah*)

hemiplegia (***hem**-ee-**PLEE**-jee-ah*)

Huntington's disease (***HUNT**-ing-tonz dih-**ZEEZ***)

intention tremor (*in-**TEN**-shun **TREM**-or*)

iris (***EYE**-riss*)

lens (*lenz*)

Lhermitte's sign (***LAIR**-mits sign*)

magnetic resonance imaging (MRI) (*mag-**NET**-ick **REZ**-oh-nans **IM**-aj-ing*)

meninges (*meh-**NIN**-jeez*)

motor nerve (***MOH**-tor nerv*)

multiple sclerosis (MS) (***MULL**-tih-pul skle-**ROH**-sis*)

myasthenia gravis (MG) (***my**-as-**THEE**-nee-ah **GRAH**-vis*)

nerve impulses (*nurv **IM**-pul-ses*)

nerves (*nurvs*)

neurons (***NEW**-ronz*)

neurotransmitter (***new**-roh-**TRANS**-mit-er*)

nystagmus (*nis-**TAG**-mus*)

ophthalmologist (***of**-thal-**MOL**-oh-jist*)

optic nerve (***OP**-tick nurv*)

paralysis (*pah-**RAL**-ih-sis*)

paraplegia (***pair**-ah-**PLEE**-jee-ah*)

Parkinson's disease (***PARK**-in-sons dih-**ZEEZ***)

peripheral nervous system (*peh-**RIF**-er-al **NUR**-vus **SIS**-tem*)

position sense (*poh-**ZISH**-un sens*)

presbycusis (***pres**-beh-**KYOU**-sis*)

presbyopia (***pres**-bee-**OH**-pee-ah*)

pupil (***PYOU**-pil*)

quadriplegia (***kwahd**-rih-**PLEE**-jee-ah*)

reflex (***REE**-flex*)

retina (***RET**-ih-nah*)

sclera (***SKLEH**-rah*)

sensory nerve (***SEN**-sor-ee nurv*)

spatial-perceptual deficit (***SPAY**-shul-per-**SEP**-tyou-al **DEF**-ih-sit*)

stroke (*strohk*)

thrombus (***THROM**-bus*)

transient ischemic attack (TIA) (***TRAN**-see-ent is-**KEE**-mick ah-**TACK***)

unilateral neglect (***you**-nih-**LAT**-er-al neh-**GLECT***)

vertigo (***VER**-tih-goh*)

COMPONENTS OF THE NERVOUS SYSTEM

The nervous system controls body functions by sending electrical messages called **nerve impulses** throughout the body. The two parts of the nervous system are the:

- **Peripheral nervous system (PNS)**—the nerves outside the brain and spinal cord
- **Central nervous system (CNS)**—the brain and spinal cord

Special sense organs and receptors receive information from the environment. The information travels along the cranial or spinal nerves to reach the brain and spinal cord, where the sensation is interpreted. Information is received by the:

- Eyes
- Ears
- Taste buds
- Receptors in the nose for smell
- Nerve endings (receptors) in the skin, muscles, joints, and tendons
- Receptors in body organs

The nerve endings in the skin pick up sensations of pain, pressure, and variations in temperature. Receptors in muscles, tendons, and joints carry information about the degree of muscle contraction and position of body parts. Receptors in the walls of body organs carry information related to hunger, thirst, and visceral (organ) pain.

Neurons

Neurons are special cells that carry messages (Figure 29-1). The neurons and other cells make up the nervous tissue of the brain, spinal cord, and peripheral nerves. Neurons are composed of:

- A central area, called the body
- One or more dendrites—structures that receive messages and carry them toward the cell body
- An axon—the structure that carries messages away from the cell body

Axons and dendrites are called nerve fibers. A message or nerve impulse begins in the dendrites and is carried along the cell body and then to the axon. It takes more than one neuron to carry the message from where it begins to where it can be carried out or interpreted. The neurons do not actually touch each other. The little space between the axon of one neuron and the dendrites of the next is called the synapse.

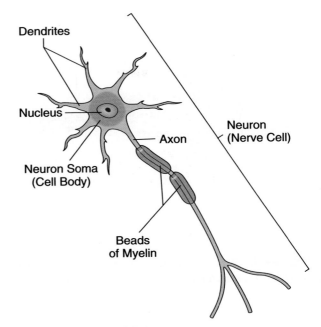

FIGURE 29-1 A neuron

Neurotransmitters

Neurotransmitters are chemicals that enable messages (nerve impulses) to pass from one cell to another (Figure 29-2). If the chemicals are not produced in adequate amounts, the message pathway becomes confused or blocked.

Nerves

Nerves are bundles of nerve fibers (axons and dendrites) that connect the body with the CNS. Nerves are named according to the type of message they carry and the direction in which they carry the message. The two general types of nerves are:

- Sensory nerves
- Motor nerves

Sensory nerves carry messages about pain, temperature change, changes in body position, taste, touch, sound, and sight. They carry messages toward the brain and spinal cord. When sensory nerves are damaged, the ability to receive messages and interpret sensations is impaired or lost.

Motor nerves carry messages from the brain and spinal cord to muscles and glands to bring about responses. When motor nerves are damaged, the person loses the ability to voluntarily control body movement. This condition is called **paralysis**. Paralysis may be complete, with no movement possible, or partial with a weaker than normal response.

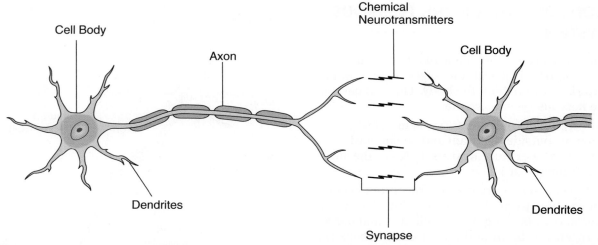

FIGURE 29-2 Chemicals called neurotransmitters help pass the nerve message across the synapse from one neuron to the next.

Peripheral nerves carry both incoming and outgoing information. These are mixed bundles of nerves carrying both sensory and motor fibers throughout the body.

CENTRAL NERVOUS SYSTEM

The CNS is made up of the brain and spinal cord. These organs are protected by the bones of the skull and vertebral column. A triple-layered membrane, the **meninges**, surrounds the brain and spinal column, providing additional protection.

Spinal Cord

The spinal cord is about 18 inches long and extends from the brain to just above the small of the back. Thirty-one pairs of spinal nerves enter and leave the spinal cord, carrying messages to and from the body. The spinal cord:

- Carries messages to and from the brain and relays them to the body through the spinal nerves (Figure 29-3).
- Handles certain special responses called reflexes.

A **reflex** occurs when an incoming message becomes an outgoing command without needing to go to a higher conscious level. For example, if you touch something hot, you immediately pull your hand back. You may then realize what you have done, but pulling back your hand was a reflex response handled by the spinal column.

The Brain

The brain is the most complex organ in the body (Figure 29-4). The neurons of the brain carry out many complex functions, including:

- Reasoning
- Thinking
- Forming and recalling memories
- Making judgments
- Controlling body functions
- Interpreting the sensations that are brought in by the nerves

Twelve pairs of cranial nerves carry messages into and out of the brain.

The **cerebrum** is the largest part of the brain. It is divided into two halves or hemispheres. The surface of the cerebrum forms lobes that have the same names as the bones under which they are located. They are the:

- Frontal lobes
- Parietal lobes
- Temporal lobes
- Occipital lobes

(Refer to Figure 29-4.)

Different parts of the cerebrum carry out specific activities:

- Motor control of one side of the body is managed by cells in the opposite side of the frontal lobe.
- Sensations originating on one side of the body are interpreted on the opposite side of the parietal lobe.
- Vision is interpreted in the occipital lobe.
- Hearing is in the temporal lobe.

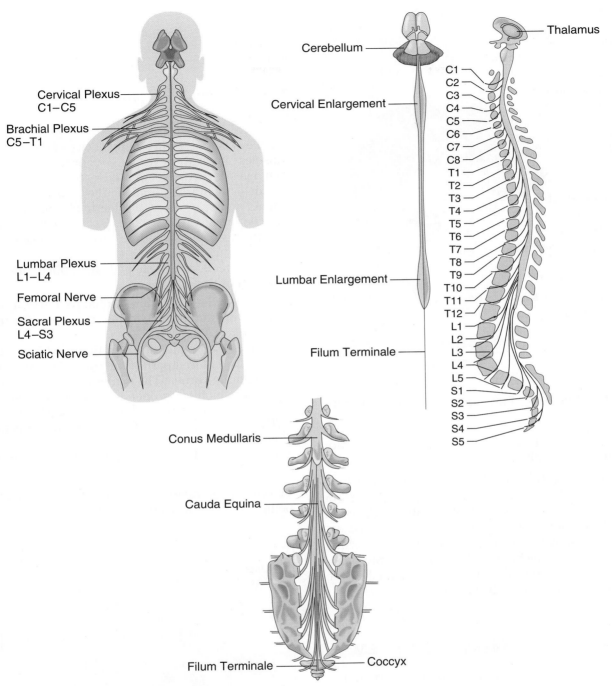

FIGURE 29-3   Spinal cord and nerves

The **cerebellum** is called the little brain. It lies beneath the occipital lobes of the cerebrum. This part of the brain coordinates muscular activities and maintains balance.

The **brain stem** is the portion of the brain that is connected to the spinal cord. It is composed of special groups of nerve cells that con-

trol the vital (living) functions of the body. These vital functions include:

- Respiration
- Heart rate and rhythm
- Size of the blood vessels
- Functioning of internal body organs such as the organs of the digestive tract

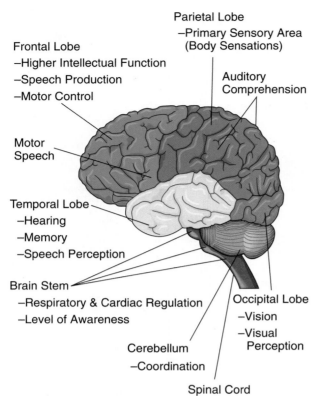

FIGURE 29-4 Functional areas of the brain

Most of the twelve pairs of cranial nerves are attached to the brain stem.

Cerebrospinal Fluid. The **cerebrospinal fluid** (CSF) is a clear, colorless fluid derived from the plasma of the blood. It fills cavities in the brain called ventricles and circulates in the central canal of the spinal cord. It acts as a watery cushion around both the brain and spinal cord. CSF is continuously produced. It is also reabsorbed at the same rate back into the bloodstream.

AUTONOMIC NERVOUS SYSTEM

The autonomic nervous system is part of the PNS. It controls heart rate, the secretions of glandular cells, and the contraction of the smooth muscular walls of organs.

SENSE ORGANS

The sense organs carry messages about the external world to the brain. Sense organs carry messages about:

- Touch
- Temperature
- Pain
- Vision
- Hearing
- Taste
- Smell
- Equilibrium

The Eye

Each eye is located in a bony cavity of the skull. Muscles move the eyes in a coordinated way. The eyelids and eye are covered by a clear mucous membrane called the **conjunctiva**. Mucus and tears from the lacrimal gland keep the eye moist (Figure 29-5). Excess tears drain into the nose and sometimes from the outside of the eyes.

The eye is a ball-shaped, fluid-filled organ made up of three layers:

- **Sclera**—the outer white protective cover. The front of the sclera forms the transparent **cornea**.
- **Choroid**—the middle layer that contains the **iris** (the colored part of the eye). The iris lies behind the cornea. The center of the iris is the **pupil**, which is an opening that changes size to control the amount of light entering the eye. The **lens** behind the iris bends and directs light rays.
- **Retina**—the innermost layer containing nerve receptors (Figure 29-6)

Vision. Light rays are reflected from the object being seen. The rays pass through the cornea and

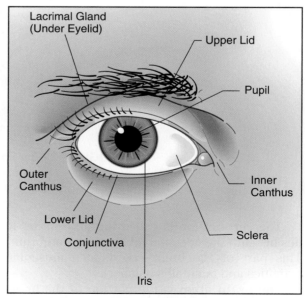

FIGURE 29-5 Tears come from the lacrimal gland and exit from the eye through the nasolacrimal duct.

FIGURE 29-6   Internal view of the eye

pupil and are bent to focus on the retina. The image on the retina is then transmitted by the **optic nerve** to the brain for vision interpretation. (The optic nerve is one of the cranial nerves.)

The Ear

The ear enables us to hear and also assists in controlling **equilibrium**. This allows us to maintain our sense of balance. The ear is made up of the:

- Outer ear
- Middle ear
- Inner ear (Figure 29-7)

Hearing.   Sound waves enter the ear and are carried toward the eardrum (tympanic membrane). This structure separates the outer and middle ear. The sound waves make the eardrum vibrate. Three tiny bones stretch across the middle ear. The first bone is attached to the eardrum. It begins to vibrate as the eardrum moves. The second bone is attached to the first and the third to the second. Each little bone vibrates in turn at the same rate as the eardrum moves. The third bone attaches to the membranous opening of the inner ear. Vibrations against this membrane

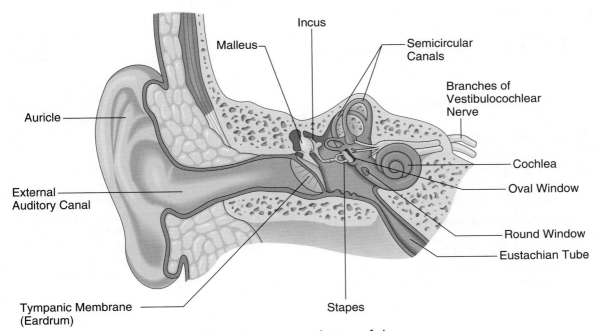

FIGURE 29-7   Internal view of the ear

set up fluid vibrations in the inner ear. The inner ear is made up of the:

- Semicircular canals
- Vestibule
- Cochlea

The three semicircular canals pick up information about starting and stopping movements. The vestibule picks up information about the position of the head. Deep within the snail-shaped cochlea are the special hearing receptors that are stimulated by the fluid vibrations. When these receptors are stimulated, the message is picked up and transmitted to the **auditory nerve** and then to the brain for interpretation of sounds that are heard.

CHANGES IN THE NERVOUS SYSTEM CAUSED BY AGING

The effects of aging on the nervous system are not as noticeable as they are on some of the other body systems. It is important to remember that intelligence does not decrease. Any change in mental status is an indication of a disease process.

Aging affects the senses of vision, hearing, taste, and smell. Most people have visual changes that make it difficult to read and see close objects. This is because the elasticity of the lens decreases with age. This condition is

called **presbyopia** (also called farsightedness). Eyeglasses will correct this problem. Many older people have glasses with *bifocal* or *trifocal* lenses. These lenses correct more than one visual impairment. Some residents are not able to care for their own glasses. You must remember to do this for them.

CAUSES OF SEVERE VISION IMPAIRMENT

Several disorders of the eye may result in severely impaired vision or blindness. These changes are not due to normal aging. Some of these disorders can be treated and are reversible. Others lead to severe vision impairment or blindness.

Cataracts

The lens is normally clear. Sometimes the lens becomes cloudy and is called a **cataract**. The cataract causes vision to become blurred and hazy. A person with a cataract has problems judging distance. Color vision may disappear and glare from bright lights is annoying.

The only treatment for a cataract is surgery to remove the lens. The surgeon will usually put in an artificial lens during the surgery. If this is not done, the person must wear very strong glasses or contact lenses.

PROCEDURE
106   Care of Eyeglasses

1. Carry out each beginning procedure action.
2. Assemble equipment:
   - Resident's eyeglasses
   - Cleaning solution
   - Clear water
   - Soft cleaning tissues
3. Provide only the assistance that the resident needs.
4. Handle glasses only by the frames.
5. Clean lenses with cleaning solution or clear water. Check the condition of the

frames and lenses. Report any damage to the frames and ear pieces and serious scratching of the lenses.
6. Dry with tissues.
7. Help resident put glasses on or return glasses to case and place in drawer of bedside table. If the resident puts the glasses on, note how well the glasses fit. Report any looseness or slipping. If the glasses have nose pieces, check that they are not irritating the resident's skin.
8. Carry out each procedure completion action.

Guidelines for

Assisting Visually Impaired Residents

1. Make sure the resident knows the location of all personal articles in the room. If the resident has a system for organizing belongings, do not attempt to make changes.
2. Always put things back where they were.
3. Do not rearrange furniture unless it is absolutely necessary. Then tell the resident what changes have been made.
4. Help orient the resident to a new room by teaching the resident to locate various objects from a point of reference. Just inside the door may be the reference point. Then say, for example, "The bathroom is to your right."
5. When you walk with a visually impaired resident, ask the resident to take your arm just above the elbow. You will walk slightly behind and to one side of the resident. Describe changes that require the resident's attention. For example, "We need to go up five steps now." Some residents may use special canes as "feelers" as they ambulate.
6. To help the person locate a chair, place the person's hand on the chair's back or

arm. The seat should be located before sitting.
7. The floor should be dry and free of clutter and throw rugs.
8. Never leave doors partially open.
9. At mealtime, the resident's dishes should always be arranged in the same way. Describe the location and type of food using a clock system. For example. "The roast beef is at 12:00, mashed potatoes and gravy are at 3:00, and there are peas at 9:00."
10. Offer to cut meat, pour beverages, butter bread, and open cartons. Some residents may be able to do this.
11. Advise the resident to sprinkle salt and pepper into the hand rather than directly on the food. It is easier to know how much is being used.
12. Advise the resident to use a small piece of bread in one hand to help push food on the fork. This also prevents the food from being pushed off the plate.

Some residents may have cataract surgery while they are in the long-term care facility. They generally return to the facility immediately after surgery. Be sure you know what to do for these residents. Pressure must not be placed on the eye. Thus, the residents should avoid bending over, coughing, or excessive physical activity.

Glaucoma

Glaucoma exists when the pressure in the eyeball is higher than normal. This occurs when the meshwork between the iris and cornea thickens, obstructing the flow of the fluid in the eyeball. If not treated, the pressure eventually damages the optic nerve, causing blindness.

Glaucoma has few symptoms. Everyone over the age of 35 years should be tested for eye pressure routinely. The disease process can be stopped by using eyedrops prescribed by the **ophthalmologist** (eye physician).

Age-Related Macular Degeneration

Age-related macular degeneration is the leading cause of visual loss in the United States. Millions of older people are affected. The cause is unknown. The macula is located on the retina. The macula is damaged when abnormal blood vessels form and leak fluid. Laser treatments may help some people with this condition.

Diabetic Retinopathy

People with diabetes are at risk for **diabetic retinopathy**. It is caused by the deterioration of small blood vessels that nourish the retina. Laser treatments may interrupt the disease process. However, vision loss that has already occurred cannot be restored.

There are many things nursing assistants can do to improve the quality of life for residents with severe visual impairments.

Review Lesson 4 for communicating with persons with vision and hearing loss.

HEARING LOSS

Hearing loss is common in later years. It usually results from progressive deterioration of the cochlea. This condition is called **presbycusis**. Some residents will wear hearing aids. The devices are expensive, so they must receive proper care.

Hearing Aids

All types of hearing aids are basically the same. A battery provides the power for the hearing aid to work. The battery is contained in a battery case. The microphone picks up the sound. The amplifier makes the sound louder. The volume control adjusts the level of sound. The receiver is a tiny speaker that conveys sound to the ear. Some models have a "T" switch. This is a telephone switch that activates a telecoil. This is used when hearing over a telephone. The telephone must be compatible with the telecoil. There are several types of hearing aids:

- The canal aid is the smallest type and fits deep into the ear canal.
- The in-the-ear aid is the most commonly used. It fills the ear and is flush with the outer part of the ear (Figure 29-8).
- The behind-the-ear aid consists of an aid worn behind the ear and an earmold that directs sound into the ear canal.
- Eyeglass types of hearing aids are similar to behind-the-ear aids except that the amplification device is contained in an eyeglass frame.
- The body aid is enclosed in a case that can be carried in a pocket or attached to clothing. The hearing aid receiver attaches directly to an earmold inserted into the ear canal. The receiver is powered through a cord connected to the case of the body aid.

Caring for Hearing Aids.
1. Store hearing aids at room temperature when not worn. Temperature extremes can damage hearing aids. They should not be worn for more than a few minutes in very cold weather. Avoid exposing them to hair dryers.
2. Keep hearing aids dry. If an aid is worn accidentally in the shower, ask the nurse how to dry it. Never try to dry the aid with a hair dryer.
3. Store extra batteries in a cool, dry place. Remove batteries from the hearing aid at

FIGURE 29-8 In-the-ear hearing aid

night or open the battery compartment. This allows air to circulate in the compartment and helps dry it out. The battery will last longer.
4. Keep hearing aids safe. They break easily if dropped on a hard floor or bumped against a hard surface.
5. Remove the hearing aid if hair spray is being used. The spray may clog the microphone, causing damage.
6. Turn the hearing aid off when not in use. Turn the aid off before removing it.
7. Wipe in-the-ear aids daily with a dry tissue.
8. Check regularly to make sure the opening of the aid or earmold is free of wax. In-the-ear types come with a cleaning tool. This should be used only by someone who has been shown how to use it to remove the wax.

Troubleshooting for Hearing Aids. If the aid is not producing sound, before inserting in resident's ear:

- Check to make sure that the "+" (positive) side of the battery is next to the "+" inside the hearing aid battery case or compartment.
- Try a new battery—the old one may be dead.
- Check the earmold to see if it is plugged with wax.
- Make sure the hearing aid is set on "M" (microphone) not "T" (telephone switch).

If the hearing aid is making squealing sounds:

- Determine if the earmold fits properly. It should be completely in the ear. If it does not fit well, report it to the nurse.
- Check the volume on the aid. If it is too high, turn it down until the squealing stops.
- Check the plastic tubing on a behind-the-ear aid. If it is cracked or split, it must be replaced.

PROCEDURE *107*   Applying and Removing In-the-Ear or Behind-the-Ear Hearing Aids   OBRA

1. Carry out each beginning procedure action.
2. Assist resident to comfortable position with head turned so that the ear needing the hearing aid is closest to you.
3. Turn the hearing aid off and turn the volume down.
4. Make sure you insert the aid in the correct ear.

Behind-the-Ear Hearing Aid

- Place the aid over the resident's ear, allowing the earmold to hang free.
- Adjust the hearing aid behind the resident's ear (Figure 29-9).

Behind-the-Ear Hearing Aid and In-the-Ear Hearing Aid

- Grasp the earmold and gently insert the tapered end into the ear canal.
- Gently twist the earmold into the curve of the ear while gently pulling on the earlobe with the other hand. The hearing aid should fit snugly but comfortably, flush with the ear.

5. Turn on the control switch. To adjust the volume, talk to the resident as you increase the volume. Stop when the resident can hear you.

Removing the Hearing Aid

1. Wash hands and explain to resident what you plan to do.
2. Turn off hearing aid.

FIGURE 29-9 Adjust the hearing aid behind the resident's ear.

3. Loosen the outer portion of the earmold by gently pulling on the upper part of the ear.
4. Lift earmold upward and outward.
5. Store in safe area.
6. Carry out each procedure completion action.

NERVOUS SYSTEM DISORDERS

Several diseases can affect the nervous system. Some of these are due to an imbalance in neurotransmitters. Other neurologic problems are caused by damage to brain cells or the spinal cord.

Diseases affecting the nervous system often have different signs and symptoms. Some common problems that may exist with these diseases include:

- Impaired mobility because of damage to the brain, spinal cord, or nerves in the legs
- Difficulty swallowing due to damage to the brain or damage to the nerves of the face and mouth
- Communication disorders due to damage to the brain or damage to the nerves of the face and mouth

Parkinson's Disease

Parkinson's disease is a chronic illness that is often progressive. It is due to a decrease in a neurotransmitter that passes messages between cells in the cerebrum and the gray matter of the brain. These cells affect movement, balance, and walking (Figure 29-10).

The signs and symptoms of Parkinson's disease include:

- Tremors
- Muscular rigidity
- Difficulty and slowness in carrying out voluntary activities

Tremors of the hands commonly affect the fingers and thumbs so that the resident appears to be rolling a pill between them. The tremors begin in the fingers, then involve the entire hand and arm, and finally affect the entire side of the body. Starting on one side, the tremors eventually involve both sides of the body.

The muscular rigidity makes the person more prone to falls and injury. The joints may develop contractures if appropriate care and treatment are not given. The rigidity also affects muscles used in breathing. This increases the risk of respiratory infections.

Persons with advanced Parkinson's typically have a shuffling walk and difficulty starting the process. Once started, they may have episodes of "freezing" when they appear unable to move.

Speech is affected, causing words to be slurred. The tone of voice is low and the sound is monotone. Rigid facial muscles cause the face to look expressionless.

The resident with Parkinson's may drool and become incontinent or constipated. Depression is a common problem. Some residents with Parkinson's may undergo mental changes known as **dementia**.

There is no specific diagnostic test for Parkinson's disease. The physician will take a history and make a thorough neurologic examination to rule out other problems.

Parkinson's disease has no cure. In some cases the disease can be controlled with medications. In other cases, the disease may be progressive, causing severe disability.

 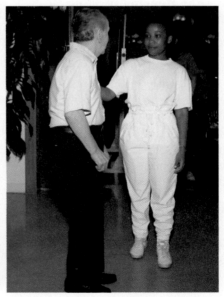

FIGURE 29-10 Note the typical posture from front and side views of the resident with Parkinson's disease.

*G*uidelines for

Caring for Residents with Parkinson's Disease

1. Give passive range of motion exercises at least twice a day. Encourage participation in active exercise if the resident is able to do so.
2. Improve walking by encouraging the resident to:
   - Bring the toes up with every step.
   - Put the foot down, heel first then toes.
   - Swing the arms.
   - Ambulate—assist by using a gait belt and walking with the resident.
3. Reposition dependent residents frequently and avoid flexion as much as possible.
4. Observe the resident closely and report:
   - Signs of respiratory infection
   - Problems with urinary elimination
   - Constipation

5. Give at least 2,000 mL fluid by mouth every day unless contraindicated.
6. Assist with activities of daily living only to the extent necessary.
7. Observe for drooling. Residents who are unable to control saliva may also have trouble swallowing. Watch for any problems during eating.
8. Give emotional support and encouragement. The disease usually affects the facial muscles. Because of this, the resident may have no facial expression. This lack of expression is not a true indication of what the resident is feeling.

Stroke

Stroke (also called brain attack) is the fourth most common cause of death in the United States. Two-thirds of stroke victims are over age 65 years. Stroke is also called **cerebrovascular accident** or **CVA**. The word *cerebrovascular* refers to blood vessels in the brain. Major risk factors for a stroke include:

- Hypertension (high blood pressure)
- **Atherosclerosis** (buildup of fatty deposits in arteries)
- History of **transient ischemic attack (TIA)**
- Smoking
- Lack of exercise
- Obesity

A TIA is not a stroke, but may be a warning that a stroke is likely to occur. During a TIA, the resident may experience speech disturbances and paralysis. These symptoms last from a few minutes to 24 hours. They are never permanent.

A stroke may occur as a result of:

- Hemorrhage—This occurs when an **aneurysm** in the brain ruptures or hypertension causes a blood vessel in the brain to rupture. An aneurysm is a thin spot on an artery wall.
- Thrombus—A **thrombus** is a blood clot. It forms when fatty deposits on the artery walls cause the walls to become roughened. This causes platelets in the blood to form a clot.

When the thrombus interrupts blood flow to the brain, a stroke occurs.

- Embolus—An **embolus** is a thrombus that develops in an artery in one part of the body, breaks loose, and travels to another part of the body. In the case of a stroke, the embolus travels to an artery in the brain and blocks the flow of blood.

Symptoms of Stroke. The symptoms of stroke depend on the part of the brain that is damaged. If the left side of the brain is damaged, these symptoms may be noted:

- Paralysis on the right side of the body. This is called right **hemiplegia**.
- **Aphasia**—an inability to express or understand speech
- Change in personality. The individual with left brain damage becomes very slow, anxious, and cautious.

If the right side of the brain is damaged, these symptoms may be noted:

- Paralysis on the left side of the body. This is called left hemiplegia (Figure 29-11).
- **Spatial-perceptual deficits**. This means it is difficult to distinguish between left and right, up and down. The world may appear "tilted" to the person with right-brain damage. The resident will have problems propelling a wheelchair, setting down items, and carrying out activities of daily living.

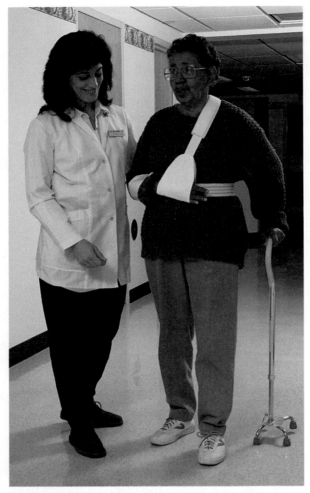

FIGURE 29-11 The resident had a stroke, resulting in paralysis of one side of the body.

• Change in personality. The individual with right brain damage becomes very quick and impulsive.

Other symptoms may be present with either right or left brain damage. These include:

• Sensory-perceptual deficits.
  • Loss of **position sense**. The individual cannot tell where the affected foot is or what position it is in.
  • The inability to identify common objects. The person who has had a stroke may not recognize a comb, a fork, a pencil, or other common items.
  • The inability to use common objects. The person may know what the object is, such as a comb, but be unable to pick it up and use it appropriately even with the unaffected arm. This is not a result of paralysis but of damage to certain cells in the brain.

• **Unilateral neglect**. The resident ignores the paralyzed side of the body. For example, the affected arm may hang over the side of the wheelchair without the resident realizing where the arm is.
• **Hemianopsia**. This is impaired vision. Both eyes only have half vision. For example, if the resident has left hemiplegia, the left half of both eyes is blind (Figure 29-12).
• **Emotional lability**. Residents who have had strokes may start to cry or laugh for no apparent reason. They have very little control over this and may be embarrassed.

Goals of Poststroke Care. Three major nursing goals for a resident who has had a stroke are:

1. Maintain the skills and abilities that the individual has left.
2. Prevent complications caused by immobility.
   • Contractures
   • Pressure ulcers
   • Pneumonia
   • Blood clots
3. Regain functional abilities (Figure 29-13).
   • Activities of daily living
   • Bowel and bladder control
   • Mobility
   • Communication skills

Communicating with persons with aphasia is presented in Lesson 4.

The recovery from stroke is different for each person. Some individuals recover with a minimal degree of disability. Others may have a

FIGURE 29-12 Hemianopsia causes a person to see only part of the visual field.

---

*G*uidelines for

Caring for Residents Who Have Had a Stroke

Complications following stroke can be prevented by several measures.

1. Proper positioning. Lesson 22 gives instructions for positioning residents with hemiplegia. Remember to support the paralyzed arm so that the shoulder does not become dislocated. Check the paralyzed leg and arm frequently. The resident may be unaware of injury to the extremities.
2. Passive range of motion exercises twice a day (see Lesson 22). The resident may learn to do self range of motion exercises. This also provides exercise for the unaffected arm.
3. Intake of an adequate amount of fluids each shift

4. Implementation of bowel and bladder programs
5. Maintenance of nutritional status
6. Encouraging and supporting the resident at all times
7. You can help the resident regain functional abilities by encouraging and allowing the resident to do as much as possible. Provide the help that is necessary for completing activities of daily living but avoid "over-helping." You can carry out restorative programs under the direction of the physical therapist, occupational therapist, and restorative nurse.
8. You can help the resident regain mobility skills by increasing the resident's mobility as directed by the nurse or physical therapist (Lessons 22 and 23).

---

greater degree of disability but learn to adapt and regain some independence. A few individuals are severely impaired and will regain very little, if any, ability for self-care.

FIGURE 29-13 The resident who has had a stroke must be retrained in activities of daily living.

Multiple Sclerosis

Multiple sclerosis (MS) is another CNS disease. The cause is unknown. The myelin sheath that covers the part of the neuron called the axon is destroyed. When the myelin sheath is destroyed, impulses are unable to travel through the axon.

MS is usually diagnosed before the age of 50. Many individuals live the usual life span even though they have this chronic disorder. Therefore, it is not unusual to see elderly residents in long-term care with this diagnosis. Most facilities also have young residents in their twenties and thirties with MS (Figure 29-14).

The symptoms are variable and may not be the same for all individuals. Symptoms may include:

- Loss of sensation with regard to temperature, pain, touch
- Feelings of numbness and tingling
- **Vertigo** (a spinning sensation)
- Loss of position sense
- **Lhermitte's sign** (a tingling, shock-like sensation that passes down the arms or spine when the neck is flexed)

Problems with vision occur in almost half of the people who have MS. This problem may be

FIGURE 29-14 Multiple sclerosis frequently affects young people.

permanent or temporary. Sometimes it is the first symptom that is noted. Symptoms may include:

- Blurriness, color blindness, or difficulty seeing objects in bright light
- Double vision
- **Nystagmus** (jerky eye movements)

Mobility is usually affected:

- Pain in the legs that disappears with rest
- **Paraplegia** (paralysis of both legs)
- Spasticity
- **Intention tremor** (shaking of the hands that gets worse as the individual tries to touch or pick up an object)

In severe MS, speech is affected because of the weakness of the muscles in the chest, face, and lips. The speech may be slow with poor articula-

*G*uidelines for
Caring for Residents with Multiple Sclerosis

1. Prevent complications.
   - Contractures can occur rapidly because of the spasticity. Range of motion exercises and position changes are important. The resident may also perform muscle-stretching exercises with the help of the rehabilitation nurse or physical therapist.
   - Spasticity affects the bladder and causes incontinence. For this reason, residents with severe MS may have indwelling catheters. Excellent catheter care is necessary to prevent bladder infections. Make sure the resident has adequate fluid intake.
   - Residents with MS are at risk for pressure ulcers. Follow all directions for pressure ulcer prevention. Because of lack of sensation, ulcers may develop without the resident feeling discomfort or pain.
2. Encourage independence.
   - The use of adaptive devices for activities of daily living may help maintain independence for a longer period of time.
   - Mobility may be prolonged if assistive devices such as canes or walkers are

used. Leg braces are helpful for some people. Many individuals (even in the facility) may use motorized scooters. This increases independence for people who are no longer able to walk.

3. Maintain a balanced schedule of rest and activity.
   - Residents with MS need exercise and activity. However, they also need rest periods to avoid becoming overtired.
   - Remember that fatigue can be a major problem. Help residents set priorities for their available energy. If a resident expects the family to visit in the evening for example, allow more rest periods during the day.

4. Provide emotional support and encouragement.
   - Residents in long-term care facilities may have access to MS support groups. Some people find these groups very helpful.
   - Not all residents with MS will be elderly. Remember the developmental stages of the residents in your care. This will allow you to be more empathic and give better care.

tion. The mind usually remains alert. Incontinence of bowel and bladder is also common.

One of the most disabling features of MS is fatigue. This very real physical symptom, not psychological, makes it impossible for the person to move about.

The diagnosis of MS is not based on a specific test. The physician takes a thorough history and performs a complete neurologic examination. **Magnetic resonance imaging (MRI)** is a test that may reveal lesions in the neurons in the brain. The person conducting the test records pictures (scans) of brain tissue beneath the bone.

MS may eventually lead to **quadriplegia** (paralysis of all four extremities). Residents with quadriplegia require total care. However, not all persons who have MS are severely impaired. At the time of diagnosis, it is seldom known what course the disease will take. It is difficult for the person to deal with this uncertainty for the future. The disease may follow one of four courses:

- *Benign course:* mild attacks with long periods of no symptoms

- *Exacerbating-remitting:* Severe attacks (exacerbations) followed by periods of partial or complete recovery (remissions). Often the periods of exacerbation get longer with shorter periods of remission.
- *Slowly progressive:* slow, steady deterioration
- *Rapidly progressive:* deterioration is rapid and progressive and may be life-threatening

Huntington's Disease

Huntington's disease is a hereditary disease. This means it is a **genetic disease** because it is passed from one generation to another through a defective gene. Either parent carrying the gene can transmit the disease to either sons or daughters. Each child of a parent with the defective gene for Huntington's has a 50% chance of receiving the defective gene from the parent.

The disease is progressive and affects the CNS as well as the mind and the emotions. Symptoms may become evident between the ages of 20 and 60 years. The most evident symptom is the body movements called choreiform

---

*G*uidelines for
Caring for Residents with Huntington's Disease

Safety is a major concern because of the constant body movements.

1. Prevent injuries by:
   - Padding side rails to avoid injury to the arms and legs
   - Using padded clothing and shoes without laces
   - Using a gait belt and having two assistants walk with the resident—providing stability and counteracting the jerky movements
   - Using alternatives to restraints, which are dangerous because of the movements

2. Prevent choking by:
   - Ensuring that all who are responsible for feeding residents are knowledgeable about the residents' abilities, if possible
   - Having all persons who feed know how to do abdominal thrusts for an obstructed airway
   - Providing a diet as tolerated

Other concerns for residents with Huntington's disease include:

3. Incontinence
   - Assist the resident to the bathroom every 2 hours or as needed. As the disease progresses, this becomes impossible with the loss of ambulatory skills.
   - Catheters usually pose a danger because of the resident's involuntary movements, which may cause tearing of the urethra.
   - Incontinent pads may be necessary.
   - Careful attention to skin care is essential.

4. Nutrition
   - Additional calories may be needed because of the energy used in the involuntary movements.

movements. These begin early in the disease with fidgeting, twitching, clumsiness, and falling. As the disease progresses, the extremities are in constant movement during waking hours. Eventually it becomes impossible for the individual to walk or perform any activities independently.

The mind is also affected, resulting in a form of dementia. The capacity to plan and organize is lost. Impulsiveness and loss of judgment are also common. Emotional disorders such as depression, antisocial behavior, and seclusion may also develop.

The disease is always chronic and progressive. There may be periods of stability. As the disease progresses, the symptoms become more severe. Eventually, death occurs, usually as a result of pneumonia or an infection.

Many residents with Huntington's disease are young people. Some of them may have young children. This is a difficult situation for families as children watch a parent become progressively worse. Whether or not the children will develop the disease is a major concern for all family members. Each family deals with this in its own way. Avoid passing judgment on families and the way they choose to cope with this problem. Referral for professional counseling should be made by the social services staff to all family members as well as the resident. It is the individual's decision whether to participate in the counseling.

Amyotrophic Lateral Sclerosis

This disease is also known as ALS or Lou Gehrig's disease. Mr. Gehrig was a famous baseball player who died of ALS. ALS generally affects persons between the ages of 50 and 70. The nerve cells in the brain and spinal cord gradually deteriorate. The disease is chronic and progressive. There is no cure. The muscles under their control weaken and waste away. The disease eventually affects all voluntary muscles. The mind stays alert and the person is able to think clearly. The first signs and symptoms include:

- Trouble with walking—stumbling and falling
- Trouble picking up objects and frequently dropping them
- Trouble completing activities of daily living, for example, lacing shoes, buttoning, or cutting meat

Persons with ALS eventually have:

- Difficulty speaking
- Difficulty swallowing (may need a feeding tube)
- Disabling fatigue
- Shortness of breath (may need a ventilator)
- Inability to move arms or legs independently

Myasthenia Gravis

Myasthenia gravis (MG) is also a chronic disease that affects the muscles. This is due to incomplete transmission of nerve impulses

*G*uidelines for
Caring for Residents Who Have Amyotrophic Lateral Sclerosis

1. Keep the resident upright as much as possible to avoid aspiration and to increase lung expansion. When lying down, position the resident on either side, turning at least every 2 hours. Place a cloth beneath the mouth to absorb saliva from the mouth.
2. Encourage coughing and deep breathing to prevent respiratory infections.
3. Encourage the resident to take frequent rest periods. Encourage the use of a wheelchair to save energy.
4. Use methods of communication as directed by the nurse or speech therapist. The resident may eventually have to communicate by blinking the eyes. Remember that even though the resident cannot speak, he can understand others.
5. Observe food and fluid intake. Residents with ALS may be too weak or too tired to eat. Try to have the resident rest for a half hour before meals and for 2 hours after meals. If the resident has to be fed, allow frequent breaks during the meal.
6. Report any signs of potential pressure ulcers.

*G*uidelines for

Caring for Residents Who Have Myasthenia Gravis

Medications can help most people with myasthenia gravis to live productive lives. The disease affects each person differently. It is important to know for a specific resident which muscles are affected and how much activity the resident can tolerate.

1. Pace the resident's activity and allow adequate time for rest between activities.
2. Use alternative methods of communication according to the care plan.
3. Review Lesson 17 for feeding residents who have swallowing problems.
4. Encourage the resident's independence but provide assistance as needed.

where the nerves and muscle join. The cause is unknown. The same muscles are not affected in all people. Signs and symptoms always involve the muscles and may include:

- Weakness of the eye muscles, causing double vision and drooping of the eyelid
- Inability to smile, frown, or pucker the lips if facial muscles are involved

- Voice weaker if larynx is involved
- Generalized muscle weakness:
  - Difficulty putting arms above head
  - Difficulty rising from chair or toilet and difficulty walking up stairs
  - Difficulty managing saliva
  - Mouth hangs open due to inability to close mouth

LESSON SYNTHESIS: Putting It All Together

*Y*ou have just completed this lesson. Now go back and review the Clinical Focus. Try to see how the Clinical Focus relates to the concepts presented in the lesson. Then answer the following questions.

1. Why might self-feeding be difficult for Mr. Raye?

2. Why is it important to carry out range of motion regularly with Mr. Raye?

3. How can ambulation be encouraged and made safer?

4. Nursing assistants must be alert to the possibility of which serious complications that could affect Mr. Raye?

5. Why do Mr. Raye and his family need the emotional support of the staff?

REVIEW

A. Select the one best answer for each of the following:

1. The brain and spinal cord make up the
   (A) central nervous system
   (B) peripheral nervous system
   (C) sensory organs
   (D) recepton system

2. Neurotransmitters are
   (A) neurons
   (B) special nerves
   (C) chemicals that help pass messages from one cell to another
   (D) brain cells

3. The brain stem controls
   (A) voluntary movements
   (B) thinking
   (C) vital functions of the body
   (D) emotions

4. When the lens of the eye becomes cloudy and impairs vision, it is called
   (A) glaucoma
   (B) macular degeneration
   (C) diabetic retinopathy
   (D) cataract

5. Hearing aids should be kept as follows, except
   (A) at room temperature
   (B) on at all times
   (C) free of wax
   (D) dry

6. Parkinson's disease is due to
   (A) a decrease in a neurotransmitter
   (B) brain injury
   (C) changes in the myelin sheath of the neuron
   (D) decreased blood flow to the brain

7. Persons with Parkinson's generally have all of these symptoms, except
   (A) tremors
   (B) rigidity
   (C) slowness of movement
   (D) high fever

8. Nursing care for persons with Parkinson's disease does not include
   (A) instructions for walking
   (B) restricting self-care
   (C) giving adequate fluids
   (D) positioning to avoid flexion

9. A person who has had a stroke on the left side of the brain will
   (A) have left hemiplegia
   (B) become quick and impulsive
   (C) have aphasia
   (D) not experience sensory changes

10. The person who has had a stroke on the right side of the brain will
    (A) have left hemiplegia
    (B) have aphasia
    (C) become slow and cautious
    (D) not experience sensory changes

11. Residents with stroke
    (A) need no support of the arm on the affected side
    (B) need passive range of motion exercises at least twice a day
    (C) should be encouraged to do as little as possible
    (D) do not require restorative care

12. Multiple sclerosis occurs because
    (A) the myelin sheath of the neuron is damaged
    (B) of a hemorrhage in the brain
    (C) of a lack of a certain neurotransmitter
    (D) muscle damage

13. Residents with multiple sclerosis may experience all of the following except
    (A) loss of sensation to temperature, pain, touch
    (B) visual impairments
    (C) tremors
    (D) chest pain

14. Spasticity of the muscles in multiple sclerosis may cause
    (A) respiratory tract infections
    (B) choking
    (C) urinary tract infections
    (D) urinary incontinence

15. Nursing care for residents with multiple sclerosis does not include
    (A) preventing contractures
    (B) preventing pressure ulcers
    (C) restricting fluids
    (D) maintaining mobility as long as possible

16. Huntington's disease is characterized by
    (A) hemiplegia
    (B) aphasia
    (C) chorea
    (D) slowness of movements

17. Amyotrophic lateral sclerosis (ALS) causes all of the following, except
    (A) inability to move independently
    (B) disabling fatigue
    (C) difficulty speaking
    (D) no change in swallowing ability

18. The person with ALS usually has
    (A) mental impairment
    (B) vision impairment
    (C) shortness of breath
    (D) hearing impairment

19. Residents with ALS should
    (A) be positioned upright as much as possible
    (B) be kept as active as possible through the day
    (C) be positioned in supine position for several hours a day
    (D) communicate by writing

20. Signs and symptoms of myasthenia gravis include all of the following, except
    (A) weakness of the eye muscles
    (B) inability to keep the mouth closed
    (C) drooling
    (D) unaffected speech

B. Fill in the blanks by selecting the correct word or phrase from the list.

age-related macular degeneration	hemianopsia hemiplegia
amyotrophic lateral sclerosis	Lhermitte's sign neurotransmitters nystagmus
aphasia	paraplegia
central nervous system	position sense presbycusis
dementia	presbyopia
equilibrium	quadriplegia
genetic	thrombus
glaucoma	unilateral neglect

21. Chemicals that help pass nerve impulses from one cell to another are called _____.

22. The brain and spinal cord make up the _____.

23. The ear is responsible for hearing and for _____.

24. Older adults often develop a vision problem called _____.

25. A condition in which the pressure within the eyeball is higher than normal is called _____.

26. The leading cause of visual loss in this country is _____.

27. Many older adults suffer hearing loss called _____.

28. Persons with Parkinson's disease may undergo mental changes referred to as _____.

29. Stroke may be caused by a blood clot called a _____.

30. Paralysis on one side of the body is called _____.

31. The inability to express or understand speech is _____.

32. If a resident with a stroke cannot tell where the affected foot is, the resident has loss of _____.

33. _____ is loss of vision of one-half of the eye in both eyes.

34. _____ means the resident ignores the paralyzed side of the body.

35. A tingling shock-like sensation that passes down the arms or spine when the neck is flexed is _____.

36. Paralysis of both legs is _____.

37. Paralysis of all four extremities is _____.

38. Jerky eye movements seen in multiple sclerosis are called _____.

39. Huntington's disease is _____.

40. The disease also known as Lou Gehrig's disease is _____.

SECTION 9

Residents with Special Needs

LESSONS

30 Alzheimer's Disease
and Related Disorders
(Caring for the
Cognitively Impaired
Resident)

31 Caring for Residents
with Developmental
Disabilities

32 Caring for the Dying
Resident

33 Caring for the Person
in Subacute Care

LESSON 30

Alzheimer's Disease and Related Disorders (Caring for the Cognitively Impaired Resident)

Clinical Focus

Think about the nursing care required by the resident who suffers from Alzheimer's disease and related disorders as you study this lesson and meet:

*G*race McGinnis, who has been a resident in your facility for almost 2 years. About 10 years ago, she realized that she could not remember details as well as she once had. Gradually, her mental and emotional status declined. Her husband employed a housekeeper to stay with her. Four years later, Mr. McGinnis had a heart attack and died. Family members felt admission to a long-term care facility was the only answer. Mrs. McGinnis suffers from Alzheimer's disease and is in stage 2.

OBJECTIVES

After studying this lesson, you should be able to:

- Define and spell vocabulary words and terms.
- List four symptoms of Alzheimer's disease.
- Identify the concerns associated with caring for people with dementia.
- Identify three approaches that are effective when working with residents with Alzheimer's disease or other dementias.
- Describe the differences between an Alzheimer's unit and a general unit.
- State three guidelines for assisting residents with dementia with the activities of daily living.
- Describe four effective techniques for communicating with residents with dementia.

VOCABULARY

Alzheimer's disease *(ALTZ-high-mers dih-ZEEZ)*

aphasia *(ah-FAY-zee-ah)*

aspiration *(ass-pih-RAY-shun)*

catastrophic reaction *(kat-ah-STROH-fick ree-ACK-shun)*

cognitive impairment *(KOG-nih-tiv im-PAIR-ment)*

delusion *(dee-LEW-zhun)*

dementia *(dee-MEN-she-ah)*

depression *(dee-PRESH-un)*

disorientation *(dis-oh-ree-en-TAY-shun)*

hallucination *(hah-loo-sih-NAY-shun)*

neurotransmitter *(new-roh-TRANS-mit-er)*

organic mental syndrome *(or-GAN-ick MEN-til SIN-drohm)*

pacing *(PAYS-ing)*

perseveration *(per-sev-er-AY-shun)*

pet therapy *(pet THER-ah-pee)*

reality orientation *(ree-AL-ih-tee oh-ree-en-TAY-shun)*

reminiscing *(reh-mih-NISS-ing)*

sensory-perceptual changes *(SEN-sor-ee-per-SEP-tyou-al CHAIN-jes)*

sundowning *(SUN-down-ing)*

validation therapy *(val-ih-DAY-shun THER-ah-pee)*

wandering *(WAN-der-ing)*

DEFINITION OF ALZHEIMER'S DISEASE

You will care for residents who have **Alzheimer's disease** or other dementia. Alzheimer's disease is a disorder of the brain that involves thinking, memory, and judgment. Alzheimer's disease is a form of **dementia**. **Organic mental syndrome** is a general term that includes all dementias. Dementia is not a disease in itself but is a group of symptoms seen in a number of different diseases. Alzheimer's is the most common form. Other types of dementias are related to cerebrovascular disease, Parkinson's disease, and Huntington's disease. The term **cognitive impairment** means that the mental or intellectual abilities of the individual are damaged (Figure 30-1).

The information in this lesson refers to Alzheimer's disease because it is the most common form of dementia. Remember that other dementias have many of the same signs and symptoms. The treatment and care are similar regardless of the medical diagnosis.

Alzheimer's disease can begin during middle age but is more common in older persons. The disease affects people of all races, intelligence levels, education, and financial status. It is progressive and has been called a "slow death" of the mind. In the past, the term *senility* was used to describe these symptoms. We now know that it is a disease of the brain cells and is not normal aging (Figure 30-2).

Research continues into the cause of Alzheimer's disease. There is no specific test to confirm the diagnosis and no cure. When symptoms appear, the individual should have a complete medical diagnostic workup.

It is important to rule out other conditions such as diabetes and other endocrine problems, vitamin deficiencies, malnutrition, brain tumors, impaired circulation, epilepsy, depression, and medication interactions. Unlike Alzheimer's disease, these conditions may be treatable and curable. The diagnostic tests commonly include:

- Blood tests
- Electroencephalogram (EEG), a study of brain waves
- Magnetic resonance imaging (MRI)
- Brain scan
- Psychological evaluation to rule out depression
- Evaluation of all medications being taken including over-the-counter drugs
- Mental status examination

The mental status examination assesses the person's:

- Orientation to time and place
- Attention span
- Ability to recall information
- Ability to use language
- Ability to follow directions
- Ability to read and write
- Ability to copy a design

FIGURE 30-1 Descriptions of major forms of dementia

Disease	Features	Course
Alzheimer's	Lack of chemical in brain causing neurofibrillary tangles, neuritic plaques	Onset age: 60–80 Slowly progressive
Multi-infarct dementia	Interference with blood circulation in brain cells due to arteriosclerosis, atherosclerosis	Onset age: 55–70 Outcome depends on rate of damage to brain cells
Huntington's	Inherited from either parent who has gene for the disease	Onset age: 25–45 Average duration 15 years
Parkinson's	Deficiency of chemical in brain (dopamine)	Onset age: 55–60 Several years duration
Creutzfeldt-Jacob	Noninflammatory virus, changes in brain	Onset age: 50–60 Rapidly progressive
Syphilis	Spirochete (bacteria) causes brain damage	Occurs 15–20 years after primary infection
AIDS dementia	HIV-1 infection	Symptoms sometimes precede diagnosis of AIDS

Changes in the Brain Leading to Alzheimer's Disease

Messages are normally passed between nerve cells (neurons) in the brain by chemicals called **neurotransmitters**. People with Alzheimer's lack one of these chemicals. If an autopsy of the brain is performed after death, distinctive changes are noted. These changes are called neuritic plaques and neurofibrillary tangles—indications of the damage that has occurred to the brain.

STAGES AND SYMPTOMS OF ALZHEIMER'S DISEASE

Little is certain about Alzheimer's disease. It is believed that changes in the brain may occur for several years before symptoms appear. The disease progresses through several stages. At first, the person appears normal to people who do not know him. In the first stage, the person is aware of the changes and realizes that something is wrong, but is helpless to change the situation. Changes in behavior are the only indication that the disease is progressing. All signs and symptoms of the person with Alzheimer's disease are related to the loss of mental abilities. The disease may last from 10 to 25 years.

Stage 1

This stage lasts between 1 and 3 years. The person loses interest in people or activities. Little attention is paid to grooming and hygiene. Personality

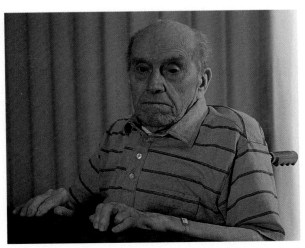

FIGURE 30-2 The symptoms of Alzheimer's disease are not normal aging.

changes in the person cause the family to feel that a stranger has entered their home. **Depression** may be present and is marked by inactivity, withdrawal, and minimal interaction with others. Anxiety related to the inability to "figure things out" may cause the person to have angry outbursts. Changes include:

- **Short-term memory loss**
  The person may:
  - Be unable to find his way around his home
  - Get lost while driving a familiar route
  - Forget information as soon as it is given to him
- **Decreased ability to concentrate, attention span shortens**
  - If setting the table, for instance, the person may place a plate on the table and then wander off without completing the task. Directions are not followed because the person is unable to concentrate on the sequence of steps.
- **Disorientation to time and place**
  - **Disorientation** to time is the inability to determine the day, date, month, year,

FIGURE 30-3 Persons with Alzheimer's disease exhibit poor judgment.

or season. Disorientation to place is the inability to know the building one is in (even one's home), the city, the county, or the state.

- **Poor judgment**
  - Poor judgment may be reflected in poor money management or inappropriate social behavior (Figure 30-3).
- **Delusions**
  - **Delusions** are fixed, false beliefs.

Stage 2

Stage 2 lasts from 2 to 10 years. All of the signs and symptoms in stage 1 continue and become more intense. Some individuals may be able to remain at home if enough family members are able to provide care 24 hours a day, 7 days a week. By the end of this stage, most families are unable to give the time, energy, and emotional resources that are required. Safety is a major concern as the person's judgment is reduced further. Additional changes include:

- **Wandering and pacing**
  - **Wandering** is an aimless walking about.
  - **Pacing** is walking the same path over and over and is a result of anxiety.
- **Sundowning**
  - **Sundowning** is a term used when the person has increased disorientation in the late afternoon, evening, or during the night. Sleeplessness is often accompanied by wandering. The person may go outside and wander several miles in the middle of the night.
- **Sensory-perceptual changes**
  - The person with **sensory-perceptual changes** is unable to recognize an object and use it appropriately. This includes common objects such as eating utensils, combs, and pencils (Figure 30-4). The person is unable to distinguish right from left, up from down, left from right, hot from cold.
- **Perseveration**
  - **Perseveration** refers to repeating an action over and over. Examples are repeating the same word or phrase, lip licking, chewing, or finger tapping.
- **Catastrophic reactions**
  - **Catastrophic reactions** are characterized by increased agitation and anxiety. They may be noted by increased pacing, verbalization, and restlessness or they may result in violent behavior (Figure 30-5).

FIGURE 30-4 Persons with Alzheimer's disease are unable to recognize and use common items appropriately.

FIGURE 30-5 Catastrophic reactions may result in violent behavior.

- **Hallucinations**
  - **Hallucinations** are false perceptions of sensory information (seeing, hearing, smelling) that is not real.
- **Gait difficulties**
  - Walking becomes more difficult. The hips may appear to be internally rotated and a shuffling type gait is present.
- **Aphasia**
  - Problems with verbal communication occur. The person is unable to understand others and is unable to express speech. The person may have perseveration of speech or use words inappropriately. Aphasia also affects the ability to read and to write.
- Bowel and bladder incontinence

Clinical Focus:

Mrs. McGinnis is in stage 2 Alzheimer's disease. Think of specific problems that might occur if she lived alone.

Stage 3

Stage 3 lasts from 8 to 12 years. Almost all persons with stage 3 Alzheimer's disease will be in a long-term care facility. Characteristics of stage 3 include:

- Total dependence for all activities of daily living
- Verbally unresponsive
- Totally incontinent
- Minimal mobility

CARING FOR RESIDENTS WITH DEMENTIA

Caring for a resident with a dementia is challenging, rewarding, and gratifying. Caregivers must be compassionate, patient, and calm and have a sense of humor.

Providing quality care to residents with Alzheimer's disease revolves around the ability of staff members to manage the behaviors of the residents. When caring for residents with

Alzheimer's disease or other dementias, it is helpful to remember:

- Residents with Alzheimer's have the same needs as anyone else—physical needs, the need to feel safe and secure, and a need for love and self-esteem. They are dependent on the caregivers to meet these needs (Figure 30-6).
- All behavior has a reason, even though we may not always know what the reason is.
- Behavior is neither good nor bad—it just is. Avoid using negative terms such as uncooperative, rebellious, or hostile to describe behavior.
- Realize that residents with a dementia are not responsible for what they do or say.
    - Their behavior is not intentional and they cannot change.
    - They are not aware of what they are doing.
    - They lose the ability to control their impulses. They may say or do whatever comes into their minds, whether or not it is appropriate (Figure 30-7).

FIGURE 30-7 People with Alzheimer's disease lose the ability to control their impulses.

- Avoid confrontation. Always allow them to "save face" and not feel belittled or embarrassed.
- Residents with Alzheimer's disease can "read" us. They respond to nonverbal communication. Their behaviors tend to reflect the behaviors of those around them. If staff members are anxious and abrupt, residents will tend to become anxious and agitated.
- Even though both short-term and long-term memory are eventually lost, "affective" memory tends to remain. This means that the resident may not remember certain individuals but will sense feelings of discomfort if that person was unpleasant, rude, or abusive to the resident. This may be reflected in increased verbalization or anxiety or attempts to hit that person.
- If a new behavior occurs, investigate the cause. The resident may have a physical illness or be agitated by the environment.
- Reconsider behaviors. Before attempting to modify a behavior, ask the questions:
    - "Is it interfering with the health or safety of the resident?"
    - "Is it interfering with the health or safety of others?"
    - "Is it infringing on the rights of other residents?"
    - "Is it causing the resident to be anxious or agitated?"

If the answer to these questions is no, then the behavior probably does not need modifying.

- No one really knows what is happening in the minds of people with dementia. Never assume that they are unaware of the environment and the people around them.

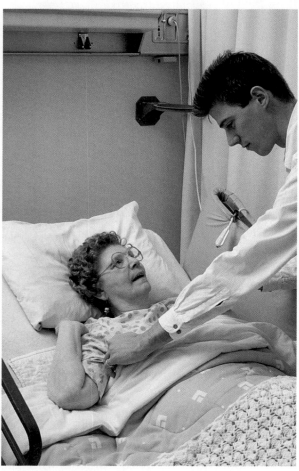

FIGURE 30-6 People with Alzheimer's disease need love and attention.

Goals for Caregiving

Always keep in mind the following goals when caring for residents with Alzheimer's disease or other dementias:

1. Protect the resident from physical injury.
2. Maintain the resident's independence as long as possible.
3. Focus on what the resident is still able to do.
4. Provide physical and mental activities within the resident's capabilities.
5. Support the resident's dignity and self-esteem at all times.

To meet these goals:

1. The care must be consistent. Procedures should be carried out in the same way, all the time. All caregivers should use the same approach.
2. The routine of care should be structured but flexible to accommodate residents when they are more responsive or less responsive.
3. The care must be given in a peaceful, quiet environment that is simple, uncluttered, and unchanged.

4. Staff members must be educated to the needs of the residents with dementia and must learn how to meet these needs.

Alzheimer's Units

Many facilities have established special Alzheimer care units. These units differ from general units in several ways:

- There is a higher staff-to-resident ratio.
- The staff has received special training in Alzheimer's care.
- Cross-training of staff may be done. For example, nursing assistants may help with activities and activity staff or social service staff may help with meals.
- The unit is a "dedicated" unit. This means that the same staff work on the unit all the time. New staff are assigned to the unit only when there is an opening that has to be filled.

This type of staffing results in:

- Staff who have a special interest in Alzheimer's residents.
- Staff who know each resident, their strengths, and their weaknesses.

---

*G*uidelines for

Caring for Residents with Alzheimer's Disease

1. Use eye contact with residents, if culturally appropriate (Figure 30-8).

FIGURE 30-8 Use eye contact, if culturally appropriate.

2. Use appropriate body language.
3. Accept residents as they are without being judgmental or critical.
4. Use touch appropriately. This can be soothing, but if a resident is surprised by the body contact, it can result in a catastrophic reaction.
5. Avoid using logic, "reasoning," or lengthy explanations. This will only increase the resident's agitation.
6. Remember that when the ability to use speech is lost, communication can still occur through nonverbal means.
   - Biting, scratching, and kicking may be the only way the resident can express displeasure.

(continues)

*G*uidelines *(continued)*

FIGURE 30-9 Observe facial expressions and body language for clues to the resident's feelings.

- Facial expressions, body language, and the resident's eyes may give clues to feelings and moods (Figure 30-9).
- Learn what triggers agitation or anger and work on preventing these situations.

7. Use techniques of diversion and distraction. These work well because of the resident's shortened attention span. Calmly take the resident by the hand and walk together or direct the resident's attention to another activity.

8. Remember that the most important qualities for caregivers are to:

FIGURE 30-10 A sense of humor is beneficial for staff and residents.

- Be creative. Be willing to look beyond the usual procedures and routines for solutions to giving care.
- Be able to laugh with the resident (Figure 30-10). Many of them retain a keen sense of humor for a long time. Laughter is beneficial for residents and staff.
- Be able to go back in time with the resident. If the resident is living in 1950, think of what life was like then.

- Staff who better understand the need to facilitate an interdisciplinary support system.
- Staff who can provide valuable input for the plan of care.

The environment is specially designed to:

- Provide calmness and serenity through the use of color and design.

- Avoid disturbing noises. For example, there is no loudspeaker system, telephones do not ring, and televisions are turned on only when appropriate.
- Be secure, so that residents may wander at will without threat of danger.
- Most activities can take place on the unit. The dining room and activities areas are incorporated into the unit.

- Families are encouraged to take part in the care and activities if they wish.

Residents must meet certain pre-established criteria before being admitted to the special unit. This is to ensure that placement will benefit the resident and also the other residents.

Residents' Rights

Residents with dementia have the same rights as other residents. They may need assistance to ensure that these rights are protected. It is important to remember that:

- Making decisions and having choices is a resident's right. However, residents with dementia may be unable to make decisions and may become overwhelmed with too many choices. This can cause the resident to become very upset.
- Staff must protect residents with dementia. Do not allow them to be taken advantage of or abused by other people.
- The rights of residents with dementia do not have priority over the rights of other residents. For example, it is upsetting to other residents to have confused residents wandering into their rooms. The resident with dementia is not aware of this. It is the staff's responsibility to

FIGURE 30-11 Always treat the resident with dignity.

resolve these issues without infringing on the rights of either resident.

- Residents with dementia have the right to have possessions that give them pleasure as long as these do not impair the health or safety of the resident or other people. For example, if a resident receives pleasure from a doll or stuffed animal, do not take it away. Above all, do not tease or make fun of the situation. The resident deserves to be treated with dignity (Figure 30-11).

*G*uidelines for

Activities of Daily Living

1. Allow the resident to do as much as possible.
   - Use hand-over-hand techniques for personal care and eating.
   - Give only one short, simple direction at a time.
2. Assist the resident to maintain a dignified, attractive appearance by helping with grooming, dressing, and hygiene. Residents may be unaware of soiled or torn clothing.
   - Help them change when necessary.
   - Pick out clothing for the resident or hold out two outfits for the resident to choose from. Residents with a dementia are unable to make decisions. If you ask the resident, "What do you want to wear today?" the resident may become agitated. She cannot remember what is in her closet. Showing the resident all

of the clothing is overwhelming and will also cause agitation.

3. Residents with dementia may not want to bathe.
   - Consider the resident's previous habits. Did the resident prefer a tub bath or shower? How often did the resident bathe? Was bathing done in the morning or evening?
   - Check the environment. Is the room warm enough? Is it light enough? Is there adequate privacy?
   - Do not ask the resident "Do you want to take a bath now?" The resident may say no every time you ask. Calmly walk with the resident to the bathroom. When you get there say, "I am going to help you with your bath now" and begin

(continues)

Guidelines *(continued)*

the bath procedure calmly and slowly. If the resident refuses, try again later.

- Do not attempt to remove the resident's clothes right away. Many residents feel unsafe when they are nude. When the resident realizes he is going to get wet, he will usually be willing to undress.

4. Monitor food and fluid intake.

- Too many foods at once are confusing.
- Place one food at a time in front of the resident.
- Do not use plastic utensils that can break in the resident's mouth.
- Provide nutritious finger foods when the resident is unable to use utensils.
- Avoid pureed foods as long as possible.
- Check food temperatures before serving.
- Prepare foods for eating by buttering the bread, cutting meat, opening cartons.
- If you are feeding the resident, watch for swallowing. Sometimes they will appear to be chewing long after they have swallowed (perseveration).
- Check the resident's mouth after eating. Squirreling food in the mouth can cause

aspiration (the food goes into the trachea or windpipe).

- Maintain adequate fluid intake. Residents with dementia may not realize when they are thirsty.
- Weigh the resident regularly to detect patterns of weight gain or loss.
- Maintain a quiet and calm environment for eating.

5. Residents with dementia eventually lose bowel and bladder control. Taking residents to the bathroom every 2 hours keeps them dry and prevents skin breakdown. For successful toileting:

- Toilet regularly.
- Evaluate wandering and pacing behavior for possible need to toilet.
- Provide privacy.
- Make sure the bathroom is warm, quiet, and calm.
- Allow the resident ample time to eliminate urine or stool.
- Provide comfort. A commode may work better than the toilet.
- Praise success.

Family Members

In most cases, family members have cared for the resident with a dementia for months or years prior to admission to the long-term care facility. By the time the decision is made to admit the individual, the family is often physically and emotionally drained. The admission is a traumatic experience. As you work with the residents with Alzheimer's or other dementias, remember:

1. The family remembers the resident as a vital family member. Acknowledge the family's presence.
2. The spouse of the resident may have no other support system. If they have children, they may be many miles away. It can be very upsetting not to be recognized by a spouse of many years. Some facilities have support groups for families.

3. Listen to the family's suggestions. They often know what will work and what will not be effective in caring for the new resident.
4. Allow the family to participate in the care, if they choose to and if it is appropriate. For example, many family members like to assist the resident at mealtime.

Recreational Activities

Residents with dementia need activities that match their level of ability.

- Avoid large groups or competitive activities.
- In later stages, use sensory stimulation with soft touching, quiet talk, familiar odors, or old time pictures.
- Puppies or kittens (**pet therapy**) bring pleasure to severely impaired residents.
- Activities with children may also be satisfying to the residents with dementia.

- Music is an appropriate activity. Residents with dementia respond to soft music from their past. Many of them like to dance. Old hymns are also a favorite.
- "Normalizing" activities are beneficial. Consider the resident's past and provide opportunities for:
  - Folding towels and washcloths
  - Dusting
  - A hand craft such as knitting (Figure 30-12)
  - Baking (with supervision)
  - Using a manual carpet sweeper
  - "Tinkering" with familiar tools (with supervision)

Daily exercise must be planned according to the resident's habits and abilities (Figure 30-13).

- The resident who wanders or paces throughout the day may need only range of motion exercises.
- Residents in the final stage will need passive range of motion exercises at least twice a day.
- Many recreational activities can be directed to the abilities of the resident:
  - Shooting baskets
  - Bowling

FIGURE 30-13 Daily exercise is important.

  - Volleyball
  - Hitting a ball with a bat

Community outings may also be enjoyable. Plan outings carefully and be sure that:

- There will be no excessive sensory stimulation. This will agitate many of the residents.
- The residents will not be fearful of wide, open spaces.
- Public places can accommodate residents with mobility problems.
- The residents will not be mistreated by others if they exhibit unusual behaviors in public.

SPECIAL PROBLEMS

Wandering and Pacing

Residents with Alzheimer's disease may wander or pace for hours at a time. No one knows why this occurs. Some reasons may be:

- They are looking for companionship, security, or loved ones.
- It is a way to handle stress.
- They realize they are in a strange environment and are looking for home.

When this behavior occurs:

1. Allow them to wander. The use of restraints increases their anxiety and frustration, resulting in other problems.
2. Adapt the environment to the residents, making it safe and secure. There are many

FIGURE 30-12 Familiar tasks bring enjoyment.

types of security systems available. Getting lost, rather than falling, may be a problem. When the resident walks off, walk with the resident, gradually returning to the direction of the facility.

3. Watch wandering residents for signs of fatigue. They may have forgotten how to sit down and will need reminders and demonstrations of how to get into the chair or bed.

4. Special chairs for residents with Alzheimer's disease allow the residents to rock without tipping over. A tray table top keeps residents secure and can be used for hand activities.

5. Nutritional needs increase with wandering. Additional food intake may be necessary.

Agitation, Anxiety, and Catastrophic Reactions

Agitation and anxiety are shown by an increase in physical activity such as pacing or perseveration. If appropriate actions are not taken in time, a catastrophic reaction is likely to occur. This is noted by any or all of the following:

• Increased physical activity
• Increased talking or mumbling
• Explosive behavior with physical violence

Not all catastrophic reactions are dramatic or violent. However, if not dealt with appropriately, the reaction may grow. To avoid catastrophic reactions:

1. Monitor behavior closely.
2. Watch for signs of increasing agitation.
3. Check to see if the resident:
   • Is hungry
   • Needs to go to the bathroom
   • Is too hot or too cold
   • Is overtired or in pain
   • Has signs of physical illness

4. Check the environment for:
   • Too much noise
   • Too many people
   • Staff anxiety
   • Television programs—people with dementia cannot distinguish fiction from reality.

5. People with dementia may not be able to make decisions. The simple question, "What do you want to wear today?" may be more than they can handle.

When agitation or catastrophic reactions occur:

1. Do not use physical restraints or force to subdue the resident. This increases agitation and can result in injury to the resident and caregivers.

2. Avoid having several staff members approach the resident at the same time. This is frightening to the resident.

3. Use a soft, calm voice. Do not try to reason with the resident. Using touch may or may not be appropriate. Some residents respond in a positive manner to the smooth stroking of the arm or back. Others may react violently if they are already agitated.

Sundowning

Sundowning means the resident has increased confusion and restlessness in the late afternoon, evening, or during the night. It may be prevented by avoiding too much activity before bedtime and by establishing a consistent bedtime routine.

1. Overfatigue may cause sundowning. Encourage the resident to nap or rest in the early afternoon for a short time.

2. Discourage the resident from sleeping too much during the day.

3. The evening meal should be eaten at least 2 hours before bedtime. Eliminate caffeine from the diet.

4. Involve the resident in quiet evening activities with a caregiver or family member.

5. At bedtime, provide a light snack that is easily chewed and digested.

6. Take the resident to the bathroom just before bedtime. Allow enough time for bladder and bowel elimination.

7. Give a slow back massage if resident accepts touch.

8. Check with family members and continue established habits such as wearing socks to bed, using two pillows, or having a nightlight.

9. Check the lighting of the room. Shadows and reflections may be disturbing.

10. If the resident wakes up during the night, repeat the bedtime routine. If this is ineffective and the resident does not remain in bed, try a recliner or Alzheimer's chair (Figure 30-14). The resident may like to sit by the nurses' station.

Delusions and Hallucinations

Delusions are fixed, false beliefs. Never argue with a resident about a delusion. This will increase the agitation and probably cause a catastrophic reaction. If the delusion is not bothering the resident, let it be. For example: A resi-

FIGURE 30-14 A recliner may be useful for a resident with sundowning.

dent tells you, "I have to take care of my babies now," and is not agitated. She may be reliving a happier, more satisfying time in her life. If the delusion is causing the resident to be anxious, then you must try to assure the resident that you will keep the resident safe.

Follow the same approach with hallucinations.

Pillaging and Hoarding

This does not present a major problem unless residents collect items from other residents' rooms (pillaging), or they hide things that are difficult to find (hoarding).

1. Label all residents' belongings.
2. If a missing item is located, note where it was found. It is likely that the resident will choose the same hiding place the next time.
3. Check the room daily for food.
4. Keep the resident's hands busy. Activities like folding washcloths or "fiddling" with keys on a ring may help.
5. Provide a "rummaging" drawer or box for the resident.

SPECIAL MANAGEMENT TECHNIQUES

Reality Orientation

Reality orientation (RO) is used for helping disoriented residents remain oriented to the environment, to time, and to themselves. When used appropriately, it decreases anxiety in the resident. RO may be effective in the first stages of dementia. In later stages, it is meaningless and increases agitation. Follow these basic guidelines for RO:

1. Always treat residents as adults, with respect and dignity, no matter how confused they may be.
2. Speak clearly and directly. Avoid the temptation to speak louder when they do not understand.
3. Give simple, brief instructions and responses.
4. Set and maintain a structured, flexible routine.
5. Be polite and sincere.
6. Allow residents to be independent as long as possible.
7. Give residents adequate time to respond.
8. Set residents' watches to the correct time.
9. Make sure they have clean eyeglasses and hearing aids if they need them.
10. Place large-numbered calendars in rooms and cross off the days as they pass.
11. Placement of large-numbered clocks around the facility helps orient residents to the time of day.
12. Call residents by name. Disoriented residents usually respond more quickly to their first names.
13. Tell residents your name, but do not expect them to remember you.
14. Use RO in conversation with residents—"It's only March fifth today, but it is very warm outside."

When using RO:

1. Do not put residents on the spot. For example, do not ask, "Do you remember who I am?" or "Do you know what day this is?" If you need to verify their orientation, ask them, "What are your plans for today?" The answer usually will tell you if the resident is oriented.
2. Answer questions honestly but avoid giving the residents information they are unable to handle. A resident whose husband is deceased may ask, "Is my husband coming today?" It is cruel to answer by saying, "Remember, your husband died 2 years ago." This response is likely to trigger a catastrophic reaction. It is better to answer by asking another question: "Emma, will you tell me about your husband?" She will receive pleasure from reminiscing and may work up to the present time on her own.
3. Never argue with a resident's reality. When a resident has a delusion, arguing increases anxiety and agitation. Many delusions are based on past life experiences. Because the

resident is disoriented, the experience seems to be happening in the present. Some residents may be much happier if they are living in the past. If this is true, do not force reality on them.

4. Residents with some forms of dementia may have moments of orientation from time to time. Do not assume the resident is disoriented because you do not understand what the resident is saying.

5. Do not reinforce the resident's confusion or tease the resident about the confusion.

6. Remember that a pleasant facial expression, relaxed body language, and caring touch are the most important aspects of caring for disoriented residents.

Reminiscing

Reminiscing is a natural activity for people of all ages. We tend to reminisce when we see old friends or get together with families.

1. Pleasant times from the past are remembered and enjoyed.

2. As people age, the tendency to reminisce increases and is more important.

3. It is an appropriate activity for residents in early stages of dementia if long-term memory is still intact.

4. Reminiscing may serve as a life review as past life experiences are remembered. This process can also bring back unpleasant memories. If this occurs, the situation must be handled skillfully and tactfully. If these experiences are resolved, peace of mind can be found. The recall of happy memories can confirm the worth and value of the individual's life (Figure 30-15).

5. Reminiscing can help people adapt to old age. It helps to maintain self-esteem and allows them to work through personal losses.

6. When we listen to residents reminisce, we understand them better.

7. Reminiscing therapy can be a group activity. The leader must be skillful and sensitive to the feelings of the members.

FIGURE 30-15 Reminiscing can help recall happy times.

Validation Therapy

Validation therapy was developed by Naomi Feil. It is based on the following assumptions:

1. The identity and dignity of the residents must be maintained.

2. We can help disoriented people with dementia feel good about themselves.

3. There is a reason for all behavior. What seems like disoriented behavior may be an acting out of memories.

4. Feelings and memories can be acknowledged.

5. Disoriented people have the right to express feelings when they are no longer able to be oriented to reality.

6. Living must be resolved to prepare for dying.

7. Elderly persons may have experienced so many losses during a lifetime that they have no coping abilities left.

8. To live in reality is not the only way to live.

9. Disoriented people have worth. We can give them joy by allowing them to express themselves.

10. Within each disoriented person is a human being who was once a child and later an adult with hopes, joys, sadness, failures, and successes. They deserve to be cared for and loved in their final years.

LESSON SYNTHESIS: Putting It All Together

You have just completed this lesson. Now go back and review the Clinical Focus. Try to see how the Clinical Focus relates to the concepts presented in the lesson. Then answer the following questions.

1. Why do people think of Alzheimer's disease as a "slow death"?

2. Why do the families of residents with Alzheimer's disease need special understanding and support?

3. Because Mrs. McGinnis is in stage 2, what special safety precautions must be observed?

4. What special characteristics are needed in a nursing assistant who cares for residents suffering from Alzheimer's disease?

REVIEW

A. Select the one best answer for each of the following.

1. Alzheimer's disease is
   (A) curable
   (B) preventable
   (C) progressive
   (D) congenital

2. Alzheimer's disease is more common in
   (A) young people
   (B) older people
   (C) middle-aged people
   (D) the white race

3. One of the first symptoms of Alzheimer's disease is
   (A) short-term memory loss
   (B) long-term memory loss
   (C) aphasia
   (D) sundowning

4. Delusions are
   (A) false perceptions of sensory information
   (B) an example of sensory-perceptual changes
   (C) false, fixed ideas
   (D) the result of catastrophic reactions

5. Goals for giving care to residents with Alzheimer's include all but
   (A) protecting the resident from physical injury

   (B) maintaining the resident's independence as long as possible
   (C) focusing on what the resident can do
   (D) limiting activities for saftey reasons

B. Answer each statement true (T) or false (F).

6. T F There are many types of dementia.

7. T F There is no specific test for diagnosing Alzheimer's disease.

8. T F Alzheimer's disease is the result of poor circulation in the brain.

9. T F Residents who wander should be restrained.

10. T F Catastrophic reactions may result from too much stimulation in the environment.

11. T F Residents with Alzheimer's disease are unable to feel emotion.

12. T F Residents with Alzheimer's disease frequently exhibit bad behavior.

13. T F The best way to manage behavior is to use logic to reason with the resident.

14. T F Many residents with Alzheimer's disease have a keen sense of humor.

15. T F Reminiscing is healthy and beneficial.

16. T F Residents' rights do not apply to residents with Alzheimer's disease.

17. T F A dignified, attractive appearance is important for residents with Alzheimer's disease.

18. T F Residents with Alzheimer's disease enjoy large group activities.

19. T F Baking is an example of a "normalizing" activity.

20. T F Some residents are happier if they are living in the past.

Caring for Residents with Developmental Disabilities

Clinical Focus

Think about the special care needs of the resident who is developmentally disabled as you study this lesson and meet:

*T*eresa Michaels, who is developmentally disabled and unable to care for herself. Her mind is bright and keen. She is unable to use her hands for self-care because of the spastic paralysis related to her cerebral palsy.

OBJECTIVES

After studying this lesson, you should be able to:

- Define and spell vocabulary words and terms.
- List the characteristics present in a developmental disability.
- List four examples of developmental disabilities.
- Describe three possible causes of a developmental disability.
- Define the classifications of mental retardation.
- Describe different types of seizures.

VOCABULARY

adaptive behavior *(ah-**DAP**-tiv bee-**HAYV**-yur)*

anoxia *(ah-**NOX**-ee-ah)*

ataxic cerebral palsy *(ah-**TACK**-sick **SER**-eh-bral **PAWL**-zee)*

athetoid cerebral palsy *(**ATH**-eh-toyd*

***SER**-eh-bral **PAWL**-zee)*

behavior modification *(bee-**HAYV**-yur mod-ih-fih-**KAY**-shun)*

cerebral palsy *(**SER**-eh-bral **PAWL**-zee)*

developmental disability *(dee-**vel**-op-**MEN**-tal dis-ah-**BILL**-ih-tee)*

VOCABULARY

diplegia   (die-**PLEE**-jee-ah)

electroencephalogram (EEG)   (ee-**leck**-troh-en-**SEF**-ah-loh-gram)

epilepsy   (**EP**-ih-**lep**-see)

grand mal seizure   (grand mahl **SEE**-zhur)

hemiplegia   (**hem**-ee-**PLEE**-jee-ah)

intelligence quotient (IQ)   (in-**TELL**-ih-jens **KWOH**-shent)

mental retardation   (**MEN**-tal **ree**-tar-**DAY**-shun)

petit mal seizure   (peh-**TEE** mahl **SEE**-zhur)

quadriplegia   (**kwahd**-rih-**PLEE**-jee-ah)

seizure   (**SEE**-zhur)

spastic cerebral palsy   (**SPAS**-tick **SER**-eh-bral **PAWL**-zee)

CHARACTERISTICS OF A DEVELOPMENTAL DISABILITY

Long-term care facilities often provide care for residents with developmental disabilities. A **developmental disability** has specific characteristics. It is:

- Caused by a mental or physical impairment or a combination of both
- Apparent before 22 years of age (some states indicate before 18 years of age)
- Likely to continue indefinitely

In addition, the disability must result in functional limitations in three or more of these life activities:

- Self-care
- Use of receptive and expressive language
- Learning
- Mobility
- Self-direction
- Independent living
- Economic self-sufficiency

Because of these limitations, the person who is developmentally disabled requires lifelong care, treatment, or services (Figure 31-1).

Some residents in your facility who have developmental disabilities did not acquire these as adults. Federal legislation forbids the admission of persons with developmental disabilities to skilled nursing facilities unless the facilities are licensed to care for them. However, there may be residents who were in the facility before this law was implemented. They may also be admitted if they have another medical problem that requires skilled nursing care.

A developmental disability may be caused by:

- A condition that impairs the development of the brain or body before birth (Figure 31-2)

FIGURE 31-1 The resident on the right has needed assistance with activities of daily living throughout his life.

- A condition that causes damage to the newborn infant during the birth process
- A disease or injury that causes damage to the brain or body after birth, before the age of 22 years, or the age specified by state regulations

At one time, people with developmental disabilities often died before reaching adulthood. Today they frequently live a normal life span. During childhood they go to school and attend classes that meet their needs and abilities. After graduating, they may work in a sheltered workshop or obtain a job that they are capable of doing. They may be able to live independently with assistance or in supervised group homes. Some people with milder disabilities may marry and have children.

People with developmental disabilities also experience the aging process. Sometimes the changes of aging combined with the disability make it increasingly difficult for them to function.

FIGURE 31-2 This child with phocomelia has no hands because a drug taken by his mother during early pregnancy interfered with limb development. (Courtesy of the March of Dimes Birth Defects Foundation)

Of the many types of developmental disabilities, some affect physical function, some affect mental function, and some affect both. Persons with mental retardation are developmentally disabled. However, not all persons who are developmentally disabled are mentally retarded (Figure 31-3).

FIGURE 31-3 This man is developmentally disabled but is not mentally impaired.

MENTAL RETARDATION

Children and adults with mental retardation are limited in their ability to learn. They are generally socially immature and sometimes have special emotional and physical needs. **Mental retardation** is a condition that occurs before age 22 and refers to significantly below average mental function. In addition, deficits in adaptive behavior exist. **Adaptive behavior** is the degree to which the person meets standards of personal independence and social responsibility appropriate for the person's age and culture. These standards apply to:

- Physical self-care
- Communication skills
- Social skills
- Economic abilities
- Holding a job
- Capability for self-direction

Causes of Mental Retardation

Some disorders in which mental retardation may be present are:

- Down syndrome (a chromosomal disorder)
- Cerebral palsy (not all people with cerebral palsy are mentally retarded)

FIGURE 31-4 Classification of levels of impairment

Characteristic	Mild	Moderate	Severe	Profound
IQ	52–67	36–51	20–35	Less than 20
Development	Slow	Slow	Motor development, speech, and language are impaired.	All areas of development are impaired.
Potential	Educable within limits; can be trained in social and vocational skills. Needs support under stress.	Can be taught ADLs. Needs sheltered environment and support.	Often physically challenged. May assist with self-care. Needs controlled environment and supervision.	Constant care and supervision required for survival.

• Phenylketonuria (PKU)—a metabolic disorder present at birth

Mental retardation may also be caused by:

• Environmental influences such as poor nutrition
• Lack of oxygen (**anoxia**) before, during, or after birth
• Complications of diseases during childhood such as encephalitis or meningitis
• Premature birth (lack of developmental maturity)

Testing for Level of Impairment

People with mental retardation do not all have the same degree of disability. Screening tests may be performed during infancy if a delay in development is noted. Later, **intelligence quotient (IQ)** tests can be given. Intelligence includes the:

• Ability to solve problems appropriate to one's age
• Ability to adapt appropriately to the demands of environment
• Ability to understand abstract relationships

The results of the IQ test alone do not confirm the absence or presence of mental retardation. Intelligence is not constant. It is variable and influenced by emotions and the environment. IQ tests are considered along with other test results.

An Adaptive Behavior Scale measures a person's behaviors as they relate to activities of daily living, self-help skills, physical and social development, language ability, and time and number concepts. The scale also examines inappropriate behaviors such as violence and self-abuse. The results are compared to the expected behavior of people of the same chronological age.

Diagnosis and evaluation should be conducted by an interdisciplinary team of specialists in the field. The IQ level used for classification varies somewhat with the test being used. Usually, mental retardation is classified as:

• mild retardation: IQ = 52–67
• moderate retardation: IQ = 36–51
• severe retardation: IQ = 20–35
• profound retardation: IQ = less than 20

Most persons with mental retardation are mildly retarded and demonstrate the following potentials to varying degrees:

• children educable within limits
• adults with training can achieve vocational and social skills for minimal stress

The lower the IQ, the less potential exists and the more support and care are needed. Those with profound retardation require constant care and supervision.

Refer to Figure 31-4 for a classification of the levels of impairment.

Many services are available to meet the needs of persons with mental retardation. Children can benefit from special education and training. A program that is started early and is consistent is most effective in meeting their special needs and helping them to enjoy a good quality of life. Remember that individuals with mental retardation have all the needs of another person of the same chronological age. They need affection, discipline, and acceptance just as all humans do. They are less able, however, to handle rejection or confusion or the demands of too high expectations.

Families, too, need support and empathy because they may be dealing with personal feelings of guilt and frustration.

If people with mental retardation are living in your facility, the care you give depends on the:

- Specific problems of the individual
- Age of the individual
- Degree of retardation
- Presence of other physical problems

Even the most profoundly retarded person responds favorably to:

- Pleasant, colorful, personalized surroundings
- The healing and comforting effect of caring persons

OTHER FORMS OF DEVELOPMENTAL DISABILITIES

Cerebral Palsy

Cerebral palsy describes a large group of movement disorders of varying symptoms and severity. *Cerebral* refers to the brain and *palsy* means disorder of movement. Figure 31-5 lists several causes of cerebral palsy. These include damage to the baby before, during, or after birth that result in damage to the nervous system.

A person with mild cerebral palsy may be only a little awkward with movements but otherwise mentally and physically capable. A person with more severe cerebral palsy may be mentally retarded, subject to seizures, or physically challenged. Several terms describe the movement disturbance and effect on the limbs, as follows:

- **Diplegia**
  - The legs are primarily affected.
- **Hemiplegia**
  - Both the arm and leg on one side are affected.
- **Quadriplegia**
  - Both arms and both legs are affected.
- **Spastic cerebral palsy**
  - The muscles are tense, contracted, resistant to movement.
  - The lower legs may turn in and cross at the ankle.

FIGURE 31-5 Causes of cerebral palsy
• Cerebral anoxia
• Hemorrhage
• Maternal infection
• Cord around infant's neck
• Meningitis
• Difficult delivery

- The movements of the legs are stiff and resemble the crossed blades of a pair of scissors (scissors gait).
- **Athetoid cerebral palsy**
  - Involuntary, slow, and incessant movements (athetosis) of the parts of the body that are affected.
  - Facial grimacing and drooling may be present.
- **Ataxic cerebral palsy**
  - The principal movement disturbance is a lack of balance and coordination (ataxia).

In some cases, symptoms of each type of palsy may be mixed. Persons with cerebral palsy may also have problems in speaking, chewing, and swallowing. They may be unable to focus their eyes. Drooling and loss of bowel or bladder control also occur.

Caring for the Resident with Cerebral Palsy. Care may include:

- Assisting with transport to special education classes
- Caring for and applying splints and braces
- Performing range of motion exercises
- Providing emotional support
- Assisting with activities of daily living

Other problems associated with cerebral palsy are seizure disorders, mental or emotional impairment, hearing loss, and visual handicaps.

Seizure Disorder (Epilepsy)

Epilepsy may be considered a developmental disability if it meets the criteria described at the beginning of this lesson. It is not a disease with a single cause. It is a set of symptoms that arise from abnormal nerve cell activity in the brain. Normally, the nerve cells (neurons) generate small bursts of electrical impulses. These impulses move between neurons, communicating with muscles, sense organs, and glands. In

FIGURE 31-6 Some causes of seizures

- Neoplasms
- Trauma
- Cerebral anoxia
- Metabolic imbalances
- Congenital malformations
- High temperature

epilepsy, the nerve cell activity is disturbed. This may result in a **seizure** (convulsion). The type of seizure that occurs depends on the part of the brain that is affected by the disrupted nerve cell activity. Some causes of seizures are listed in Figure 31-6.

Partial or generalized seizures may occur. Partial seizures are classified as follows. For each type, the general symptoms are listed:

1. Simple partial (sensory type) seizure
   - Feelings are distorted
   - Seeing flashing lights, hallucinations
   - Smelling foul odors
   - Dizziness
   - Tingling sensations
2. Simple partial (jacksonian motor type) seizure
   - Localized motor seizure
   - Tingling, jerking in one extremity
   - No loss of consciousness
   - May progress to generalized tonic-clonic convulsions
3. Complex partial (psychomotor or temporal lobe) seizure
   - Signs and symptoms vary
   - Purposeless behavior such as chewing movements and uncontrolled speech
   - Glassy stare
   - Aimless wandering
   - Mental confusion
   - Loss of memory following episode
4. Secondary generalized partial seizure
   - Either simple or complex
   - May experience an aura
   - Immediate loss of consciousness

Generalized seizures are classified as follows, with general symptoms listed:

1. Generalized tonic-clonic seizure (**grand mal seizure**) (Figure 31-7)

FIGURE 31-7 Generalized seizures may be accompanied by: A. Rigid posturing. B. Uncontrolled movements.

- Early changes in sensation (aura)
- Entire body involved
- Sudden cry
- Loss of consciousness
- Involuntary contraction of the muscles producing contortions of body and limbs
- Saliva forms around the mouth causing the appearance of "foaming at the mouth"
- Incontinence of bowel or bladder or both may occur during the seizure
- Person generally sleeps after the seizure
- Lasts 2 to 5 minutes

2. Absence seizure (**petit mal seizure**)

- No convulsion
- Occurs most often in children without warning
- Lasts 1 to 10 seconds
- Vacant facial expression, staring eyes
- No recall of episode

3. Myoclonic seizure

- Brief involuntary jerking movements of body and extremities
- Convulsions may occur in rhythmic waves.
- No loss of consciousness

4. Akinetic seizure

- Uncommon
- General loss of postural tone may cause resident to "drop" to the floor.
- Temporary loss of consciousness
- Lasts 1 to 2 minutes

When seizure activity occurs so frequently that consciousness is not gained between seizures, it is called status epilepticus.

In some people, epilepsy begins during adulthood. This may be the result of:

- An accident causing brain injury
- Brain tumor
- Stroke
- Dementia

The diagnosis of epilepsy is made by performing an **electroencephalogram (EEG)**. A computed tomography (CT) scan or magnetic resonance imaging (MRI) is also performed during the EEG. Electrodes are attached to the scalp to record the brain's electrical activity. The test can determine the presence and type of seizures. The test is painless. The CT scan and MRI permit visualization of the brain structures.

Many medications are able to control seizures. Sometimes the medication dosage has to be readjusted.

Care of the resident who is experiencing a seizure is covered in Lesson 9.

CARING FOR RESIDENTS WITH DEVELOPMENTAL DISABILITIES

Residents with developmental disabilities may be placed in a long-term care facility for the following reasons:

- The resident may have lived in a facility most of his or her life because family members were not able to provide care.
- The resident may have been admitted as an adult to the facility when the parent(s) became elderly or died (before federal laws were changed).
- The resident may have a medical problem that cannot be treated in the resident's home.

Young adult residents are often admitted for medical problems. Their parents may have devoted all their energies to the lifelong care of their child. It is difficult in these situations for the parents to "turn over" the care of the resident to staff members. It is important to:

- Acknowledge that the parents have learned much about how to care for their child in the years they have provided care.
- Listen to the parents' suggestions and their concerns.
- Answer their questions.
- Allow the parents to participate in the care as much as possible and as much as they wish.

In some cases, the resident may be admitted after one parent has died and the other is no longer able to provide total care. In these situations, the remaining parent may be suffering from guilt for placing the child in the facility. Feelings of anger at the deceased spouse may exist for "leaving" them with this problem. Attempt to understand what the parent is going through. Be kind, considerate, and nonjudgmental.

The care you give depends on the types of problems experienced by the residents with developmental disabilities. These residents are at risk for many physical complications:

- Respiratory tract infections
- Urinary tract infections
- Contractures
- Pressure ulcers

You must study the care plan to learn exactly what approach and procedures you must use.

Physical therapy and occupational therapy may be a part of the plan of care (Figure 31-8).

You may have residents who go out of the facility every day to attend a sheltered workshop. These workshops:

- Train persons with a developmental disability to acquire job skills within their abilities

FIGURE 31-8 Residents with developmental disabilities may need physical therapy.

- Train persons with developmental disabilities to get around in the community by adapting their abilities to the situation
- Provide opportunities for socializing with other people of the same age

Behavior problems may occur. **Behavior modification** is an approach to overcoming these problems that is based on:

- Rewarding positive behaviors
- Initiating corrective actions for negative behaviors

The care plan provides specific approaches and directions regarding the use of behavior modification. Behavior modification will succeed only if all staff members are consistent and follow the plan exactly as it is written.

Persons with developmental disabilities have the same physical and emotional needs as everyone else. When they are in the long-term care facility, it is the responsibility of the staff to provide for these needs so that persons with developmental disabilities will enjoy a life of quality.

LESSON SYNTHESIS: Putting It All Together

*Y*ou *have just completed this lesson. Now go back and review the Clinical Focus. Try to see how the Clinical Focus relates to the concepts presented in the lesson. Then answer the following questions.*

1. How do you think Teresa's disability affects the way people view her until they get to talk with her and know her?

2. Do all people with cerebral palsy have a low IQ?

3. What parts of Teresa's body are affected by her condition?

4. How are Teresa's special needs being met?

REVIEW

A. Fill in the blanks by selecting the correct word or phrase from the list.

cerebral palsy
developmental
  disability
diplegia

hemiplegia
mental
  retardation
twenty-two

1. A severe, chronic disorder present before the age of _____ best describes a _____.

2. When a person has mental function that is significantly below average, with deficits in adaptive behavior, he is said to have _____.

3. A person with mild _____ may be only a little awkward with movements but otherwise be mentally and physically capable.

4. _____ describes the fact that the legs of a person with cerebral palsy are affected.

5. A person with cerebral palsy whose arm and leg on one side are affected has _____.

B. Provide brief answers for each of the following.

6. List three characteristics a disorder must have to be classified as a developmental disability.

7. List seven functional limitations, three of which must be present in addition to those characteristics listed in question 6.

8. Name three possible causes of developmental disabilities.

9. Name four examples of developmental disabilities.

10. List the IQ values for each level of mental retardation: mild, moderate, severe, profound.

11. Describe five activities that may occur during a grand mal seizure.

C. Select the one best answer for each of the following.

12. Children and adults with mental retardation are
   (A) socially mature
   (B) emotionally secure
   (C) persons over 25 years of age when the disability developed
   (D) limited in their ability to learn

13. Mental retardation is not associated with
   (A) Down syndrome
   (B) phenylketonuria
   (C) premature birth
   (D) normal physical development

14. A person with mild mental retardation
   (A) has an IQ of 52 to 67
   (B) requires constant care and attention
   (C) is always physically challenged
   (D) is not able to be educated

15. During a generalized tonic-clonic seizure, the resident
   (A) loses consciousness
   (B) remains conscious
   (C) may wander aimlessly
   (D) remembers the event clearly

D. Clinical Experience

16. Rachel is 37, has spastic paralysis, and an IQ of 20. She has been a resident in your facility since her mother died. Her father visits infrequently and seems very upset when he sees her. What can you do to help reduce his stress?

17. Lea is a teenage girl who is acting out her frustration with the staff who are following the care plan. The team decides that a behavior modification approach is the way to handle the situation. On what principles is this approach based?

18. Brett is 14 and recently admitted to your facility. His mother, his primary caregiver, died and his father is unable to provide care. Brett was injured when hit by a car 11 years ago. What can you do to ease the anxiety expressed by Brett's father?

Caring for the Dying Resident

Clinical Focus
Think about the very special sensitivity the nursing assistant needs as he or she assists residents and their families during the period when death is drawing near as you study this lesson and meet:

*E*rnie Sperling and his family. Mr. Sperling, a Roman Catholic, suffers from terminal cancer. His malignancy originated in his prostate gland and quickly spread throughout his pelvis and into his vertebral column. Despite surgery, radiation, and a course of chemotherapy, the progress of the disease could not be stopped. Mrs. Sperling had been separated from her husband for several years, but since his illness has visited him regularly. Mr. Sperling is often angry and uncooperative with the staff and his wife.

OBJECTIVES
After studying this lesson, you should be able to:

- Define and spell vocabulary words and terms.
- Describe hospice and hospice care.
- Define a terminal diagnosis.
- Identify the stages of grieving as described by Elizabeth Kübler-Ross.
- Describe how different people handle the death/dying process.
- Respect the resident's cultural and religious practices during the dying process.
- Recognize at least five signs of approaching death.
- Demonstrate the following:
  Procedure 108 Giving Postmortem Care

VOCABULARY

acceptance   *(ack-**SEP**-tans)*

anger   *(**AYN**-ger)*

bargaining   *(**BAR**-gan-ing)*

code blue   *(kohd bloo)*

comatose   *(**KOH**-mah-tohs)*

denial   *(dih-**NIGH**-al)*

depression   *(dee-**PRESH**-shun)*

hospice   *(**HAHS**-piss)*

last rites   *(last rights)*

moribund   *(**MOR**-ih-bund)*

mottling   *(**MOT**-ling)*

no-code order   *(know-kohd **OR**-der)*

palliative   *(**PAL**-ee-uh-tihv)*

postmortem   *(post-**MOR**-tem)*

postmortem care   *(post-**MOR**-tem kair)*

resuscitation   *(ree-**sus**-eh-**TAY**-shun)*

rigor mortis   *(**RIH**-gor **MOR**-tis)*

Sacrament of the Sick   *(**SACK**-rah-ment of the sick)*

terminal illness   *(**TER**-mih-nal **ILL**-ness)*

INTRODUCTION

Death is a universal experience that we all share, yet we find it very difficult to talk about it or even to think about its possiblity for ourselves or those we know or love. Our attitudes toward death and dying are influenced by our culture, religion, experience, age, and the support systems we have available to us. The grieving process and how to cope with death and dying are learned through experience.

Young children before the age of five years may see death as a punishment. By the age of seven, children know that death is final, although they do not believe that they themselves will die. They may also associate death with punishment and body mutilation. Adults have more fears related to pain, suffering, and invasion of their privacy and final abandonment. They also fear the loss of relationships and experience concerns about the welfare of those who will be left behind. Older people, for the most part, have fewer fears. They may even look forward to release from pain and to joining those who have gone on before (if that is part of their belief system).

The residents you care for may live in the long-term care facility for several months or years. As you get to know them, you may develop special relationships and friendships. Losing a friend through death is a sad experience.

Death, however, is a universal experience. As a nursing assistant in long-term care, you will often work with dying residents and their families. For the elderly with significant health problems, death is not unexpected. The death of younger residents may be more difficult to accept because they are closer in age to the caregivers. It is especially difficult when a young child dies.

The role you play in providing care to dying residents is important and one you can perform with dignity.

Death occurs in various ways:

- A resident may be unresponsive for a long time before dying.
- Some residents develop an acute illness and are unable to recover and die suddenly.
- Others die quietly in their sleep.

HOSPICE CARE

Hospice care is given to persons with a **terminal** (life-ending) **illness**, usually with a life expectancy of six months or less. This time is variable because no one can accurately predict the exact time of death.

The care may be provided in a long-term care facility or in the person's own home. The guiding philosophy of hospice care is to provide a continuity of care that will assure pain control and physical, emotional, and social comfort for a person during the dying period. This is known as **palliative** care.

Both the family and the client experience anticipatory grief when a terminal diagnosis is made. They may experience a variety of feelings ranging from helplessness to guilt, confusion, rage, and fear. During this period the emotions may be very intense. Patience and understanding are needed. Some may see the diagnosis as a chance to correct old hurts or problems. Others begin to withdraw from the pain of the impending loss.

Members of a hospice team plan for the client's needs. Each team member contributes special skills and expertise to assure the comfort of the client and family (Figure 32-1).

FIGURE 32-1   The hospice team
• **Home health aide/nursing assistant:** provides direct personal care and emotional support to both family and client
• **Registered nurse:** develops the care plan and coordinates resident's care
• **Physician:** prescribes treatments
• **Social worker:** assists family and resident with financial and social needs
• **Spiritual advisor:** assists resident and family in meeting their spiritual and religious needs

FIGURE 32-3   Some residents are unable to talk about their feelings and prefer to be left alone to work things out.

Clients are encouraged to be as independent as possible for as long as possible. The nursing assistant providing hospice care in a facility is expected to give excellent physical care. In addition, the nursing assistant must have well-developed interpersonal skills to help residents and their families during this difficult period. Hospice services are usually funded through Medicare, Medicaid, or other health insurance.

THE DYING PROCESS

Nursing assistants provide continuing care to residents through the dying (**moribund**) period and into the after-death period (**postmortem**). Accepting the idea that death is the natural result of the life process may help you respond to the resident's and family's needs more generously.

Each person will have a different response to the dying process and death (Figures 32-2 and 32-3). Reactions to the diagnosis of a terminal (life-ending) illness include the following:

• Some residents may have had time to prepare psychologically for death. They may accept or be resigned to it (Figure 32-4).
• Some may look forward to relief from the pain and emotional burden of a long illness. They may await death calmly.
• Some may be fearful or angry and demonstrate behavior that swings from denial to depression (Figure 32-5).
• Others may reach out, trying to verbalize feelings and thoughts of an uncertain future.

FIGURE 32-2   People react differently as they deal with approaching death.

FIGURE 32-4   Even though the resident seems to have accepted her diagnosis, she still needs support and caring.

FIGURE 32-5 Depression and withdrawal are a natural part of the grieving process.

- In others, despair and anxiety may give way to moments of active hostility or periods of searching questions.

The residents will not all react in the same way to the prospect of death. They will not all follow the same progression of steps in the grieving process. You must accept the resident's behavior with understanding (Figure 32-6). You must also understand the dying resident's need for support, both from caregivers and family. Finally, you will need to support the family in

FIGURE 32-6 When coming to terms with the diagnosis of a terminal illness, the resident needs the support and understanding of the nursing assistant.

meeting their own needs during the adjustment period.

All staff members should know what the resident has been told about his or her condition. The amount of information given to the resident is a medical decision, with family input where possible. All staff members must abide by it.

Resuscitation

Unless otherwise ordered, every effort must be made to keep the resident alive. Be prepared to assist with cardiopulmonary **resuscitation** (CPR). In some facilities, nursing assistants who have had appropriate training are permitted to start this technique.

A resident may specify through a living will or durable power of attorney that resuscitation efforts are not to be made. This is referred to as a **no-code order**. However, if a no-code order does not exist for the resident, a **code blue** is called and resuscitation is started. Staff work quickly to attempt to revive the resident. Unless you have specific responsibilities in the resuscitation effort, you should:

- Stay out of the way.
- Be prepared to assist, if asked.
- Help keep other residents calm and out of the way.

Stages of Grieving

After a terminal diagnosis is made and the resident and the family are advised of the diagnosis, they will usually progress through a series of steps known as the stages of grieving* (Figure 32-7). These are:

- Denial
- Anger
- Bargaining
- Depression
- Acceptance

Both the resident and family members will experience the grieving process. Some people will progress through all steps and reach an acceptance of death as a natural part of the life experience. Other people will not reach acceptance but will stop at some intermediate step. Some people may go back and forth between steps before moving on to acceptance. The experience is not the same for all people.

As an example of the grieving process, Mrs. Bloomberg has been told of her terminal

*Elizabeth Kübler-Ross has done much of the pioneer work in the understanding of the grieving process. See her book *On Death and Dying*, published by Macmillan.

FIGURE 32-7 Remember that residents with a terminal diagnosis move back and forth from one stage to another and may never progress to final acceptance before death.

Stages of Grief	
Denial	Resident refuses to accept the truth.
Anger	Resident may act out feelings, directing anger to caregivers and family.
Bargaining	Resident attempts to "make deals" for more livable time.
Depression	Resident comes to full realization that situation cannot change and feels saddened over things that will be left unfinished.
Acceptance	Resident recognizes that death is part of the natural progression of life.

diagnosis. In the beginning she refuses to accept it. She seems cheerful and says, "I know that there are other therapies that could help. I'm too young to die. I still have much to accomplish." She may even tell you about her future plans. She is in the stage of **denial**.

As time passes and her health does not improve, she says, "It's all so unfair. I don't deserve this!" In **anger** Mrs. Bloomberg strikes out verbally at you and her family. Then, the anger gives way to **bargaining**. She spends time in prayer and visiting the chapel. You hear her say, "If only God (nature, or the doctors) can do something, I will be a better person from now on."

When the bargaining fails, then **depression** sets in. Mrs. Bloomberg speaks of past errors and says how sorry she is that there was not time to do or say certain things. She reviews her life, mourns the losses, and is saddened by things that will be left unfinished. The last step is **acceptance**. She seems calmer and more in control. She starts to put her affairs in order and may begin giving personal possessions away.

Residents at any stage of the grieving process need the emotional support of a caring, understanding staff.

Family Dynamics

Remember that the family and friends of the resident are also going through a grieving process of their own. The relationships that exist between them and the resident are strained by the recognition that little time is left to enjoy each other or to resolve problems.

Each person may have feelings of guilt, anger, frustration, and powerlessness over the inability to avoid the final separation. Feelings that were hidden in everyday activities escape when peo-

ple must also deal with the stress of terminal illness and death (Figure 32-8).

The death of a partner can result in profound grief. The remaining partner may lose the will to live, attempt suicide, and experience serious mental and physical problems. Bereaved persons experience initial feelings of shock and numbness as they go through a period of yearning for the lost loved one. Depression follows and then a final resolution and acceptance that life must go on. There is no timetable for griev-

FIGURE 32-8 These responses may be experienced by anyone coping with grief: resident, staff, family, or other residents.

Coping Techniques to Protect Self-Esteem in Response to Grief
• Anger
• Irritability
• Crying
• Withdrawal
• Agitation
• Restlessness
• Sleep disturbance
• Weight gain
• Chronic complaining
• Muscle aches

ing. Some people may work through their grief in a matter of weeks or months. Others may take much longer to move beyond their grief.

As a nursing assistant, you must:

- Read the care plan thoroughly. A statement of family problems may be included
- Be aware that this is a stressful period for family and friends as well as the resident
- Know that sometimes unexpected interactions occur
- Not offer advice or take sides
- Listen quietly and be supportive
- Remember not to repeat to either the resident or the family or friends information that has been shared with you
- Be supportive, courteous, and respectful
- Maintain eye contact and use the resident's name
- Offer physical comfort to visitors by advising them of the location of rest areas, rest rooms, and nutrition sources
- Permit family members to participate in simple caregiving activities if they desire. This gives them a sense of being needed and assisting in the resident's comfort.

Caregivers and the Grieving Process

The staff must deal with their feelings about death, the loss of the resident, and their own mortality at the same time that they must be providing support to the resident and the family. Staff members who have developed close relationships with residents will also experience the grieving process.

When caregivers first encounter the process of dying and death, the experience can be frightening and stressful. This is especially true if the caregiver has a close relationship with the resident or if the resident is young. The loss of a young person is especially difficult to understand and accept. With experience, the caregiver realizes that supporting and caring for the dying resident is an important service.

There is no one way to prepare yourself completely for the first experience of death, but some things you can do may help:

- Discuss your feelings about life and death with colleagues in a private setting.
- Discuss your thoughts about death with a member of the clergy of your faith.
- Give yourself permission to feel the grief and sadness that accompanies the loss of a resident.
- Believe that the tasks will become easier with experience.

On the Job

You will feel grief when a resident you have cared for dies at a time when others are looking to you for support.

Religious Practices Related to the Dying Process and Death

Many residents who have a terminal illness gain strength and peace through the practice of their religious beliefs. Each religion has practices related to death. For example, for gravely ill Roman Catholic residents a priest will be summoned to perform **last rites**, also known as the **Sacrament of the Sick** (Figure 32-9).

Residents of other religious groups may desire the spiritual support of the clergy of their own faith. Spiritual readings may provide some comfort. Be open to their needs and requests.

Figure 32-10 shows a sampling of practices related to death and dying for major religions.

Nursing Assistant Responsibilities

You have a special opportunity to be of service to the resident with a terminal diagnosis and to his or her family. Because of your day-to-day contact, you are in a position to provide the emotional and physical support needed. Make an effort to build

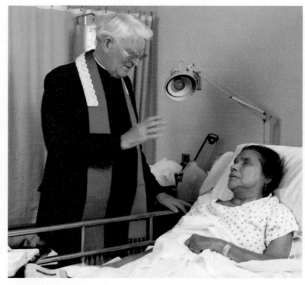

FIGURE 32-9 The Sacrament of the Sick is administered to gravely ill Roman Catholic residents.

FIGURE 32-10   Beliefs and practices related to dying and death for major religions

Different religions vary in beliefs and practices related to dying and death

Religion	Autopsy	Organ Donation	Beliefs and Practices
Judaism (Orthodox)	Only in special circumstance	With consultation of rabbi	Visits to the dying are a religious duty. Witness must be present if death occurs, to protect family and commit soul to God. Torah and Psalms may be read and prayers recited. Conversation is kept to a minimum. Someone should be with the body after death until burial, usually within 24 hours. Body must not be touched 8–30 minutes after death. Medical personnel should not touch or wash body unless death occurs on Jewish Sabbath; then care may be given by nurse wearing gloves. Water is emptied from the room. Mirrors may be covered at family's request.
Hinduism	Permitted	Permitted	Priest ties thread around neck or wrist of deceased and pours water in the mouth. Only family and friends touch body.
Buddhism	Personal preference	Permitted	Buddhist priest is present at death. Last rites are chanted at the bedside.
Islam (Muslim)	Only for medical or legal reasons	Not permitted	Before death, read Koran and pray. Resident confesses sins and asks forgiveness of family. Only family touches or washes body. After death, body is turned toward Mecca.
Roman Catholic	Permitted	Permitted	Sacrament of Sick administered to ill residents, to residents in imminent danger, or shortly after death.
Christian Scientist	Unlikely	Not permitted	No ritual is performed before or after death.
Church of Christ	Permitted	Permitted	No ritual is performed before or after death.
Jehovah's Witness	Only if required by law	Not permitted	No ritual is performed before or after death.
Baptist	Permitted	Permitted	Clergy ministers through counseling and prayers.
Episcopalian	Permitted	Permitted	Last rites are optional.
Lutheran	Permitted	Permitted	Last rites are optional.
Eastern Orthodox Christian	Not encouraged	Not encouraged	Last rites are mandatory and handled by ordained priest.

and maintain a trusting relationship with each resident. Make sure the resident feels secure and knows you will not abandon him. Watch carefully for verbal and nonverbal clues as to what the resident feels and needs. Use your own special touch and listening skills to comfort the resident.

You can help the moribund resident by:

- Making frequent contact with the resident
- Increasing contact as death approaches
- Keeping the resident comfortable and clean
- Changing resident's position every 2 hours
- Providing proper mouth care
- Using moistened applicators on the lips and inside the mouth
- Meeting basic physical needs
- Monitoring vital signs carefully
- Keeping the room quiet but well lit

You can help the family by:

- Giving proper care to the resident
- Treating the resident with respect and ensuring the resident's dignity
- Listening quietly to their concerns
- Providing privacy

SIGNS OF APPROACHING DEATH

Approaching death is signaled by a slowing of body functions and a loss of control. Signs and symptoms include:

- The body seems to relax and the jaw drops.
- Breathing becomes labored.
- Control of bowels and bladder or both may be lost (incontinence).
- Circulation slows.
- Blood pressure drops.
- Extremities become colder.
- Profuse perspiration is common.
- Respirations become labored (dyspnea) or temporarily cease (apnea).
- Periods of dyspnea followed by apnea, known as *Cheyne-Stokes respirations*, may occur.
- The pulse becomes more rapid and weaker.
- The skin pales and **mottling** (discoloration) may occur.
- The eyes do not respond to light.
- Hearing is the last sense to be lost. Do not assume that the resident can no longer hear. You must be careful in what you say. Always remember to treat the dying person with dignity and respect. This also holds true for handling the body after death.

Continue to talk to the resident in a normal tone even if the resident is **comatose** (unconscious).

Gradually, breathing becomes more labored and then stops. If the nurse is away from the bedside, note the time that breathing ceases and inform the nurse when the vital signs are lost. If the resident's family is present at the time of death, they will be asked to step outside while the nurse examines the resident and then calls the physician. Under no circumstances is the nursing assistant to inform the family that death has occurred. This is the responsibility of the nurse or physician.

Provide a comfortable, private area for the family and stay with them unless they prefer to be alone. It is appropriate to let the family know how much the resident meant to you, so do not be embarrassed if you feel like crying. Do, however, try to control your emotions because the family members will need your support.

POSTMORTEM CARE

The care given immediately after death is called **postmortem care**. The changes in the resident's body after death are listed in Figure 32-11. Make sure the resident is positioned naturally, with limbs straightened. This is important because **rigor mortis** (stiffening of the body muscles) will occur some hours after death. Return dentures to the mouth if they were normally worn. Make sure the linen is clean. Family members may want to spend a little time with the body. Stay with them, if requested, but provide privacy otherwise.

After the death of a resident, your behavior should be dignified and restrained. Death in the facility is upsetting to other residents. Residents are informed of the deaths of other residents. Some will experience feelings of the loss of a friend; others will be reminded that their own

FIGURE 32-11 Postmortem signs
Postmortem signs include:
• Gradual cooling of body temperature
• Loss of circulation
• Body discoloration with pressure
• Evacuation of bowel or bladder or both
• Rigor mortis (stiffening of muscles and joints) beginning with head and neck and progressing downward

PROCEDURE
108   Giving Postmortem Care

1. Carry out each beginning procedure action.
2. Assemble equipment:
   - Disposable gloves
   - Shroud or clean sheet
   - Basin with warm water
   - Washcloth
   - Towels
   - Pads as needed
3. Put on disposable gloves.
4. Remove all appliances, tubing, and used articles, if instructed to do so.
5. Work quickly and quietly; maintain an attitude of respect.
6. With bed flat, position the body on the back, head and shoulders elevated on a pillow.
   - Close the eyes by grasping the eyelashes, gently pulling the eyelids down, and holding shut for a few seconds.
   - Remove watch and all jewelry except a wedding band, according to facility policy.
   - Straighten arms and legs and place arms by sides.

   - Make itemized list of watch and jewelry. Ask family member to check the list and sign it.
   - If used, replace dentures in the resident's mouth. If used, replace artificial eye.
7. Bathe body as necessary. Remove any soiled dressings and replace with clean ones. Groom hair.
8. Place a disposable pad underneath the buttocks.
   - Put clean gown on resident.
   - Replace top bed linen.
9. If the family is to view the body:
   - Make sure the room is neat.
   - Adjust the lights to a subdued level.
   - Place chairs around the bed for family members.
   - Remove disposable gloves. Dispose of them according to facility policy. Wash hands.
   - Allow the family to visit in private.
10. Collect all belongings and make a list. Wrap properly and label.
11. Carry out each procedure completion action.

---

lives are limited. Some residents withdraw and others may openly grieve. Let the residents know that you understand their feelings and that such feelings are natural. Be willing to listen. Be patient if a resident seems irritable or angry. Report the resident's reactions to the nurse so the care plan will reflect the proper staff response.

As residents grieve for their deceased friend, they may want to recall their relationship. Be supportive as they express their feelings of grief (Figure 32-12).

Some facilities hold memorial services for deceased residents. Members of the family, residents, and staff are invited to celebrate the life of the resident. The services help to bring closure.

FIGURE 32-12   Remember that residents often form close friendships. When one dies, you must be prepared to offer comfort to those who remain.

LESSON SYNTHESIS: Putting It All Together

*Y*ou have just completed this lesson. Now go back and review the Clinical Focus. Try to see how the Clinical Focus relates to the concepts presented in the lesson. Then answer the following questions.

1. Why do you think Mr. Sperling is behaving the way he is?

2. How do you think the marital history of Mr. and Mrs. Sperling might affect their emotional response to this terminal condition and death?

3. How could the nursing assistant be supportive?

4. What special sacrament would be appropriate when Mr. Sperling is moribund?

REVIEW

A. Match each term (items a.–e.) with the proper definition.

a. comatose
b. mottling
c. moribund
d. postmortem
e. Sacrament of the Sick

1. _____ discoloration
2. _____ dying
3. _____ last rites
4. _____ unconscious
5. _____ after death

B. Provide brief answers for each of the following.

6. List five signs of approaching death.

7. List the five stages of grieving.

8. List six ways the nursing assistant can help the moribund resident.

C. Answer each statement true (T) or false (F).

9. T F Death is a natural part of the life cycle.

10. T F Everyone responds to the thought of death in the same way.

11. T F A terminal illness is curable.

12. T F Given time, residents can move steadily forward through each stage of grieving.

13. T F Rigor mortis develops immediately after death.

D. Select the one best answer for each of the following.

14. Signs of approaching death include
(A) blood pressure rises
(B) circulation speeds up
(C) extremities become warmer
(D) breathing becomes labored

15. When a resident is dying,
(A) other residents are not affected
(B) staff members are not upset
(C) family members are not concerned
(D) other residents may be deeply affected

16. The Sacrament of the Sick is administered to
(A) Buddhist residents
(B) Jewish residents
(C) Roman Catholic residents
(D) residents who are members of the Church of Christ

17. After the death of a resident who belongs to the Muslim faith,
    (A) the nursing assistant may wash the body
    (B) the body is turned toward Mecca
    (C) the Bible is read
    (D) an autopsy is always performed

18. When a resident is comatose, he
    (A) may be able to see
    (B) may be able to hear
    (C) cannot hear
    (D) is able to speak

E. Clinical Experience

19. Juan is working in the hospice unit of a long-term care facility. Mrs. Sophen, who has metastatic pancreatic cancer, is one of his residents.
    a. How would Mrs. Sophen's prognosis be described?
    b. What word best describes the kind of care Mrs. Sophen is receiving?
    c. What is the focus of this care?
    d. Who, besides Juan, provides this care?
    e. Where else might this care be given?

20. Liza is caring for Mr. Simms, who has been comatose for 12 hours. His breathing has just ceased. The nurse is away from the bedside.
    a. What action should Liza take?
    b. Should Liza inform the family members who are in the waiting room?
    c. When the family returns to the resident's room, what should Liza do to offer them support?
    d. Mr. Simms was a resident in the facility for 18 months. Liza liked him and feels very sad about his death. Is it appropriate for her to let the family know that she will also miss him very much?

Caring for the Person in Subacute Care

Clinical Focus

Think about the care that is required by residents in subacute units as you study this lesson and meet:

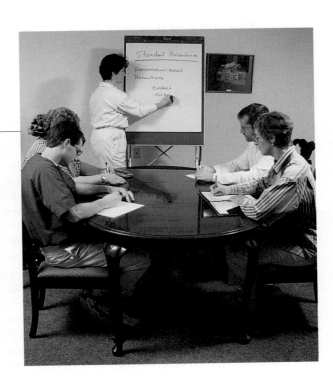

*S*teven Goldstein, who has been a nursing assistant for several years. He has just been hired to work in a subacute care unit of a long-term care facility. Steven will need to participate in additional inservice education to fulfill the requirements of his new job. He is looking forward to the challenge of learning and acquiring new skills.

OBJECTIVES

After studying this lesson, you should be able to:

- Define and spell vocabulary words and terms.
- Describe the purpose of subacute care.
- List the differences between acute care, subacute care, and long-term care.
- Describe the responsibilities of the nursing assistant when caring for residents receiving the special treatments discussed in this lesson.

VOCABULARY

alopecia *(al-oh-PEE-shee-ah)*

anorexia *(an-oh-RECK-see-ah)*

central venous (CV) catheter *(SEN-tral VEE-nus KATH-eh-ter)*

chemotherapy *(kee-moh-THER-ah-pee)*

dialysis *(dye-AL-ih-sis)*

enteral feedings *(EN-ter-al FEED-ings)*

epidural catheter *(ep-ih-DOO-ral KATH-eh-ter)*

fistula *(FIS-tyou-lah)*

VOCABULARY

graft *(graft)*

hemodialysis *(**he**-moh-dye-**AL**-ih-sis)*

hyperalimentation *(**high**-per-**al**-ih-men-**TAY**-shun)*

intravenous (IV) therapy *(**in**-trah-**VEE**-nus **THER**-ah-pee)*

narcotic *(nar-**KAH**-tick)*

oncology *(ong-**KOL**-oh-jee)*

patient-controlled analgesia (PCA) *(**PAY**-shent kon-**TROLD an**-al-**JEE**-see-ah)*

peripheral intravenous central catheter (PICC) *(per-**IH**-fer-al **in**-trah-**VEE**-nus **SEN**-tral **KATH**-eh-ter)*

peritoneal dialysis *(**per**-ih-toh-**NEE**-al dye-**AL**-ih-sis)*

piggyback *(**PIG**-ee-bak)*

pulse oximetry *(puls ox-**IM**-ih-tree)*

radiation therapy *(**ray**-dee-**AY**-shun **THER**-ah-pee)*

subacute care *(sub-ah-**KYOUT** kair)*

total parenteral nutrition (TPN) *(**TOH**-tal pah-**REN**-ter-al new-**TRIH**-shun)*

tracheostomy *(**tray**-kee-**OS**-toh-mee)*

transcutaneous electrical nerve stimulation (TENS) *(**trans**-kyou-**TAN**-ee-us ee-**LEK**-trih-kal nerv stim-you-**LAY**-shun)*

transitional care *(tran-**ZIH**-shun-al kair)*

DESCRIPTION OF SUBACUTE CARE

Subacute care is a type of "step-down" care given to persons who have been acutely ill. These individuals are out of the acute phase of illness but still need monitoring and ongoing treatment and services. Subacute care is sometimes called **transitional care**. The purpose of subacute care is to provide the care a person needs but at a lower cost than care given in an acute care facility (hospital). Subacute care units are usually located in a section of a skilled nursing facility. Most residents in subacute care units are there for 3 to 4 weeks. Residents with terminal illness or with acquired immune deficiency syndrome (AIDS) may be there for a longer time. Residents who can be discharged may go to:

- Their homes
- A skilled care or intermediate care facility
- An assisted living facility

On a subacute care unit there are:

- Highly trained nurses and nursing assistants
- More medications and treatments to administer than on a regular skilled unit
- More frequent physician's visits
- More sophisticated types of equipment

Types of Care Provided in a Subacute Care Unit

Most subacute care units provide specialized care in one or two areas. Some examples are:

- Rehabilitation—all therapies are provided and the resident participates in rehabilitation for 5 hours a day, 6 or 7 days a week.
- Peritoneal dialysis—a method of ridding the body of wastes for a person who has kidney failure
- Ventilator weaning and tracheostomy care—for persons who have been unable to breathe without the help of a ventilator
- Cardiac monitoring—for persons who have had a myocardial infarction or acute heart failure
- Pain management and control—for persons who have acute or chronic pain
- Oncology—the care of persons with cancer who are receiving treatments such as chemotherapy or radiation
- Wound management—for persons with severe stage 3 or stage 4 pressure ulcers, ulcers related to peripheral vascular disease, or burns
- Brain injury—for persons who have suffered brain damage resulting from trauma
- AIDS—for persons in the terminal stages of AIDS who need 24-hour-a-day care
- Hospice care—for persons in the terminal stages of any disease
- Postoperative care (care given to individuals who have had surgery) for persons who have other complicating conditions—for example, a person who has had repair of a hip fracture and who also has chronic obstructive pulmonary disease

If you work on a subacute care unit you will participate in special in-service training to meet the needs of the residents in your care. A nursing assistant on a subacute unit will be expected to:

- Work closely with registered nurses who are specialists in critical care or in a specific area of nursing such as rehabilitation or wound care
- Have extensive knowledge of the types of residents cared for on the subacute care unit
- Care for residents receiving complicated treatments
- Have excellent observational skills because of the complex conditions of the residents on the unit
- Be a member of an interdisciplinary health care team that includes highly trained professionals in areas like physical therapy, occupational therapy, speech therapy, respiratory therapy, and social services

It is important that the staff on a subacute care unit be able to provide for the resident's emotional well-being. Many of the residents on the unit will be able to return to their homes. For them, this is a time for rejoicing and for making plans for the future. Some of the residents, however, will have an uncertain future. For example:

- Will the resident receiving dialysis receive a kidney transplant in time?
- Will the cancer be cured in the resident receiving radiation or chemotherapy?
- Will the resident on the ventilator be able to be weaned off the ventilator or will it be a life-long need?
- Will the resident receiving rehabilitation recover enough independence to be able to go home?

SPECIAL PROCEDURES PROVIDED IN THE SUBACUTE CARE UNIT

You may care for residents who are receiving special treatments because of their health problems. These treatments may require the use of equipment that is unfamiliar to you. As a nursing assistant you will not be expected to be responsible for these procedures. However, you will be providing the same personal care and procedures that you would with any residents. In addition you will need to know what observations to make for these residents.

CARE OF THE SURGICAL PATIENT

It is possible that you may care for a resident who was admitted or readmitted to the facility shortly after surgery. Be sure you know what nursing care is expected. You may find that:

- Vital signs are taken more frequently
- The resident has devices connected to drainage tubes
- Intravenous feedings are running

When caring for a resident who has had surgery:

- Encourage the resident to breathe deeply, cough, and move in bed. The position should be changed every 2 hours.
- Turn the resident's head to one side and support if vomiting. Have an emesis basin ready, as well as tissues and a wet cloth.
- Report any signs of drainage from the operative area.
- Report complaints of pain promptly.

PULSE OXIMETRY

Residents receiving oxygen may be monitored with pulse oximetry. (See Lesson 25 for oxygen therapy.) **Pulse oximetry** is used to monitor the level of oxygen in the arterial blood. Red and infrared light are sent through an artery in the fingertip. A photodetector is placed over the finger. The photodetector measures the transmitted light as it passes through the blood (Figure 33-1). The nurse is responsible for this procedure.

FIGURE 33-1 Pulse oximetry monitors the level of oxygen in arterial blood. (Courtesy of Ohmeda, Louisville, CO)

INTRAVENOUS THERAPY

Intravenous (IV) therapy refers to medication or solutions administered directly into a vein. Standard intravenous therapy is given into a peripheral vein (a large vein in the arm) (Figure 33-2). This is called an IV. The IV may consist of a single bag of solution connected to a simple tubing with a needle or small catheter on the end. Sometimes an additional small bag of fluid is attached to tubing that is connected to the main (primary) tubing. This is called a **piggyback**. This small bag contains medication such as an antibiotic that is given intermittently into the vein (Figure 33-3).

Central Venous Insertion

Intravenous therapy can also be administered through a **central venous (CV) catheter**. A special catheter is inserted into a vein near the resident's collar bone (Figure 33-4). The catheter tip ends in or near the heart chamber. CV therapy is used to administer medications or to provide total parenteral nutrition.

FIGURE 33-3 The small bag (piggyback) contains medication.

Peripheral Intravenous Central Catheter Line

A **peripheral intravenous central catheter** or **PICC** line consists of a catheter that is inserted into a peripheral vein and threaded upward

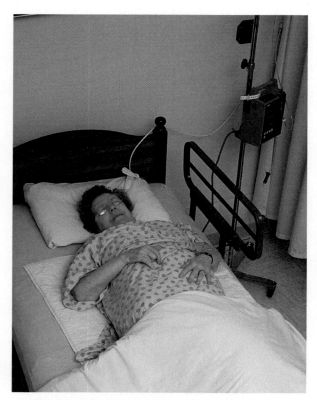

FIGURE 33-2 Intravenous therapy is most often given through a peripheral vein in the resident's arm.

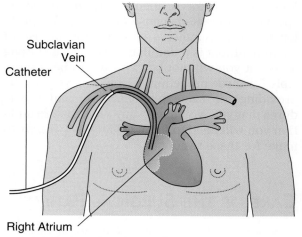

FIGURE 33-4 Central venous insertion

through the vein to the jugular or subclavian vein. It is used to administer medications or to provide total parenteral nutrition.

Total Parenteral Nutrition

Total parenteral nutrition (TPN) is also called **hyperalimentation.** TPN is given to a resident whose bowel needs complete rest. All required nutrients (carbohydrates, proteins, and fats) are given directly into the vein so the bowel does not have to work to digest food. Residents receiving TPN may need to be weighed daily or every other day. This should be done at the same time of day with the resident wearing the same type of clothing. The resident may be gradually changed to **enteral feedings.** With an enteral feeding, liquid nourishment is administered through a tube inserted into the resident's stomach (Figure 33-5).

PAIN MANAGEMENT PROCEDURES

Pain management may be the major reason why some residents are on a subacute unit. Other residents may be undergoing pain management related to other conditions such as

recent surgery or pain related to cancer. Both drug and nondrug treatments can be successful in helping to prevent and control pain. Various types of relaxation techniques are frequently used for pain management.

Patient-Controlled Analgesia

Patient-controlled analgesia (PCA) is used for acute, chronic, or postoperative pain. *Analgesia* means pain relief. A device is inserted into the resident's vein. It is connected to a solution that contains a **narcotic.** A narcotic is a drug such as morphine that is used for pain relief. The dosage is controlled by equipment that has been preset. The patient or the nurse pushes the PCA button at times of discomfort.

Report to the nurse if you note any change in the resident's:

- Level of consciousness
- Rate and pattern of respirations
- Pupil size
- Skin color

Pain Management with an Epidural Catheter

An **epidural catheter** is implanted beneath the resident's skin. It is inserted near the spinal cord at the first lumbar (L1) space. A local

FIGURE 33-5 Nourishment may be given through a tube inserted into the resident's stomach.

*G*uidelines for

Caring for Residents with Intravenous Lines

The nursing assistant tasks include the following:

1. Know the drip rate in the drip chamber. Observe drip chamber for drip rate. If rate changes or drip chamber is full, notify the nurse.
2. Avoid pulling or twisting tubing. Make sure resident is not lying on tubing.
3. Observe area of needle insertion for signs of swelling, redness, or warmth.
4. Note signs of moisture that may indicate the tubing is leaking.
5. Make sure that all junctions in the tubing are securely connected.

6. Report immediately to the nurse:
   * Signs of dyspnea, cyanosis, chest, or back pain
   * Complaints of pain or burning at site of needle insertion
7. Remember that all IV procedures are sterile. If you are assisting a nurse with any of these procedures, you must never contaminate the sterile field or supplies.
8. When caring for residents with any type of intravenous therapy, *NEVER:*
   * Change drip rate
   * Disconnect any tubing
   * Manipulate needle or tubing
   * Remove, change, or manipulate dressing over site

PROCEDURE
109

Changing a Gown on a Resident with a Peripheral Intravenous Line in Place

Note: This procedure is to be used only when the IV is not run through an electronic pump. When a pump is used, the resident may wear a gown that snaps at the shoulder. In this case, the gown can be removed without touching the IV bag or tubing. If the resident is wearing a nonsnap gown, call the nurse if the gown is to be changed. Never disconnect the tubing from the pump.

1. Carry out each beginning procedure action.
2. Assemble equipment:
   * Clean gown
3. Make sure windows and door are closed to prevent chilling the resident.
4. Remove gown from the arm without the IV and bring gown across resident's chest to other arm.

5. Place clean gown over resident's chest to avoid exposure.
6. On the arm with the IV, gather material of gown in one hand so there is no pull or pressure on the line, and slowly draw gown over tip of fingers (Figure 33-6).
7. With free hand, lift IV free of standard and slip gown over bag of fluid (Figure 33-7), removing gown from resident's body. **Never allow the bag of fluid to be lower than the resident's arm.**
8. Take sleeve of clean gown and slip it over the bag of fluid, the tubing, and up the resident's arm.
9. Replace bag of fluid on IV standard.
10. Remove soiled gown and place at end of bed. Finish putting clean gown on resident's other arm. Secure neck ties.

(continues)

PROCEDURE *109* *(continued)*

FIGURE 33-6 Gather material of gown in one hand so there is no pull or pressure on the line. Slowly draw gown over tips of fingers.

11. Place soiled gown in laundry hamper.
12. Make sure IV is dripping and that tubing is not kinked or twisted.
13. Carry out each procedure completion action.

FIGURE 33-7 With free hand, lift IV free of standard and slip gown over bag of fluid.

Note: If you are changing a gown for a resident with a centrally inserted line, you will not need to lower the fluid container. Change the gown in the usual manner, taking care not to manipulate the tubing.

anesthetic is administered either intermittently or continuously through the catheter. The resident may have leg numbness and weakness for the first 24 hours after the catheter is inserted. Report to the nurse at once if:

- Catheter becomes dislodged from the insertion site
- You note changes in respiration rate and pattern
- Resident complains of itching
- Resident vomits or complains of nausea

Transcutaneous Electrical Nerve Stimulation

Transcutaneous electrical nerve stimulation (TENS) is a nondrug method of pain relief. Mild, harmless electrical current stimulates nerve fibers to block the transmission of pain to the brain. Electrodes are taped to the resident's skin. The location of the electrodes depends on the areas related to the pain. The electrodes are attached to wires that are attached to a control box (Figure 33-8). The intensity of the stimulation is set on the control box by the nurse.

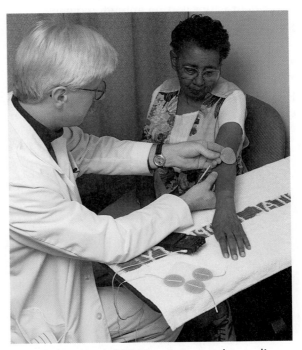

FIGURE 33-8 A TENS unit is used to relieve pain.

CARING FOR RESIDENTS WITH TRACHEOSTOMIES

You may care for a resident with a tracheostomy. A **tracheostomy** is a tube that is inserted into a surgical opening in the resident's trachea (windpipe). A tracheostomy is performed when the resident is unable to breathe in air through the nose. The tube allows the resident to "breathe" as air goes directly into the trachea and then into the lungs. A person who is on a ventilator for a long time will have a tracheostomy that is connected to the ventilator. The resident may have secretions coming from the chest and through the tube. The nurse will need to use suction to remove the secretions.

The tube may be made of plastic or metal. Tracheostomy tubes consist of an inner removable tube called a cannula and an outer tube called a neckplate that is held in place with neck ties. The neckplate rests between the clavicles (breastbones). There is a slot on each side. Tracheostomy ties are inserted here to secure the tube in place (Figure 33-9). Residents with tracheostomies can usually take a bath or shower but must keep the water away from the opening. Avoid using powders, sprays, or shaving cream around the tube. When you care for a resident with a tracheostomy, observe for:

- Changes in respiratory rate, depth, quality
- Changes in mental status such as confusion, restlessness, or irritability that indicate the resident is not getting enough oxygen

Report to the nurse immediately if the:

- Tube becomes dislodged from the opening
- Resident is having trouble breathing
- Resident needs suctioning

Be sure you know how the resident communicates. The incision in the trachea will interfere with the resident's ability to talk.

FIGURE 33-9 Ties hold the tracheostomy tube in place.

CARING FOR THE RESIDENT RECEIVING DIALYSIS TREATMENTS

Dialysis is a process by which the blood is cleansed of liquid wastes artificially when the kidneys are unable to remove the wastes. This procedure is needed when a person has kidney failure. Without dialysis the person would die as the waste products accumulated in the bloodstream. Dialysis is usually considered a temporary treatment that is used until a suitable kidney is found for a kidney transplant. The two types of dialysis are hemodialysis and peritoneal dialysis.

Hemodialysis

During **hemodialysis** treatment the resident's blood is circulated outside of the body into an artificial kidney machine. In the dialysis machine, the blood is cleansed with a liquid substance called dialysate and then returned to the resident's body. Most persons needing hemodialysis treatments are treated in a dialysis center. However, you may care for residents in the subacute unit who go as outpatients to the dialysis center for their treatments. Dialysis is usually done three to four times a week. Each treatment takes several hours. To do dialysis, a connection must be made between the resident's circulatory system and the artificial kidney machine. Minor surgery is done to create either a fistula or a graft. The **fistula** (Figure 33-10) is created when a vein is attached to an artery either in an arm or leg. When a **graft** is used (Figure 33-11), synthetic material is inserted to form a connection between an artery and a vein. Two needles are inserted for treatment with either the fistula or graft. The needles are connected to tubes that go to and from the artificial kidney machine. As a nursing assistant, you are not expected to care for the

A.V. Fistula

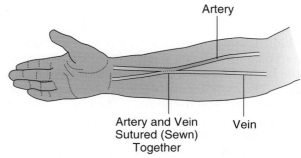

FIGURE 33-10 Fistula used for hemodialysis

Graft

Radial Artery

Graft

Basilic Vein

FIGURE 33-11   Graft used for hemodialysis

fistula or graft. You need to be aware that the resident will:

- Have fluid restrictions
- Have dietary restrictions for calories, sodium, protein, potassium, calcium, and phosphorus
- Need all fluid intake and output measured and recorded
- Need to be weighed regularly at the same time of day and with the same type of clothing
- Need to be monitored and have blood pressure taken frequently after dialysis. Remember that blood pressure should not be taken in the arm used for dialysis.

Report to the nurse if the resident has:

- Swelling (edema) of the hands or feet
- Changes in vital signs (blood pressure, temperature, pulse, or respirations)
- A change in weight
- A change in intake and output measurements
- Shortness of breath
- Complaints of pain at the site of the fistula or graft

Peritoneal Dialysis

Peritoneal dialysis is also a process of cleansing the blood. In peritoneal dialysis, the process takes place within the resident's body in the peritoneal (abdominal) cavity, rather than outside the body in a machine. During dialysis the dialysate is introduced into the abdominal cavity, allowed to stay in for some time, and then drained out. As blood flows through the vessels in the peritoneum, waste products are filtered and excess fluids are removed. The nurse instills the dialysate through a catheter that is surgically implanted through the wall of the abdomen into the abdominal cavity. This is done using sterile technique.

Nursing assistants are not expected to administer peritoneal dialysis. You may be responsible for monitoring the resident's vital signs every 10 to 15 minutes for the first 1 to 2 hours after a treatment and then every 2 to 4 hours. Notify the nurse if there are any changes in vital signs.

ONCOLOGY TREATMENTS

Oncology is the care and treatment of persons with cancer. Cancer may be treated with surgery, radiation, chemotherapy, or a combination of any of these.

Radiation Therapy

Residents receiving radiation therapy in the long-term care facility will be transported to a special cancer treatment center or to a hospital to receive the therapy as an outpatient. **Radiation therapy** is the use of high-energy radiation to kill cancer cells. It is considered a local therapy because it kills only the cancer cells in the area being treated. Residents receiving radiation may complain of fatigue and lack of appetite. When caring for residents receiving radiation therapy:

- Report signs of redness, pain, or peeling of the skin in the area being treated.
- Do not remove markings made on the skin for treatment purposes.
- Do not use any heat or cold treatments on the area being treated.
- Wash the area only with tepid water and a soft washcloth. Do not apply any soaps, powders, deodorants, perfumes, makeup, lotions, or skin preparations to the area.
- Instruct resident to avoid wearing tight clothing over area.

Chemotherapy

Chemotherapy is the use of drugs to kill cancer cells within the body. The drugs may be given by mouth (orally), through the vein (IV), or in the muscle (intramuscular [IM]). The nurse or physician administers the drugs. The person receiving chemotherapy may have side effects including nausea, vomiting, **anorexia** (loss of appetite), or **alopecia** (loss of hair). Modern treatment techniques have minimized the side effects of chemotherapy. However, loss of hair is still common. The hair will usually come back after the treatments are completed. Some persons prefer to wear wigs during this time. Respect the resident's wishes regarding personal appearance.

LESSON SYNTHESIS: Putting It All Together

*Y*ou have just completed this lesson. Now go back and review the Clinical Focus. Try to see how the Clinical Focus relates to the concepts presented in this lesson. Then answer the following questions.

1. Consider the different types of care that subacute units provide. If Steven works in a unit with residents receiving dialysis, what should he know about kidney function and kidney disease?

2. Using the knowledge presented in earlier lessons in this text, what differences would you expect between acute care, subacute care, and long-term care?

3. What challenges would you expect to accept if you work in a subacute care unit?

4. How would you prepare yourself for meeting these challenges?

REVIEW

A. Select the one best answer for each of the following.

1. Subacute care is given to persons who
   (A) have been acutely ill
   (B) have had a long, progressive illness
   (C) require only custodial care
   (D) require intensive care

2. The purpose of subacute care is to
   (A) increase the population of long-term care facilities
   (B) discharge patients from the hospital as quickly as possible
   (C) provide the care a person needs at a lower cost
   (D) provide pre-operative care

3. Examples of the type of persons treated in subacute care include all of the following except those
   (A) requiring dialysis
   (B) being held for observation
   (C) receiving wound care
   (D) requiring high levels of rehabilitation

4. A nursing assistant working in subacute care would need to
   (A) learn how to start intravenous feedings
   (B) have excellent observational skills
   (C) learn how to administer chemotherapy
   (D) instruct residents in pain management techniques

5. If you accept a position in a subacute care unit, you will not be required to learn
   (A) why hyperalimentation is given
   (B) your responsibilities for residents receiving dialysis
   (C) more about the rehabilitation process
   (D) advanced burn care

6. The procedure to measure the level of oxygen in arterial blood is called
   (A) hemodialysis
   (B) pulse oximetry
   (C) total parenteral nutrition
   (D) intravenous therapy

7. A central venous catheter is inserted into
   (A) a vein in the resident's arm
   (B) an artery in the resident's arm
   (C) the jugular or subclavian vein
   (D) the epidural space

8. Total parenteral nutrition (TPN) is used for residents
   (A) who need to lose weight
   (B) who are unconscious
   (C) who refuse to eat
   (D) whose bowel needs complete rest

9. The nursing assistant's responsibility for caring for residents with intravenous feedings is to
   (A) insert the needle into the vein
   (B) add medication to the bag of fluid when it is due
   (C) observe for complications
   (D) change the drip rate if it is going too fast or too slow

10. Patient-controlled analgesia is used for all of the following, except
    (A) to allow the patient to receive as much medication as he or she wants at any time
    (B) for administering narcotics for pain
    (C) to allow the resident to receive the medication when he or she needs it
    (D) for acute, chronic, or postoperative pain

11. An epidural catheter is used for
    (A) pain management
    (B) administering nutrition
    (C) emptying the bladder
    (D) intravenous feedings

12. When caring for residents with tracheostomies, you should
    (A) not allow the resident to take a bath or shower
    (B) observe for changes in respiratory rate, depth, and quality
    (C) maintain the resident on a liquid diet
    (D) be responsible for changing the tracheostomy tube

13. Dialysis is a procedure for
    (A) cleansing the blood of liquid wastes
    (B) relieving postoperative pain
    (C) administering oxygen
    (D) giving total parenteral nutrition

14. A resident on dialysis will have all of the following, except
    (A) fluid restrictions
    (B) dietary restrictions
    (C) frequent weights taken
    (D) unchanged blood pressure

15. When caring for residents on dialysis, you should report
    (A) edema of the hands and feet
    (B) stable vital signs
    (C) muscle aches
    (D) no change in weight

16. Oncology is the care and treatment of residents with
    (A) severe wounds
    (B) kidney failure
    (C) cancer
    (D) terminal illness

17. When caring for residents receiving radiation therapy, you should
    (A) remove the markings made on the skin for treatment purposes
    (B) apply cold treatments to the area
    (C) avoid applying soaps, powders, lotions, deodorants, or other substances to the treated area
    (D) wrap the treatment area with an elastic bandage

B. Fill in the blanks by selecting the correct word or phrase from the list.

dialysis	pulse oximetry
enteral	transcutaneous
hyperalimentation	electrical nerve
narcotic	stimulation
piggyback	transitional care

18. Subacute care is also called _____.

19. A procedure for removing liquid wastes from the blood is called _____.

20. _____ is used for measuring the oxygen level in arterial blood.

21. A _____ refers to a small bag of fluid containing intravenous medication that is connected with a tube to the primary tubing.

22. Total parenteral nutrition (TPN) is also called _____.

23. A feeding administered through a tube into the resident's stomach is called an _____ feeding.

24. A _____ is a potent drug used for pain relief.

25. The use of electrical current to treat pain is done with a procedure called _____.

SECTION 10

Employment

LESSON

34 Seeking Employment

Seeking Employment

Clinical Focus

Think of the process involved in successfully seeking employment as you study this lesson and meet:

*R*uby Stepp, who has just completed a program that has prepared her to work in a long-term care facility. She has passed all tests. Ruby is now ready to enter a field of service and personal satisfaction as she seeks her first full employment.

OBJECTIVES

After studying this lesson, you should be able to:

- Define and spell vocabulary words and terms.
- List objectives to be met in obtaining and maintaining employment.
- Develop a process for self-evaluation.
- List sources of nursing assistant employment.
- Get set for a successful interview.
- Prepare a résumé and letter of resignation.

VOCABULARY

cross-training *(kros-**TRAYN**-ing)*
interview *(**IN**-ter-vue)*
networking *(**NET**-werk-ing)*

references *(**REF**-er-en-ses)*
résumé *(**REH**-zoo-may)*

CONGRATULATIONS ARE IN ORDER

You have done it! You have passed the certification tests and have proven your ability in the clinical area. You are now certified and are ready to make your contribution to the care of residents in a long-term care facility.

You will now begin the search for available positions and prepare yourself to apply for them. You can do several things to make the search easier and more productive.

Step I—Self-Appraisal

The first step is a self-appraisal—an honest look at your own strengths and limitations (Figure 34-1). You can do this by making a list.

On one side of a sheet of paper, list all the things you have to offer an employer. Be as specific as you can about personal as well as educational assets or strengths. For example, write statements about:

- Your sense of responsibility—Are you a punctual person?
- Your nursing assistant skills—How well trained and prepared are you?
- Your attitude—Are you caring and patient?
- Your personal appearance—Are you clean and neat at all times?

These are important characteristics in a successful nursing assistant.

On the other side of the paper, list any restrictions to your employment. Write statements about:

- Your availability for work—Are there hours when you cannot work (for example, when you must be home to care for children)?
- Preferred location of work—Do you have to work within a specific area because you rely on public transportation?
- Personal responsibilities you may have—Do you have any responsibilities that may interfere with the performance of a job?

Think of ways to manage your responsibilities so they will not interfere with your employability. For example, if you have an elderly parent living with you and must be home to prepare meals, is there a neighbor or other family member who could prepare meals on the days or hours that you work?

Put the list away and then review it in a day or two. There may be items you will want to add or revise.

Step II—Possibility Search

You have listed your strengths and limitations. Now it is time to search for job possibilities. Where do you look?

- Start with the newspapers.
  - The classified advertisements are your best bet here (Figure 34-2). Circle those that list positions located within your desired work area and that have openings for the shift you need to work.
  - Look in the telephone book for facilities in your area.
  - List names, numbers, and addresses. Follow up and contact them.
- Investigate the facility in which you had your clinical experience. Nursing administrators often will invite nursing assistants who have trained in their facilities to join the staff on completion of training. There are advantages to this policy. For one thing, you have already spent time in the facility so less time is needed to orient you as a new employee. Also, the staff has had time to evaluate you while observing you during your training period.
- **Networking** is a valuable technique that can reveal opportunities (Figure 34-3). Let friends

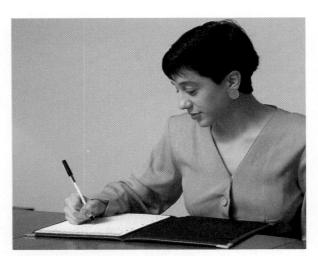

FIGURE 34-1 Nursing assistant listing strengths and limitations

FIGURE 34-2 The classified ads are a good place to start your job search.

FIGURE 34-3 Friends, classmates, and colleagues are valuable sources of information about potential jobs.

and colleagues know that you are looking for employment. Jobs are often located on the recommendation of a network of friends. Making connections and learning of opportunities through people one meets is called *networking*. Networking means gathering a group of people with similar needs and interests to learn about:

- Working conditions
- Job openings
- Special ways of carrying out your responsibilities

Registry

A *registry* is a private agency that employs health care workers, including CNAs. Health care facilities contact the registry when they need workers. The registry then sends workers to the facilities. The worker is free to accept the assignment or not. The worker's salary is usually higher than those of facility-employed workers because no benefits are included. The registry takes a percentage of the worker's salary for the placement service. Registry employment offers flexibility in hours, variety of experience, and higher income, but requires constant adjustment to the routines of different facilities.

STEP III—THE RÉSUMÉ

A **résumé** is a summary of your education and prior work experience. The résumé should be neatly prepared, preferably typed. It is helpful to a prospective employer to have the résumé before and after your interview is held.

When an employer interviews many applicants, it is sometimes difficult to remember all the information given during a particular conversation. A note on your résumé by the interviewer can make all the difference between being hired and not being hired.

The résumé should include:

- Your name, address, and telephone number
- Your educational background. List your most recent education first, giving dates and a brief summary of the content.
- Your work history, especially if it shows successful experience in the same or related areas as the position for which you are applying. Include your work history over the past 5 years. List your most recent experience first.
- Other experiences you have had can be valuable. Jobs in which you have shown initiative, reliability, and trustworthiness are a plus and should be included. If you have not had paid employment, indicate how you spent your time. Worthwhile endeavors that might be included are:
  - Taking care of children
  - Finishing school
  - Doing volunteer work for your church or community
- List three references (people who know you and can comment on your character and abilities). *Note:* You must get permission from your references before using their names.
- Include some personal information, such as hobbies and other interests. It is not necessary to include your:
  - Ethnic origin
  - Religion
  - Age
  - Marital status

Note: Some people feel that to include personal information such as height, weight, sex, marital status, or religious affiliation is an invasion of privacy. Some of this information may be discussed in the interview, but it is not necessary to include it on your résumé.

Make several copies of your résumé. Always keep the original so that you can make more copies if necessary. Put a copy in your own file. Carry a copy of your résumé whenever you seek employment. It is a ready reference as you fill out forms.

Step IV—References

References are people who know you and who are willing to comment, either in writing or over the telephone, about you and your abilities. The references need to know you well enough to make an honest evaluation, but they should not be part of your family. Always get permission to use their names before listing references in your résumé. This is a matter of courtesy and ethics.

You may want to refresh the memory of your references about dates of employment or experiences that you have listed in your résumé. When listing these references be sure to include:

* Names
* Accurate titles
* Addresses
* Telephone numbers

Step V—Taking the Step

You have made your assessment of your strengths, limitations, and needs. You have searched the market for opportunities and prepared your résumé. Now you must apply for a job:

* Select three facilities that you are most interested in.
* Call and ask for the Director of Nursing or Personnel Department (Figure 34-4).
* If you are responding to advertisements in the newspaper, follow the printed instructions

FIGURE 34-4 Call for an appointment for an interview.

about the person to contact and if your résumé must be mailed or personally delivered to the facility.

* Ask if there are any openings for a nursing assistant. If yes, ask what application procedure is to be followed.

The person in charge of hiring may ask you some questions about your education and experience, so be prepared to answer in a positive manner. He or she may set up an appointment for an **interview**. This is a specific time to meet and discuss your possible employment. Before you call, it is helpful if you know when you will be available and how you would reach the facility to keep the appointment.

Before hanging up:

* Obtain the name of the person to whom you are speaking.
* Thank this person by name.

Step VI—The Interview (Putting Your Best Foot Forward)

You must sell yourself during the interview. Prepare carefully for the interview by:

* Planning what you will wear
    * Do not overdress.
    * Be sure your clothes are neat and clean.
    * Polish your shoes.
    * Check your clothes for loose or lost buttons or stains; repair hems if necessary.
* Being sure to use deodorant
* Making sure your hair is clean and neat
* Making sure a beard or mustache is trimmed
* Avoiding the use of heavy makeup or strong perfume or aftershave

Next, make a list of information you want to share with the interviewer (Figure 34-5). You will of course share your background and answer questions the interviewer will ask. The interviewer will want proof of citizenship. Many facilities require drug testing and a criminal background check. Information from the certified nursing assistant registry of each state in which you were previously employed will be gathered. Be honest.

You will be asked to complete an employment application. Be sure you have a copy of your résumé for reference. Also have with you your nursing aide certificate, CPR card, proof of continuing education, and some form of identification such as your driver's license.

FIGURE 34-5 Be prepared for the interview. Know what you want to learn and what you want to share with the interviewer.

Be prepared to answer questions from the interviewer. Typical questions include:

- Why do you want to work in this facility?
- Why are you leaving your present employment, or why did you leave your last position?
- What do you feel are your strongest skills?
- What are your weakest skills and how have you tried to improve them?
- How well would your coworkers and supervisors feel you related to them?
- How do you feel about people who need much care and are often demanding?

In turn, you will want to learn the following:

- Starting salary
- Schedule of raises
- Fringe benefits
  - Retirement
  - Tuition reimbursement
  - Availability of credit union
  - Holiday pay or overtime
  - Health benefits
- Hours of work
- Responsibilities (ask for a job description)
- Uniform regulations
- Opportunities for growth (in-service, education, and orientation)

Make sure your interview is a success:

- Be on time for your interview. Promptness indicates interest and dependability.
- Stand until you are invited to sit down—then do so.
- Let the interviewer lead the discussion.
- Answer all questions honestly and frankly, but avoid negative comments about others.
- Emphasize your reasons for wanting to be part of the staff.

On the Job

It sometimes takes multiple interviews before you find the right job for you.

- Explain how you can contribute to the facility.
- Question the interviewer about salary and benefits toward the end of the interview.
- Thank the interviewer(s) at the end of the interview, whether you are hired or not.
- Leave a copy of your résumé, if you have not already done so. If an opening occurs in the near future, your file is available and you will be remembered.

After the interview:

- Go home and congratulate yourself if you were hired.
- If you were not hired, do not be discouraged. Think through the interview. Consider changes you may want to make in your answers in future interviews.
- Send a short thank-you note to the person who interviewed you. Thank the person for giving you the opportunity to be interviewed for the job (Figure 34-6).

Job hunting is not easy. It is emotionally stressful and can be physically exhausting. Keep trying and you will find a position to challenge you. Good luck!

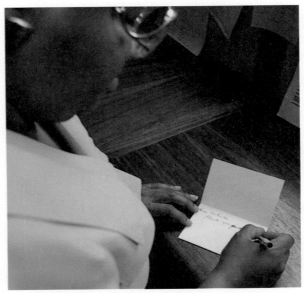

FIGURE 34-6 Send a thank-you note after the interview. It is considerate and helps the interviewer remember you.

KEEPING THE JOB

Getting the job was only the beginning; now you must keep it. You can secure your position if you:

* Arrive on time (Figure 34-7).
* Perform your work as taught, and be flexible about change.
* Follow the rules of ethical and legal conduct.
* Maintain an open positive attitude; be ready to learn and grow. *Remember:* Learning is a life-long challenge.

GROWING

You will continue to grow if you take advantage of each new experience and the opportunities you find.

* Watch experienced staff members and learn by their example.
* Do not be afraid to ask questions at the appropriate times.
* Use the nursing and medical literature that is available to learn more about the conditions of the residents (Figure 34-8).
* Participate in the care plan conferences with an open mind so that each can become a learning experience for you.
* Listen to your periodic evaluation with an open mind and follow the suggestions for improvement.

Investigate ways of advancing your education, such as:

FIGURE 34-7 Secure your new job by being prompt.

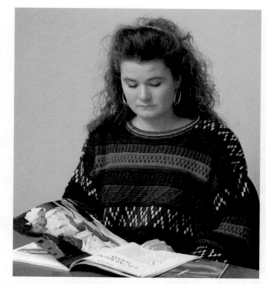

FIGURE 34-8 Take every opportunity you can to increase your knowledge.

* A general education course offered at the high school or college in your area
* Courses in communication, listening, English, and psychology. These can be helpful in your career.
* **Cross-training** courses to increase your skills in related work. For example, you may be trained to draw blood or perform specific respiratory care procedures. Such a program may be available in your facility, at a local community college or vocational school, or in an acute care hospital.
* Courses offered for continuing education credit for nurses. These are sometimes available, without credit and at a reduced price, for nonlicensed persons.
* Courses offered by hospitals or public health facilities on subjects of general public interest, such as hypertension, weight control, and diabetes
* Selecting books at the library about aging and the aging process
* Programs that can prepare you for professional development as a licensed practical nurse or registered nurse
* Learning about advanced positions in your own facility for which you may be qualified now or could study to qualify for at a later time

In-Service Education

All staff members are expected to participate in in-service education programs. This is called *staff development*. Some of the programs will be attended by all members of the interdisciplinary team. Other programs may be presented for nursing assistants only (Figure 34-9). OBRA requires that all nursing assistants participate in a minimum of 12 hours of in-service education each year. At these programs, you will learn:

- New or revised state and federal regulations
- New facility policies
- New procedures for resident care
- Use of new equipment
- Care of residents with unusual diagnoses or unique problems
- Issues in health care

The more you learn, the better you can care for residents and the more you will enjoy your work.

RESIGNING

The time may come when you find it necessary to leave your current job. To do this properly, check your facility policy before making your resignation plans. Then give notice as early as possible and submit a letter of resignation. Appropriate notice is usually equal to the time of a pay period, or 2 weeks on the average.

Your letter of resignation should include:

- The date
- A salutation to the Director of Nursing
- A brief explanation of your reasons for leaving. *Note:* Even if you feel upset by something that happened, make your reasons positive in nature.

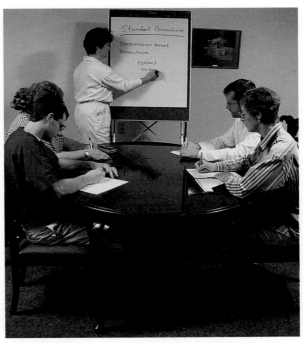

FIGURE 34-9 In-service education helps the staff grow in their understanding of residents and residents' needs.

- The date your resignation is to be effective
- A thank-you for the opportunity to have worked and learned as an employee of the facility
- Your signature

Remember that if you do not work as a nursing assistant in long-term care for 24 months, you must recertify before you can be re-employed.

LESSON SYNTHESIS: Putting It All Together

You have just completed this lesson. Now go back and review the Clinical Focus. Try to see how the Clinical Focus relates to the concepts presented in the lesson. Then answer the following questions.

1. Why is honest self-appraisal the first step a nursing assistant must take when seeking employment?

2. Why should a reference be someone who is unrelated to the applicant?

3. Why is it important to dress "appropriately" for an interview?

4. Why is it important to be truthful during the initial interview about any limitations or restrictions related to employment?

REVIEW

A. Match each term (items a.–d.) with the proper definition.

a. interview   c. references
b. networking   d. résumé

1. _____ gathering a group of people with similar needs and interests to learn about work-related opportunities

2. _____ specific time to meet and discuss possible employment

3. _____ summary of education and work experiences

4. _____ people who know you and are willing to comment about you and your abilities

B. Answer each statement true (T) or false (F).

5. T   F   The first step in preparing to find a job is to call for an interview.

6. T   F   A positive attitude is important in a person who is seeking a job.

7. T   F   Personal appearance is important in making a first impression on a prospective employer.

8. T   F   After giving a person's name as a reference, you should always obtain permission from that person.

9. T   F   During the interview you should learn about the responsibilities of the job.

10. T   F   Thank the interviewer whether you are hired or not.

11. T   F   Being prompt to an interview indicates interest.

12. T   F   Before the interview, you should make a list of the information you want to share with the interviewer and the information you want from the interviewer.

13. T   F   When giving a person as a reference, it is not necessary to ask permission first.

C. Provide brief answers for each of the following:

14. List two factors that may limit the location where you can work.

15. Name three places to start looking for job opportunities.

D. Select the one best answer for each of the following.

16. When completing a résumé, include your
(A) ethnic origin
(B) religion
(C) educational background
(D) marital status

17. A person listed as a reference should be able to comment on your
(A) character and abilities
(B) age and marital status
(C) religion and ethnic origin
(D) height and weight

18. When listing a reference, be sure to include the person's
(A) place of employment
(B) ethnic origin
(C) marital status
(D) accurate telephone number

19. You can grow in your career if you
(A) never ask questions
(B) attend related educational courses
(C) do not attend care plan conferences
(D) read books on flower arranging

20. During the interview you will want to learn about all of the following, except
(A) salary
(B) benefits
(C) hours of work
(D) public transportation schedule

21. If you have not had paid employment recently, you should:
(A) give a detailed explanation of your hobbies
(B) list worthwhile endeavors
(C) list your least recent experience first
(D) make up something and hope the employer will not check

E. Clinical experience

22. Sarah has been employed by her facility for a year. She enjoys her work and the people she works with but she would like to be more challenged. What actions can she take to help her meet her needs?

23. Tilly has just received her evaluation. Her supervisor suggested several ways she can improve her performance. Tilly is upset by the evaluation and complains about her supervisor to her friend during lunch. What do you think of Tilly's response? Is it a productive response? How would you respond?

24. Charlie is going to his first in-service education meeting. What kinds of information might he learn? How many hours of in-service education must Charlie have each year?

25. Marie is a single mother with two small children. She is thinking of working through the registry in her town. Why might this be a good plan for her?

Glossary

abbreviation shortened form of a word or phrase

abdominal area area of trunk between thorax and pelvis

abdominopelvic cavity the body cavity extending between the diaphragm and the floor of the pelvis

abduction movement away from midline or center

accelerated increased motion, as in pulse or respiration

acceptance favorable reception

accuracy completing assignments carefully, without mistakes

acetone a colorless liquid produced in the body; found in small quantities in normal urine and larger amounts in diabetic urine

active assistive range of motion carrying out of specific exercises by the resident with some help from the care provider; exercises are designed to move each joint through its range of motion

active range of motion resident carries out exercises without help; all joints are moved through their full range of motion

activities of daily living (ADL) the activities necessary for resident to fulfill basic human needs

acupressure therapy that uses pressure at specific points to cure illness or relieve pain

acupuncture therapy from Chinese medicine that uses insertion of small needles in specific areas of the skin to cure illness or relieve pain

adaptive behavior the degree to which a person meets standards of personal independence and social responsibility appropriate for the person's age and culture

adaptive device ordinary items that are modified or changed in some way so that the device can be used by individuals with specific disabilities

adduction movement toward midline or center

adjunctive (complementary) therapy a treatment that goes with and supplements primary medical care

ADL *See* activities of daily living

administrator one who manages a facility

adrenal glands two glands, located one on top of each kidney, that produce hormones

adrenaline epinephrine—hormone produced by adrenal glands

advance directive a document signed before the diagnosis of a terminal illness, when the individual is still in good health, indicating the person's wishes regarding care during dying

advocate one who speaks and acts on behalf of another

age-related macular degeneration cause of blindness in elderly

agitation an increase in physical activity usually accompanied by anger and irritation

aiding and abetting not reporting dishonest acts that are observed

AIDS acquired immune deficiency syndrome; a condition caused by the HIV virus

airborne precautions techniques to prevent transmission of airborne organisms

akinesia abnormal absence or poverty of movement

alignment proper position

allergen substance that causes sensitivity or allergic reactions

alopecia hair loss

alternative therapy a regimen or treatment that is not a part of conventional Western medicine

alveoli tiny air sacs that make up the bulk of the lungs

Alzheimer's disease a disorder of the brain that involves thinking, memory, and judgment; a form of dementia

ambulate to walk

amenorrhea abnormal cessation or absence of the menses

amputation removal of a limb or other body appendage

amulet protective charm

anastomose surgical connection made between two body structures (such as blood vessels) that are not normally joined

anatomic position standing erect, facing observer, feet flat on the floor; arms extended, palms forward

anatomy study of the structure of the human body

anemia deficiency of red blood cells in the blood

aneurysm a sac formed by dilation of the wall of a blood vessel (usually an artery) and filled with blood; a weak spot in an arterial wall

anger feeling of hostility or rage

angina pectoris acute pain in the chest caused by interference with the supply of oxygen to the heart

ankle-foot orthosis assistive device that provides medial lateral support for an unstable ankle

anorexia loss of appetite

anoxia lack of oxygen

anterior in anatomy, in front of the coronal or ventral plane

antibiotic medication to fight infection caused by bacteria

antibody protein formed in the body that protects a person against a specific infectious organism

antidepressant medication effective against depressive illness

antigen a foreign or pathogenic substance that enters the body and stimulates the production of antibodies

antihypertensive medication effective against hypertension (high blood pressure)

antioxidant a substance that inhibits oxidation and cellular damage from free radicals

anuria absence of secretions of urine by the kidneys

anus the outlet of the rectum lying in the fold between the buttocks

aorta the great artery arising from the left ventricle

apathy indifference; lack of emotion

apex the top of a cone-shaped structure, such as the heart

aphasia language impairment; loss of ability to comprehend normally

apical pertaining to the apex of a structure such as the heart

apical pulse pulse rate taken by placing stethoscope over tip of heart

apnea period of no respirations

approach steps to be taken to reach a goal

Aquamatic K-Pad® commercial unit for applying heat or cold

aromatherapy inhalation treatment using oils and scent to relieve pain and promote healing

arteriosclerosis general term meaning a narrowing of the blood vessels, which can result in subsequent tissue hypoxia; degeneration and hardening of the walls of arteries and sometimes of the valves of the heart

artery a vessel through which the blood passes away from the heart to various parts of the body

arthritis joint inflammation

articulation point where two bones meet

artificial nutrition ways other than eating to provide nutrition for a resident

ascites fluid accumulation in the abdomen

asepsis without infection

asepto syringe glass syringe with rubber ball used to perform moist treatments

aspiration drawing foreign material into the respiratory tract

assault violent act; an unlawful threat or attempt to harm another physically

assessment act of evaluating

assignments a designated list of duties

assistive device equipment used to help people be more effective in their physical activity; helps promote and maintain independence in performing activities of daily living

asthenia weakness

asthma a chronic respiratory disease characterized by bronchospasms and excessive mucus production

ataxic cerebral palsy form of cerebral palsy in which the principal disturbance is a lack of balance and coordination

atherosclerosis degenerative process involving the lining of arteries, in which the lumen eventually narrows and closes; a form of arteriosclerosis; primarily associated with some degree of atheroma development

athetoid cerebral palsy form of cerebral palsy characterized by involuntary, slow, incessant movements of the parts of the body that are affected

atrium (pl. *atria*) one of the upper heart chambers

atrophy shrinking or wasting away of tissues

attitude the state of mind that is indicative of feelings or opinions

audiologist physician specializing in hearing problems

auditory nerve nerve carrying sound from the ear to the brain

aura a peculiar sensation preceding the appearance of more definite symptoms in a convulsion or seizure

aural pertaining to the ear

autoclave a sterilizing machine

autoimmune antibodies against components of the body

automatic external defibrillator nonintrusive device that restores the heartbeat and rhythm by means of electric shock

axilla the armpit

Ayurveda Eastern Indian system of medicine that uses body types *(doshas)* as the basis for prevention, diagnosis, and cure of disease

bacteremia the presence of bacteria in the blood

bargaining attempting to make a "deal" to influence the final outcome of a situation

battery an unlawful threat or attempt to harm another physically

behavior modification an approach that is based on rewarding positive behaviors and initiating corrective action for negative behaviors

benign prostatic hypertrophy noncancerous enlargement of the prostate gland

bile a secretion of the liver needed to prepare fats for digestion

biofeedback therapy that trains the user to gain voluntary mental control over normally involuntary bodily responses

biohazard contaminated with blood or body fluids and having the potential to transmit disease

bladder a membranous sac containing fluid, such as the urinary bladder

blood pressure pressure of blood exerted against the vascular walls

body alignment correct and straight body position

body language nonverbal communication signaled by behavior, facial expressions, body stance

body mechanics using muscles correctly to move or lift heavy objects properly

body work   hands-on therapies that involve manipulation, massage, and realignment of the body

bowel   intestine

Bowman's capsule   tubule surrounding the glomerulus of the nephron in the kidney

bradycardia   unusually slow heartbeat

Braille   system of raised dots representing letters A through Z and numbers 0 through 9 that allows sight-impaired residents to "read" through the sense of touch

brain stem   part of the brain including the medulla oblongata, diencephalon, pons, and midbrain

bridging   technique used to reduce pressure on ischemic areas by use of pillows and pads

bronchi   primary divisions of the trachea

bronchioles   one of the finer subdivisions or branches of the bronchial tree

bronchitis   inflammation of the bronchi

burnout   loss of enthusiasm and interest in an activity

bursae   small synovial-filled sacs located around joints that help reduce friction

bursitis   inflammation of a bursa

calculi   stones or concretions

calorie-restricted diet   a diet that limits the intake of calories

cancer   a malignant tumor; malignancy

cannula   a small tube that may be inserted into a cavity to allow the passage of fluid

capillary   hairlike blood vessel; the link between arterioles and venules

carbohydrates   energy foods; used by the body to produce heat and for work

carbon dioxide   gas that is a waste product in cellular metabolism

cardiac arrest   sudden heart stoppage

cardiac cycle   all the events (mechanical and electrical) that occur between one contraction and the next; the series of movements through which the heart passes in performing one heartbeat

cardiac muscle   special tissue making up the muscular wall of the heart

cardiogram   a record of cardiac pulsation produced by cardiograph

cardiopulmonary resuscitation (CPR)   emergency medical procedure undertaken to restart and sustain heart and respiratory function

cardiovascular   pertaining to the heart and blood vessels

care plan   plan developed by the interdisciplinary health care team that describes the goals and approaches that all team members are to use in caring for the resident

care plan conference   a meeting of team members to plan resident care

caries   dental cavities

carrier   a person who harbors infectious organisms that can be transmitted to others but who shows no sign of illness personally

cartilage   type of connective tissue

cast   rigid covering to keep a joint or other body part immobile

cataract   opacity of the lens, resulting in loss of vision

catastrophic reaction   response characterized by increased agitation and anxiety

catheter   tube for evacuating or injecting fluids

cavity   an enclosed area

cell   basic unit in the organization of living substance

cellular respiration   physiologic process that takes place in the cells by which cellular energy is derived

cellulose   a basic substance of all plant foods, which can supply the body with roughage

Celsius   scale for measuring temperature

centimeter   one-hundredth of a meter

central nervous system (CNS)   brain and spinal cord

central venous catheter   small tube placed in a major vein, such as the subclavian vein

central venous pressure (CVP)   measurement of blood pressure in the large central veins

cerebellum   part of the brain responsible for balance and muscle coordination

cerebral   pertaining to the brain

cerebral palsy   motor disorder that results in inability to control body movement

cerebrospinal fluid   watery, clear fluid that surrounds the brain and spinal cord

cerebrovascular accident (CVA)   interference with the cerebral blood flow

cerebrum   largest and main portion of the brain responsible for sensory interpretation and voluntary muscle activity

certification   official recognition of successful completion of education, learning, and testing; also, the qualification of a health care facility for government funding

character (of pulse)   rhythm and volume of pulse

chart   record of information concerning resident

cheeking   storing food in one side of the mouth

chemical restraint   drugs used to influence or control a resident's behavior

chemotherapy   treatment with drugs or chemicals

Cheyne-Stokes respiration   periods of apnea alternating with periods of hyperpnea

CHF   congestive heart failure

Chinese medicine   traditional Chinese system of medicine and therapies, based on balancing of *yin* and *yang* elements in the body

chiropractic   system of therapy that uses manipulation and adjustment of bodily structures, particularly the spinal column, to relieve pain and promote health and healing

chlamydia   rod-shaped microbes that can cause trachoma, a serious eye infection, and sexually transmitted infections

choroid   the vascular layer, or coat, of the eye

chronic   persisting over a long period

chronic bronchitis   condition in which there is excessive mucus secretion in the bronchi

chronic disease   a condition that continues over a long period

chronic obstructive pulmonary disease (COPD)   any condition that causes interference with normal respirations over a prolonged period, such as emphysema

chux   disposable pads sometimes placed under residents as a linen saver

circadian   daily biorhythmic functions and cycle

clear liquid diet   a diet in which all nutrients must be in the form of liquid that is clear

clergy   ministers, priests, rabbis; religious leaders

client   resident

climacteric   menopause; the combined phenomena accompanying the cessation of the reproductive function in the female or diminution of testicular activity in the male

clitoris   a small, cylindrical mass of erotic tissue; part of the external female reproductive organs analogous to the penis in the male

CNS   central nervous system

code blue   a signal given when a resident is in danger of dying so that lifesaving techniques can be used

cognitive impairment   a term used to describe any form of dementia

colon   large intestine

colonized   establishment of a population of micro-organisms growing on body surfaces but not necessarily causing an infection

colostomy   a surgically established opening between the colon and the surface of the abdomen to allow elimination of feces

comatose   unconscious; in a coma

combining form   part of word that may be arranged in different ways to form new words

comminuted fracture   fracture in which the bone is broken or crushed into small pieces

commode   a portable toilet

communal   pertaining to something that is shared with others

communicable   capable of being transferred from one person to another directly or indirectly, such as infectious disease

communicate   to make known

communication   transmission of a message from a sender to a receiver

community services   special services provided outside of the facility

compensation   in psychology, the act of seeking a substitute for something unacceptable or unattainable

compliance   obedience; following directions; doing what one is supposed to do

compound fracture   fracture in which the broken bone protrudes through the skin

comprehension   the capacity of the mind for understanding

concentration   an increase in strength by evaporation

condom   a rubber sheath used to cover the penis

confidential   keeping what is said or written to oneself; private; nonsharing

congestive heart failure (CHF)   a chronic inability of the heart to maintain an adequate output of blood from one or both ventricles, resulting in an inadequate blood supply to the body tissues

conjunctiva   mucous membrane that covers the eye and lines the eyelids

connective tissue   special body tissue that holds other tissues together and provides support for organs and other structures of body

connective tissue cell   cell that produces connective tissue

constipation   difficulty in defecating

constricting   making narrower

constriction   narrowed or compressed area

consultant   one who offers professional advice

contact precautions   practices used to prevent the spread of pathogens by direct or indirect contact

contagious   communicable or easily spread

contaminated   unclean; impure; soiled with germs

continent   able to control elimination of feces and urine

contract   an agreement between two or more people, especially one that is written; to shorten, to decrease in size

contracture   permanent shortening or contraction of a muscle because of spasm or paralysis

convalescent home   long-term care facility

convulsion   involuntary muscle spasm

COPD   chronic obstructive pulmonary disease; for example, pulmonary emphysema

cornea   clear (transparent) anterior covering of the eye

coronary occlusion   closing off or blockage of a coronary artery

corporal punishment   use of painful treatment to correct behavior

cortex   the outer covering or portions of an organ

cortisone   hormone produced by the adrenal cortex

Cowper's gland   two small glands located besie the male urethra, below the prostate gland, which secrete a fluid into the semen

CPR   *See* cardiopulmonary resuscitation

cross-training   education and instruction in a field or area different from one's primary employment

cubic centimeter (cc)   a measurement of volume equal to 1000 cubic millimeters

culture and sensitivity   taking a sample from an infected area to discover the cause of the infection and then determine the proper antibiotic therapy; the organisms are grown and their reactions to different antibiotics determined

cutaneous   relating to the skin

cutaneous membrane   skin

cuticle   area around the base of a fingernail or toenail

CVA   cerebrovascular accident

CVP   central venous pressure; measurement of blood pressure in the large central veins

cyanosis   bluish skin discoloration from lack of oxygen

cyanotic   pertaining to blueness most commonly observed under the nails, lips, and skin as a result of lack of oxygen

cystocele   bladder hernia

cystoscopy   procedure using cystoscope for visualization of the urinary bladder, ureter, and kidney

day care center   a place where senior citizens may go for various services

day room   a room in a long-term care residence where residents can meet for activities and socialization at times other than meal time

debilitating   weakening

debridement   removal of foreign matter or devitalized tissue from a wound

decline   deterioration or negative change in a resident's condition or abilities

deconditioned   condition in which tissue and organs become weakened from lack of use

decubiti   pressure sores; bedsores; decubitus ulcers

defamation of character   making false or damaging statements about another person that harm that person's reputation

defecation   bowel movement that expels feces

defense mechanism   psychological reaction or technique for protection against a stressful environmental situation or anxiety

defibrillation   artifical restoration of the heartbeat and heart rhythm by means of electric shock

dehydration   excessive loss of fluid from the body

delegation   passing on of orders or responsibilities

delirium   disordered mental condition in which speech is incoherent, fever may occur, and illusions, delusions, and hallucinations may be experienced

delusion   a false belief

dementia   progressive mental deterioration caused by organic brain disease

dendrite   the branch of a neuron conducting impulses toward the cell body

denial   an unconscious defense mechanism in which an occurrence or observation is refused recognition as reality to avoid anxiety or pain

dental hygienist   a person licensed and specially trained to perform oral hygiene, including cleaning of teeth

dentist   a person licensed and specially trained to practice dentistry and/or dental surgery

dentures   false teeth

deoxygenated   to have lost oxygen

dependability   trustworthiness; reliability

depressant   something (a drug, for example) that decreases functional activity

depression   feelings of sadness and unresponsiveness

dermal ulcer (decubitus)   pressure sore or bed sore

dermis   corium; true skin; the layer of skin beneath the epithelium

deteriorate   to progressively break down or disorganize

developmental disability   a severe, chronic disorder apparent before age 22, caused by mental or physical impairment

developmental disease   condition or disease that is present at birth or early childhood and limits a person's ability to provide self-care in an independent way

developmental tasks   in psychology, tasks that are normally carried out as steps in personality development

diabetes mellitus   a disorder of carbohydrate metabolism

diabetic coma   a comatose state of acidosis caused by diabetes mellitus

diabetic ketoacidosis   state of acidosis caused by diabetes mellitus

diabetic retinopathy   damage to the eye and vision as a result of diabetes mellitus

diagnosis   determination of the specific disease or condition causing a patient's symptoms

diagnostic-related group   classification that limits the number of days resident can stay in facility

dialysis   treatment when kidneys fail to remove accumulated wastes from the blood

diaphoresis   profuse sweating

diaphragm   dome-shaped muscle that divides the ventral cavity into a thorax and an abdominopelvic cavity

diarrhea   watery stool

diarthrotic   pertains to freely movable joints

diastole   period during which the heart muscle relaxes and the chamber fills with blood

diastolic   pertains to the relaxation phase of the cardiac cycle

diathermy   treatment with heat

diet   the food and drink necessary for body nourishment

dietetics   systematic regulation of the diet for therapeutic purposes

dietician   a person specially trained in the field of nutrition and the science of dietetics (diets)

dificiencies   lacks; absence of or lessened abilities; areas of noncompliance with relevant standards

digestion   the process of converting food into an assimilable form

dilating   enlarging

diplegia   movement disturbance that primarily affects the legs

directive   serving or qualified to direct; a statement (document) that allows families, physicians, and nurses to follow the wishes of the individual when death occurs or is imminent

dirty contaminated with microbes

disability persistent physical or mental defect or handicap

discharge planner person who arranges for care after discharge from facility and helps resident make the transition from the facility to the community

discharge planning planning for care after resident leaves facility

disinfected cleaned to destroy pathogens

disinfection process of destroying pathogenic organisms or agents on articles or surfaces

dislocation one bone displaced from its normal alignment with another

disorientation loss of recognition of time, place, location, or persons

displacement an unconscious defense mechanism in which an emotion such as anger is directed at the wrong person

distal farthest away from a central point, such as point of attachment of muscles

distended to be stretched

diuretics drugs that increase urine output

diverticuli small blind pouches that form in the lining and wall of the colon

diverticulitis inflammation of diverticula

diverticulosis presence of many diverticula

DNR *See* do not resuscitate order

document the process of recording observations and data about a resident's condition

documentation substantiating statements

do not resuscitate (DNR) order physician order indicating that resident is not to be revived when cardiac and respiratory arrest occur

dorsal posterior or back

dorsal cavity the posterior body cavity consisting of the cranium and vertebral canal

draw sheet a sheet folded under resident and extending from above the shoulder to below the hips

DRG diagnosis-related grouping

drip chamber part of the equipment used to administer parenteral fluids

droplet precautions practices used to prevent the spread of microbes transmitted by droplets in the air produced by laughing, talking, singing, sneezing, or coughing

dry sterile dressing (DSD) a sterile dressing that is applied dry to a wound

duodenum the first part of small intestine

durable power of attorney a document that permits a person to delegate to someone else the power to make any health care decisions that the person is unable to make

dyspepsia indigestion

dysphagia difficulty in swallowing

dyspnea difficult or labored breathing

dysuria painful urination

ECG *See* electrocardiogram

edema excessive accumulation of fluid in the tissues

ejaculation forcible, sudden expulsion of semen from the penis

ejaculatory duct part of the male reproductive tract extending from the seminal vesicles to the urethra

electrocardiogram (ECG or EKG) a recording of the electrical activity of the heart

electroencephalogram graphic recording of the electrical activity of the brain

electrolytes compounds that play an essential role in body function

elimination excretion; discharge from the body of indigestible materials and of waste products of body metabolism

embolus blood clot that moves through the vascular system

emergency unexpected occurrence that requires immediate action

Emergency Medical Services (EMS) services provided by specially trained people at the scene of the emergency and in the ambulance

emesis vomitus

emesis basin utensil for catching vomitus

emotional lability easily upset, emotionally unstable

empathy intellectual understanding of something in another person that is foreign to one's self

emphysema chronic obstructive pulmonary disease in which the alveolar walls are destroyed

empowerment power or authority

EMS *See* Emergency Medical Services

endocrine gland gland that secretes hormonal substances directly into bloodstream; ductless gland

endometrium lining of the uterus

endotracheal within the trachea

endotracheal tube a tube placed in the trachea to assist respiration

enema the introduction of liquid into the bowel or the rectum to be returned or retained

enteral feeding feeding that bypasses the mouth and goes directly into the intestinal tract

enteric pertaining to the alimentary canal; intestinal

environment surroundings

environmental services department and workers responsible for maintaining clean and comfortable surroundings for residents and staff

enzymes organic catalysts produced by living cells but capable of acting independently of the cells producing them

epidermis the top layer of skin

epididymis an elongated, cordlike structure along the posterior border of the testes in the ducts of which the sperm is stored

epidural catheter tube inserted into spinal area for delivery of medication

epilepsy a noninfectious disorder of the brain manifested by episodes of motor and sensory dysfunction, which may or may not be accompanied by convulsions and unconsciousness

epithelial cells   cells that produce and form epithelial tissue

epithelial tissue   tissue that forms the skin and parts of the secreting glands and that lines the body cavities; specialized in its ability to absorb, secrete, excrete, and protect

epithelium   tissues characterized by tightly packed cells with a minimum of intracellular material; forms epidermis and lines all hollow organs and passages of respiratory, digestive, and genitourinary systems

equilibrium   sense of balance

ergonomics   techniques used by workers to avoid injuries

erythrocyte   red blood cell

esophagus   a tube extending from the pharynx to stomach

estrogen   hormone produced by ovaries

ethical code   rules governing the right or wrong of professional behavior

ethics   the study of standards of conduct or moral judgement

evaluation   judgment; critical review of a situation or condition; determination of how the resident's plan of care is working

exacerbation   period of increased severity of symptoms

excreta   excretions, such as feces

expectorant   medication to aid in expectoration (spitting up phlegm)

expectorate   spit

expiration   exhalation

exposure incident   a situation in which an individual has been in possible contact with infectious material

extended care facility   long-term care facility

extension   movement by which the two ends of any jointed part are drawn away from each other

external fixation   method of stabilizing fractured bones

Fahrenheit (scale)   scale for measuring temperature

fallopian tube   *See* **oviduct**

false imprisonment   detaining an individual without a reason and against the individual's will

fantasizing   imagining

fasting   the act of going without food over a definite and prolonged period

fats   nutrient used to store energy

fecal impaction   feces firmly wedged in the rectum

feces   semi-solid waste eliminated from the body

femur   thigh bone

fiber   nondigestible part of food that adds bulk to intestinal waste

financial abuse   misuse or unauthorized use of a resident's money

fistula   abnormal tubelike passageway within body tissue

flaccid   soft, not firm; incapable of independent movement

flatulence   excessive gas in the stomach and intestines

flatus   gas or air in the stomach or intestines; air or gas expelled via any body opening

flexed   bent

flora   community of organisms living in or on a particular body area

flow meter   an instrument for controlling gas flow in oxygen equipment

flow rate   the speed at which a fluid such as glucose and water flows into an intravenous infusion, or a gas such as oxygen flows into an oxygen mask to a resident

folk medicine   traditional treatments and therapies developed over many years by various cultures

fomite   inanimate objects or sufaces on which disease-producing and infectious agents may be conveyed

footboard   appliance placed at the foot of the bed so the feet rest firmly against it; maintains feet at 90° angle to the legs

forced fluids   notation meaning that resident must be encouraged to take as much fluid as possible

foreskin   prepuce; loose tissue covering the penis and clitoris

Fowler's position   head of bed is rolled up and resident is in semi-sitting position

fracture   break in the continuity of bone

frequency   occurrence often repeated

friction   rubbing of one surface against another surface

full liquid diet   a diet in which all nutrients must be in liquid form

functional ability   ability to carry out activities of daily living

functional changes   decrease in ability to carry out activities of daily living

gait   manner of walking

gait belt   belt placed around the resident's waist to assist in ambulation

gait training   teaching the resident to walk

gallbladder   small, saclike organ, found on the underside of the liver, that stores bile

gangrene   the death and putrefaction of body tissue, caused by stoppage of circulation of blood to an area

gastritis   inflammation of the stomach

gastrointestinal tract   intestinal or digestive tract

gastrostomy   surgical opening into the stomach

gastrostomy tube (GT)   tube surgically placed through the abdomen into the stomach for feeding

gatch bed   bed fitted with a jointed back rest and knee rest; resident can be raised to a sitting position and kept in that position; special bed that can be raised or lowered, and allows the head and knee areas to be elevated to different positions

gavage   feeding through a tube

genetic disease   condition caused by problems with the genes

genital   pertaining to reproduction

genitalia   the reproductive organs

geriatric   pertaining to the elderly

germs   pathogenic microorganisms

gerontology   study of the aging process

glaucoma   increased intraocular pressure, which ultimately results in loss of vision

glomerulus   a ball-like bed of capillaries that forms part of the nephron

glucagon   a hormone formed by the islets of Langerhans in the pancreas; raises the glucose level of blood

glucometer   instrument used to measure blood sugar levels

glucose   simple sugar; also called dextrose

glycosuria   sugar in the urine

goal   objective outcome or result

goiter   enlargement of the thyroid gland

gonads   reproductive organs; ovaries (female) and testes (male)

goniometer   instrument for measuring angles, used in assessing range of motion and contractures

gonorrhea   a sexually transmitted disease characterized by a purulent drainage from the mucous membranes of the genital organs

gossip   talking about residents at lunch time or on a break

graft   body tissue used for transplantation

grand mal seizure   a convulsion that involves the whole body; the person loses consciousness and may be incontinent

grievance   a circumstance felt to be unjust or about which there are grounds for complaint

GT   *See* gastrostomy tube

halitosis   bad breath

hallucination   idea or perception that is not based on reality

harmony   friendly, pleasant relations

heart   hollow, muscular organ lying slightly to the left of the midline of the chest

heart attack   condition that makes the heart unable to function properly or at all

heart block   partial or complete inhibition of the speed of electrical impulse conduction from the atrium to the ventricle of the heart

Heimlich maneuver   technique used to dislodge food from the throat of a choking person

hematuria   blood in the urine

hemianopsia   blindness in one-half of the visual field of one or both eyes

hemiplegia   paralysis on one side of the body

hemodialysis   removal of toxic products and excess fluid from the blood through a membrane

hemoptysis   expectoration of blood

hemorrhage   escape of blood from blood vessels

hemorrhoids   varicose veins in the rectum

hepatitis   inflammation of the liver

hernia   protrusion or projection of an organ or a part of an organ through the wall of a cavity that normally contains it

herniorrhaphy   surgial operation for hernia

hiatal hernia   protrusion of a portion of the stomach through the esophageal hiatus of the diaphragm

high density   concentrated

high Fowler's position   position in which the resident is sitting almost upright with knees flexed

high-protein diet   a diet in which the protein content is increased beyond the usual

HIV   *See* human immunodeficiency virus

holistic   applying to the whole; seeing a person as a complete, integrated entity with many aspects

home health services   help provided after an acute hospitalization

homeopathy   controversial alternative medicine system that relies on similarities, individualism, and infinitesimals to restore health and promote healing

homeostasis   a state of balance or equilibrium

hormone   secretion of endocrine gland; substance produced by endocrine gland

hospice   special facility or arrangement to provide care of terminally ill persons

hot-line number   a toll-free number residents may use to reach authorities outside the facility to register complaints

hot soak   a treatment in which a part of the body, such as a hand, is placed in warm water as a method of applying heat

human immunodeficiency virus (HIV)   microorganism that causes HIV disease, which may progress to AIDS

Huntington's disease   progressive degenerative disease of the brain that results in uncontrolled movements and mental deterioration

hydrotherapy   treatment that uses water for healing purposes

hygiene   a system of principles or rules designed for the promotion of health

hyperalimentation   parenteral nutrition; nutrition delivered directly into the bloodstream

hyperglycemia   excessive level of blood sugar

hypertension   high blood pressure

hyperthyroidism   a condition in which the thyroid gland is enlarged

hypertrophy   increase in size of an organ or structure, which does not involve tumor formation

hypoglycemia   abnormally low level of sugar in the blood

hypotension   low blood pressure

hypothermia   greatly reduced temperature

hypothyroidism   inadequate functioning of the thyroid gland

hypoxia   lack of adequate oxygen supply

hysterectomy   surgical removal of the uterus

IADL *See* instrumental activities of daily living

I&O intake and output

ice bag a plastic or rubber bag filled with small pieces of ice. The bag is covered with cloth and placed against a resident's body to apply cold

IDDM *See* insulin-dependent diabetes mellitus

ileostomy surgically made opening in the ileum through the abdominal wall

ileum the lower three-fifths of the small intestine, lying between the jejunum and cecum

illusion a mental impression derived from misinterpretation of an actual sensory stimulus

IM intramuscular

immunity ability of the body to fight off disease caused by microbes

immunization process of making a person more resistant to infectious agents

immunosuppression failure of the body to respond to the challenge of infectious disease organisms

impaction condition of being tightly wedged or stuck (as feces in the bowel)

impairment disability

implementation put into action; process of carrying out a plan

impotence inhability to perform sexually

incident something of consequence that happens unexpectedly. An event that might result in harm to a resident

incontinence inability to predict and control elimination of body wastes

incontinent unable to control elimination

indwelling catheter a small tube that remains in the patient for an extended period to provide continuous drainage

infarction death of tissue

infection the invasion and multiplication of any organism and the damage caused by this in the body

inferior below another part

inferior vena cava large vein that returns blood to the right atrium of the heart

inflammation process that brings blood and white blood cells to the area of injury or infection, characterized by heat, redness, swelling, and pain

inflammatory response tissue reaction to injury whether direct or referred

influenza viral disease spread by droplets

informed consent permission given by one who fully understands all the facts relating to what is going to happen

infusion introduction of a solution into a vein by gravity such as an intravenous infusion (IV)

inguinal hernia condition in which intestines push through abdominal wall in the groin area

inhibition that which restrains an action, emotion, or thought

insertion distal point of attachment of skeletal muscle

inspiration the drawing of air into the lungs (inhalation)

instrumental activities of daily living (IADL) higher-level tasks performed by adults, such as money management and driving

insulin the active antidiabetic hormone secreted by the islets of Langerhans in the pancreas; promotes utilization of sugar in the body

insulin-dependent diabetes mellitus (IDDM) a condition in which the person must rely on insulin injections to metabolize glucose

insulin shock hypoglycemia (a decrease in blood sugar), attended by anxiety, excitement, perspiration, delirium, or coma

intake refers to any nourishment or fluid taken into the body; frequently refers to intake of everything that is liquid at room temperature

intake and output (I&O) measurement of all fluids the resident ingests and excretes, in whatever form

integumentary system body system consisting of the skin, its various layers, and its accessory structures (hair, nails, and skin glands)

intelligence quotient (IQ) the ability to solve problems, adapt to the demands of the environment, and to understand abstract relationships appropriate to one's age

intention tremor trembling of hands that increases with efforts to control trembling

intercourse interchange or communication between individuals; an alternate term for sexual relations

interdisciplinary health care team group of health care providers in different specialties who act together to plan and implement the plan of care for each resident

intermittent positive pressure breathing (IPPB) a technique in which a machine is used to deliver air or oxygen and medication under pressure to a person's lungs; technique for assisting breathing

interpersonal relationships how people interact with each other

intervention actions that influence the eventual outcome of a situation

interventricular septum dividing portion between the ventricles of the heart

interview meeting with a prospective employer and discussion regarding a position

intramuscular (IM) between muscles

intravenous infusion nourishment given through a sterile tube into the veins

intravenous therapy (intravenous infusion) nutrition or medication injected by means of a sterile needle and tubing directly into a vein

invasion of privacy revealing information of a private nature regarding a resident

involuntary muscle type of muscle forming the walls of organs; also known as visceral or smooth muscle

involuntary seclusion   being kept without care and apart from others against one's will

IPPB   *See* intermittent positive pressure breathing

IQ   *See* intelligence quotient

iris   colored portion of eye

ischemia   deficient blood supply to body tissues

islets of Langerhans   special cells in the pancreas that produce insulin

isolation   place where resident with easily transmitted diseases is separated from others

isolation technique   special procedures carried out to prevent the spread of infectious organisms from infected persons

jaundice   yellowing of the skin

jejunum   portion of the small intestine between the duodenum and the ileum

job description   the duties and responsibilities involved in a position

joint   point of articulation between bones

Kardex   a type of file in which nursing care plans are kept

keratoses   roughened, scaly, wartlike lesions

ketones   products from fat metabolism

ketosis   abnormal levels of ketones in the blood; a complication of diabetes mellitus

kidney dialysis   *See* **hemodialysis**

kidneys   glandular organs that secrete urine

kilogram   1,000 grams; 2.2 pounds

kyphosis   extreme dorsal curvature of the spine in the thoracic area (hunchback)

labia majora   two large, hair-covered, liplike structures that are part of the vulva

labia minora   two hairless liplike structures found beneath the labia majora

laceration   an injury or wound made by tearing or cutting of the flesh

lactose   a form of sugar found in milk

larynx   part of the respiratory tract found on the top of the trachea just below the root of the tongue. It is the organ of voice

last rites (Sacrament of the Sick)   special service of confession and blessing practiced by clergy for Catholic residents when gravely ill

lateral   to the side; away from the midline

lateral position   side-lying position

laxative   medicine to relieve constipation

legal guardian   one who has the legal authority to make decisions and act on behalf of another

leisure   time free from engagement

lens   portion of the eye that bends light rays

lentigines   elevated yellow or brown spots or patches that occur on exposed skin; "liver spots"

lesion   abnormal change in tissue formation

leukemia   malignant disease of the blood-forming organs, characterized by abnormal proliferation and distortion of the leukocytes in the blood and bone marrow

leukocyte   white blood cell

Lhermitte's sign   seen in multiple sclerosis; a feeling of tingling and pain in the spinal column when head is flexed

libel   any oral or written defamatory statement

libido   sex drive

licensed practical nurse (LPN)/licensed vocational nurse (LVN)   a person licensed by the state who provides direct care under the supervision of a registered nurse

licensure   permission to operate or practice from a state agency that regulates a business or profession

life care facility   apartment homes that offer health care and recreational facilities for the elderly

ligaments   bands of fibrous tissue that hold joints together

light therapy   treatment regimen that uses controlled light to influence and regulate bodily processes

lipase   a fat-splitting enzyme produced by the pancreas

lipodystrophy   any disturbance in fat metabolism

living will   a written statement, usually by those who are terminally ill, requesting not to be kept alive on life support systems when faculties have failed

long-term care facility   a facility that provides care for residents with long-standing disabilities; can be terminal care

lower extremities   pertains to the legs and feet

low-fat diet   a diet in which the amount of fat has been reduced

low-sodium diet   a diet that limits the amount of sodium chloride, a mineral salt

LPN   *See* licensed practical nurse

lumen   channel (opening) within a tubelike organ

LVN   licensed vocational nurse. *See* licensed practical nurse

lymph   fluid found in lymphatic vessels

lymph node   a mass of lymphatic tissue along lymph vessels; mainly acts as a filter

magnetic resonance imaging (MRI)   procedure using computer and magnetic fields to visualize inner body organs

magnetic therapy   use of magnets in treatments to relieve pain and promote healing

malignancy   cancerous condition which, if left untreated, leads to death

malpractice   poor or improper medical treatment; for example, when assistant gives improper care or gives care in which he or she has not been instructed

manipulative behavior   actions designed to control the responses of others

mastication   the act of chewing food with the teeth in preparation for swallowing

masturbation   sexual gratification by self-manipulation of the genitals

Material Safety Data Sheets (MSDS)   information sheets on chemicals used in facility that list the health hazards, safe use, and emergency procedures for chemical exposure

maturity state of full development, physically, mentally, and psychologically

MDS 2.0 *See* Minimum Data Set

meatus an opening or channel

mechanical lift a device used to move residents who are unable to bear weight or are very heavy

mechanical soft diet a diet in which the foods are specially prepared to make them easier to chew

medial close to the midline of a body or structure

mediastinum the space between the lungs

Medicaid federal- and state-funded program that pays for medical costs for those whose income falls below a certain level

medical asepsis procedures followed to keep germs from being spread from one person to another

medical chart record of pertinent legal information relating to the resident, the resident's progress, and care

medical terminology specialized words, phrases, and abbreviations used in the field of medicine

Medicare federal program that assists those over 65 years of age with hospital and medical costs

medulla the internal portion of a gland; also refers to the lowest part of the brain stem where the vital centers for respiratory, cardiac, and vasomotor control are located

membrane a thin lining or covering of cells

memo brief written or electronic communication

meninges three-layered serous membrane covering the brain and spinal cord

menopause period when ovaries stop functioning and menstruation ceases; climacteric

menstruation periodic shedding of the endo-metrium

mental abuse making verbal threats to hurt, punish, or humiliate a resident

mental retardation a condition that occurs before age 22 and refers to significantly subaverage mental functioning and deficits in adaptive behavior

mercury a silvery metal that is liquid at room temperature; most frequently used in clinical thermometers

metabolism the sum total of the physical and chemical processes and reactions taking place in the body

metastasis spreading of cancer to other body parts

meter metric distance measurement equaling 39.371 inches

methicillin-resistant *Staphylococcus aureus* (MRSA) a common infectious microbe that is resistant to the effect of methicillin, an antibiotic

metric system a system of weights and measurements based on the meter and having all units based on some power of ten

microbe tiny organism that can only be seen with a microscope; some may cause disease

micturition urination

midplane an imaginary line that divides the body evenly into a right and left side

milliliter (mL) a measurement of capacity—volume of 1 g of water at standard temperature and pressure

mineral inorganic chemical compound found in nature; many minerals are important in building body tissues and regulating body fluids

Minimum Data Set (MDS 2.0) assessment completed for all residents admitted to a skilled care facility

mitered corner a bedmaking technique in which the top sheet is tucked in at the front of the bed, forming a 45° angle with the perpendicular edge of the mattress

mitosis division of the cytoplasm and nucleus in the cell

mobility ability to move or to be moved easily from place to place

mobility skills ability to move easily from place to place

morbidity state of being diseased; conditions inducing disease

moribund dying

mortality rate the proportion of deaths to population

motor nerve nerve that carries messages to muscles from the brain

mottling discoloration of skin or irregular areas

MRI *See* magnetic resonance imaging

MRSA *See* methicillin resistant *Staphylococcus aureus*

MSDS *See* Material Safety Data Sheets

mucolytic destroying or dissolving mucus

mucous pertaining to or resembling mucus; also, secreting mucus

mucous membrane special tissues that secrete a sticky substance called mucus; these membranes line body cavities that open to the outside

mucus secretion of mucous membranes; thick, sticky fluid

multiple sclerosis (MS) disease characterized by hardened patches scattered throughout the brain and spinal cord that interfere with the nerves in these areas

muscle tissue composed of contractile (contracts and relaxes) fibers or cells

muscle cell cells characterized by their ability to contract and bring about movement

muscle tissue tissue that forms the body wall and organs and is specialized for movement

myasthenia gravis (MG) disease characterized by muscular weakness caused by inadequate neurotransmitters

myocardial infarction area of dead heart tissue caused by lack of blood flow

myocardial ischemia lack of blood flow to the heart muscle

myocardium heart muscle

myth fixed idea about a group of people

narcosis a stuporous state produced by drugs

narcotic drug that produces abnormally deep sleep

nasogastric (NG) tube soft rubber or plastic tube that is inserted through a nostril and into the stomach

naturopathic medicine a holistic alternative medicine system based on holistic principles and stressing self-healing

necrosis tissue death

neglect failure to attend to duties properly; lack of proper care

negligence failure to give care that is reasonably expected of an assistant

nephron microscopic kidney units that produce the urine; made up of the glomerulus, Bowman's capsule, and the convoluted tubules

nerve a bundle of nerve processes (axons and dendrites) that are held together by connective tissue

nerve cell characterized by the ability to conduct a bioelectrical current called the nerve impulse

nerve impulse an electrical wave that transmits a message

nervous tissue highly specialized tissue capable of conducting a nerve impulse

networking a line of communications among individuals with a common interest or goal

neuron cell of the nervous system

neurotransmitter chemical compound that transmits a nervous impulse across cells at a synapse

NG tube *See* nasogastric tube

NIDDM *See* non–insulin-dependent diabetes mellitus

NIOSH-approved respirator a type of personal protective equipment for breathing that is approved by the National Institute for Occupational Safety and Health

nitroglycerin a vasodilator drug used mainly in angina pectoris

no-code (DNR) order order not to resuscitate (revive) a resident

nocturia excessive urination at night

non–insulin-dependent diabetes mellitus (NIDDM) relative insulin deficiency or resistance to insulin action; does not necessarily require insulin replacement

nonverbal communication sending messages without the use of words

non-weight bearing no weight to be borne by hip(s)/leg(s)

nosocomial infection infection that occurs while the resident is in facility care

nurse's notes documentation in the resident's medical record done by nursing staff

nurses' station area on a resident unit where medical records and care plans are kept

nursing assistant nurse's aide or orderly

nursing diagnosis nursing statement of a patient problem

nutrient food that supplies heat and energy, builds and repairs body tissue, and regulates body functions

nutrition the process by which the body uses food for growth and repair and to maintain health

nystagmus involuntary and jerky repetitive movements of the eyes

obesity the condition of being overweight

objective observation observations made by seeing, hearing, feeling, touching, and smelling; sign

OBRA Omnibus Budget Reconciliation Act of 1987; a law that set many standards for the health care industry, including for licensure, certification, and regulation

observation something that is noticed

occupational exposure opportunity to come in contact with a hazard while carrying out assignments

Occupational Safety and Health Administration (OSHA) federal government agency responsible for developing and enforcing health and job safety standards to protect employees

occupational therapist person licensed to provide rehabilitative services to evaluate and treat persons with physical injury or illness, psychosocial problems, or developmental disabilities

occupied bedmaking bedmaking while the resident is in the bed

O.D. as used in text, pertains to right eye

oil gland sebaceous gland that is found in the skin and secretes an oily substance into the follicles

olfactory pertaining to the sense of smell

oliguria scant urine

ombudsman a public official designated to investigate complaints objectively

oncology study of neoplasms or tumors

open reduction/internal fixation method of stabilizing fractures

ophthalmologist a physician who specializes in the treatment of defects and diseases of the eye

optic nerve nerve carrying messages from eye to brain

optometrist health care provider who specializes in measuring visual acuity

oral pertaining to the mouth

oral hygiene proper care of the mouth and teeth

orally through the mouth

organ any part of the body that carries out a specific function or functions, such as the heart

organic mental syndrome a general term that includes all dementias

origin proximal point of attachment to skeletal muscle

orthopnea condition in which there is difficulty breathing except when sitting or standing upright

orthopneic position sitting supported in an upright position to relieve respiratory distress

orthosis device used to maintain the position of an extremity

orthotic device   device such as a brace or splint that restores or improves function and prevents deformity

O.S.   as used in text, pertains to left eye

OSHA   *See* Occupational Safety and Health Administration

osteoarthritis   degenerative joint disease caused by disintegration of the cartilage that covers the ends of the bones

osteoporosis   the most common metabolic disease of bone in the United States; characterized by a decrease in the mass of bony tissue; most commonly affects women past middle age

ostomy   suffix word ending meaning to create a new opening, as colostomy

output   the measured amount of fluid excreted in a given period

ovaries   endocrine glands located in female pelvis; female gonads

oviduct; fallopian tube   part of the female reproductive tract that carries ova from ovaries to uterus

ovulation   a discharge of an egg from the ovary

ovum (pl. *ova*)   the female egg

oxygen   gas essential to cellular metabolism and all life

oxygen mask   a cuplike appliance attached to an oxygen source that is placed over a resident's nose and mouth to deliver oxygen

oxygenated   carrying oxygen

pacemaker (pacer)   an artificial device placed in the body to regulate heartbeat

pacing   repeatedly walking back and forth

palliative   relieving symptoms but not curing disease

pallor   less color than normal of the skin

pancreas   a gland located behind the stomach. It secretes several enzymes necessary for digestion, plus insulin and glycogen

paralysis   loss or impairment of the ability to move parts of the body

paranoia   a state in which one has delusions of persecution and/or grandeur

paraplegia   paralysis of both legs

parathormone   a hormone produced by the parathyroid glands; important in managing the level of body calcium

parathyroid glands   several small glands located on the posterior thyroid gland that produce the hormone parathormone

Parkinson's disease   progressive disease of the brain, characterized by stiffness of muscles and tremors, occurring later in life

paroxysmal   abrupt in onset and termination

partial weight bearing   limited amount of weight can be borne on one or both legs

passive range of motion   movement of joints by caregiver

pathogen   microorganism or other agent capable of producing a disease

pathology   disease

patient   person unable to provide self-care; resident

patient controlled analgesia (PCA)   device used by patient (resident) to control when pain medication is administered

pelvic cavity   that portion of the ventral cavity shaped like a basin surrounded by the pelvic bones

pelvis   the lower portion of the trunk of the body; a basin-shaped area bounded by the hip bones, the sacrum, and the coccyx

penis   male organ of copulation

pension   retirement income or fund

perceptual deficit   an inability to reason, think systematically, make judgments, or use common items

perceptual process   interpretation of information

pericardial   pertaining to the pericardium (the sac enclosing the heart)

pericardium   membrane that surrounds the heart

perineal care   specific cleaning of the area between the resident's legs

perineum   in the male, the area between the anus and scrotum; in the female, the area between the anus and vagina

peripheral   away from the center

peripheral intravenous central catheter (PICC)   small tube inserted into a vein in the arm and threaded through to a larger vein, such as the superior vena cava

peripheral nervous system (PNS)   nerves that carry messages to and from the brain and spinal cord

peripheral vascular disease (PVD)   disease resulting from decreased blood supply to the extremities

peristalsis   a progressive, wavelike movement that occurs involuntarily in hollow tubes of the body, especially in the alimentary canal

peritoneal cavity   that portion of the abdomino-pelvic cavity that is enclosed within the membranous peritoneum

peritoneal dialysis   procedure used to remove liquid wastes from blood stream

peritoneum   delicate serous membrane that lines the abdominal pelvic cavity and covers the organs

perseveration   the constant repetition of an action such as finger tapping or lip licking

personal inventory   list of resident's personal belongings

personal protective equipment   coverings such as masks, aprons, gloves, and glasses that protect the caregiver against the transmission of infectious organisms

personality   sum of the ways we react to the events in our lives

petit mal seizure   a type of epilepsy attack, generally short in nature; absence attack

pet therapy   providing animals to bring pleasure to severely impaired residents

phalange any bone of a finger or toe

phantom pain pain that seems to exist in an amputated limb

pharynx the muscular and membranous tube between the mouth and the esophagus

phlebitis inflammation of a vein

phlebotomy incision of a vein for the purpose of withdrawing blood

phlegm thick mucus found in the throat or respiratory tract

physical abuse any physical contact that intentionally causes pain or discomfort

physical needs needs that include maintaining hygiene and cleanliness and maintaining nutrition and fluid intake

physical restraint device used to inhibit body movement; also prevents personal access to body

physical therapist a person licensed by the state to provide rehabilitation sources to evaluate and treat persons with neuromuscular and musculoskeletal problems caused by disease, injury, or developmental disability

physician a licensed medical doctor

physiology the science that deals with the functioning of living organisms

physiotherapist a trained professional who provides therapy and exercise to maintain mobility

PICC *See* peripheral intravenous central catheter

piggyback procedure used to administer medication through a vein

piles hemorrhoids

pineal body glandular structure found in the cranium connected to the thalamus; produces some hormones thought to delay puberty until an appropriate age

pitting edema a condition in which the tissue remains indented when pressure is applied to an edematous area

pituitary gland the gland located beneath the brain that serves a variety of functions, including regulation of the gonads, thyroid, adrenal cortex, and other endocrine glands

plane imaginary line used to describe the relationship of one body part to another

plaque irregular patch or flat lesion that forms on an artery lining in atherosclerosis

plasma liquid portion of blood

platelet thrombocyte; involved in the blood clotting mechanism

pleura the membranes that surround the lungs

pleural pertaining to the pleura

pneumonia inflammation of the lungs

PNS peripheral nervous system

podiatrist a physician specializing in foot problems

podigeriatrics a medical specialty that deals with treatment and care of aging feet

point of attachment areas where arms and legs are attached to the torso

policy book a book that outlines the rules governing the facility and explains what will be done for the residents

polydipsia excessive thirst

polyphagia excessive ingestion of food

polyuria excessive excretion of urine

pore opening of one of the ducts leading from the sweat glands to the surface of the skin

position sense ability to tell how one's extremities are positioned without looking at them

posterior back or dorsal

postmortem after death

postmortem care care of the body after death

postural drainage positioning a patient to encourage drainage from the respiratory tract

postural support pads, pillows, or rolls used to help residents remain in proper alignment

potassium an element essential to the body; an electrolyte

potency power; especially the ability of the male to perform coitus

potentially infectious materials material that might possibly cause infection

power of attorney for health care legal document that authorizes someone other than the resident to carry out the health care wishes of the resident

prefix a term placed before a word that changes or modifies the meaning of the word

prepuce foreskin, a fold of skin covering the glans penis

presbycusis progressive loss of hearing due to normal aging

presbyopia impaired vision as a result of the aging process (farsightedness)

pressure ulcer also called dermal ulcers or decubitus ulcers; ulcerations that form as the result of ischemia of tissues due to pressure

procedure a series of steps outlining how to do something and in what order and manner

procedure book a reference for procedures

professionalism a knowledgeable, compassionate, responsible manner of delivering health care

progesterone hormone produced by ovaries

prognosis probable outcome of a disease or injury

progressive mobilization a process used to increase a resident's mobility skills

projection an unconscious defense mechanism in which an individual sees his or her own defects as belonging to another

prolapse the falling down or downward displacement of a body part or organ

prone turning the forearm so the palm is facing downward

proprioception information received from internal stimuli

prostatectomy removal of all or part of the prostate gland

prostate gland gland of male reproductive system that surrounds the neck of the urinary bladder and the beginning of the urethra

prosthesis artificial substitute for a missing body part, such as a denture, hand, leg

protein the basic material of every body cell; an essential nutrient

protocol plan of treatment; a particular stated or standard method or procedure

protraction to be brought forward

proximal closest to the point of attachment

pruritus itching

psychosocial relating social conditions to mental health

psychotic completely out of touch with reality

puberty the condition or period of becoming capable of sexual reproduction

pubic pertaining to the pubis or pubic bone, which forms the center bone of the front of the pelvis

pulmonary artery blood vessel that carries deoxygenated blood from the right ventricle to the lung

pulmonary emphysema a chronic lung disorder in which the terminal bronchioles become plugged with mucus and lung elasticity is lost

pulmonary veins large veins that return blood from the lungs to the left atrium of the heart

pulse wave of pressure exerted against the walls of the arteries in response to ventricular contraction

pulse deficit difference between contractions of the heart and pulse expansions of the radial artery

pulse oximetry procedure used to determine oxygen levels in bloodstream

pulse pressure the difference between the systolic and diastolic pressure

pulse rate number per minute of impulses transmitted to the arteries by contraction of the left ventricle

pupil opening in the center of the iris of the eye that allows light to enter the eye

PVD *See* peripheral vascular disease

pylorus the narrow, tapered end of the stomach opening into the duodenum

pyorrhea periodontitis; loosening of the teeth caused by gum disease

quadrant one section when imaginary lines are drawn over the abdomen, dividing it into four equal areas

quadriplegia paralysis of all four limbs

quality assurance program measurement of care provided to residents

RACE acronym for a series of activities to take during a fire; r = remove all residents, a = activate alarm, c = contain, e = extinguish

radial artery blood vessel carrying oxygenated blood located on the lateral anterior wrist at the base of the thumb; most often used to determine pulse rate

radiation therapy diagnosis and treatment using radiation

rales abnormal respiratory sound heard in auscultation of the chest

range of motion (ROM) exercises series of exercises specifically designed to move each joint through its range

rapport understanding between two people

rationalization an unconscious defense mechanism in which one devises a logical, self-satisfying but incorrect explanation for one's behavior or feelings

reaction a response to a stimulus; opposite action or counteraction

reality orientation (RO) techniques used to help residents remain oriented to the environment, to time, and to themselves

receptor peripheral nerve ending; specialized for response to a particular type of stimuli

recovery position body position used for persons who are breathing but unresponsive

rectocele protrusion of part of the rectum into the vagina

rectum the lower part of large intestine, about 5 inches long, between the sigmoid flexure and the anal canal

references in a résumé, statements about abilities and characteristics; persons who give such statements

reflex involuntary response to a stimulus

registered nurse (RN) a person who has completed a 2-, 3-, or 4-year program in a nursing school and is licensed by the state to assess, plan for, and evaluate the nursing care needs of residents

regular diet a routine or balanced diet; sometimes called a house diet

regularity routinely eliminating waste products from the body

regurgitate (air) swallowing air and expelling it in a controlled manner for speech

regurgitating "throwing up" undigested food from the stomach

regurgitation backward flow of fluids in the body

rehabilitation pertaining to a return to a former improved state

rehabilitation aide specially trained nursing assistant who helps residents regain lost skills or teaches new skills

reminiscing recalling past events

remission period of decreased severity of symptoms in chronic disease

renal calculi kidney stones

renal pelvis the portion of the kidney that collects the urine and directs it into the ureter

reprisal retaliation

resident patient in a long-term care facility

resident care plan statement of the resident's medical diagnosis, problems, and directions for resolving the problems

Resident Council group of residents who meet regularly; the councils give residents a method for communication with each other and with staff

resident unit room occupied by resident and his or her personal possessions; may be shared by other residents

residual limb portion of a limb left after part has been removed

respiration process of taking oxygen into the body and expelling carbon dioxide

respiratory arrest when breathing stops

rest home long-term care facility

restoration to remedy or bring up to a normal state

restorative care describing care in which the inter-disciplinary health-care team assists the resident to reach an optimal level of ability

résumé a short account of one's career and qualifications that is prepared by an applicant for a job

resuscitation restoration to life of one who has cardiac and respiratory arrest

retention the inability to excrete urine that has been produced

retina innermost or third layer of the eye, which receives images

retinopathy noninflammatory disease of the retina

retirement period after leaving employment

retraction to be brought backward

retroperitoneal space area of the anterior cavity behind the peritoneum; in it are the kidneys, aorta, inferior vena cava

rheumatoid arthritis autoimmune response that results in inflammation of the joints

rhythm regularity

ribs the 24 long, flat bones forming the wall of the thorax

rigor mortis a stiffening of the body some hours after death

RN *See* registered nurse

RO *See* reality orientation

ROM *See* range of motion exercises

rotation the act of turning about the axis of the center of a body, as rotation of a joint

rubra unusual redness or flushing of skin

rupture the bursting of a part

Sacrament of the Sick (last rites) given by a clergyman to a Catholic person who is terminally ill (dying)

safety device a device that in some way restricts the activity of a resident to protect that resident or others

saliva digestive secretion produced by the salivary glands and found in the mouth

sclera white of the eye

scrotum saclike pouch that holds the male gonads

sedative medication that has calming effect; used to control nervousness, irritability, and excitement

seizure sudden attack of a disease; an epileptic fit

self-care (functional) deficit an inability to care for oneself in one or more areas of activities of daily living

Self-Determination Act a federal law passed in 1990 stating that competent adults have the right to be adequately informed about their medical conditions and the options of treatment available to them, and then to make their own decision as to their degree of participation

self-esteem feelings of confidence about oneself

self range of motion exercises done by the resident

seminal vesicles pouchlike sacs found on the posterior wall of the bladder that produce the bulk of the seminal fluid

semiprone position modified prone position in which body is supported on pillows to relieve pressure on most of the bony prominences

semisupine position lying partially on the back and side

senescent growing old

senescent changes normal aging changes

senile affected with the infirmities of age

senile keratosis roughened, scaly, slightly elevated wartlike lesions, believed to be related to sun damage in fair-skinned individuals

senile lentigines yellow or brown spots that occur on exposed skin surfaces

senior person over the age of 65

senior citizen center place where seniors can meet for social and other activities

sensitivity the state of acute or abnormal responsiveness to stimuli

sensory deprivation lack of stimulation to the sense of vision, hearing, smelling, taste, or touch

sensory nerves nerves that carry messages—about pain, temperature change, changes in body position, taste, touch, sound, and sight—toward the brain for interpretation

sensory-perceptual changes an inability to recognize and use common objects such as eating utensils, combs, or pencils

sensory stimulation activities that increase the resident's awareness of the surroundings

sensual pertaining to the senses or sensation

sensuality quality or state of being sensual

sepsis infection

septicemia infection in the bloodstream

septum wall or partition dividing a body cavity or space

seropositive HIV positive

serous membrane a special tissue that secretes a serous fluid; covers organs and lines cavities that do not open to the outside

serum the clear liquid portion of the blood remaining after removal of the solid components and blood clotting elements

sexual abuse using physical or verbal threats to force a resident to perform any sexual act; tormenting or teasing a resident with sexual gestures or words

sexuality the attitude of a person in relation to sex and sexual behavior

sharps needles, razor, or any sharp or cutting item

shearing (force) occurs when any part of the supported body is on a gradient; the deeper tissue near the bone slides toward the lower gradient while the skin remains at its point of contact; the tissues between become ischemic

sheath covering

shift report information regarding resident status given to on-coming shift from those going off duty

sign observation apparent to examiner or viewer

signing using hands and facial expression to communicate without speaking words

simple fracture fracture that does not produce an open wound in the skin

sitz bath bath providing moist heat to the genitals or anal area

skeletal muscle muscle tissue that is attached to bone; sometimes called voluntary

skilled nursing facility long-term care facility

skin external covering of the body

skin tear small breaks that occur in fragile skin

slander a false and damaging oral statement that injures the reputation of another person

sliding board a smooth waxed board used for a sitting transfer, such as bed to wheelchair

sling a bandage used for support

smooth muscle type of tissue that forms the walls of organs—involuntary or visceral

social worker a person licensed by the state to assess and provide services for nonmedical, psychosocial needs of the residents

society a group of people who have common interests

spastic cerebral palsy a form of cerebral palsy in which the muscles are tense, contracted, and resistant to movement

spasticity a condition of rigidity or spasm of muscle

spatial-perceptual deficit difficulty in distinguishing between left and right, up and down

specimen sample of body secretion, excretion, or tissue used for diagnosis or determination of condition

speech-language pathologist person trained and educated to diagnose and treat swallowing problems and speech and language disorders

sperm the male reproductive cell

sphincter a circular muscle that constricts a passage or closes a natural orifice; when relaxed, it allows passage of materials

sphygmomanometer instrument for determining arterial pressure; blood pressure gauge

spinal column backbone or vertebral column

spiritual healing treatment through prayer and invocation of supernatural forces to achieve healing and unity with a higher power

spirituality the state of being spiritual-minded or religious

splint rigid device applied to maintain a body part in a specific position

spouse a marriage partner; husband or wife

sprain an injury to a ligament caused by sudden overstretching

sputum expectorated matter, composed of saliva and mucus from the lungs and throat

square corner a bedmaking technique in which the top sheet is tucked in at the bottom of the bed by forming a line parallel to the perpendicular edge of the mattress

standard precautions infection control practices used for all people receiving care

status condition or state of health

stereotype characteristic assigned to entire groups of people; rigid, biased ideas about people as a group

sterile free from bacteria or other microorganisms; incapable of reproducing sexually

sterilization process that renders an individual incapable of reproduction

steroids a group name for certain compounds that include progesterone, the adrenocortical and gonadal hormones, bile acid, and sterols such as cholesterol

stethoscope instrument used in auscultation to make audible the sounds produced in the body

stimulant agent that produces stimulation

stoma an artificial, mouthlike opening

stool an evacuation of the bowel

strain an excessive stretching of a muscle resulting in pain and swelling of the muscle

strengths activities that an individual can perform

stress feelings that cause a person to be anxious about his or her well-being

stroke cerebrovascular accident; damage to the blood vessels of the brain

stump the distal end of a limb remaining after amputation

subacute care care provided to patients with stable conditions who require skilled care

subcutaneous beneath the layers of the skin

subcutaneous tissue tissue that attaches the skin to the muscles

subjective observation observation based on reports of the resident (symptom)

subluxation incomplete dislocation of a joint

suffix a term added to the end of a word that changes or modifies the meaning of the word

sundowning a resident has increased confusion and restlessness in late afternoon, evening, or during the night

superior toward the head; upward

superior vena cava large blood vessel that drains the blood from the upper part of the body into the right atrium of the heart

supine turning the forearm so the palm is facing upward, lying in a face-up position in the back

supine position lying on the back, face up

supportive care providing comfort measures

support services services not directly involved in resident care; for example, building and ground maintenance, housekeeping, kitchen work, administration duties

suppository medication inserted in the rectum used to help the bowels eliminate the feces

suppression consciously refusing to acknowledge unacceptable feelings and thoughts

survey to examine, inspect, observe, or scrutinize; the inspection performed by licensing authorities

surveyor one who conducts a survey

sweat gland sudoriferous glands, found in the skin, that produce perspiration

symbol a mark or character that represents some quality, relationship, or word

symptom subjective observation

synapse space between the axon of one cell and the dendrites of others

synarthrotic pertains to an immovable joint

syncope faint; sudden loss of consciousness or strength

synovial membrane special membrane that lines movable joint cavities

synovium joint lining

syphilis a sexually transmitted disease that may cause lesions in almost all tissues of the body and seriously affect the nervous septum

system group of organs organized to carry out a specific body function or functions, as respiratory system

systole contraction, or period of contraction, of cardiac muscle

systolic applies to the contraction phase of the cardiac cycle

tachycardia an unusually rapid heartbeat

tachypnea respiratory pattern of rapid, shallow respirations

tact sensitive mental perception

tactile pertaining to touch

tai chi an ancient Chinese form of meditative movement practiced through a series of exercises and breathing techniques; thought to improve the life energy flow

talisman engraved stones, rings, or other objects used to ward off evil

task segmentation breaking down a complex task into a series of single steps

TED hose support hose

tendon fibrous band of connective tissue that attaches skeletal muscle to bone

TENS *See* transcutaneous electrical nerve stimulation

terminal the end

terminal cleaning cleaning and sterilization of a room after resident's death or departure

terminal condition an illness, injury, or condition that will result in death

terminal illness life-ending condition

testes male sex glands (gonads) found in the scrotum; produce sperm and the hormone testosterone

testicles testes

testosterone male sex hormone produced by the testes

theft taking that which does not belong to you; stealing

therapeutic pertaining to results obtained from treatment; a healing agent

therapeutic diet a planned intake of food and fluid to treat a specific disease condition

therapeutic recreational specialist person trained and educated to use physical recreation as a rehabilitation therapy

therapy treatment designated to eliminate disease or other bodily disorder

thermal blanket fluid-filled blanket, the temperature of which can be raised or lowered

thermometer instrument used to determine temperature

thoracic pertaining to the chest

thoracic cavity chest cavity

thorax the chest, the part of the body between the neck and the abdomen, encased by the shoulder girdle, ribs, and diaphragm

thrombocyte blood platelet that is formed in the bone marrow and is important in blood clotting

thrombophlebitis inflammation of a vein as a result of a blood clot

thrombus (pl. *thrombi*) blood clot

thyroid gland an endocrine gland located in anterior neck in front of and on either side of the trachea. Produces hormones thyrocalcitonin and thyroxine

thyroxine hormone of the thyroid gland that contains iodine

TIA *See* transient ischemic attack

tilt table a table used to secure patients during position changes to improve chest drainage

tipping giving money as a reward or thanks for service rendered; not salary-connected

tissue a group of similar cells and fibers forming a distinct structure; piece of paper used for cleansing (e.g., toilet tissue, facial tissue, Kleenex)

toe pleat a bedmaking technique in which an extra fold of the top sheet is made at the foot of the bed to provide extra room for the resident's feet

torso the body, exclusive of the head and limbs

total care health care that takes into account the physical and psychosocial needs of individual residents

total parenteral nutrition (TPN) a technique in which high-density nutrients are introduced into a large vein

touch therapy treatment in which a healer moves his or her hands above an individual's body to promote self-healing and restore energy balances

trachea the windpipe, a tube extending from the larynx to the bronchi

tracheostomy opening in the anterior trachea

traction technique that pulls the ends of bones into normal position or alignment

tranquilizer agent used to calm or quiet anxious person without causing drowsiness

transcutaneous electrical nerve stimulation (TENS) method of pain relief

transfer move from one place to another

transfer belt (gait belt) a webbed belt 1½ to 2 inches wide, about 54 to 60 inches long; used as a safety device to assist residents during transfers

transient ischemic attack (TIA) drop attacks caused by vertebrobasilar insufficiency; temporary decrease in blood flow to brain

transitional care care provided between acute care and discharge

transmission transfer from one place or person to another

transurethral prostatectomy removal of the prostate through the urethra

transverse plane an imaginary line that divides the body into a superior and inferior part

trapeze a horizontal bar suspended overhead down the length of the bed

trauma mechanical injury

trichomonas vaginitis an infection of the vaginal tract by a parasitic protozoan

trochanter roll a rolled bath blanket positioned under the resident extending from well above to well below the hips; the roll prevents external hip rotation

tubal ligation tying off a fallopian tube

tubercle small, rounded nodule formed by infection with *Mycobacterium tuberculosis*

tuberculosis disease condition occurring when tuberculosis organism causing tuberculosis infection begins to spread and is not restrained

tuberculosis infection occurs when tuberculosis germs enter the body. The organisms may be walled off, forming a tubercle and causing the person to be unaware of the process

tumor neoplasm; new uncontrolled growth of cells

tunica intima the inner coat of the blood vessels

turning sheet a flat bed sheet folded in half used to move dependent residents in bed

tyloma a callus

tympanic pertaining to the eardrum

ulcer open sore caused by inadequate blood supply and broken skin

ulceration development of an ulcer

umbilicus the navel; marks site that gave passage to umbilical vessels in the fetal stage

unilateral neglect inability to recognize the existence of one side of the body

unoccupied bedmaking bedmaking when the resident is out of the bed

upper extremity the arm and hand

uremia the presence of excessive amounts of urea, a waste product, in the blood

uremic frost (snow) secretions of perspiration containing substances normally found in urine

ureter narrow tube that conducts urine from the kidney to the urinary bladder

urethra mucus-lined tube conveying urine from the urinary bladder to the exterior of the body; in the male, the urethra also conveys the semen

urgency the need to urinate

urinalysis laboratory analysis of urine

urination the act of discharging urine from the bladder

urosheath a condomlike appliance that is used to collect urine when attached to drainage tubing

USDA United States Department of Agriculture

uterine tubes fallopian tubes or oviducts; tubes through which the ova travel from the ovary to the uterus

uterus muscular, hollow organ where fetus develops in the female

vaccine suspensions or products of infectious agents used chiefly for producing active immunity

vagina the tube that extends from the vulva to the uterine cervix; the female organ of copulation that receives the penis during sexual intercourse

vaginitis inflammation of the vagina

validation therapy a way of relating to residents that helps them feel secure and oriented within their own reality

value system setting priorities of what is important in life

valve a fold of membrane in a passage or tube permitting the flow of contents in one direction only

vancomycin-resistant enterococci (VRE) microbes resistant to the effects of vancomycin, an antibiotic

varicose veins weakened veins usually found in lower extremities

vas deferens the tube that carries sperm from the epididymis to the junction of the seminal vesicle; ductus deferens

vasectomy excision of part or all of the vas deferens; bilateral vasectomy results in sterility

vasoconstriction decrease in the caliber of the blood vessels

vasodilation increase in the caliber of the blood vessels

vasodilator a neuron or medication that causes dilation of the blood vessels

vein a vessel through which blood passes on its way back to the heart

venereal warts verruca condyloma; lesions are reddish brown and have a rough, cauliflower type surface caused by the human papilloma virus

ventilation process of admitting fresh air and expelling stale air; the movement of gases into and out of the lungs

ventral front; anterior

ventricle a small, bellylike cavity such as one of the lower chambers of the heart

venule small vein

verbal abuse using words to mistreat another, such as using sarcasm, slang, or foul language

verbal communication messages sent using words

vertigo dizziness

violence sudden and intense exertion of physical force to cause injury, destruction, or abuse

visceral muscle smooth muscle; makes up walls of internal organs

vital capacity the volume of air a person can forcibly expire from the lungs after a maximal inspiration

vital signs measurements of temperature, pulse, respiration, and blood pressure

vitamin a general term for various, unrelated organic substances found in many foods in minute amounts that are necessary for normal metabolic functioning of the body

vocal cords membranes that stretch across the inside of the larynx and function in voice production

voiding the release of urine from the bladder

volume the capacity or size of an object or of an area; the measure of the quantity of a substance

voluntary muscle any part of the skeletal muscle that is under direct control

volunteerism the contribution of one's time and energy to helping others

vomitus the material vomited or brought up from the stomach

VRE *See* vancomycin-resistant enterococci

vulva the external female genitalia

wandering aimless walking about

warm soak warm water at a specific temperature applied to a body part

water liquid essential for life

weight bearing an ability to stand on one or both legs

wet compress pieces of gauze that have been moistened and wrung out, then placed against the resident to apply cold or heat

withdrawal the retreat from reality or from social contact that is associated with severe depression and other psychiatric disorders

withhold order to refrain from serving a resident certain foods or all food

womb another term for the female uterus

word root word form whose basic meaning can be used in forming new words by combining it with prefixes and suffixes

work practice controls specific procedures to prevent the spread of infection

Index

A

Abbreviations, 69, 72–76
Abdominal quadrants, 78
Abduction, 433
Abduction pillow, 560
Abuse, 103–104
Acceptance stage of grief, 619
Accommodation of needs, right to, 105–108
Accuracy, 35
Acquired Immune Deficiency Syndrome (AIDS), 163–165, 204, 591, 628
Active listening, 56–57
Active range of motion exercises, 441, 558
Activities director, 23
Activities of daily living (ADLs)
adaptive devices, 426, 427–429
approaches used, 425–426
dementia and, 597–598
description of, 423–424
nursing assistant responsibilities, 40, 41
stroke and, 578–579
task segmentation, 424, 425
Acupressure, 229, 230
Acupuncture, 230
Acute care, 5, 35
Acute care hospital, 7
Acute myocardial infarction, 510–511
Adaptation. See Adjustment
Adaptive behavior, 607
Adaptive device, 26, 426, 427–429
Adduction, 433
Adjunctive therapies, 228, 230
Adjustment
to admission, 395
challenges to, 219
to chronic illness, 220
defense mechanisms, 220–221
to loss of independence, 220
to loss of loved one, 219–220
to loss of voice, 520
to terminal illness, 617–618
in younger resident, 208
ADLs. See Activities of daily living (ADLs)
Administrative organization, 28–29
Administrator, 23, 28
Admission to facility
adaptation, helping with, 395
anxiety about, 390–391
assessments, 392
day of admission, 391–392
nursing assistant responsibilities, 392–393
personal inventory, 393–395
preadmission activities, 391
procedure for, 393
reasons for, 390
Adrenal glands, 531
Advance directives, 109
Advance practice nurse, 25
Advocacy groups, 116
Age-related macular degeneration, 573
Aggressive behavior triggers, 64
Aging
cardiovascular system and, 501
changes caused by, 200–203
digestion and, 295
endocrine system and, 532
infection and, 521
musculoskeletal system and, 553–555
nervous system and, 572

normal, process of, 200
overview of, 200
reproductive system and, 544
respiratory system and, 519, 520
skin and, 257
stereotypes and myths of, 205–207
urinary system and, 340–341
Agitation and Alzheimer's disease, 600
AIDS (Acquired Immune Deficiency Syndrome), 163–165, 204, 591, 628
Airborne precautions, 178–180
Airborne transmission of infection, 157, 158
Air circulation, 240
Alcoholic beverages, 299
Alternating air pressure mattress, 263–264
Alternative therapies, 228–232
Alzheimer's disease
agitation, anxiety, and catastrophic reactions, 600
care for resident with, 595–596
care units for, 595–597
changes in brain and, 591
definition of, 590–591
delusions and hallucinations, 600–601
management techniques, 601–602
pillaging and hoarding, 601
stages and symptoms of, 591–593
sundowning, 600
wandering and pacing, 599–600
Ambulation
Alzheimer's disease and, 593
assessment of, 482
assisting, with cane or walker, 486–487
assistive devices, 26, 483–485
gait, 481–483
gait training, 483
guidelines for, 485
of resident, 486
See also Wheelchairs
Amputation, 455, 561–562
Amyotrophic lateral sclerosis, 582
Anatomic terms, 76–78
Anemia, 505
Aneurysm, 470, 577
Anger stage of grief, 619
Angina pectoris, 511
Ankle range of motion exercises, 440
Ankle stirrup, 446
Answering telephone, 55
Anterior, 77
Antibiotic, 160
Antibody, 159–160
Anticipatory grief, 616
Antigen, 159–160
Antioxidants, 229
Anxiety
about admission, 390–391
Alzheimer's disease and, 600
causes and symptoms of, 210
subacute care and, 629
Aphasia
Alzheimer's disease and, 593
communicating with resident with, 63
stroke and, 577
Apical pulse, 373–374
Appearance, 36–37
Application for job, 644

Approach, 95
Aquamatic K-Pad®, 407, 408
Aromatherapy, 230
Arteries, 503, 504, 506–507
Arteriosclerosis, 506, 507
Arthritis, 450, 559–561
Articulation, 53
Ascites, 512
Asepsis, 170
Aspiration, 135, 142–143, 521
Assault, 117
Assessment
ambulation, 482
of bladder control, 461, 462–463
by interdisciplinary team, 94
mental status, 90, 590
Minimum Data Set (MDS 2.0), 15–16, 94, 419
Assignments, 40, 42, 54
Assistant director of nursing, 25
Assisted living facility, 9–10
Assisted standing transfer
one assistant, 472–473
two assistants, 474–475
Assistive device for ambulation, 26, 483–485
Asthma, 522
Atherosclerosis, 506, 507, 577
Atrophy, 421, 553
Attitude, 35–36
Audiologist, 23, 27
Auditory nerve, 572
Aura, 150
Autoclave, 193
Automated external defibrillator (AED), 141, 144, 148
Autonomic nervous system, 570
Autopsy, 621
Ayurveda, 229

B

Backrub, 264, 265
Back support, 125
Bacteria, 156
Bacterial infections, 160–162
Bargaining stage of grief, 619
Baseline observation, 87
Basic human needs, 214–216
Bathing
adaptive devices for, 427
in bed using basin and water, 267–269
in bed using rinse-free cleanser and moisturizer, 270–271
overview of, 264, 266
partial bath, 272–273
perineal care, 273–276
restorative program for, 430
safety issues, 266
task segmentation, 425
therapeutic bath, 273
transferring resident to tub or shower chair, 476–477
tub bath or shower, 271–272
waterless bed bath, 270
Bath mitt, making, 268
Battery, 117
Bed
assisting independent movement in, 459–460
bath in, 267–269, 270–271
bringing resident to sitting position at edge of, 471–472
changing linens, 246–252
linens for, 245
in long-term care facility, 10, 239
making, 246

measuring and weighing resident in, 385–386
moving resident in, 446–450
safety of, 128
transferring nonstanding resident from wheelchair to, 477–478
transferring resident from chair to, 473–474
waterless bed bath, 270
Bed cradles, 262, 263, 444
Bedpan, 322, 323–324
Bedside commode, 322, 325–326
Bedside stand, 10–11, 171
Beginning procedure actions, 243–244
Behavior
Alzheimer's disease and, 599–601
demanding type, 222
dementia and, 594
ethical type, 118
maladaptive type, 223
manipulative type, 222
observations of, 90–91
reactive type, 222–223
reporting, 92
Behavior modification, 612
Benign prostatic hypertrophy, 545
Bereavement, 219–220
Biofeedback, 230
Biohazardous waste, 176, 190–191
Bladder, 340
Bladder Retraining Assessment, 462–463
Blood
components of, 503–504
disorders of, 504–509
hemodialysis, 634–635
peritoneal dialysis, 635
Bloodborne pathogens, 174
Blood pressure
equipment, 376, 377
factors influencing, 376
gauge, reading, 376, 377
normal, 509
preparing to take, 378
taking, 379–380
See also Hypertension
Blood spills, 176, 177
Blood vessels
heart, 502
types of, 503
Body alignment, 434
Body flora, 158
Body language. See Nonverbal communication
Body mechanics, 124–127, 446, 447
Body parts, abbreviations for, 73
Body sciences, 76
Body work, 230
Bones, 552
Bowel and bladder management programs, 460–463
Bowel movement. See Feces
Bowman's capsule, 340
Bradycardia, 374
Braille, 62–63
Brain, 568–570, 591
Brain stem, 569–570
Breast self-examination, 544–545
Breast tumors, 544
Breathing exercises, 524
Breathing patterns, 375
Bridging, 264, 455–456
Bronchitis, 522–523
Brushing teeth
assisting with, 283
for resident, 281, 282, 284

Burnout, 43
Burns, 151–152
Bursae, 553
Bursitis, 555

C
Call light, 11, 128, 239–240
Calorie-restricted diet, 304, 305
Cancer
 digestive system, 313
 leukemia, 504–505
 reproductive system, 544–545
 respiratory system, 520
 treatment of, 204, 628, 635
Canes, 484, 485, 486–487
Capillaries, 503
Carbohydrates, 294, 295
Carbon dioxide, 518
Cardiac arrest, 141
Cardiac chair, 458
Cardiac cycle, 503
Cardiac muscle, 79
Cardiopulmonary resuscitation
 (CPR)
 cardiac arrest and, 141, 142
 nursing assistant
  responsibilities, 618
 one-rescuer, adult, 147
 resident rights and, 109
Cardiovascular system
 aging and, 202, 203
 blood, 503–506
 blood disorders, 506–509
 blood vessels, 503, 506–509
 complications from inactivity,
  422
 description of, 80, 500–501
 diabetes and, 534
 diseases of, 501
 heart, 501–503
 heart disease, 510–514
 lymph, 503
 observation of, 88, 91
Career health, 43
Care for resident
 after open reduction/internal
  fixation (ORIF), 557–559
 after stroke, 578–579
 with amyotrophic lateral
  sclerosis, 582
 with cerebral palsy, 609
 with chronic obstructive
  pulmonary disease, 523–526
 with dementia, 593–599
 with developmental disability,
  611–612
 with diabetes mellitus, 535
 during dialysis treatments,
  634–635
 with hip prosthesis, 559–560,
  561
 with Huntington's disease, 581
 with intravenous line, 632
 with multiple sclerosis, 580
 with myasthenia gravis, 583
 with Parkinson's disease, 577
 during radiation therapy, 635
 with skin breakdown, 260, 262
 with tracheostomy, 634
Caregiver and grief, 620
Care plan
 alternative practices and, 232
 description of, 56, 57
 interdisciplinary team and, 22,
  94–95
 nursing assistant
  responsibilities, 94, 95
 Post-Discharge Plan of Care,
  400–401
 resident participation, 103
Carriers, 158
Cartilage, 553
Cast, 556
Cataracts, 572–573

Catastrophic reactions, 592, 593,
 600
Catheter
 ambulating with, 344, 349
 care of, 342–344
 disconnecting, 344–346
 leg bag drainage, 349–350
Cavities of body, 81–82
Cells, 78–79, 503–504
Central nervous system, 567,
 568–570
Central venous insertion, 630
Cerebellum, 569
Cerebral palsy, 609
Cerebrospinal fluid, 570
Cerebrovascular accident (CVA).
 See Stroke
Cerebrum, 568
Certification
 of long-term care facilities,
  16–17
 of nursing assistants, 14–15
Chair positioning, 456–457
Chair scale, 381, 384, 385
Chaplain, 23
Charge nurse, 25
Charting guidelines, 93–94
Chemical hazards, 127–128
Chemical restraints, 104
Chemotherapy, 635
Chi, 229
Chinese medicine, 229–230
Chiropractic, 230–231
Chlamydia infection, 547
Choice, right to, 103
Choking
 aspiration and, 142–143
 feeding and, 310
 Heimlich maneuver, 143–144
 preventing, 135
 unconscious person, 145–146
Choroid, 570
Chronic disease
 adjustment to, 220
 description of, 204, 420
Chronic heart failure, 513–514
Chronic obstructive pulmonary
 disease (COPD), 522–526
"Clean," 170
Clean-catch urine specimen,
 collecting, 352–353
Cleanliness and order, 240, 242
Clear liquid diet, 303–304
Client, 6
Clinical thermometers
 glass, 365–368
 reading, 363–364
 safety issues, 364
 types of, 363
Clinitron bed, 264
Clitoris, 543
Clostridium difficile, 161
Clothing, 286
Code blue, 618
Cognitive impairment, 590
Cold applications
 commercial preparations,
  406–407
 dry, 409–412
 moist, 412
 safety issues, 406, 409
 uses of, 409
Colon, 295, 326
Colostomy, 333–336, 470
Combing hair, 277
Combining form, 69–71
Comfort, 209–210
Communal setting, 12
Communicating with resident
 after laryngectomy, 520
 with aphasia, 63
 guidelines for, 56–60
 with hearing impairments, 61
 touch, 218

 with visual impairments, 61–63
 who is disoriented, 63–64
 who is potentially violent, 64
Communication process
 description of, 52
 nonverbal, 53
 organizational chart and, 53, 54
 touch and, 60–61
 verbal, 52–53, 53–55
 written, 55–56
 See also Communicating with
  resident
Community activities, 115, 599
Community health care facilities,
 4–8
Community nursing center, 7–8
Community services, 398
Compensation, 221
Complaint, filing, 116
Complementary therapies, 228, 230
Computers in health care facilities,
 12–13
Condom for urinary drainage,
 353–354
Confidential information, 12, 105
Conflicts between staff members,
 42
Confusion, 210
Congestive heart failure, 511–512
Connective tissue, 79
Constipation, 312, 327–328
Consultant, 26
Contact precautions, 180–182
Contact transmission of infection,
 157, 158
Contaminated, 170
Continuing education, 646–647
Contractures, 421, 431–432, 553,
 561
COPD (chronic obstructive
 pulmonary disease), 522–526
Coughing, 526
Cowper's glands, 541
CPR. *See* Cardiopulmonary
 resuscitation (CPR)
Creutzfeldt-Jacob dementia, 591
Cross-training, 646
Crutches, 484–485
Cryptosporidiosis, 165
Cultural awareness
 admission procedures, 392
 aging, 208
 beliefs, 103
 eye contact, 58
 food, 304
 health care practices and
  remedies, 228–229
 illness, 216
 isolation procedures, 178
 personal space, 238–239
 symptom expression, 87
 touching others, 60
 working with staff and, 28
Culture, 214
Culture and sensitivity test, 160
Cutaneous membrane, 81
Cyanotic, 374
Cystocele, 354, 545

D
Daily hair care, 276–277, 278
Day room, 12
Death
 postmortem care, 622–623
 of resident, 616, 620
 signs of approaching, 622
Deconditioning of heart, 422
Decubiti. *See* Pressure ulcer
Defamation of character, 118
Defense mechanisms, 220–221
Defibrillation, 143–144, 148
Dehydration, 300–301
Delusions, 592, 600–601
Demanding behavior, 222

Dementia
 ADLs, 597–598
 care for resident with, 593–599
 communicating with resident
  with, 63–64
 family members of resident
  with, 598
 forms of, 591
 Huntington's disease and, 582
 Parkinson's disease and, 576
 recreational activities, 598–599
 resident rights and, 597
 See also Alzheimer's disease
Demonstration, 426
Denial, 221
Denial stage of grief, 619
Dental hygienist, 23, 27–28
Dentist, 23, 27–28
Dentures, 282, 285
Dependability, 35
Depression
 Alzheimer's disease and, 592
 care for resident with, 223
 grief and, 619
 terminal illness and, 617, 618
Dermis, 256–257
Developmental disability
 aging and, 606–607
 care for resident with, 611–612
 causes of, 606
 cerebral palsy, 609
 characteristics of, 606
 community facilities for, 6, 7
 description of, 204
 mental retardation, 607–609
 seizure disorder, 609–611
Developmental tasks, 215–216
Diabetes mellitus
 causes of, 532
 coma, 534
 complications of, 533–535
 diet, 304, 305
 ketoacidosis, 534
 nursing assistant
  responsibilities, 535–536
 retinopathy, 573
 signs of, 533
 treatment of, 535
 types of, 533
Diagnoses, abbreviations for, 73
Diagnosis-related group, 390
Dialysis, 634–635
Diarrhea, 327
Diastole, 503
Diastolic pressure, 379
Diathermy, 407
Dietary manual, 56
Dietitian, 23, 26
Diets
 diabetes and, 535
 food groups, 297–299
 standard, 303–304
 therapeutic, 304–305
 See also Eating
Digestive process, 293–295
Digestive system. *See*
 Gastrointestinal system
Dining room, 12, 305–306
Director of nursing, 25
"Dirty," 170
Disability, 203–205, 420
Disaster manual, 56
Discharge planner, 390, 391
Discharge planning, 398
Discharging resident, 398–403
Disconnecting catheter, 344–346
Disinfection of equipment, 171,
 193, 240
Dislocation, 152, 445
Disorientation
 Alzheimer's disease and, 592
 causes of, 210
 communicating with resident
  with, 63–64

management techniques, 601–602
sensory deprivation and, 423
symptoms of, 223
Disposable cold pack, 409–410
Distal, 78
Distraction, 596
Diversion, 596
Diverticulosis, 313
DNR (do not resuscitate), 109, 142, 618
Documentation
description of, 56
of observations, 92–94
overview of, 41
See also Medical terminology
Dorsal, 77
Dorsal cavity, 81
Doshas, 229
Drainable fecal incontinence collector, 337
Draw sheet, 245
Dressing
adaptive devices for, 428
resident, 286–288
restorative program for, 430
task segmentation, 425
Droplet precautions, 180, 181
Droplet transmission of infection, 157, 158
Dry cold applications, 409–410, 412
Dry sterile dressing, 260
Dry warm applications, 407, 408
Duties of nursing assistant, 40–41
Dying process
adjustment to terminal diagnosis, 617–618
caregivers, 620
family dynamics, 619–620
nursing assistant and, 620, 622
religious practice and, 620, 621
resuscitation, 618
stages of grieving, 618–619
Dysphagia, 312
Dyspnea, 511, 521
Dysuria, 354

E
Ear, 571–572
Eating
adaptive devices for, 429
restorative program for, 430
task segmentation, 425
See also Feeding
Edema, 296, 442, 512
Educational services, 29
Efficiency, 42
Ejaculatory duct, 541
Elasticized stockings, 512–513
Elbow protectors, 262, 263
Elbow range of motion exercises, 436
Electrocardiogram, 503
Electrolyte balance, 296
Electronic speech, 520
Electronic thermometer, 364–365, 369–370
Elimination needs
bowel aids, 328–332
constipation, 327–328
continent resident, 321–326
external urinary drainage, 353–354
fecal incontinence, 336–337
internal urinary catheter drainage, 342–346
lower digestive tract, 326–327
ostomies, 333–336
overview of, 320–321
rectal tube and flatus bag, 332–333
routine or clean-catch urine specimen, collecting, 351–353

stool specimen, collecting, 337–339
urinary retention and incontinence, 341–342
urinary system, 339–341
Embolus, 422, 577
Emergency
burns, 151–152
cardiac arrest, 141
choking, 142–143
defibrillation, 143–144, 148
description of, 140
fainting, 152
hemorrhage, 148, 149
orthopedic injury, 152
poisoning, accidental, 152
recovery position, 143, 148
responding to, 140–141
seizures, 148, 150–151
Emesis basin, 10
Emotional health, 43–44
See also Adjustment; Depression; Psychosocial needs
Empathy, 35, 208, 209
Emphysema, 523
Employee personnel handbook, 56
Employee safety, 124–127
Employment search
applying for job, 644
interviewing for job, 644–645
job possibilities, finding, 642–643
references, 643, 644
résumé, preparing, 643
self-appraisal, completing, 642
Endocrine system
aging and, 202, 532
components of, 530, 531
description of, 80
glands of, 530–532
Endotracheal tube, 526
Enemas
commercially prepared solution, 328, 329
oil-retention type, 328, 329
overview of, 328
soapsuds type, 330–332
Enteral feeding, 311–312, 631
Enterococci, 160–161
Environment
Alzheimer's unit, 596–597
description of, 238
extended, caring for, 240–242
personal space, 238–239
restorative type, 426, 431
Environmental needs, accommodation of, 108
Environmental procedures, 176–177
Enzymes and digestion, 292, 293
Epidermis, 256
Epididymis, 541
Epidural catheter, 631, 633
Epilepsy, 609–611
Epithelial cells, 78
Epithelial tissue, 79
Equilibrium, 571
Equipment
disinfection of, 171, 193, 240
safety issues, 128–129
Ergonomics, 124, 125
Erythrocytes, 503
Escherichia coli (E. coli), 161
Esophageal speech, 520
Estrogen, 531
Ethical behavior, 118
Evaluation of care plan, 95
Eversion, 434
Excreta, 320
Exercise
diabetes and, 535
range of motion, 431–441, 558
resident with dementia and, 599
warm-up, 127

Exposure control, 174
Exposure incident, 174
Extension, 433
External fixation, 557, 558
External urinary drainage, 353–354
Extremities, 77
Eye, 570–571
Eye contact, 58
Eyeglass care, 572

F
Face shield, 175
Facial hair, 277–279
Fainting, 152
Fallopian tubes, 543
Falls, preventing, 134–135, 150
False imprisonment, 117
Family
admission to facility and, 391
anticipatory grief of, 616
discharge planning and, 399
grieving process of, 619–620
resident with dementia and, 598
resident with developmental disability and, 611
right to access to, 116
spouse, right to share room with, 116
Family and resident groups, 114
Fats, 294, 296
Fax machine, 13
Fear, 215, 220
Fecal impaction, 327–328
Fecal incontinence, 336–337
Feces, 292, 326–327
Feeding
assisting resident with, 306, 307–308
choking and, 310
dependent resident, 309–310
enteral type, 311–312
resident, 306
total parenteral nutrition, 312
See also Aspiration
Feeding restrictions, 109
Female perineal care, 274–275
Female reproductive system, 541–544
Fiber, 295
Financial abuse, 104
Fingernails
caring for, 268, 279–280
handwashing and, 173
of nursing assistant, 36
Fingers range of motion exercises, 437–438
Fire extinguishers, 136
Fire safety, 135–136
First-degree burn, 151
Fistula, 634
Flaccid paralysis, 442
Flatus bag, 332–333
Flexion, 432–433, 554
Flossing teeth, 284
Flotation mattress, 264
Fluid intake
calculating, 301–302
dehydration, 300–301
measuring and recording, 302–303
Fluid output, measuring and recording, 346–349
Foam pads or pillows, 262–263
Folk medicine, 231
Fomites, 157
Food groups, 297–299
Food Guide Pyramid, 297–299
Food thickeners, 308
Footboards, 443–444
Foot care, 280–281, 562
Foot problems, 562
Foot supports, 444
Foreign body airway obstruction.
See Choking

Foreskin, 540
Fowler's position, 454–455, 512, 523
Fracture
of hip, 557–559
treatment of, 152, 556–557
types of, 555–556
Free radicals, 229
Friction, 258
Frustration, 222
Functional ability, 424
Functional changes with aging, 201–203
Fungi, 157, 165

G
Gait, 481–483, 593
Gait belt, using to transfer resident, 469–470
Gait training, 483
Gangrene, 534
Gastrointestinal system
aging and, 201, 202
complications to from inactivity, 423
description of, 80, 292–293
disorders of, 312–313
observation of, 89
Gastrostomy (G) tube, 311–312
Gel-filled mattress, 264
Generalized seizure, 150, 151, 610–611
Genetic disease, 581
Genitalia
female, 541
male, 540
washing, 269
Genitourinary system, 89–90, 91
See also Urinary system
Geriatric care, 8
Geriatric chair, 458
Geriatrics, 200
Gerontology, 200
Giardiasis, 165
Glass thermometer, using
axillary temperature, 368
oral temperature, 365–366
rectal temperature, 367
Glaucoma, 573
Glomerulus, 340
Gloves
contact precautions and, 181
disposing of, 240
putting on, 183
removing contaminated, 183–184, 185–187
standard precautions and, 175
using, 172
Glucose, 532
Glucose metabolism, 532
Goal, 95
Goggles, 175
Gonads, 531
Goniometer, 431
Gonorrhea, 546
Gown
changing on resident with IV line, 632–633
putting on, 184–185
removing contaminated, 185–187
Grab bars, 475
Graft, 634, 635
Grief
anticipatory type, 616
of family and friends, 619–620
loss of loved one and, 219–220
of residents, 622–623
stages of, 618–619
Grievances, 114
Grooming
adaptive devices for, 427
of nursing assistants, 36
restorative program for, 430
task segmentation, 425

Growth in job, 646–647
Gums, cleaning, 285

H

Hair care, 276–277, 278
Hallucinations, 593, 600–601
Hand and nail care, 268, 279–280
Hand-over-hand technique, 426
Handwashing, 156, 170, 172–173
Health care
  community facilities, 4–8
  delivery problems, 4
  scientific (Western) approach to,
    228
Hearing, 571–572
Hearing aids, 574–575
Hearing impairment,
  communicating with resident
    with, 61
Hearing loss, 574–575
Heart, 501–503
Heart attack (myocardial
  infarction), 507, 510–511
Heart block, 514
Heart disease, 510–514
Heart failure, 511–512, 513–514
Heart rate, 373–374
Heel protectors, 262, 263
Height, measuring, 380–381, 383,
  385–386
Heimlich maneuver, 143–144
Hematuria, 355
Hemianopsia, 578
Hemiplegia, 424, 577
Hemodialysis, 355, 634–635
Hemoptysis, 512
Hemorrhage, 148, 149
Hemorrhoids, 313
Hepatitis, 163
Herbal remedies, 229, 230
Hernias, 312–313
Herpes, 546–547
High-efficiency particulate air
  (HEPA) filter mask, 179
High-protein diet, 304, 305
Hip fracture, 557–559
Hip prosthesis, 559–560, 561
Hip range of motion exercises,
  439–440
HIV (human immunodeficiency
  virus), 163–164
Hoarding, 601
Holistic care, 228
Home health care, 4, 6
Homeopathy, 231
Homeostasis, 296
Home setting, modifications to,
  399, 402
Hormones, 530
Hospice care, 6, 616–617, 628
Hot-line number, 116
Human immunodeficiency virus
  (HIV), 163–164
Human sexuality. *See* Sexuality
Humidifier bottle, refilling, 525
Huntington's disease, 581–582, 591
Hydrotherapy, 230
Hyperalimentation, 312, 631
Hyperglycemia, 532, 534
Hypertension, 376, 507, 508–509
Hyperthyroidism, 532
Hypoglycemia, 532, 534–535
Hypotension, 376
Hypothermia blanket, 411–412
Hypothyroidism, 532
Hypoxia, 512
Hysterectomy, 545

I

Ice bag, 409, 410–411
Ileostomy, 336
Immunity, 159–160
Immunization, 160
Immunosuppression, 160

Impairment, 203–204
Implementation of care plan, 95
Inactivity, preventing
  complications from, 421–423
Incident, 124, 130
Incontinence
  bowel and bladder programs,
    460–463
  fecal, 336–337
  urinary, 341–342
Independence
  adjustment to loss of, 220
  admission to facility and,
    390–391
  restorative care and, 420–421
Independent bed movement,
  459–460
Indwelling catheter, 342–346
Ineffective cough, 526
Infarction, 501
Infection
  aging and, 521
  bacterial type, 160–162
  breaking chain of, 159
  chain of, 157–158
  description of, 156
  detection of in elderly, 166
  fungal type, 165
  natural body defenses against,
    158–159
  parasitic type, 165
  prevention of, 166–167
  respiratory system, 520–521
  risk of in elderly, 165–166
  types of, 158
  viral type, 162–165
Inferior, 77
Inflammation
  description of, 159
  of gastrointestinal tract, 313
Influenza, 162–163, 520–521
Informed consent, 117
Inguinal hernia, 313
In-service education, 29, 44–45,
  646–647
Instrumental activities of daily
  living (IADLs), 205, 424
Insulin, 532
Insulin-dependent diabetes
  mellitus, 533
Insulin shock, 534
Intake and output (I&O), 301–303,
  346–349
Integumentary system
  aging and, 201
  complications from inactivity,
    422
  description of, 80, 256–257
  observation of, 89
  See also Skin
Intelligence quotient (IQ), 608
Intention tremor, 580
Interdisciplinary team
  assessments by, 392
  care plan process, 94–95
  consultants, 27–28
  dietitian, 26
  discharge planning, 398, 399,
    402–403
  members of, 22–25
  nursing staff, 25
  physician, 26
  restorative care, 419–420
  social services, 25–26
  special therapists, 26–27
  staff relations, 39–40
  support services, 28
International time, 94
Intervention, 95
Interviewing for job, 644–645
Intravenous (IV) therapy, 630–631,
  632–633
Invasion of privacy, 117
Inventory List form, 394

Inversion, 434
Ischemia, 501, 510
Islets of Langerhans, 532
Isolation unit
  caring for linens in, 188
  measuring vital signs in, 188–189
  preparing, 182
  psychological aspects of, 178
  purpose of, 178
  serving meal tray in, 189–190
  specimen collection from,
    190–191
  transferring nondisposable
    equipment outside, 192
  transporting resident to and
    from, 192–193
IV (intravenous) therapy, 630–631,
  632–633

J

Jewelry, 37
Job
  applying for, 644
  growing in, 646–647
  interviewing for, 644–645
  keeping, 646
  position description, 37–39
  possibilities, finding, 642–643
  resigning from, 647
Joint movements, 432–434
Joints, 553, 555, 561

K

Kaposi sarcoma, 164
Kardex, 12
Keeping job, 646
Kidneys, 79, 339, 634
Kidney stones, 354–355
Knee range of motion exercises,
  439
Kyphosis, 555

L

Lap robe, 241
Large intestine, 295
Larynx, 519, 520
Lateral, 77
Lateral position, 442, 452–453
Laundry, 14
Leg bag drainage, 349–350
Lesions on skin, 257–264
Leukemia, 504–505
Leukocytes, 503
Level of impairment in mental
  retardation, 608
Lhermitte's sign, 579
Libel, 118
Lice, 165
Licensed practical nurse (LPN),
  23, 25
Licensure of facilities, 16–17
Lifting, rules for, 125–126
Lifting sheet, 457, 492
Ligaments, 553
Lighting, 240–241
Light therapy, 230
Linens, caring for
  bed linens, 245
  changing, 246–252
  in isolation unit, 188
Listening actively, 56–57
Living will, 109, 110–111
Logrolling, 449–450
Long-term care facility
  administrative organization,
    28–29
  admission to, 390
  dining room/day room, 12
  financing in, 15–16
  functional areas in, 10–14
  functions of, 8
  kitchen, 14
  laundry, 14
  licensure of, 16–17

nurses' station, 12
  placement in, 8, 9
  rehabilitation areas, 13–14
  resident unit, 10–12
  services provided in, 5
  types of, 8–10
Loss of loved one, 219–220
Lou Gehrig's disease, 582
Lower extremity amputation,
  561–562
Low-fat diet, 304, 305
Low-residue diet, 305
Low-sodium diet, 304, 305
Lungs, 518–519
Lymph, 503

M

Magnetic resonance imaging
  (MRI), 581
Magnetic therapy, 230
Maladaptive behavior, 223
Male perineal care, 275–276
Male reproductive system,
  540–541, 544
Malnutrition, 299–300
Manipulative behavior, 222
Manuals, 56
Mask
  putting on, 183
  removing contaminated, 185–187
  standard precautions and, 175
  types of, 179–180
Maslow's hierarchy of needs,
  214–215
Masturbation, 217–218
Material Safety Data Sheets
  (MSDS), 127–128
Maturity, 34–35
Mealtime, 305–306
  See also Diets; Eating; Feeding
Meal tray, serving in isolation unit,
  189–190
Measurements, abbreviations for,
  75–76
Mechanical lift
  transferring resident with,
    478–480
  weighing resident with, 381, 382,
    385–386
Mechanical soft diet, 303, 304
Medial, 76, 77
Medicaid, 15, 115
Medical asepsis, 170–172, 322
Medical chart
  components of, 56
  documentation guidelines, 93–94
  purpose of, 58
Medical record practitioner, 23
Medical terminology
  abbreviations, 69, 72–76
  anatomic, 76–78
  combining forms, 69–72
  description of, 68
  prefixes, 69, 71–72
  suffixes, 69, 72
  word parts, 68–69
Medical treatment, right to refuse,
  114
Medicare, 15–16, 115
Medication
  control and dispensing of, 12
  diabetes and, 535
  epidural catheter, 633
  intravenous therapy, 630
  patient-controlled analgesia,
    631
Medicine cart, 12
Meltaway bag, 188
Membranes, 79, 81
Memo, 55
Meninges, 81, 568
Menopause, 544
Menstrual cycle, 543–544
Mental abuse, 104

Mentally ill, community facilities for, 7
Mental retardation, 607–609
Mental status, 90
Mental status examination, 590
Mercury in thermometers, 363–364
Message, taking, 55
Metabolism, 532
Methicillin-resistant *Staphylococcus aureus* (MRSA), 160
Metric system, 362
Microbes, 156–157, 158
Midline or midsagittal line, 76, 77
Minerals, 294, 296
Minimum Data Set (MDS 2.0), 15–16, 94, 419
Mitered corner, making, 247, 248
Mobility
    definition of, 468
    multiple sclerosis and, 580
    progressive mobilization, 431
    restorative care and, 420
    task segmentation, 425
    See also Ambulation
Modifications to home setting, 399, 402
Moist cold applications, 412
Moist warm applications, 407–408
Moribund period, 617
Motor nerves, 567
Mouth
    digestion and, 293, 294
    oxygen therapy and, 525
    See also Oral hygiene
Moving resident in bed
    logrolling onto side, 449–450
    turning sheet, 446–447
    turning to side, 448–449
Mucous membranes, 81
Multiple sclerosis (MS), 579–581
Muscle cells, 79
Muscles, 552–553, 554
Muscle tissue, 79
Musculoskeletal system
    aging and, 201, 202, 553–555
    complications to from inactivity, 421–422
    components of, 552
    conditions affecting, 555–562
    description of, 80
    observation of, 90, 91
    skeletal muscles, 79
    skeleton, 552, 553
Myasthenia gravis, 582–583
Mycobacterium tuberculosis, 161
Myocardial infarction, 507, 510–511
Myths of aging, 205–207

N

Narcotic, 631
Nasogastric (NG) tube, 311–312
National Nurse Aide Assessment Program, 14–15
Naturopathic medicine, 231–232
Negative air pressure, 179
Neglect, 104, 118
Nerve cells, 79
Nerves, 567
Nervous system
    aging and, 201, 572
    components of, 567–568
    description of, 80
    disorders of, 576–583
    observation of, 90
Nervous tissue, 79
Networking, 642–643
Neurons, 567
Neurotransmitters, 567, 568, 591
Nitroglycerin, 511
No-code, 109, 142, 618

Nocturia, 341
Noise, controlling, 241, 242
Nondisposable equipment, transferring outside isolation unit, 192
Non-insulin-dependent diabetes mellitus, 533
Nonverbal communication, 53, 58, 59
Nosocomial infection, 156
Notification of change in condition, right to, 117
Nourishments, 310
N95 respirator mask, 179, 180
Nurse's notes, 92, 93
Nurses' station, 12
Nursing assistant
    acute care setting, 5
    appearance, 36–37
    attitude, 35–36
    certification, 14
    duties, 23, 40–41
    home health care setting, 6
    job description, 4, 37–39
    long-term care setting, 5
    personal characteristics, 34–35
    personal hygiene, 36
    professionalism, 34
    resident rights and, 102
    self-care, 43–44
    survey and, 17
Nursing diagnosis, 94
Nursing facility (NF), 9
Nursing policy manual, 12, 56
Nursing staff, 25
Nutrients, 294, 295–296
Nutrition
    total parenteral nutrition, 312, 631
    See also Diets
Nutritional status, 299–300, 305–306
Nystagmus, 580

O

Objective observation, 86
OBRA legislation, 14–15
Observation
    baseline, 87
    body systems, 88–90
    description of, 86
    documenting, 92–94
    pain and behavior, 90–91
    reporting, 91–92
    signs and symptoms, 86–87, 88–90
    skin lesions, 257–258
Obstructed airway, 143–146
    See also Choking
Occupational exposure, 174
Occupational Safety and Health Administration (OSHA), 124, 128
Occupational therapist, 23, 26–27, 402–403
Occupational therapy department, 13
Occupied bed, changing linens for, 250–252
Odor, controlling, 241–242, 264
Oil glands, 257
Oil-retention enemas, 328–329
Ombudsman, 116
Oncology treatment, 628, 635
Open reduction/internal fixation (ORIF), 557–559
Ophthalmologist, 28, 573
Opposition, 434
Optic nerve, 571
Optometrist, 23, 28
Oral communication, 53–55
Oral hygiene
    brushing teeth, 281, 282, 284
    denture care, 282, 285

flossing teeth, 284
    for unconscious resident, 286
Oral temperature, 363, 364, 365–366, 369
Organ donation, 621
Organic mental syndrome. *See* Dementia
Organization of time, 41–42
Organs, 79
Orthopedic injury, 152
Orthopnea, 511
Orthopneic position, 512, 523–524
Orthosis, 444–445
Orthotic device, 26–27, 444–445, 556
Orthotist, 23
Osteoarthritis, 559–560
Osteopathy, 232
Osteoporosis, 422, 555, 559
Ostomies, 333–336
Output, recording, 346–349
Ovaries, 531, 543
Overbed table, 10–11
Oxygen, 518
Oxygen concentrator, 525
Oxygen safety, 129, 524, 525
Oxygen therapy, 512, 524–525, 629

P

Pacemaker, 470, 514
Pacing, 592, 599–600
Pain
    assessment of, 92
    management of, 628, 631, 633
    observations of, 90–91
    signs and symptoms of, 88
Palliative care, 616
Pancreas, 79, 530
Paralysis, 567
Paraplegia, 424, 580
Parasites, 157, 165
Parathyroid glands, 532
Parkinson's disease, 204, 576–577, 591
Partial bath, 272–273
Partial seizure, 148, 610
Passive range of motion exercises, 432, 434–441
Pathogens, 156
Patient, 7
Patient-controlled analgesia, 631
Penis, 540
Perceptual deficits, 424
Pericardium, 81
Perineal care, 273–276
Peripheral intravenous central catheter line, 630–631
Peripheral nerves, 568
Peripheral nervous system, 567
Peripheral vascular disease, 507, 508–509
Peritoneal dialysis, 628, 635
Peritoneum, 81
Perseveration, 592
Personal equipment, 10–11
Personal funds, 115
Personal hygiene, 36
Personality, 215–216
Personal possessions
    inventory of, 393–395
    labeling and storage of, 171
    right to, 116–117, 118
Personal protective equipment (PPE)
    emergency procedures and, 142
    gloves, 172, 175, 181, 183–184, 185–187, 240
    gown, 184–187
    mask, 175, 179–180, 183, 185–187
    standard precautions and, 178
Personal space, 238–239
Pet therapy, 598
PFR95 respirator mask, 179, 180

Phantom pain, 562
Pharmacist, 23
Phocomelia, 607
Physical abuse, 104
Physical needs
    accommodation of, 106–107
    comfort, rest, and sleep, 209–210
    description of, 214–215
Physical restraints
    description of, 104, 130
    guidelines for, 132–134
    reducing need for, 130–131
Physical therapist, 23, 26, 27, 399, 402
Physical therapy
    after open reduction/internal fixation (ORIF), 557–558
    developmental disability and, 611, 612
Physical therapy department, 13
Physician, 24, 26
Physician orders, abbreviations for, 73–75
Physician's office, 7
Piggyback for IV therapy, 630
Pillaging, 601
Pillows for positioning, 264
Pineal body, 531
Pituitary gland, 530–532
Planning work, 42
Plasma, 503
Platelets, 504
Pleura, 81, 518
Pneumonia, 422, 521
Podiatrist, 24, 28, 280, 562
Poisoning, accidental
    emergency treatment, 152
    preventing, 131
Policy book, 12, 56
Pores, 256
Positioning resident
    with arthritis, 450
    in bed, 262
    bridging, 264, 455–456
    in chair or wheelchair, 456–457, 491–493
    with COPD, 523–526
    Fowler's position, 454–455, 512, 523
    guidelines for, 442–443
    lateral position, 452–453
    with lower extremity amputation, 455
    orthopneic position, 512, 523–524
    with paralysis, 455
    purposes of, 442
    semiprone position, 454
    semisupine position, 452
    skin breakdown and, 258
    steps in, 442
    supine position, 451
    supportive equipment, 443–446
Position sense, 578
Post-Discharge Plan of Care, 400–401
Posterior, 77
Postmortem care, 622–623
Postmortem period, 617
Postoperative care in subacute unit, 628, 629
Postural supports, 443
Power of attorney for health care, 109, 112–113
Prefix, 69, 71–72
Presbycusis, 574
Presbyopia, 572
Pressure ulcer
    causes and signs of, 259–260, 422
    observation of, 87
    preventing, 262–264
    treatment of, 260, 262

Preventing
accidental poisoning, 131
choking, 135
complications from inactivity, 421–423
falls, 134–135, 150
heart disease, 510
infection, 166–167
injuries, 128–129, 134, 176, 257
sexually transmitted disease, 547
skin breakdown, 261, 262–264
Privacy, right to, 105, 117
Procedure book, 12, 38, 56
Procedure completion actions, 243–244
Procedures, description of, 242–244
Professionalism, 34
Progesterone, 531
Progressive diet, 305
Progressive mobilization, 431
Projection, 221
Prolapsed uterus, 545
Pronation, 433
Prone position, 442
Prostate, 541, 545
Prosthesis, 559–560
Prosthetist, 24
Protective isolation, 182
Proteins, 294, 296
Protraction, 453
Proximal, 77
Pruritus, 545
Pseudomonas aeruginosa, 161
Psychosocial needs
accommodation of, 107–108
description of, 215
inactivity and, 423
meeting, 221–222
reactive behavior and, 222–223
religion, 217
sexuality and intimacy, 217–219
spirituality, 216–217
Puberty, 543
Pulse
apical type, 373–374
description of, 372
radial type, 372–373
Pulse oximetry, 629
Pulse sites, 373
Pureed diet, 303–304

Q
Qi, 229
Qigong, 230
Quadriplegia, 424, 581
Quality assurance manual, 56

R
Radial deviation, 434
Radial pulse, 372–373
Radiation therapy, 635
Range of motion
active exercises, 441, 558
contractures, 431–432
joint movements, 432–434
passive exercises, 432, 434–441
self exercises, 441
Rationalization, 221
Reactive behavior, 222–223
Reality orientation, 601–602
Records, 12
Recovery position, 143, 148
Recreational activities for resident with dementia, 598–599
Rectal suppositories, 328
Rectal temperature, 363, 364, 367, 369–370
Rectal tube, 332–333
Rectocele, 354, 545
References, 643, 644
Reflex, 568

Registered nurse (RN), 24, 25
Registry, 643
Regular diet, 303
Rehabilitation aide, 24, 27
Rehabilitation areas, 13–14
Rehabilitation clinic, 7
Rehabilitation compared to restoration, 419–420
Rehabilitation nurse, 25, 419
Religion
dying process, death, and, 620, 621
as psychosocial need, 217
Religious activities, 115
Remain in facility, right to, 116
Reminiscing, 602
Renal calculi, 354–355
Renal failure, 355
Reporting for duty, 42, 118
Reporting on observations, 91–92
Reporting periods for Resident Assessment Instrument (RAI), 16
Reproductive system
aging and, 202, 203, 544
description of, 80, 540
diseases of, 544–545
female, 541–544
male, 540–541
sexually transmitted disease, 545–547
Resident
behavior of, 42–43, 64
description of, 8
discharging, 398–403
interdisciplinary team and, 24
meeting new, 392–393
transferring, 395–398
See also Admission to facility
Resident Assessment Instrument (RAI), 15–16
Resident Assessment Protocols (RAP), 16
Resident care plan. *See* Care plan
Resident council, 114
Resident rights
access to family, 116
accommodation of needs, 105–108
advance directives, 109
advocacy group information, 116
benefits information, 115
cardiopulmonary resuscitation, 109
complaints, 116
confidentiality, 105
dementia and, 597
feeding restrictions, 109
free choice, 103
freedom from abuse and restraints, 103–104, 117
grievances, 114
hospitalization, 109
manage personal funds, 115
medication and treatment restrictions, 114
notification of change in condition, 117
nursing assistant responsibilities, 38
organize and participate in groups, 114
participate in activities, 114–115
personal possessions, 116–117
privacy, 105
remain in facility, 116
share room with spouse, 116
survey result information, 115
work for facility, 116
Residents' Rights document, 102, 117–118
Resident Transfer Form, 396–397
Resident unit, 10–12, 239–240

Resigning from job, 647
Respect
for personal space of resident, 238–239
treating resident with, 238, 597, 601
Respiration, 374–376
Respiratory arrest, 141
Respiratory system
aging and, 202, 519, 520
chronic obstructive pulmonary disease, 522–526
complications from inactivity, 422
description of, 80
gases, 518, 519
infections, 520–521
malignancies, 520
observation of, 88
organs of, 518–519
Respiratory therapist, 24
Respiratory therapy department, 14
Rest and sleep, 210
Restorative nursing assistant (RNA), 24, 27
Restorative (rehabilitative) care
ambulation, 481–487
description of, 8–9
environment for, 426, 431
interdisciplinary team and, 419–420
nursing assistant responsibilities, 430
potential for, 426
preventing complications from inactivity, 421–423
principles for, 421
programs for, setting up, 424–426
purposes of, 204–205, 420–421
transfers, 468–481
Restraints
false imprisonment and, 117
guidelines for, 132–134
reducing need for, 130–131
types of, 104
Résumé, preparing, 643
Retina, 570
Retraction, 453
Reverse isolation, 182
Rheumatoid arthritis, 559, 560–561
Rigor mortis, 622
Rotation, 433

S
Safety and security needs, 215
Safety of employees
body mechanics, 124–127, 446, 447
ergonomics, 124, 125
mechanical lift, using, 478
overview of, 124
during transfers, 469
Safety of residents
assistive devices for ambulation, 483–485
bathing, 266
choking, preventing, 135
clinical thermometers, 364
falls, preventing, 134–135
fire safety, 135–136
nursing assistant responsibilities, 38–39
overview of, 130
oxygen use, 524, 525
poisoning, preventing accidental, 131
risk factors for incidents, 130
skin injuries, preventing, 134, 257
thermal injuries, preventing, 134
toileting, 322

warm and cold applications, 406, 407, 409
wheelchairs and, 135, 488
Salmonella, 161
Salt, adding to food, 299
Scabies, 165
Scales, 380–381, 382
Sclera, 570
Scrotum, 532, 540
Second-degree burn, 151
Seeking employment. *See* Employment search
Seizure disorder, 609–611
Seizures, 148, 150–151
Self-appraisal, 642
Self-care, 43–44
Self-care deficit, 205, 423–424
Self-Determination Act, 109
Self-esteem, 215, 217, 221
Self range of motion exercises, 441
Self-stimulation, 217–218
Semiprone position, 454
Semisupine position, 452
Sending message, 58–59
Senescent changes, 200–203
Senile lentigines, 258
Sense organs
changes in with aging, 201–202, 203
ear, 571–572
eye, 570–571
Sensitivity, 34–35
Sensory deprivation, 423
Sensory nerves, 567
Septicemia, 341
Serous membranes, 81
Setup, 425, 426
Sexual abuse, 104, 219
Sexual harassment, 44
Sexual intercourse, 218
Sexuality
aging and, 203, 206–207, 217
expression of, 217–219
resident rights and, 107–108
sense of identity and, 540
younger resident and, 209
Sexually transmitted disease (STD), 545–547
Shampooing hair, 277
"Sharps," preventing injury from, 128–129, 176
Shaving, 277–279
Shearing, 258, 259, 442
Sheepskin pads, 262, 263
Shift report, 42, 53–55
Shingles, 162
Shoulder range of motion exercises, 434–436
Shower, 271–272
Side, turning resident onto, 448–450
Side rails, 10, 134
Sign, 86, 88–90
Sign language, 61, 62
Sitting transfer, 469, 480–481
Skeletal muscle, 79
Skeletal system, 80
Skeleton, 552, 553
Skilled nursing facility (SNF), 8–9
Skin
aging and, 257
breakdown of, 258–259, 261
functions of, 257
injuries to, preventing, 134, 257
lesions on, 257–264
See also Pressure ulcer
Skin cancer, 258
Skin tears, 258
Slander, 118
Sleep, 210
Sliding board transfer, 480–481
Slings, 445–446
Small intestine, 294–295

Smooth muscle, 79
Soapsuds enemas, 330–332
Social activities, 114–115
Social services department, 25–26, 391
Social worker, 24, 26
Sodium-restricted diet, 304, 305
Soiled linen, 245, 247
Spasticity, 442
Special procedures, 41
Specimen collection
   from isolation unit, 190–191
   sputum, 521–522
   stool, 337–339
   urine, 351–353
Speech and multiple sclerosis, 580–581
Speech-language pathologist, 24, 27
Speech therapy department, 13
Sperm, 540
Sphincter (rectal), 328
Sphygmomanometer, 376, 377, 378
Spinal cord, 568, 569
Spiritual healing, 230
Spirituality, 216–217
Splints, 26–27, 444–445, 556
Spouse, right to share room with, 116
Sprain, 152
Sputum, 521–522
Square corner, making, 247, 249
Staff development, 29, 44–45, 646–647
Staff nurse, 25
Staff relations, 39–40
Standard precautions, 174–175, 177–178
Standing transfer
   assisted, 472–473, 474–475
   description of, 468–469
Staphylococcus aureus, 160, 161
STD (sexually transmitted disease), 545–547
Stereotype
   dangers of, 206
   description of, 205
   positive, 207
Sterile package, opening, 194–195
Sterile procedures, 194
Sterilization of equipment, 193–194
Stethoscope, 376, 377, 378
Stoma, 333, 334
Stoma care, 334–336
Stomach, 294
Stool. *See* Feces
Stool specimen, collecting, 337–339
Strain, 152
Streptococcus pyogenes, 161
Stress
   reducing, 43–44
   signs of, 42
   symptoms of, 222
Stroke, 506–507, 577–579
Subacute care
   description of, 8, 628–629
   dialysis, 634–635
   intravenous therapy, 630–631, 632–633
   nursing assistant responsibilities, 629
   oncology treatment, 635
   pain management procedures, 631, 633
   pulse oximetry, 629
   surgical patients in, 629
   tracheostomy, 634
Subcutaneous tissue, 256
Subjective observation, 86–87
Subluxation, 445
Suffix, 69, 72
Sugar, 299

Suicide, signs of, 223
Sundowning, 592, 600, 601
Superior, 77
Supervisor, 25
Supination, 433–434
Supine position, 442, 451
Supplements, 310
Support services, 28, 41
Suppression, 221
Surgical asepsis, 194
Surgical patient, care of, 629
Survey for licensure and certification, 16–17, 115
Sweat glands, 256–257
Symptoms, 86–87, 88–90
Syncope, 152
Synovial membranes, 81
Syphilis, 546, 591
Systems, 79, 80
Systole, 503
Systolic pressure, 379

T
Tachycardia, 374
Tai chi, 230
Task segmentation, 424, 425
Tears, 570
TED hose, 512–513
Teeth. *See* Brushing teeth
Telephone, answering, 55
Temperature
   of facility, 240
   measuring, 363–372
Tendons, 553
Terminal condition
   adjustment to, 617–618
   description of, 109, 616
Terminal stage, 8
Terminology. *See* Medical terminology
Testes, 532, 540
Testosterone, 532, 540
Tests
   abbreviations for, 75
   for Alzheimer's disease, 590
   for epilepsy, 611
   for heart disease, 510
   level of impairment in mental retardation, 608
   to monitor diabetes, 536
   for multiple sclerosis, 581
Theft, 118
Therapeutic bath, 273
Therapeutic diets, 26, 304–305
Therapeutic recreational specialist, 24, 27
Therapeutic relationship, 35–36
Thermal blanket, 409, 411–412
Thermal injuries, preventing, 134
Third-degree burn, 151
Thorax, 519
Thrombus, 422, 577
Thrush, 157
Thumb range of motion exercises, 438
Thyroid gland, 530, 532
Tilt position, 452
Time
   abbreviations for, 75
   documentation of medical chart and, 94
   organization of, 41–42
Tissue breakdown, 259–260
Tissues, 79, 262
Toenail care, 269, 280–281
Toe range of motion exercises, 440–441
Toileting
   bathroom, 326
   bedpan, 322, 323–324
   bedside commode, 322, 325–326
   elevated toilet seat, 321
   grab bars, 321–322
   safety issues, 322

task segmentation, 425
transferring resident from wheelchair to toilet and back, 475–476
urinal, 324–325
Total care, 22
Total parenteral nutrition, 312, 631
Touch
   communicating through, 60–61, 218
   restorative care and, 431
Touch therapy, 230
Tracheostomy, 520, 634
Traction, 556–557
Transcutaneous electrical nerve stimulation (TENS), 633
Transfer belt use, contraindications to, 470
Transferring resident
   assisted standing transfer, 472–473, 474–475
   bringing to sitting position at edge of bed, 471–472
   from chair to bed, 473–474
   guidelines for, 469
   with mechanical lift, 478–480
   nonstanding, from wheelchair to bed, 477–478
   within and outside facility, 395–398
   purpose of, 468
   sliding board transfer, 480–481
   transfer (gait) belt, using, 469–470
   to tub or shower chair, 476–477
   types of, 468–469
   wheelchair to toilet and back, 475–476
Transient ischemic attack (TIA), 507–508, 577
Transitional care. *See* Subacute care
Transmission-based precautions
   airborne, 178–180
   contact, 180–182
   droplet, 180, 181
   isolation and, 178–182
   overview of, 178
Transmission of infection, 157, 158
Transporting resident to and from isolation unit, 192–193
Transurethral prostatectomy, 545
Transverse line, 77
Trauma, 204
Treatment, right to refuse, 114
Tremors, 576, 580
Trichomonas vaginitis, 546
Triggers, 16
Trochanter roll, 443, 444
Tub bath, 271–272
Tuberculosis, 161–162
Tui ma, 230
Turning resident to side, 448–450
Turning schedule, 261
Turning sheet, 446–447
Tympanic temperature, 363
Tympanic thermometer, 365, 370–372

U
Ulnar deviation, 434
Umbilicus, 78, 79
Unconscious resident, oral hygiene for, 286
Undressing. *See* Dressing
Unfinished assignment, 40
Uniforms, 36–37
Unit secretary, 24, 25
Unoccupied bed, changing linens for, 246–250
Upper respiratory tract, 518

Upright scale, 381, 383
Uremia, 355
Ureters, 339
Urethra, 340, 540
Urinal, 324–325
Urinary incontinence, 341
Urinary retention, 341
Urinary system
   aging and, 201, 202, 340–341
   complications from inactivity, 423
   components of, 339–340
   conditions of, 354–355
   description of, 80
   internal catheter drainage, 342–346
Urine specimen, collecting, 351–353
Uterus, 543, 545

V
Vaccine, 160
Vagina, 543
Vaginitis, 545
Validation therapy, 602
Vancomycin-resistant enterococci (VRE), 160–161
Varicose veins, 507
Vas deferens, 541
Vasoconstriction, 409
Vasodilation, 407
Vasodilator, 511
Vectors, 158
Veins, 503, 505, 507, 508
Venereal warts, 547
Ventilation, 240
Ventral, 77
Ventral cavity, 81
Verbal abuse, 104
Verbal communication, 52–53
Verbal cues, 425
Vertigo, 579
Violence in workplace, 42–43
Violent resident
   Alzheimer's disease and, 592, 593, 600
   communicating with, 64
   dealing with, 42–43
Viral infections, 162–165
Viruses, 156–157
Vision
   diabetes and, 533–534
   impairment in, causes of, 572–573
   multiple sclerosis and, 579–580
   overview of, 570–571
   stroke and, 578
   See also Visual impairment
Visitor, violence by, 43
Visual impairment
   assisting resident with, 573
   communicating with resident with, 61–63
   See also Vision
Vital signs
   measuring, 362–363
   measuring in isolation unit, 188–189
   recording, 386
Vitamins, 294, 296
Vocabulary, expanding, 69
Vocal cords, 519
Voice, loss of, 520
Vomiting, 142–143
Vulva, 541, 543

W
Walkers, 485, 487
Wandering, 592, 599–600
Warm applications, 406–408
Warm-up exercises, 127
Water as nutrient, 294, 296
Waterless bed bath, 270
Weight, measuring, 380–386

Weight bearing, 468
Weight loss, unintended, 299–300
Wheelchairs
    curbs, 489–490
    fit of, 487–488
    positioning resident in, 457,
      491–493
    preventing falls from, 134
    ramps and inclines, 489
    relieving pressure while in, 458,
      493
    safety measures for, 135, 488
    stairs, 490–491
    tilting backward, 488–489
    transferring resident from,
      475–478
Wheelchair scale, 381, 384
Whirlpool tub, 266
Word parts, 68–69
Word root, 69
Work at facility, right to, 116
Wrist range of motion exercises,
    437
Written communication, 55–56

Y
Younger resident, 208–209